GLOBAL HEALTH NURSING
IN THE 21ST CENTURY

Suellen Breakey, PhD, RN, is assistant professor at the MGH Institute of Health Professions, in Boston, Massachusetts, where she teaches accelerated BSN students. She completed her BS in biology at Salem State University, an MSN in critical care nursing at the MGH Institute of Health Professions, and a PhD in nursing at Boston College Connell School of Nursing. Her research area is the nurse's role in treatment decision making in seriously ill adults. Her clinical interests are cardiac surgical and critical care nursing. Dr. Breakey's global nursing efforts are focused on prevention and treatment of rheumatic heart disease in resource-limited settings. She is a leader in Team Heart, a nonprofit organization that works in Rwanda. Dr. Breakey led a team that developed the teaching modules, both written materials and videos, which were translated into Kinyarwanda language for their patients. She has also organized and participated in ongoing nursing professional development for the Rwandan nursing community. Dr. Breakey was a member of a screening team to study the prevalence of rheumatic heart disease in school-age children in Rwanda.

Inge B. Corless, PhD, RN, FAAN, is a professor at the MGH Institute of Health Professions, School of Nursing and served as an honorary research fellow at the University of KwaZulu-Natal in 2003. She completed a BSN at Boston University, an MA in sociology from the University of Rhode Island, and a PhD from Brown University. Dr. Corless completed postdoctoral work as a Robert Wood Johnson Clinical Scholar at the University of California, San Francisco. She is a fellow of the American Academy of Nursing. She served as president of the Association of Nurses in AIDS Care in 1997. Earlier in her career, she left the University of Michigan, where she had been researching the hospice movement, to cofound St. Peter's Hospice in Albany, New York. She was also a member of the first board of directors of the New York State Hospice Association, and served as chair of the Research Committee for the National Hospice Organization and, subsequently, for the National Hospice and Palliative Care Organization. Her career includes extensive work in South Africa on adherence to HIV/AIDS treatment and care. Dr. Corless has led a number of groups of students and alumni of the School of Nursing on international health courses to southern Africa. Dr. Corless was inducted into the International Nurse Researcher Hall of Fame by the Honor Society of Nursing, Sigma Theta Tau International (STTI), in 2011.

Nancy L. Meedzan, DNP, RN, CNE, is associate professor of nursing at Endicott College in Beverly, Massachusetts, where she teaches in the BSN, RN to BSN, and MSN programs. She completed her BSN at Boston College Connell School of Nursing, an MSN at Salem State University, and a DNP at Regis College. Dr. Meedzan developed an undergraduate course, Intercultural Nursing, and along with Dr. Nicholas, developed a master's level track in global health nursing. Dr. Meedzan has been teaching nursing for the past 10 years, and prior to that, practiced clinically in medical and surgical nursing in the acute care setting and in the community. Her clinical emphasis is on cardiovascular nursing care. Dr. Meedzan's passion for global health began when she visited Haiti in 1987 as a senior nursing student at Boston College. She rekindled this passion during her DNP program and now travels with students to Guatemala, the Dominican Republic, and Mississippi for cultural immersion experiences.

Patrice K. Nicholas, DNSc, DHL (Hon), MPH, MS, RN, ANP, FAAN, is director of Global Health and Academic Partnerships at Brigham and Women's Hospital in the Division of Global Health Equity and the Center for Nursing Excellence. She is professor at the MGH Institute of Health Professions. She completed a BSN at Fitchburg State University, and MS and DNSc degrees at Boston University. Dr. Nicholas completed a postdoctoral fellowship and master's of public health degree at the Harvard School of Public Health. She received an honorary Doctor of Humane Letters degree from Fitchburg State University in 2010. Dr. Nicholas served on the Board of Directors of Sigma Theta Tau International (STTI) Honor Society of Nursing (2009–2013) and currently serves on the STTI Leadership Succession Committee (2013–2015). She was a Fulbright Senior Scholar in Germany (2003) and South Africa (2006–2007) and served on Fulbright Senior Review panels for the U.S. Council for International Exchange of Scholars. Dr. Nicholas is a fellow of the American Academy of Nursing. Her area of research is HIV/AIDS and quality of life.

GLOBAL HEALTH NURSING IN THE 21ST CENTURY

Suellen Breakey, PhD, RN

Inge B. Corless, PhD, RN, FAAN

Nancy L. Meedzan, DNP, RN, CNE

Patrice K. Nicholas, DNSc, DHL (Hon), MPH, MS, RN, ANP, FAAN

EDITORS

SPRINGER PUBLISHING COMPANY
NEW YORK

Springer Publishing Company, LLC
11 West 42nd Street
New York, NY 10036
www.springerpub.com

Acquisitions Editor: Joseph Morita
Composition: diacriTech

ISBN: 978-0-8261-1871-4
e-book ISBN: 978-0-8261-1872-1
Test Bank: 978-0-8261-2826-3
Instructors PowerPoints: 978-0-8261-2827-0

Instructors Materials: Qualified instructors may request supplements by emailing textbook@springerpub.com

15 16 17 18 / 5 4 3 2 1

The author and the publisher of this Work have made every effort to use sources believed to be reliable to provide information that is accurate and compatible with the standards generally accepted at the time of publication. Because medical science is continually advancing, our knowledge base continues to expand. Therefore, as new information becomes available, changes in procedures become necessary. We recommend that the reader always consult current research and specific institutional policies before performing any clinical procedure. The author and publisher shall not be liable for any special, consequential, or exemplary damages resulting, in whole or in part, from the readers' use of, or reliance on, the information contained in this book. The publisher has no responsibility for the persistence or accuracy of URLs for external or third-party Internet websites referred to in this publication and does not guarantee that any content on such websites is, or will remain, accurate or appropriate.

Library of Congress Cataloging-in-Publication Data
Global health nursing in the 21st century / Suellen Breakey, Inge B. Corless, Nancy Meedzan, Patrice K. Nicholas, editors.
    p. ; cm.
Includes bibliographical references and index.
ISBN 978-0-8261-1871-4 — ISBN 978-0-8261-1872-1 (e-Book) — ISBN (invalid) 978082612826-3
(test bank) — ISBN (invalid) 978-0-8261-2827-0 (instructors PowerPoints)
I. Breakey, Suellen, editor. II. Corless, Inge B., editor. III. Meedzan, Nancy, editor. IV. Nicholas, Patrice K., editor.
[DNLM: 1. Nursing — trends. 2. Internationality. 3. Nurse's Role. 4. World Health. WY 16.1]
RT51
610.73 — dc23
                                                      2014042828

Special discounts on bulk quantities of our books are available to corporations, professional associations, pharmaceutical companies, health care organizations, and other qualifying groups. If you are interested in a custom book, including chapters from more than one of our titles, we can provide that service as well.

For details, please contact:
Special Sales Department, Springer Publishing Company, LLC
11 West 42nd Street, 15th Floor, New York, NY 10036-8002
Phone: 877-687-7476 or 212-431-4370; Fax: 212-941-7842
E-mail: sales@springerpub.com

Printed in the United States of America by Bradford & Bigelow.

We dedicate this book to Ange, Shabani, Felix, and all of those we have met through our work in global health. Their rich lives were taken prematurely and tragically as a result of the inequities in health that exist globally, the lack of access to health care, and the need for a more robust global nursing workforce to address the pressing health needs of the world's people.

We are better for having known you, for your deaths remind us that issues of global health are not theoretical; they are in fact very real and continue to cut short the lives of countless individuals whose only flaw was that they were born into poverty.

We also dedicate this book to Professor Leana Uys, who contributed a chapter with Professor Hester Klopper on advancing professional nursing in South Africa. Upon completion of their chapter, Professor Uys died after a long illness and a rich and productive career in nursing and nursing education.

Contents

Contributors

Ansuya Bengre, RN, RM, MSc(N)   Manipal College of Nursing, Manipal University, Karnataka, India

Busisiwe Rosemary Bhengu, PhD, RN   Chairperson, South African Nursing Council; Honorary Associate Professor, School of Nursing and Public Health, University of KwaZulu-Natal, Howard Campus, Durban, South Africa

Noella Bigirimana, BS   Project Manager, Team Heart Inc., Newton, Massachusetts

Regina Szylit Bousso, RN, MS, PhD   Associate Professor, School of Nursing, University of Sao Paulo, Sao Paulo, Brazil

Suellen Breakey, PhD, RN   Assistant Professor, MGH Institute of Health Professions, Boston, Massachusetts

Elizabeth J. Brown, RN, MSN, MBA   Director, Global Nursing Programs, Partners Healthcare International, Boston, Massachusetts

Julie Carragher, MS, RN, ACNP   Clinical Instructor, Northeastern University, Boston, Massachusetts

Puangtip Chaiphibalsarisdi, PhD, RN   Associate Professor and Dean, School of Nursing, Shinawatra University, Pathumthani, Thailand

Karen A. Conley, DNP, RN   Associate Chief Nurse, Connors Center for Women and Newborns, Brigham and Women's Hospital, Boston, Massachusetts

Inge B. Corless, PhD, RN, FAAN   Professor, MGH Institute of Health Professions, Boston, Massachusetts

Sheila Davis, DNP, RN, FAAN   Chief Nursing Officer, Partners In Health, Boston, Massachusetts

Carol Dawson-Rose, PhD, RN, FAAN   Associate Professor, School of Nursing, University of California, San Francisco, San Francisco, California

Mary de Chesnay, PhD, DSN, RN, PMHCNS-BC, FAAN   Professor, WellStar School of Nursing, Kennesaw State University, Kennesaw, Georgia

Tabatha Dye   Graduate Research Assistant, University of Alabama, Tuscaloosa, Alabama

Linda A. Evans, PhD, RN   Assistant Professor, MGH Institute of Health Professions; Nurse Researcher, Brigham and Women's Hospital, Boston, Massachusetts

Paul Farmer, MD, PhD   Koloktrones University Professor, Harvard Medical School; Chair of Department of Global Health and Social Medicine, Harvard Medical School; Chief of the Division on Global Health Equity, Brigham and Women's Hospital, Boston, Massachusetts

Susan E. Farrell, MD   Program Director, Partners Healthcare International, Boston, Massachusetts

Joyce J. Fitzpatrick, PhD, MBA, BSN, RN, FAAN   Professor of Nursing, Case Western Reserve University, Cleveland, Ohio

Julio Frenk, MD, MPH   Dean of the Faculty, Harvard School of Public Health; T & G Angelopoulos Professor of Public Health and International Development, Harvard School of Public Health and Harvard Kennedy School, Boston, Massachusetts

Holly Fulmer, RN, MSN   Brigham and Women's Hospital, Boston, Massachusetts

Erin George, MSN, CNM, RN   Nurse Midwife, Brigham and Women's Hospital, Boston, Massachusetts

Diane E. Hazel, MSN, MPH, RN   School Nurse, Canton Public Schools, Canton, Massachusetts

Patricia A. Hickey, PhD, MBA, RN, FAAN   Vice President, Cardiovascular and Critical Care Services, Boston Children's Hospital; Assistant Professor of Pediatrics, Harvard Medical School, Boston, Massachusetts

Nancy Hoffart, PhD, RN   Founding Dean and Professor, Alice Ramez Chagoury School of Nursing, Lebanese American University, Byblos, Lebanon

Pamela Hoyt-Hudson, BSN, RN   Global Nursing Coordinator, Dreyfus Health Foundation, The Rogosin Institute, New York, New York

Lily Hsu, MS, RN   Director, Project Hope Education, China

Carol L. Huston, PhD, RN, FAAN   Past President, Sigma Theta Tau International; Director, School of Nursing, California State University, Chico, California

Avril Kaplan, MSc   Senior Analyst, Abt Associates, Washington, DC

James Kiarie, MBChB, MMed, MPH   University of Nairobi, Center for HIV Research and Prevention, Nairobi, Kenya

Hester C. Klopper, PhD, RN, RM, MBA, FANSA President, Honor Society of Nursing, Sigma Theta Tau International; Professor, Northwest University and University of the Western Cape, Pretoria, South Africa

Ann Kurth, PhD, RN, FAAN Professor and Executive Director, New York University College of Nursing Global; Associate Dean for Research, New York University Global Institute of Public Health, New York, New York

Elissa C. Ladd, PhD, RN, FNP-BC Associate Professor, MGH Institute of Health Professions, Boston, Massachusetts

Rana Limbo, PhD, RN, PMHCNS-BC, CPLC Bereavement and Advance Care Planning Services, Gundersen Health System, LaCrosse, Wisconsin

Teri Lindgren, PhD, MPH, RN Assistant Professor, Rutgers the State University of New Jersey, Newark, New Jersey

Jianhua Lou, RN Chief Nursing Officer, Shanghai Children's Medical Center, Shanghai, China

Antonia Makosky, MS, MPH, ANP-BC Clinical Assistant Professor, School of Nursing, MGH Institute of Health Professions, Boston, Massachusetts

R. Kevin Mallinson, PhD, RN, AACRN, FAAN Associate Professor, Assistant Dean Doctoral Division, School of Nursing, College of Health and Human Services, George Mason University, Fairfax, Virginia

Bridget E. Meedzan, BS Clinical Research Coordinator, AED Pregnancy Registry, Pediatrics Department, Massachusetts General Hospital, Boston, Massachusetts

Nancy L. Meedzan, DNP, RN, CNE Associate Professor, School of Nursing, Endicott College, Beverly, Massachusetts

Jayden Nadeau, RN, MSN, PMHNP-BC Nurse Practitioner, ConnectionsAZ, Phoenix, Arizona

Busisiwe P. Ncama, PhD, RN Associate Professor, Dean and Head of School, Nursing and Public Health, University of KwaZulu-Natal, Howard College Campus, Durban, South Africa

Patrice K. Nicholas, DNSc, DHL (Hon), MPH, MS, RN, ANP, FAAN Director of Global Health and Academic Partnerships, Brigham and Women's Hospital; Senior Nurse Scientist, Division of Global Health Equity and Center for Nursing Excellence; Professor, MGH Institute of Health Professions School of Nursing, Boston, Massachusetts

Annie Lewis O'Connor, PhD, MPH, NP-BC Director, Women's C.A.R.E. Clinic, Brigham and Women's Hospital, Boston, Massachusetts

John Palen, PhD, MPH   Senior Human Resources for Health (HRH) Advisor, Abt Associates, Washington, DC

Ceeya Patton-Bolman, MSN, RN   Program Coordinator, Team Heart, Inc., Newton, Massachusetts

Suzanne S. Prevost, PhD, RN, COI, FAAN   Dean, University of Alabama School of Nursing, Tuscaloosa, Alabama

Eleonor Pusey-Reid, RN, DNP, MS, MEd, CCRN   Clinical Assistant Professor, MGH Institute of Health Professions, Boston, Massachusetts

Sally Rankin, PhD, RN, FAAN   Professor and Associate Dean, Global Health and International Programs, University of California, San Francisco, San Francisco, California

Kim Rochon, MSN, RN   MGH Institute of Health Professions, Boston, Massachusetts

Ellen Schell, PhD, RN, FAAN   International Programs Director, Global AIDS Interfaith Alliance; Associate Adjunct Professor, School of Nursing, University of California, San Francisco, San Francisco, California

Michele Shedlin, PhD   Professor, College of Nursing, New York University, New York, New York

Anne Sliney, RN, ACRN   Chief Nursing Officer, Clinton Health Access Initiative; Faculty, Brown University AIDS Program; Chief Nursing Officer, Clinton Foundation, Boston, Massachusetts

Barry H. Smith, MD, PhD   President and Chief Executive Officer, The Rogosin Institute; Director, The Rogosin Institute of Dreyfus Health Foundation; Director, Research, The Rogosin Institute Xenia Division; Professor of Surgery, Weill Medical College of Cornell University; Attending Surgeon, New York-Presbyterian Hospital/Weill Cornell, New York, New York

Allison Squires, PhD, RN   Assistant Professor, Deputy Director, International Education and Visiting Scholars, New York University College of Nursing, New York, New York

Susan Stevens, DNP, MEd, MSN, PMHNP-BC   Clinical Instructor, MGH Institute of Health Professions, Boston, Massachusetts

Hsin-Ling Tsai, MHA   Dreyfus Health Foundation of the Rogosin Institute, Taipei, Taiwan

Lynda Tyer-Viola, PhD, RNC, FAAN   Director, Women's Services, Texas Children's Hospital; Adjunct Faculty, Texas Woman's University–Houston Campus, Houston, Texas

‡ **Leana R. Uys, PhD, RN** Professor Emerita and Fellow of the University of KwaZulu-Natal, South Africa

Ana M. Viamonte-Ros, MD, MPH Associate Dean for Women in Medicine and Science, Herbert Wertheim College of Medicine; Associate Professor, Department of Humanities, Florida International University; Director of Medical Staff Development, Baptist Health South Florida, Miami, Florida

Gary White Chief Executive Officer and Cofounder, Water.org, Kansas City, Missouri

Shira Winter, BA MGH Institute of Health Professions, Boston, Massachusetts

Denise Kelsey Wishner, MSN, RN Ethicist, Department of Veterans Affairs, Long Beach, California

Karen Anne Wolf, PhD, ANP-Bc, DFNAP Nurse Consultant, Oakland, California

Deborah von Zinkernagel Acting U.S. Global AIDS Coordinator, Office of the U.S. Global AIDS Coordinator, Washington, DC

‡ Deceased

Preface

The genesis of this book occurred when the editors posed the following question, "Is there a need for a text on global nursing that encompasses the work of nursing, the complex issues that affect the health of the world's people, and nursing's contributions to interprofessional efforts to achieve global health?" So began the journey that has culminated in this text, *Global Health Nursing in the 21st Century*. When we set out to answer this question, we discovered a paucity of nursing texts related to global nursing and embraced the idea that the literature would be enriched by the contribution of this book. During our review of existing scholarly works, we discovered several contributions to the global health literature from the fields of public health, international health, and global health. However, most texts were written by experts from other disciplines and few explored the unique contributions of the nursing profession to the interprofessional landscape of global health.

In retrospect, this observation should not have been unexpected. While it is widely understood that nurses represent the vast majority of the global health workforce, and that nurses and midwives play a critical role in health care delivery, their expertise is often overlooked or—at the least—undervalued. Indeed, nurses have been late in being invited to join other key stakeholders, such as health scientists, physicians, economists, public health professionals, and international development experts, in the discussions that shape global health. However, there is a growing recognition that nurses and midwives are essential to providing quality, people-centered care, and improving the cost effectiveness of that care. The World Health Organization (WHO) publication, *Nursing and Midwifery Services: Strategic Directions 2011–2015* (2010), acknowledges nursing's absence and strongly advocates that "…governments, civil society and professional associations must work together with educational institutions, nongovernmental organizations (NGOs) and a range of international and bilateral organizations to remedy the situation so that the input of nurses and midwives is actively sought and acknowledged" (p. 3).

Likewise, Frenk et al. (2010) have shifted the paradigm of those educated in the health professions and have enlisted not only educators and universities, students and young health professionals, but also NGOs, international philanthropic organizations, and foundations to promote the reform needed for the health professions to address the health of the world's people in the 21st century. These authors contend that both institutional and instructional reforms are needed to achieve a model transformative professional education. As they state: "The result will be more equitable and better performing health systems than at present, with consequent benefits for patients and populations everywhere in our interdependent world" (p. 4). One of the hallmarks of Frenk et al.'s mandate—*interdependence*—requires a shift to interprofessional and transprofessional education, as it is well understood that collaboration and teamwork result in better patient outcomes. Along with the strategic directions recommended by the WHO (2013), Frenk et al.'s mandate strengthens the argument that nurses are integral members of the global health team. They suggest that past laudable efforts to reform the health professions to suit contemporary needs have "...mostly floundered, partly because of the so-called tribalism of the professions—that is, the tendency of the various professions to act in isolation from or even in competition with each other" (p. 1). Nurses worldwide must embrace and advocate for Frenk et al.'s vision that:

> all health professionals in all countries should be educated to mobilize
> knowledge and to engage in critical reasoning and ethical conduct
> so that they are competent to participate in patient and population-
> centred health systems as members of locally responsive and globally
> connected teams. (pp. 2–3)

To realize this vision, it is critical that nurses worldwide understand and strengthen their professional scope so that they can practice to the full extent of their education and training. This goal will make nurses more effective members of an interdisciplinary team and build what is required to address the comprehensive needs for population health globally.

The underlying assertion of *Global Health Nursing in the 21st Century* is that global health encompasses the health problems of both rich and poor countries and implies a shared responsibility for achieving health and eradicating inequities (Birn, Pallay, & Holtz, 2009). It takes into account the social, political, cultural, economic, and environmental factors—including climate change—that may impact health. We developed the text to account for this unique and critical conceptualization. The book comprises three units and includes contributions from nurses with global health expertise, as well as global health experts from other disciplines. It is structured to provide a layered understanding of the complexities surrounding global health.

Unit I offers an overview of the foundations of global health. This is the first global nursing text to include the emerging concept of climate justice and its relationship to climate change and environmental health consequences. Additional tenets that underlie global health and global nursing are explored. These include an analysis of the distinctions that relate to public health, international health, and global health; the ethical context of global health, human rights, and social justice; and the importance of interprofessional education to achieve global health and global health equity. Globalization and the significant impact on the health of people worldwide is discussed not only in Unit I, but also more broadly in several chapters throughout the book. Taken together, these tenets form the basis for understanding and undertaking effective bidirectional global health partnerships.

Unit II highlights issues of global health and the effects on the most poor and vulnerable worldwide—particularly women, children, and those living in areas of conflict. The physical and mental health sequelae related to violence that occur both within and outside personal relationships and country-specific conflicts are explored. The likelihood that women and girls will experience negative health effects related to violence is also examined within the scope of their vulnerability to HIV/AIDS and their forced participation in sex trafficking. The impact of HIV/AIDS and its detrimental effects on the nursing workforce in sub-Saharan Africa, which experiences a disproportionate burden of the disease, are also explored in this unit. Maternal mortality and childhood malnutrition are additional health risks experienced by women and children that are discussed in Unit II.

Finally, while much work toward achieving global health is underway and there have been notable accomplishments, Unit III addresses areas where efforts must be redoubled to achieve success. This unit focuses on seeking and implementing solutions necessary to realize this overarching goal. The work of critical stakeholders working within governmental organizations, NGOs, and foundations is described. Collectively, their efforts are centered on increasing access to primary health care; increasing access to services that would otherwise be unavailable (e.g., surgical services); improving clinical practice by expanding educational opportunities for both students and practicing nurses and midwives; and engaging interdisciplinary researchers in the discovery of viable solutions to these challenges. At the core of *achieving global health*—and the overarching goal of the text—is the understanding that many of the initiatives highlighted are strategies aimed at strengthening health systems and achieving global health equity. The goals are achievable in the 21st century and represent a contemporary human rights obligation.

We are proud of the development of *Global Health Nursing in the 21st Century*. The chapters provide nurses and those interested in nursing's contribution to the field of global health, a comprehensive survey of the range of issues. This knowledge is essential to understanding how to best influence the health and attainment of human rights for people worldwide. In closing, we offer a quote from Nelson Mandela, who espoused the issues of equity during his journey toward achieving justice for the people of South Africa and, more broadly, the world. His vision embraced equity in all aspects of life and has relevance for social justice, human rights, and global health.

> Let there be justice for all. Let there be peace for all. Let there be work, bread, water, and salt for all. Let each know that, for each, the body, the mind, and the soul have been freed to fulfill themselves. The sun shall never set on so glorious a human achievement.
>
> —Nelson R. Mandela
> Statement of the President of the African National Congress
> at his inauguration as president of the
> Democratic Republic of South Africa, 1994

Suellen Breakey
Inge B. Corless
Nancy L. Meedzan
Patrice K. Nicholas

REFERENCES

Birn, A.E., Pillay, Y., & Holtz, T.H. (2009). *Textbook of international health: Global health in a dynamic world.* (3rd ed). New York, NY: Oxford University Press.

Frenk, J., Chen, L., Bhutta, Z. A., Cohen, J., Crisp, N., Evans, T., ... Zurayk, H. (2010). Health professionals for a new century: Transforming education to strengthen health systems in an interdependent world. *The Lancet, 376,* 1923–1958. Retrieved from http://www.healthprofessionals21.org/docs/HealthProfNewCent.pdf

World Health Organization. (2010). *Strategic directions for strengthening nursing and midwifery services (SDNM) 2011–2015.* Geneva, Switzerland: Author. Retrieved from http://www.who.int/hrh/resources/nmsd/en

Foundations of Global Nursing

Suellen Breakey and Patrice K. Nicholas

Globalization has had an enormous impact on health worldwide and, as a result, has had a significant influence on global medicine and global nursing. Ease of transportation and the expansion of communication borne out of rapid technological innovation have broken down borders, bringing continents and people closer together. Moreover, this has led to an increased awareness of health inequities—both resource-rich countries experiencing a growing understanding of the needs of the vulnerable and underserved, and those in resource-limited settings having a growing recognition of their inability to benefit from access to the most basic human needs. This realization has shifted the paradigm of how health care and the health professions view their ethical, moral, and professional responsibilities. Health professionals are increasingly engaged in and committed to addressing health inequities and sharing bidirectional knowledge worldwide.

In Chapter 1, we explore the concepts related to global health, the emergence of global medicine, and the birth of contemporary global nursing. Together these concepts bring global nursing full circle to the early, prescient views of Florence Nightingale and her wisdom on the environment and the importance of access to clean water, sanitation, air, and light. In Chapter 2, we, along with Winter, Pusey-Reid, and Viamonte-Ros, address the effects of climate change and the nascent concept of climate justice associated with climate change. There is a growing recognition and body of science that reveals the effects of climate change not only have health consequences, but also disproportionately affect the most vulnerable, who have contributed least to the causes of the denigration of our planet. In his interview in Chapter 3, Dean Julio Frenk of the Harvard School of Public Health describes our increasingly interdependent world and the importance of interprofessional education. He also discusses the key professional competencies necessary to truly transform care delivery and improve the health of the world's people. In Chapter 4, global health ethics within the context of globalization, and economic globalization in particular, are explored. Traditional Western bioethical principles and the need to reimagine these principles in the broader global context are discussed. Chapter 5 is an interview with Paul Farmer and Sheila Davis, who address the intersection of health, human rights, and social justice, and offer an interprofessional perspective on providing preferential care for the poor. Wolf examines the relationships between global health and community-public health nursing and the conceptual overlap of the disciplines in Chapter 6. In the last chapter of this unit, Sliney discusses the importance of bidirectional relationships for the success of global health partnerships and that the wisdom of those in resource-limited settings must be respected and embraced. In summary, Unit I provides the foundation for understanding the sociopolitical, economic, and cultural complexities that factor into the landscape of global health.

CHAPTER 1

Global Health and Global Nursing

Patrice K. Nicholas and Suellen Breakey

WHAT IS GLOBAL HEALTH?

The burgeoning discipline of global health has increased in scope and complexity since the beginning of the new century. Despite these advances, Farmer, Kleinman, Kim, and Basilico (2013) contend that identifying global health as a discipline is premature. Rather, they view global health as a collection of problems that affect the health of the world's people. Transformation from professional commitment to a unique discipline will require interdisciplinary efforts aimed at rigorously analyzing and solving the areas of concern for global health (Farmer et al., 2013). Global health emerged as a new concept arising from the earlier disciplines of public health and international health. Koplan et al. (2009), writing on behalf of the Consortium of Universities for Global Health Executive Board, note that:

> Global health is fashionable. It provokes a great deal of media, student, and faculty interest, has driven the establishment or restructuring of several academic programs, is supported by governments as a crucial component of foreign policy [Institute of Medicine, 2008] and has become a major philanthropic target. (p. 1993)

These authors advocate for the adoption of a common definition of global health that encompasses a broad range of health challenges (for example, maternal child health, infectious diseases, noncommunicable and chronic diseases, and environmental health issues). They argue that establishing and agreeing on a common definition is critical to prioritizing and advancing the work of global health. The authors also discuss the scope of global health in terms of both the problems to be addressed and its geographical reach. Koplan et al. contend that global health should not be restricted to health issues that cross international borders. Moreover, they suggest that:

> Global refers to any health issue that concerns many countries or is affected by transnational determinants, such as climate change or urbanization, or solutions, such as polio eradication. Epidemic infectious diseases such as dengue, influenza A (H5N1), and HIV

> infection are clearly global. But global health should also address tobacco control, micronutrient deficiencies, obesity, injury prevention, migrant-worker health, and migration of health workers. The global in global health refers to the scope of problems, not their location. (p. 1994)

Based on this rationale, Koplan et al. (2009) propose the following definition: "Global health is an area for study, research, and practice that places a priority on improving health and achieving health equity in health for all people worldwide" (p. 1995).

Global health—like public health but unlike international health—must address domestic health disparities as well as cross-border issues (Farmer et al., 2013; Koplan et al., 2009). As noted by Farmer et al. (2013), global health's antecedent term was international health, which emphasized the nation-state as the important focus. In their view, global health includes the role of nonstate institutions, including international nongovernmental organizations (NGOs), private philanthropies, and community-based organizations. Koplan et al. (2009) recommend that global health must also address the "training and distribution of the health-care workforce in a manner that goes beyond the capacity-building interest of public health" (p. 1994). They offer a view on global health that is relevant for global medicine and nursing:

> Global health can be thought of as a notion (as in the current state of global health), an objective (a world of healthy people which is a condition of global health) or a mix of scholarship, research, and clinical practice (with many questions arising as well as issues and competencies that must be addressed). (p. 1993)

Critical to a robust definition of global health, they argue, is agreeing on the goals, strategies, approaches, and skills needed by health professionals to achieve global health outcomes. Birn, Pillay, and Holtz (2009) suggest that while international health primarily focused on health issues in underdeveloped countries and the efforts by industrialized countries and international agencies to address these problems, to preserve their self-interests, the concept of global health reconceptualizes and depoliticizes international health to rise above the past ideological underpinnings of colonialism. This shift is also embedded in the recent Institute of Medicine (IOM, 2009) report on *The U.S. Commitment to Global Health: Recommendations for the Public and Private Sectors.* This report resulted from the convening of the Committee on the U.S. Commitment to Global Health to investigate the U.S. commitment to global health and articulate a vision for U.S. involvement in global health issues. The report identified five areas for action:

1. Scale-up of existing interventions to achieve significant health gains
2. Generate and share knowledge to address health problems prevalent in low- and middle-income countries

3. Invest in people, institutions, and capacity building with global partners
4. Increase U.S. financial commitments to global health
5. Set the example of engaging in respectful partnerships (IOM, 2009, p. 1)

Finally, this report notes that: "The United States has the responsibility as a global citizen, and an opportunity as a global leader, to contribute to improved health around the world. U.S. leadership in global health is a reflection of American values: generosity, compassion, optimism, and a wish to share the fruits of our technological advances with others around the world" (p. 3). This responsibility and commitment are also embraced by countries around the world. However, it is important to note that some argue that one of the negative aspects related to global health is that the United States attempts to assert unilateralism and dominate the international health agenda to meet its own national interests at the expense of international interests (Birn et al., 2009). Other industrialized countries may also need to closely examine the motivations behind their efforts.

EMERGENCE OF THE FIELD OF GLOBAL HEALTH

The field of global health emerged from the 19th-century work in public health in the United Kingdom, Europe, and the United States. Public health was influenced by the growing understanding of communicable diseases as well as the ability to gather data; to focus on population health rather than individuals; social justice and equity; and an emphasis on prevention rather than curative care (Koplan et al., 2009). Further, the IOM (1988) embraced the importance of public health in *The Future of Public Health* report, which formalized the mission, goals, and organizational framework for public health and defined the mission as "fulfilling society's interest in assuring conditions in which people can be healthy" (IOM, 1988), thus setting the stage to move public health to a global arena for societies worldwide. Fried et al. (2010) suggest that "public health has unique, and critically important, roles in creating global health and well-being" (p. S7 and original); further, they note that public health principles are foundational to global health approaches. Fried et al. also support the following key principles for global health leadership.

- Core values that include commitment to the public good and health as a human right
- A frame of reference that prevention is cost-effective and critical to accomplishing health for all
- Health promotion accomplished through a combined platform that engages science, evidence, experience, matching solutions to needs, shared knowledge, and a commitment to equity that is translated into practice
- Health systems and global public health leadership that includes a commitment to the most effective, evidence-based approaches to prevention and care in integrated health systems and with an approach to continual learning
- A continuum of prevention, treatment, and care (Fried et al., 2010, p. S8)

Fried et al.'s focus on global health also espouses a critical understanding of how population health is changing globally and that health professionals will confront old and new public health challenges in the years from 2030 to 2050 that include "the health challenges related to longevity and aging; chronic diseases (noncommunicable and communicable); the physical environment and climate change; the built environment and urbanization; disasters and conflicts shifting food sources and water and food security; population migration; and disparities and vulnerable populations" (Fried et al., 2010, p. S9). Similar to Koplan et al. (2009) and their call for a consistent definition of global health, Fried et al. suggest that clarity is needed in finding solutions to these health challenges. Their views are shared by Farmer et al. (2013) in that they propose engaging in science, technology, and practice for success in global health leadership.

International health emerged within the science of public health. Merson, Black, and Mills (2006) describe a framework that applies the principles of public health to challenges that affect low- and middle-income countries. However, this framework does not address the bidirectional issues that occur across countries or consider the fact that international health should also address the health needs of people in all countries. The Global Health Education Consortium (2009) explored the concepts of global versus international health and suggested that international health is more focused on health systems, policies, and practices with a lens on differences between countries rather than common health challenges shared across countries. Koplan et al. (2009) discuss the overlap of public health, international health, and global health. Specifically, they discuss the three areas as sharing certain characteristics that include "priority on a population-based and preventive focus; concentration on poorer, vulnerable, and underserved populations; multidisciplinary and interdisciplinary approaches; emphasis on health as a public good and the importance of systems and structures; and the participation of several stakeholders" (pp. 1993–1994). Most notably, they argue that global health is highly interdisciplinary and multidisciplinary across the health professions and extends to other disciplines and the unique and overlapping contributions that may occur. This aspect of global health further extends the scope and impact of the work from domestic health issues to crossing borders and continents, the distribution and competencies of health professionals, and capacity building and policy issues that are fundamental to the health of the world's people. Koplan and colleagues' definition of global health, as described previously, encompasses the knowledge, resources, and impact of societies in addressing health challenges. They note that global health engages in transnational solutions and engages many disciplines in promoting the goals of health. The profession of nursing, as the largest number of global health professionals worldwide, has a critical contribution to offer in global health.

THE CONTEXT OF GLOBALIZATION AND EMERGENCE OF 21st-CENTURY GLOBAL MEDICINE AND GLOBAL NURSING

The World Health Organization (WHO, 1946) defines health as "a state of complete physical, mental and social well-being and not merely the absence of disease or infirmity" (p. 100). This definition is universally accepted as the gold standard for health worldwide. Nurses and other health professionals play a key role in addressing the health of those living in our global village. There is both a professional duty as well as an ethical obligation for the nursing profession to advance this enduring vision of health for the world's people.

One of the most significant events that launched the focus on global health and subsequently global medicine and global nursing efforts was the Alma Ata conference. This conference was held in 1978 at the International Conference on Primary Health Care at Alma Ata, Kazakhstan, and was cosponsored by WHO and the United Nations Children's Fund (UNICEF). A major achievement of the conference was the adoption of a resolution, the Declaration of Alma-Ata (WHO, 1978), aimed at attaining Health for All by the Year 2000; subsequently, Health for All in the 21st Century (Health 21) was developed.

The U.S. Healthy People 2020 objectives are the U.S.-specific recommendations that address the important health goals similar to the goals of HFA 21. In 1990, the U.S. Department of Health and Human Services offered the first version of Healthy People 2000, with subsequent recommendations offered in 2010 and 2020. These reports address health promotion, health protection, and preventive services. The goals of Healthy People 2020 are shown in Figure 1.1.

Applying a Framework for Global Health and Global Nursing

Our world is becoming increasingly global. As Crigger, Brannigan, and Baird (2006) note: "Globalization is reshaping the world and its people. Nursing, likewise, is in the process of expanding its worldview to one that accommodates global care" (p. 15). In their paper on compassionate nursing professionals as good citizens of the world, they emphasize the importance of two key concepts—world citizenship and the nursing role as compassionate professional. World citizenship is a concept first developed by Nussbaum (1997) in her text *Cultivating Humanity*. Crigger et al. (2006) view nursing as integrally linked with globalization and world citizenship because of the profession's altruistic focus, engagement with social justice, and ethical framework. The second concept of compassionate professional is aimed at nurturing partnerships of mutual respect.

Austin (2001) poses a fundamental question related to the concept of compassionate professional: "What does a shift to a global frame of reference mean to the ethical practice of the 11 million nurses [now over 19.3 million] providing care around the world?" (p. 1). She contends that the global context of nursing is linked to the advancement of technology and transportation. She describes the international focus of nursing since 1870 and the work of nursing in the International Red Cross as early examples of nursing's global influence. Austin's (2001) focus is on three key ethical issues: the influence of biotechnological advancement on the business industry, the demands of equity and justice in global resource allocation, and the importance of an ethic that respects diverse cultures and values.

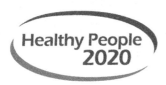

Framework

The Vision, Mission, and Goals of Healthy People 2020

The vision, mission, and overarching goals provide structure and guidance for achieving the Healthy People 2020 objectives. While general in nature, they offer specific, important areas of emphasis where action must be taken if the United States is to achieve better health by the year 2020. Developed under the leadership of the Federal Interagency Workgroup (FIW), the Healthy People 2020 framework is the product of an exhaustive collaborative process among the U.S. Department of Health and Human Services (HHS) and other federal agencies, public stakeholders, and the advisory committee.

Vision—A society in which all people live long, healthy lives.

Mission—Healthy People 2020 strives to:

- Identify nationwide health improvement priorities;
- Increase public awareness and understanding of the determinants of health, disease, and disability and the opportunities for progress;
- Provide measurable objectives and goals that are applicable at the national, state, and local levels;
- Engage multiple sectors to take actions to strengthen policies and improve practices that are driven by the best available evidence and knowledge; and
- Identify critical research, evaluation, and data collection needs.

Overarching Goals

- Attain high-quality, longer lives free of preventable disease, disability, injury, and premature death.
- Achieve health equity, eliminate disparities, and improve the health of all groups.
- Create social and physical environments that promote good health for all.
- Promote quality of life, healthy development, and healthy behaviors across all life stages.

FIGURE 1.1 Vision, mission, and goals of Healthy People 2020.

Most importantly, health challenges such as epidemics and infectious and chronic diseases, as well as human distress caused by ethnic conflicts, wars, famine, and lack of access to safe water, are drivers for the expanding role of nursing to engage in our global world. Most troubling is the fact that globalization is increasing the marginalization and poverty of the world's most vulnerable. Austin (2001)

Healthy People 2020 Framework

The Importance of an Ecological and Determinants Approach to Health Promotion and Disease Prevention

Health and health behaviors are determined by influences at multiple levels, including personal (i.e., biological, psychological), organizational/institutional, environmental (i.e., both social and physical), and policy levels. Because significant and dynamic inter-relationships exist among these different levels of health determinants, interventions are most likely to be effective when they address determinants at all levels. Historically, many health fields have focused on individual-level health determinants and interventions. Healthy People 2020 should therefore expand its focus to emphasize health-enhancing social and physical environments. Integrating prevention into the continuum of education—from the earliest ages on—is an integral part of this ecological and determinants approach.

The Role of Health Information Technology and Health Communication

Health information technology (IT) and health communication will be encouraged and supported as being an integral part of the implementation and success of Healthy People 2020. Efforts will include building, and integrating where feasible, the public health IT infrastructure in conjunction with the Nationwide Health Information Network; the *ONC-Coordinated Federal Health IT Strategic Plan: 2008–2012* and any updates developed by the HHS Office of the National Coordinator; the various aspects of IT to meet the direct needs of Healthy People 2020 for measures and interventions; and health literacy and health communication efforts.

Addressing "All Hazards" Preparedness as a Public Health Issue

Since the 2000 launch of Healthy People 2010, the attacks of September 11, 2001, the subsequent anthrax attacks, the devastating effects of natural disasters such as hurricanes Katrina and Ike, and concerns about an influenza pandemic have added urgency to the importance of preparedness as a public health issue. Being prepared for any emergency must be a high priority for public health in the coming decade, and Healthy People 2020 will highlight this issue. Because preparedness for all emergencies involves common elements, an "all hazards" approach is necessary.

FIGURE 1.1 Vision, mission, and goals of Healthy People 2020. (*continued*)

notes, "The shocking fact is that, according to the 1996 United Nations Human Development Report (1996), 358 people have more wealth than the combined incomes of 45% of the world population (i.e., 358 rich people own more than 2.3 billion poor people)" (p. 7). The trend that a very small number of people own the majority of the world's wealth continues today. Poverty is directly associated with

Healthy People 2020 Framework

Graphic Model of Healthy People 2020

The FIW developed a graphic model to visually depict the ecological and determinants approach that Healthy People 2020 will take in framing the national health objectives. This particular graphic was designed to emphasize this new approach, and is not meant as a comprehensive representation of all public health issues and societal domains. The graphic framework attempts to illustrate the fundamental degree of overlap among the social determinants of health, as well as emphasize their collective impact and influence on health outcomes and conditions. The framework also underscores a continued focus on population disparities, including those categorized by race/ethnicity, socioeconomic status, gender, age, disability status, sexual orientation, and geographic location.

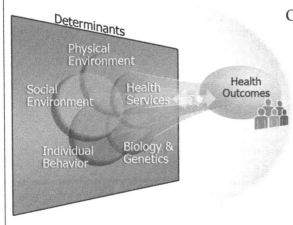

Healthy People 2020

A society in which all people live long, healthy lives

Determinants

Physical Environment

Social Environment

Health Services

Individual Behavior

Biology & Genetics

Health Outcomes

Overarching Goals:

- Attain high quality, longer lives free of preventable disease, disability, injury, and premature death.

- Achieve health equity, eliminate disparities, and improve the health of all groups

- Create social and physical environments that promote good health for all.

- Promote quality of life, healthy development and healthy behaviors across all life stages.

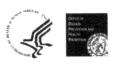

U.S. Department of Health and Human Services
Office of Disease Prevention and Health Promotion

www.healthypeople.gov

FIGURE 1.1 Vision, mission, and goals of Healthy People 2020. (*continued*)

poorer health outcomes. The resulting myriad acute and chronic health problems are frequently addressed in wealthier countries—although less effectively for the poor. However, poorer communities continue to struggle. Also, many of these communicable and chronic diseases such as measles, mumps, rubella, polio, severe acute respiratory syndrome (SARS), H1N1, and hepatitis, as well as HIV and malaria, are endemic in poorer countries.

Austin (2001) also discusses the shift of the nursing profession toward global engagement, as well as societal actions and the role of organizations, both nursing and world health organizations. Perhaps the most powerful question that she poses is the following: "Should we be tinkering with genes when, for many parts of the world, the most acute biotechnological problem is a safe water supply?" (p. 7). There are numerous issues that affect the health of the world's people and are global mandates for the nursing profession to address. These include lack of access to water, emerging infectious diseases, chronic illnesses, lack of access to natural resources, war and conflict, and climate change. As Nelson (2011) suggests: "Climate change poses challenges on a new scale for humanity, particularly for the populations of lower income countries" (p. vi). Further, women, children, and the elderly are noted to have unique vulnerabilities with respect to climate change—particularly related to "existing power inequalities and social norms, [thus] the impacts of climate change will not be felt evenly, but will be overlaid onto existing patterns of vulnerability within rural and urban populations and communities—and may make patterns of inequality more pronounced" (Nelson, 2011, p. vii).

Upvall, Leffers, and Mitchell (2014) address the intersection of international health, public health, and global nursing and define global nursing as "individual and/or population-centered care addressing social determinants of health with a spirit of cultural humility, deliberation, and reflection in true partnership with communities and other health care providers" (p. 6). Their conceptual model for partnership and sustainability for global nursing reflects the key components, the partnering process, and goal of sustainability of interventions in global efforts. Their model includes partner factors for global nurses and host partner nurses, which enriches the global projects. Mutual goal setting, collaboration, empowering, and capacity building are infused in the model since global nursing efforts should be bidirectional rather than U.S. centric.

GLOBAL HEALTH ORGANIZATIONS

This section provides an overview of several global organizations that influence the health of the world's people, including the United Nations (UN), WHO, the World Bank, the Centers for Disease Control and Prevention (CDC) in the United States, and nursing organizations such as the International Council of Nurses, which advances the work of nursing and the health needs of our global population. Although not an exhaustive review of the many organizations that contribute to global health, this section offers an overview of the contributions of global health organizations.

Global or international organizations are generally multilateral, bilateral, or nongovernmental in nature. Multilateral organizations cross several countries and borders and receive funding from multiple organizations and sources. Examples of these organizations include the UN, WHO, the Pan American Health Organization (PAHO), and the World Bank. Bilateral global organizations address country-specific needs through a single agency. The U.S. Agency for International Development (USAID) is an example of a bilateral global organization. NGOs or private voluntary organizations (PVO) are a third type of organization that addresses pressing global health needs. Examples of NGOs include Partners In Health (PIH), Project Hope, Doctors Without Borders, Oxfam, and the International Red Cross.

WHO was established in 1946 to address the international health needs and the comprehensive organization required of a health agency to address the scope of the world's health problems and the design of initiatives aimed at mitigating these problems. The organization is led by a director general and five assistant directors general with three major divisions: the World Health Assembly to address policy initiatives; an Executive Board that links the Assembly and the Secretariat; and the Secretariat, which supports the implementation of policy work and strategic initiatives with day-to-day operations. It is arguably the most important global organization to address the health of people worldwide. However, van de Pas and von Schaik (2013) suggest that there has been "a progressive erosion of the democratic space [that] appears as one of the emerging challenges in global health today" (p. 195), and that there are key challenges that WHO faces due to the power and money of which key decision makers have control. Hoffman and Rottingen (2013) argue that WHO has not been able to fully achieve its mission in

> serving as the world's pre-eminent public health authority and intergovernmental platform for global health . . . this forces [WHO] staff to walk uncomfortably along many fine lines: advising but never directing; guiding but never governing; leading but never advocating; evaluating but never judging. The result is mediocrity on both fronts. Instead, WHO should be split in two—separating its technical and political stewardship into separate entities. (p. 188)

Such a division, as Hoffman and Rottingen suggest, may strengthen WHO's political decision making and the organization's ability to secure independent scientific advice. The profession of nursing could benefit directly from this proposal if WHO's role in global nursing is strengthened and there is an emergence of strong nursing leadership within the organization and in countries worldwide.

As a global organization, in 2000 the UN promulgated the Millennium Development Goals (MDGs) in response to the 21st-century needs of the world's population. These goals look to address eight important health and development goals that aim to be achieved by 2020. The eight goals are

Goal 1: Eradicate extreme poverty and hunger
Goal 2: Achieve universal primary education

Goal 3: Promote gender equality and empower women

Goal 4: Reduce child mortality

Goal 5: Improve maternal health

Goal 6: Combat HIV/AIDS, malaria, and other diseases

Goal 7: Ensure environmental sustainability

Goal 8: Global partnership for development (UN, n.d.)

We present examples of successful global programs that address achievement of the UN MDGs in Table 1.1.

The UN has other initiatives that address global health issues, including UNICEF and global human rights initiatives. UNICEF was formed after World War II to address the health challenges of children worldwide.

TABLE 1.1 Examples of Millennium Development Goal (MDG) Programs in Global Locations

#	GOAL	TARGET	EXAMPLE
1	Eradicate extreme poverty and hunger	• Halve the proportion of people whose income is less than $1/day • Full employment and decent work for all • Halve the proportion of people suffering from hunger	Yemen: Since 2007, the World Food Programme's Food for Girls' Education Program gives wheat and vegetable oil to families who send their girls to school.
2	Achieve universal primary education	• Ensure that children are able to complete primary schooling	Guatemala: Since 2004, Abriendo Oportunidades has helped more than 4,000 girls from isolated Mayan communities build self-esteem and develop literacy.
3	Promote gender equality and empower women	• Eliminate gender disparity in education	Rwanda: UN Women is working with 15 cooperatives to teach women budgeting skills, and to encourage male farmers to include women in making financial and agricultural decisions.
4	Reduce child mortality	• Reduce the under-5 mortality rate by two thirds	Nigeria: Saving One Million Lives campaign, launched by the Nigerian government in 2012, expands access to health services by providing bed nets, supplying equipment to reduce mother–child HIV transmission, and providing health workers with telephones.
5	Improve maternal health	• Reduce maternal mortality ratio by three fourths • Universal access to reproductive health	India: UNICEF and its partners are working to provide conditional cash transfers to women who deliver in health facilities to encourage them to access appropriate medical care at time of delivery.

(continued)

TABLE 1.1 Examples of Millennium Development Goal (MDG) Programs in Global Locations (*continued*)

#	GOAL	TARGET	EXAMPLE
6	Combat HIV/AIDS, malaria, and other diseases	• Halt and begin to reverse spread of HIV/AIDS • Universal access to HIV/AIDS treatment • Halt and begin to reverse incidence of malaria and other major diseases	Thailand: In 2008, malaria parasites showed resistance to artemisinin, the most effective single malaria treatment drug. The WHO provided smartphones to community health workers who were monitoring and treating patients with the artemisinin-resistant malaria infection, facilitating the development of an electronic medical information system to track the disease and its progression. Zambia: The Zambian Ministry of Health, with support from UNDP, is creating 68 new antiretroviral therapy sites for HIV/AIDS treatment, and supplying drugs to existing sites to give 400,000 people access to free treatment.
7	Ensure environmental sustainability	• Integrate principles of sustainable development into country policies and reverse loss of environmental resources • Reduce biodiversity loss • Halve the proportion of the population without sustainable access to safe drinking water and sanitation • Achieve significant improvement in lives of at least 100 million slum dwellers by 2020	West Africa: Funding from the Global Environment Facility, along with the UN Environment Program and UNESCO, established in 2002 a transnational biosphere covering reserves in Benin, Burkina Faso, Cote d'Ivoire, Mali, Niger, and Senegal, to reduce desertification and promote biodiversity. Panama: The UN and the Panamanian government joined to bring safe water to nine indigenous communities in Panama. The communities are responsible for designing and constructing infrastructure and conducting maintenance.
8	Global partnership for development	• Further develop an open, rules-based trading and financial system • Address the needs of the least developed and landlocked countries • Deal with the debt of developing countries • Cooperate with pharmaceutical companies to provide access to essential drugs • Cooperate with the private sector to make new technologies available	South Africa: There exist over six billion mobile phone subscriptions around the world. In South Africa, more than 25,000 students have used interactive exercises and quizzes on mobile phones provided with government assistance to improve math skills. World Bank Group (WBG): In 2013, the WBG committed $52.6 billion in loans, grants, and equity investment guarantees to spur economic growth and fight extreme poverty.

PAHO was established in 1902 to address the health of people who lived in the Americas. As the oldest public health agency in the world, its aim is to develop partnerships to address health and quality of life of the people in these areas. PAHO is identified as the Regional Office for the Americas of WHO and is a member of the UN system.

The World Bank's focus as a multilateral agency is to lend money to resource-limited countries to address the health needs of populations. The mission of the World Bank is to "end extreme poverty within a generation and boost shared prosperity" (World Bank, 2013). Health-related and environmental programs are funded to support health through actions such as provision of electricity, access to safe water, communication systems, and addressing sexual and gender-based violence.

The mission of the USAID is to address extreme poverty globally and to promote democratic societies while preserving security and prosperity. The mission statement is aimed at embracing three key goals:

> We fundamentally believe that ending extreme poverty requires enabling inclusive, sustainable growth; promoting free, peaceful, and self-reliant societies with effective, legitimate governments; building human capital and creating social safety nets that reach the poorest and most vulnerable. (USAID, n.d., para 1)

Numerous NGOs provide support for global health and nursing initiatives worldwide. The International Red Cross is an example of one of the most comprehensive NGOs with a major focus on disaster relief. A wide variety of NGOs have a presence in many resource-challenged settings that focus on areas such as health care, education, and infrastructure development. Faith-based organizations have a large role in working with the marginalized and vulnerable. Clearly, as interest in global health increases, there are and will continue to be a large number of organizations offering aid and assistance. These same organizations will continue to compete for the limited existing material, financial, and human resources. A persistent challenge that will require ongoing dialogue is how to allocate these resources in a fair and equitable way.

NURSING AS PROFESSIONAL AND INTERPROFESSIONAL EDUCATION: GLOBAL ISSUES

Another critical aspect of global nursing that has emerged is the importance of interprofessional collaboration. This issue is key to global nursing since the roles of health professionals are inextricably intertwined to achieve the health of populations to accomplish global health goals (Frenk et al., 2010; IOM, 2010; WHO, 2014). In fact, the lack of interprofessional collaboration and education has yielded poorer outcomes for individuals and populations in resource-limited and resource-rich settings. In *The Lancet* report, Frenk et al. (2010) reflect on the critical need for interprofessional collaboration in the education of health professionals. This report was completed at the juncture of the 100-year anniversary of the Flexner, Goldmark, and Welch-Rose reports. The Flexner Report (1910) addressed the need to improve standards in medical education and was supported by the Carnegie Foundation. The Goldmark Report (Report of the Committee on Nursing Education; Goldmark, 1923) was funded by the Rockefeller Foundation and was the culmination of a 3-year examination of nursing education, with contemporary thought leaders in nursing—Annie W. Goodrich, M. Adelaide Nutting, and Lillian Wald—leading the study. The Welch-Rose Report (1915), also supported by the Rockefeller Foundation, focused on the need for public health education and leadership in the development of schools of public health. Notably, these reports focused on the emerging needs of health professions education in the early 20th century. However, no intersection or integration of the work across the health professions was detailed in these early reports. *The Lancet* report embarked upon an ambitious effort to address the pressing needs of our global society for advancing education of interprofessionals. As Frenk et al. (2010) noted:

> 100 years ago, a series of studies about the education of health professionals, led by the 1910 Flexner report, sparked groundbreaking reforms. Through integration of modern science into the curricula at university-based schools, the reforms equipped health professionals with the knowledge that contributed to the doubling of life span during the 20th century. (p. 1)

Thus, both Nightingale's urgent call to professionalize nursing and these reports ushered in the most productive time for advancing the health professions to address urgent global health problems.

The Lancet report spurred a call to action for 21st-century health professions educators and health care leaders to transform education to address the rapidly evolving health challenges impacting global health. Challenges identified in the document include emerging infectious diseases, environmental risks, and complex problems associated with chronic illnesses. In addition, war and conflict situations are associated with health security issues and alarming rates of morbidity and mortality. Shifting demographic patterns of low birth rates in many resource-rich countries and high birthrates in resource-limited countries underlie additional challenges. Chapter 20 addresses the complex issues of developing a robust global workforce amid the challenges of nurse migration.

Moreover, the fact that professional education has not kept pace with 21st-century health needs is a significant challenge for leaders in education and health care. Frenk et al. (2010) describe systemic problems that include

> . . . a mismatch of competencies to patient and population needs; poor teamwork; persistent gender stratification of professional status; narrow technical focus without broader contextual understanding; episodic encounters rather than continuous care; predominant hospital orientation at the expense of primary care; quantitative and qualitative

imbalances in the professional labour market; and weak leadership to improve health-system performance. (p. 1)

Frenk et al. (2010) urge that substantive efforts be made to address the deficiencies in health professions education since the *so-called tribalism* of the health professions has led to competition rather than collaboration in achieving global health outcomes.

U.S. IOM AND ROBERT WOOD JOHNSON FOUNDATION INITIATIVES: IS THERE A GLOBAL INFLUENCE FOR NURSING?

The U.S. IOM (2010) joined the collaborative effort to address these challenges with its landmark report, *The Future of Nursing: Leading Change, Advancing Health.* Although primarily a U.S.-centric focus on leading change, which was inspired by the enactment of the 2010 Affordable Care Act, the report describes the nursing profession as the largest segment of the health care workforce, and as vital in overhauling the current burdened health system. Culminating from a 2-year initiative, the report recommended a blueprint and action plan for the future of nursing. Common challenges and a call to action identified the following foci:

- Nurses should practice to the full extent of their education and training.
- Nurses should achieve higher levels of education and training through an improved education system that promotes seamless academic progression.
- Nurses should be full partners, with physicians and other health care professionals, in redesigning health care in the United States.
- Effective workforce planning and policy making require better data collection and an improved information infrastructure. (IOM, 2010)

These four recommendations have important global implications in addition to their relevance for U.S. health care reform. As Frenk et al. (2010) describe:

Redesign of professional health education is necessary and timely, in view of the opportunities for mutual learning and joint solutions offered for global interdependence due to flows of knowledge, technologies, and financing across borders, and the migration of both professionals and patients. What is clearly needed is a thorough and authoritative re-examination of health professional education, matching the ambitious work of a century ago. (pp. 1–2)

Recommendation One: Global Practice to the Full Extent of Education and Training

In our view, a comprehensive agenda for global nursing could tackle the challenges in educational systems worldwide, including differing entry and exit points for nursing education (e.g., secondary school, postsecondary school, diploma, and associate/baccalaureate, as well as entry-level programs at the graduate level) that currently exist. These complex and often conflicting entry and exit pathways are challenging for nursing professionals, as well as consumers worldwide, to understand; thus, this recommendation remains an elusive one. A more uniform global voice by nursing could extend the goal of practicing to the full extent of one's education and training, built upon a more uniform approach to global nursing education and practice. Shaffer (2014) calls for "a harmonization of education and educational portability" (p. 2) to address this. Shaffer examines the Bologna Accords (Bologna Process, 2010), which aim to harmonize educational processes and standardize the educational mobility of nurses across 47 participating countries throughout Europe. This was accomplished through the development of the European Higher Education Area (EHEA), which Shaffer (2014) notes has

> . . . made academic degree and quality assurance standards more comparable and compatible across [nursing] programs and academic institutions throughout Europe with the intent of facilitating the mobility of students, graduates, and higher education staff; preparing students for their future careers and for life as active citizens in democratic societies and supporting their personal development; and offering broad access to high-quality higher education based on democratic principles and academic freedom. (p. 2)

Recommendation Two: Achievement of Higher Education and Training Through Seamless Academic Progression

The global implications for recommendation two are compelling. Most of the global nursing workforce is ill prepared to care for the complex challenges of their patients, populations, and institutions. Whether in resource-rich settings like the United States, the United Kingdom, Canada, and other areas, or in resource-limited settings like sub-Saharan Africa, challenges exist in achieving higher education to meet the needs of patients and health systems. In one author's (PKN) experience teaching in South Africa, nurses were required to travel from Rwanda to South Africa to pursue master's level and certificate educational programs in psychiatric/mental health nursing since no programs were available in their home country. These nurses were Rwandan genocide survivors who had pursued education (secondary/postsecondary school) in nursing and were practicing in mental health facilities where many in Rwanda struggle with posttraumatic stress disorder. Traveling from one's home country for extended periods of time for advanced education is extremely challenging, particularly for nurses who are primarily women and may have familial responsibilities. Another author (SB), along with a physician, nurse, pharmacy colleagues, and others, is part of a team working toward building a sustainable cardiac surgical program; this author is engaged in an ongoing partnership with Rwandan colleagues to provide comprehensive care, including screening, surgical intervention, postoperative care, and comprehensive follow-up with patients. These are two examples of bidirectional efforts in global nursing.

Another paradox noted by Shaffer (2014) is that the United States has been slow to move toward potential changes in nursing education—particularly at the entry to practice level. Meanwhile, the international nursing community is forging ahead with baccalaureate entry for professional nursing practice, including the Philippines, India, and Mexico. Of note is that some countries that are considered resource limited are more progressive in their adoption of a standard of baccalaureate degree for practice entry and consistent approaches to seamless education. This remains an ongoing controversy for professional nursing education in the United States. The plethora of new pathways for entry to practice and confusion over degree nomenclature in the United States are additional areas for harmonization. Much can be learned across borders, countries, and continents.

Recommendation Three: Nurses Should Be Full Partners, With Physicians and Other Health Care Professionals, in Redesigning Health Care in the United States (and in Global Settings)

Perhaps one of the most remarkable challenges related to care provision globally and the notion of full partnership of those on the health professions team is the complex issue of gender since nursing is primarily a female profession and medicine historically, and in many global locations today, is a male profession. It is critical to address the gender inequity that often positions the nursing profession in a secondary role to medicine in every country of the world—what *The Lancet* report (Frenk et al., 2010) describes as persistent gender stratification by professional status. This is despite the fact that there are more than 35 million nurses worldwide and they are largely responsible for providing the vast majority of direct care in nearly every global location. Currently, our colleagues, Paul Farmer, MD, PhD, founder of Partners In Health, and Sheila Davis, DNP, RN, ANP, FAAN, have developed a collaborative interprofessional partnership that fully engages the entire team of health professionals—physicians, nurses, pharmacists, respiratory therapists, as well as nonprofessional/lay community health workers—in the redesign of care in Haiti and Rwanda. Achieving a full partnership in the health care team requires visionary interprofessional leadership. As the IOM report (2010) suggests:

> Being a full partner involves taking responsibility for identifying problems and areas of system waste, devising and implementing improvement plans, tracking improvement over time, and making necessary adjustments to realize established goals. In the health policy arena, nurses should participate in, and sometimes lead, decision making and be engaged in health care reform–related implementation efforts. Nurses also should serve actively on advisory boards on which policy decisions are made to advance health systems and improve patient care. (p. 3)

As we move toward a new, emerging paradigm of global nursing leadership in the 21st century, the full partnership of nurses worldwide is a social, cultural, and political imperative to advance the health of the world's people.

Recommendation Four: Effective Workforce Planning and Policy Making Require Better Data Collection and an Improved Information Infrastructure

Workforce planning and policy are key issues for the nursing profession in every country in the world. Historically, resource-rich countries encouraged migration of nurses from resource-limited countries to resource-rich countries to address the inadequate number of nurses, primarily for acute care settings. As described earlier, the issues of nurse migration are discussed in depth later in the text with an overview of historical, contemporary, and future challenges. However, nursing professionals are in agreement that nurses must become more engaged in workforce planning worldwide and engaged at the policy table so that the needs of populations are addressed from the nursing lens as well as an interprofessional perspective.

Another looming challenge is the breadth and scope of both workforce data and the influence of health information technology (HIT) for nursing and the health professions. Embracing HIT is another pressing global health imperative. In many settings, nursing is a key driver in the development of HIT, while in other resource-limited settings, little technology is available and progress toward advancing the promise of technology in meeting global health care needs remains a lingering challenge. A global initiative aimed at addressing HIT initiatives in resource-limited and resource-rich countries is urgently needed in the 21st century.

The IOM (2010) report primarily addresses the need to collect and analyze workforce data and projections for workforce requirements in the United States; however, there is an urgent need to do so globally. WHO collects and analyzes global workforce data for nursing, physicians, community health workers, and other roles. In 2006, the World Health Report addressed the global health workforce in the report, *Working Together for Health*. The report includes data and recommendations on the following: a global profile on health workers; responding to urgent health needs; education and preparation of the health workforce; maximizing the health workforce; managing exits from the workforce; formulating national health workforce strategies; and working together in and across countries.

THE UN MDGs AND THE ROLE OF WHO IN ADVANCING GLOBAL NURSING

WHO held a Global Forum for Government Chief Nursing and Midwifery Officers at WHO headquarters in May 2014 to address the UN MDGs and the key strategic and operational role of the nursing profession in achieving the MDGs. WHO plays a critical role, along with ministries of health, in increasing awareness of the importance of proactively addressing the requirements for the global health care workforce.

In 2010, WHO developed the Strategic Directions for Strengthening Nursing and Midwifery Services (SDNM) 2011 to 2015. This initiative was promulgated in partnership with the Commonwealth Secretariat, the Global Advisory Group on Nursing and Midwifery, the Global Network of WHO Collaborating Centers for Nursing and Midwifery Development, the International Confederation of Midwives, the International Council of Nurses, the International Labor Organization, the Honor Society of Nursing Sigma Theta Tau International, and colleagues within WHO. These strategic directions build upon the 2002 to 2008 SDNM and offer a framework for addressing broad, collaborative action to facilitate the capacity of nurses and midwives to contribute to furthering universal health care coverage; people-centered health care; policies affecting their practice and working conditions; and the scaling up of national health systems to meet global goals and targets. As noted in the SDNM document, "WHO has long acknowledged the crucial contribution of nurses and midwives to improving the health outcomes of individuals, families, and communities" (WHO, 2010, p. 2). Yet, the SDNM also points out that nurses are often not acknowledged as key stakeholders in health policy development. As such, these directions were designed to foster collaborative action as well as to ensure that they abide by the core values that underlie primary health care (PHC), including equity, solidarity, social justice, universal access to health care, and community participation.

The SDNM for 2011 to 2015 offer specific activities related to 13 objectives in five key results areas (KRAs): health system and service strengthening; policy and practice; education, training, and career development; workforce management; and partnership. The 13 objectives are linked to specific KRAs. For example, KRA 1 addresses the role of nursing in strengthening health systems and services, stating that, "nursing and midwifery services-led models form the basis of PHC reforms, especially in the areas of universal coverage and leadership for health" (p. 12). The objectives focus on nurses' and midwives' roles in people-centered care and their having a greater role in the design, delivery, and performance of health systems. The key importance of empowering nurses to provide leadership in health systems is also addressed in KRA 1 (WHO, 2010).

KRA 2 focuses on the need for proactive roles for nurses in health policy, planning, and decisions that affect the nursing profession and their role in ensuring country-specific approaches that are inclusive of nurses in leadership, governance, and regulation of practice. Three objectives are linked to KRA 2: the need to ensure that nursing and midwifery policies are viewed as integral to overall health policy making; the need to enhance the professional standing of nursing and midwifery; and the importance of building the evidence-based clinical practice of nursing and midwifery through research that will then further support the integration of evidence-based clinical practice worldwide (WHO, 2010).

KRA 3 addresses the need for developing institutional capacity and the development of appropriately skilled nurses and midwives who can fully engage in providing people-centered services. The first objective addresses the workforce supply and the need for educational programs at every level of nursing, as well as continuing education for nurses' and midwives' careers. The second objective focuses on the importance of having adequate teaching resources in order to achieve teaching objectives in both nursing and midwifery programs. Finally, the third objective for KRA 3 addresses career development and the need to develop nursing and midwifery expertise through postentry education, as well as mentoring and other development activities (WHO, 2010).

KRA 4 focuses on the need for policy makers to provide supportive environments for the nursing and midwifery workforce to meet current and emerging needs for people-centered care. Two objectives identified relate to the following: (1) workforce management and that ensures national development plans address nursing and midwifery human resources and the promotion of equitable access to nursing and midwifery services; and (2) performance enhancement, which aims to foster positive work environments through leadership support aimed at enhancing optimal nursing and midwifery performance and outcomes (WHO, 2010).

Finally, KRA 5 emphasizes the importance of including nurses and midwives as key stakeholders. Specifically, it addresses the need for active, systematic collaboration of nursing and midwifery in professional organizations and with community-based organizations, other groups of health professionals (e.g., physician organizations and NGOs), and governments (e.g., ministries of health). Three objectives are aimed at stewardship and governance, implementation and monitoring of SDNM, and effective networking and partnerships. Regarding stewardship and governance, the importance of government support to strengthen health systems is identified. Encouraging stakeholders to become involved in the implementation and monitoring of the SDNM is urged to strengthen resources, awareness, and advocacy of issues that affect the nursing and midwifery profession. The third objective is aimed at improving nursing and midwifery services through networking and partnerships with like-minded organizations and practice communities. This objective also addresses the importance of the integration of new technologies (e.g., health information technologies; WHO, 2010).

Along with developing the five KRAs and their accompanying objectives, the SDNM also provide more specific expected results and activities related to each objective within a given KRA. Additionally, indicators have been developed that can be used to assess progress toward the overarching goal of strengthening the nursing and midwifery workforce. These indicators provide more specific measures to evaluate progress in each area. And while the document states that countries may develop their own measures based on their individual priorities, they recommend that baseline data be collected in a standardized format in order to best evaluate ongoing performance and progress toward meeting the objectives of the SDNM (WHO, 2010).

CONCLUSION

This chapter provides an overview of global health, the emergence of the field of global health, a background and context of globalization, and a framework for global nursing. Florence Nightingale first addressed many of the challenges that remain lingering obstacles to achieving WHO's definition of health. The context of globalization and emergence of 21st-century nursing are critical areas to consider in achieving health goals worldwide. The UN MDGs and their relevance for nursing, as well as nursing's contribution to WHO, are discussed. Contemporary challenges and opportunities are addressed related to the global nursing workforce, nursing education, and the important reports that have implications for nursing worldwide.

REFERENCES

Austin, W. (2001). Nursing ethics in an era of globalization. *Advances in Nursing Science, 24*(2), 1–18.

Birn, A. E., Pillay, Y., & Holtz, T. H. (2009). *Textbook of international health: Global health in a dynamic world* (3rd ed.). New York, NY: Oxford University Press.

Bologna Process. (2010). *Focus on higher education in Europe: The impact of the Bologna Process.* Retrieved from http://eacea.ec.europa.eu/education/eurydice/documents/thematic_reports/122en.pdf

Crigger, N. J., Brannigan, M., & Baird, M. (2006). Compassionate nursing professionals as good citizens of the world. *Advances in Nursing Science, 29*(1), 15–26.

Farmer, P., Kleinman, A., Kim, J. Y., & Basilico, M. (Eds.). (2013). Introduction: A biosocial approach to global health. In *Reimagining global health.* Oakland, CA: University of California Press.

Flexner, A. (1910). *Flexner Report: Medical education in the United States and Canada.* New York, NY: Carnegie Foundation for the Advancement of Teaching.

Frenk, J., Chen, L., Bhutta, Z. A., Cohen, J., Crisp, N., Evans, T., . . . Zurayk, H. (2010). Health professionals for a new century: Transforming education to strengthen health systems in an interdependent world. *The Lancet, 376,* 1923–1958. Retrieved from http://www.healthprofessionals21.org/docs/HealthProfNewCent.pdf

Fried, L. P., Bentley, M. E., Buekens, P., Burke, D. S., Frenk, J. J., Klag, M. J., & Spencer, H. C. (2010). Global health is public health. *The Lancet, 375*(9714), 535–537. doi:10.1016/S0140-6736(10)60203-6

Goldmark, L. (1923). *Report of the Committee on Nursing Education.* New York, NY: Rockefeller Foundation.

Hoffman, S. J., & Rottingen, J. A. (2013). Split WHO in two: Strengthening political decision-making and securing independent scientific advice. *Public Health, 128,* 188–194.

Institute of Medicine. (1988). *The future of public health.* Washington, DC: The National Academies Press. Retrieved from http://iom.edu/Reports/1988/The-Future-of-Public-Health.aspx

Institute of Medicine. (2009). *The U.S. commitment to global health: Recommendations for the public and privates sectors.* Washington, DC: National Academies Press. Retrieved from http://www.iom.edu/Reports/2009/The-US-Commitment-to-Global-Health-Recommendations-for-the-Public-and-Private-Sectors.aspx

Institute of Medicine. (2010). *The future of nursing: Leading change, advancing health.* Washington, DC: The National Academies Press. Retrieved from http://thefutureofnursing.org/IOM-Report

Koplan, J. P., Bond, T. C., Merson, M. H., Reddy, K. S., Rodriguez, M. H., Sewankambo, N. K., & Wasserheit, J.N. (2009). Toward a definition of global health. *The Lancet, 373,* 1993–1995.

Merson, M. H., Black, R. E., & Mills, A. J. (2006). *International public health: Diseases, programs, systems, and policies* (2nd ed.). Sudbury, MA: Jones and Bartlett Publishers.

Nelson, V. (2011). *Gender, generations, social protection & climate change: A thematic review.* University of Greenwich, UK: Natural Resources Institute/Overseas Development Institute. Retrieved from http://www.odi.org/resources/docs/7283.docx

Nussbaum, M. C. (1997). *Cultivating humanity.* Cambridge, MA: Harvard University Press.

Shaffer, F. (2014). Ensuring a global workforce: A challenge and opportunity. *Nursing Outlook, 62,* 1–4.

United Nations. (n.d.). *Millennium Summitt, September 6–8, 2000.* Retrieved from http://www.un.org/en/events/pastevents/millennium_summit.shtml

United Nations. (2013). *Millennium development goals and beyond 2015.* Retrieved from http://www.un.org/millenniumgoals/partners.shtml

United Nations Development Program. (1996). *Human development report 1996.* New York, NY: Oxford University Press. Retrieved from http://hdr.undp.org/sites/default/files/reports/257/hdr_1996_en_complete_nostats.pdf

Upvall, M. J., Leffers, J. M., & Michell, E. M. (2014). Introduction and perspectives of global health. In M. J. Upvall & J. M. Leffers (Eds.), *Global health nursing: Building and sustaining partnerships* (pp. 1–20). New York, NY: Springer Publishing Company.

U.S. Agency for International Development. (n.d.). *Mission, values, and vision.* Retrieved from http://www.usaid.gov/who-we-are/mission-vision-values

U.S. Department of Health and Human Services, Office of Disease Prevention and Health Promotion. (n.d.). *Healthy People 2020.* Washington, DC. Retrieved from http://www.healthypeople.gov/2020/default.aspx

van de Pas, R., & von Schaik, L. G. (2013). Democratizing the World Health Organization. *Public Health, 128,* 195–201.

Welch, W. H., & Rose, W. (1915). *Institute of hygiene: A report to the General Education Board of the Rockefeller Foundation.* New York, NY: Rockefeller Foundation.

World Bank. (2013). *Ending extreme poverty and promoting shared prosperity.* Retrieved from http://www.worldbank.org/en/news/feature/2013/04/17/ending_extreme_poverty_and_promoting_shared_prosperity

World Health Organization. (1946). Preamble to the Constitution of the World Health Organization as adopted by the International Health Conference, New York, June 19 to July 22, 1946; signed on July 22, 1946, by the representatives of 61 states (Official Records of the World Health Organization, no. 2, p. 100).

World Health Organization. (1978). *The Declaration of Alma-Ata.* Retrieved from http://www.who.int/publications/almaata_declaration_en.pdf

World Health Organization. (2010). *Strategic directions for strengthening nursing and midwifery services (SDNM) 2011–2015.* Retrieved from http://www.who.int/hrh/resources/nmsd/en

CHAPTER 2

Climate Change, Climate Justice, and Environmental Health Issues

Patrice K. Nicholas, Suellen Breakey, Shira Winter,
Eleonor Pusey-Reid, and Ana M. Viamonte-Ros

Were there none who were discontented with what they have, the world would never reach anything better.

—Florence Nightingale

While the issue of climate change remains controversial from a political perspective, there is growing consensus that "the twentieth century witnessed an era of unprecedented, large-scale, anthropogenic changes to the natural environment" (Institute of Medicine, 2014, p. 1). Moreover, there is a burgeoning body of evidence that describes the negative aspects of climate change. This chapter provides an overview of the issues of climate change, climate justice, and the environmental health issues linked with climate change. Global warming is the most dramatic and devastating aspect of climate change. Gillis (2014), in his review of the draft of a United Nations (UN) report on climate change that was released in November 2014, reports that climate warming and shifts in climate such as "higher seas, devastating heat waves, torrential rain, and other climate extremes" will slow economic growth, erode food security, increase poverty, and limit access to water. Since the early contributions of Florence Nightingale (1860), nurses have always engaged in promoting a healthy environment as a way to ensure good health. Now, more than ever, a nursing focus on the environment is an essential component of nursing's professional mandate.

NIGHTINGALE'S INFLUENCE ON GLOBAL NURSING

The contributions of Florence Nightingale are noteworthy for her prescience in envisioning the role of nursing globally—where conflict, war, infectious diseases, increased urbanization, and lack of access to education were linked with high rates of morbidity and mortality. She was the innovator of professional nursing despite living in the 19th century and at a time when germ theory was not yet well understood. Her influence on global nursing is as strong in contemporary times as when she began writing about the importance of clean water, air, food, and light. Nightingale's visionary thinking on the essential aspects of a healthy environment for global health provides a framework for 21st-century global nursing. More than 100 years have passed since Nightingale influenced global nursing; however, some of the basic tenets of her views remain elusive for many of the world's people. The global work of nurses is often aimed at achieving the most basic of care needs—access to clean water, fresh air, medicines, and safe environments for providing care in hospitals and homes. Nightingale accomplished the goals of nursing and public health in part by developing partnerships with not only early nurse leaders, but also physicians, policy makers, engineers, government officials, and world leaders. Modeling this visionary leader's approach is critical for contemporary global nursing.

CLIMATE CHANGE VIEWED THROUGH THE LENS OF CLIMATE JUSTICE

There is an increasing body of literature that addresses emerging global health challenges and the role of health professionals—particularly nurses worldwide. The ethical framework that undergirds the nursing profession as well as the codes of ethics (American Nurses Association, 2001; International Council of Nurses, 2006) that nurses embrace necessitates a collective call to action. Among the major challenges we face are climate change and its impact on the health of the world's people.

The Fifth Assessment Reports by the Intergovernmental Panel on Climate Change (IPCC, 2014) were issued in March 2014 and Working Group II addressed the urgent health problems related to global warming. The report details that ill health due to the impact of climate change has increased rates of injury, disease, and death due to lack of access to water and food and increases in water-borne diseases; extreme heat that leaves elderly and young populations most vulnerable to health challenges; fires due to extreme heat with resulting air pollution as well as loss of shelter; floods and droughts; undernutrition due to diminished food production and food insecurity; and a host of diseases that are increasing as a result of climate change ranging from respiratory ailments to women's health issues including adverse birth outcomes.

A right to health is not the only basic human right that is endangered as a result of climate change. A recent volume of the journal *Health and Human Rights* focused solely on climate change, health, and human rights. Mary Robinson, former president of Ireland and president of the Mary Robinson Foundation—Climate Justice, offered the foreword to the volume and described climate justice as "a discipline that addresses the interlinked challenges of climate change, human rights, and development" (Robinson, 2014, p. 4). She notes that climate change has had a deleterious effect on basic human rights, including access to food, water, and shelter as well as health, and that the negative effects of extreme weather events resulting from climate change disproportionately affect the poor and vulnerable. She states that it is a grave injustice since those most affected by climate change are the least responsible for the problem. Further, Lemery, Williams, and Farmer (2014) argue that it is imperative to engage in immediate action to slow the rate of global warming since reversal may not be attainable. They discuss the importance of acknowledging the science linking climate change to damaging effects on human health. They also suggest that:

> The people who will suffer most are those who were most vulnerable to begin with, living in regions of the world with perilous human security, pervasive poverty, little fulfillment of human rights, geographic disadvantage, and contributing the least to greenhouse gas emissions. It is in these places that the threat-multiplying effects of climate change will denigrate human dignity, health, and potential the most. It is in these same disadvantaged settings that fragile health systems are least able to cope with the increased demands they will face. (Lemery et al., 2014, p. 2)

Cameron, Bevins, and Shine (2013) further the argument that issues of climate change are an injustice for the world's marginalized and vulnerable—particularly women and children—that undermines the attainment of human rights. They highlight the principle of equity and its operationalization as a means to achieve climate justice. Moreover, they advocate that the following elements are a necessary part of an effective and equitable international climate agreement: ensuring that the voices of the most vulnerable are heard; ensuring transparency and accountability in decision making, protecting the rights of all; emphasizing intergenerational equity; and ensuring that all countries benefit from a new form of economic growth that would be created (Cameron et al., 2013).

Violence, Conflict, and War

Violence poses an enormous challenge globally for nursing and is widely identified as a threat to public health. Nurses have important roles in addressing and intervening with victims of violence. In many resource-rich countries, there is an epidemic of violence—from gun violence in cities and schools to violent crime that is endemic. Poor communities struggle disproportionately with violence in their communities; however, it is a problem that is an urgent issue for all citizens of the world.

Conflict and war are major threats to human health; thus, they are critical issues for nurses to address. Florence Nightingale's role in conflict and war launched professional nursing globally. In addition to addressing soldiers' health, the human toll for those who are affected by being forced to leave their homes and communities, their health and human rights threatened, and lack of access to the rights to food, water, sanitation, and health care are all areas for the nursing profession to address. In addition, a recent National Public Radio program noted that the spark that may have ignited the violence and war in Syria was due to climatic changes that were related to a severe drought between 2006 and 2010 that transformed nearly 60% of the country into desert and killed as many as 80% of the cattle. Further, Levy and Sidel (2014) noted that "hundreds of thousands of farmers migrated to cities, seeking work, and many felt they were mistreated by the government. The dislocation and difficult conditions of the farmers helped to create the first spark of the civil war" (pp. 34–35). The resulting war in Syria has also led to instability in other countries throughout the Middle East. Conflicts related to lack of access to water and rainfall pose a looming global danger.

Water-Related Effects of Climate Change

There is no more pressing issue for global health and nursing than the challenges that occur due to lack of access to water. For the nursing profession, the lack of access to water in many regions of the world is an urgent humanitarian issue—particularly in areas of sub-Saharan Africa, Asia, and smaller island nations, for example, Haiti and the Marshall Islands (Ahlgren, Yamada, & Wong, 2014; Varma et al., 2008). With rising oceans and less rainfall in some areas, we are confronted with sea levels and saltwater intrusion that are occurring rapidly and extreme weather events due to storms, floods, and heat waves. In Haiti, the lack of access to clean water is one of the most pressing health-related and human rights challenges. Varma et al. (2008) discuss the enormous challenges that the people of Haiti face related to the lack of clean water. Problems with Haiti's water system, the lack of access to the needed quantity and quality of water, and the resulting health consequences due to water-borne illnesses are major risks for negative health outcomes. The reemergence of cholera was likely introduced into the Artibonite River by UN peacekeepers from Nepal who arrived after the devastating earthquake in 2010. The U.S. Centers for Disease Control and Prevention (CDC, 2014b) estimate that more than 470,000 cases of cholera and 6,631 deaths have occurred in the population due to diarrheal disease—representing the worst cholera outbreak in recent history and a modern public health emergency.

Ahlgren et al. (2014) discuss the grave challenges faced by the entire population of the Marshall Islands due to rising oceans and the need for international food aid. The Marshall Islands have experienced climatic changes that have led to drought periods and flooding that have yielded a significant need for food aid with unhealthy products imported. This has subsequently resulted in poorer health outcomes, including an alarming rise in the rates of diabetes in the population. Ahlgren et al. (2014) report that the people of the island nation are experiencing epidemics of child malnutrition, diabetes, obesity, and other chronic diseases due to lack of healthy foods that are sent as imported international food aid.

Both flooding and droughts are emerging water-related challenges that are important for global nursing. Whether a humanitarian disaster such as Hurricane Katrina in New Orleans in the United States or severe droughts that limit crop production in sub-Saharan Africa and other global locations, the overabundance or lack of water are looming threats to the health of the world's people. The vulnerability of the world's children was the focus of a recent World Health Organization/United Nations Children's Fund (WHO/UNICEF) (2014) report. The most recent estimates of the WHO/UNICEF Joint Monitoring Program (JMP) for Water Supply and Sanitation from data collected in 2011 suggest that:

> [Thirty-six] percent of the world's population—2.5 billion people—lack improved sanitation facilities, and 768 million people still use unsafe drinking water sources. Inadequate access to safe water and sanitation services, coupled with poor hygiene practices, kills and sickens thousands of children every day, and leads to impoverishment and diminished opportunities for thousands more. (UNICEF, 2014, para 1)

EMERGING INFECTIOUS ILLNESSES

Malaria, Dengue, Chikungunya, and Ebola as Exemplars of Global Illnesses

Many longstanding as well as emerging illnesses are becoming global health urgencies due to climate change and mobility of populations. Mosquito-borne illnesses are increasing due to shifts in temperature, rainfall, frequency of natural disasters, and shifts in population growth, migration, urbanization, and international trade and travel (Chang, Fuller, Carrasquillo, & Beier, 2014). Chang et al. (2014) note that "the speed of mosquito reproduction, the speed of viral incubation, the distribution of dengue virus and its vectors, human migration toward urban areas, and displacement after natural disasters" (p. 93) all increase health risks, particularly of the poor. Four illnesses are addressed as examples and are considered global nursing priorities.

Malaria

Malaria has been a lingering challenge for thousands of years and first erupted in Africa. Malaria spreads via two types of hosts: *Anopheles* mosquitoes and humans (WHO, 2013). When humans are infected, the malaria parasite travels to the liver and subsequently to the red blood cells, where these cells are destroyed and release daughter parasites known as merozoites (WHO, 2013).

The blood stage parasites are those that cause the symptoms of malaria; when certain forms of blood stage parasites (gametocytes) are picked up by a female *Anopheles* mosquito during a blood meal, they start another, different cycle of growth and multiplication in the mosquito (WHO, 2013). The mosquito acts as a vector since when the mosquito bites an infected human, and a subsequent human, the mosquito's salivary glands—where the parasites reside—are transmitted from one human to another (WHO, 2013).

In the annual, *World Malaria Report 2013*, WHO (2013) noted that since 2000, more than half of the countries that face ongoing challenges due to the incidence of confirmed malaria have recorded decreases in reported cases and deaths. Additionally, WHO noted that morbidity rates fell globally by 42% between 2000 and 2012 in all age groups, and by 48% in children younger than the age of 5. Further, WHO notes that if the annual rate of decrease in incidence that has occurred over the past 12 years is maintained, then malaria mortality rates may decrease by as much as 52%. However, an estimated 3.4 billion people globally were at risk of malaria in 2012 (WHO, 2013, p. xi). Dr. Margaret Chan, the director-general of WHO, stated in the *World Malaria Report 2013* (WHO, 2013) that progress has been made as a result of vector control interventions, increased access to diagnostic testing, and artemisinin-based combination therapies (ACTs).

Dengue Fever

Dengue fever is a *flavivirus* with four serotypes that are carried by two types of mosquitoes—*Aedes aegypti* and the *Aedes albopictus* mosquitoes. In humans, the virus causes an acute febrile illness accompanied by malaise, retroorbital pain, and bone pain that give dengue fever the name "breakbone fever" (Chang et al., 2014). Up to 5% of those who acquire dengue fever will develop severe dengue, which results in shock, pleural effusions, ascites, and often severe bleeding. While the dengue epidemic originated in Africa, it has spread more widely to Latin America and Asia; its spread began during World War II and spread due to population mobility (Chang et al., 2014).

Chikungunya

Chikungunya is a reemerging mosquito-borne disease that was recently documented in the Caribbean. According to the U.S. CDC (2014a), this was the first time chikungunya was found in the Americas. Symptoms include headache, muscle pain, joint swelling, or rash, as well as fever and joint pain (CDC, 2014a). Mortality is not high, but the symptoms of chikungunya may be severe and disabling, and last for months or years, although most who acquire this illness improve in approximately one week. Meason and Paterson (2014) suggest that "extrapolation of [the] regional pattern [of weather patterns], combined with known climate factors impacting the spread of malaria and dengue, summate to a dark picture of climate change and the spread of this disease [chikungunya] from south Asia and Africa into Europe and North America" (p. 105). The challenge of chikungunya has been present in episodic outbreaks in Africa, India, and Southeast Asia for many decades. In 2014, the CDC (2014a) indicated that the following Caribbean countries have reported cases of chikungunya: Anguilla, Antigua, British Virgin Islands, Dominica, the Dominican Republic, French Guiana, Guadeloupe, Guyana, Haiti, Martinique, Puerto Rico, Saint Barthelemy, Saint Kitts, Saint Lucia, Saint Martin (French), Saint Vincent and the Grenadines, Saint Maarten (Dutch), Turks and Caicos Islands, and the U.S. Virgin Islands.

Ebola Virus Disease

Ebola virus disease (EVD) (formerly known as Ebola hemorrhagic fever) is an emerging world health challenge that first appeared in 1976 in two simultaneous outbreaks in the Sudan and the Democratic Republic of the Congo; the name of the virus was taken from its outbreak in a village near the Ebola River. The case fatality rate is estimated at up to 90% and there is no known treatment (WHO, 2014b). The outbreaks were formerly in Central and West Africa; the virus is transmitted to people from wild animals and spreads to the human population through human-to-human transmission (WHO, 2014b). The CDC (2014c) recently noted that the 2014 outbreak is one of the largest in history, affecting multiple countries in West Africa, including widespread transmission in Guinea, Liberia, and Sierra Leone and infection in Nigeria and Senegal. The most recent CDC statistics, as of February 2015, indicate that the total cases are: total cases (suspected, probable, and confirmed), 22,560; laboratory-confirmed cases, 13,888; and total deaths, 9,019. The CDC (2014c) also noted that ZMapp, an experimental treatment with limited trials for safety and efficacy, has decreased the mortality rate of EVD; ZMapp is composed of three monoclonal antibodies that bind with the Ebola virus and is currently being tested in humans affected by EVD.

Recently, advanced molecular detection (AMD) methods have been utilized by the CDC to examine whether mutations are occurring in the virus during the outbreak (CDC, 2014c). The genetic sequence information confirmed the Liberian viral samples were 99% identical to the virus circulating in Guinea and Sierra Leone; critically important to the CDC was that the virus in the 2014 epidemic is 97% similar to the virus that first emerged in 1976 (CDC, 2014c).

ENVIRONMENTAL HEALTH ISSUES

Air Pollution

The health threats posed by air pollution due primarily to the burning of fossil fuels are a global challenge. While many countries have rallied to reduce air pollution and the negative health sequelae that occur as a result of long-term exposure to air pollutants, other countries have been slow to engage in addressing this enormous health risk. As a result, respiratory ailments, cardiovascular disease, and other chronic illnesses are becoming more common worldwide and many countries have not addressed the need to limit exposure to the aftereffects of burning fossil fuels. Most countries in the world continue to rely on fossil fuel energy despite the need to reduce the use and limit greenhouse gases (GHG).

Because of the urgency associated with environmental pollution and climate change, the Kyoto Protocol to the UN Framework Convention on Climate Change (UNFCCC) was adopted in Kyoto, Japan, in 1997 and entered into force in February 2005 (UN, 2014). The Kyoto Protocol is an international treaty that sets binding obligations specifically for industrialized countries to reduce emissions of greenhouse gases. The protocol is an environmental treaty with the goals of limiting anthropogenic (or human-induced) interference on the climate system. In Article 2 of the UNFCCC, the important goal of allowing ecosystems to adapt naturally to climate change and ensuring that food security is not threatened, as well as supporting economic development, are discussed. Unfortunately, this international agreement did not gain the necessary support of a large number of countries—including the United States, which signed but did not ratify the treaty. Since the Kyoto Protocol expires in 2020, representatives from several countries and agencies have agreed to meet in 2015 in Paris to address the need for international consensus on the issues and to attract support in addressing the enormous challenges caused by emissions of greenhouse gases.

The UNFCCC website states that the Protocol:

> recognizes that developed countries are principally responsible for the current high levels of GHG [greenhouse gas] emissions in the atmosphere as a result of more than 150 years of industrial activity, and places a heavier burden on developed nations under the principle of common but differentiated responsibilities. (UN, 2014, para 1)

Air pollution resulting from environmental conditions related to industry and automobile use are responsible for an increasing prevalence of acute and chronic respiratory and cardiovascular problems. In fact, the United States was the largest contributor to carbon pollution, but since 2000, emissions have decreased substantially. Both China and India have highly coal-intensive economies, and China has a substantial problem with sulfur dioxide particulate pollution (Shaw, 2014). Both carbon and sulfur dioxide pollution have a highly deleterious impact on health with high morbidity and mortality, particularly from respiratory and cardiovascular diseases.

Other contributing factors to poor health include household air pollution, which is the inhalation of acrid smoke and particulates often related to indoor cooking smoke (Bruce, Perez-Padilla, & Albalak, 2000). WHO (2014c) has identified indoor cooking smoke as linked to acute respiratory infections, chronic obstructive pulmonary disease (COPD), chronic bronchitis and emphysema, lung cancer, heart disease, blindness, and low birth weight. In addition, the risk of severe burn injuries for women and particularly children is a major public health issue because of the dangers associated with open-fire cookstoves that are widely used in resource-limited countries.

Tobacco Use and Health Consequences

Another of the greatest health challenges of the 20th and 21st centuries is tobacco use and its association with a host of complex illnesses. Most notably, lung cancer and cardiovascular complications including coronary heart disease and stroke/cerebrovascular disease, as well as chronic respiratory problems including COPD and exacerbation of asthma, are linked to tobacco use. Tobacco use has been identified as a major global public health problem. It is known that not only firsthand smoke, but also exposure to secondhand smoke by a nonsmoker and exposure to thirdhand smoke (e.g., exposure to the clothing of a smoker even if not directly exposed to the tobacco smoke) are associated with negative health outcomes. Early efforts in the 1960s to address this problem included public health campaigns aimed at reducing the incidence of smoking, bans on advertising in certain media, a warning label on tobacco products, and a ban on smoking in many settings. In the United States and other countries, bans on smoking exist both inside buildings and in public areas; this has reduced exposure to secondhand tobacco smoke in an effort to ameliorate the effects of tobacco exposure. Unfortunately, the tobacco industry has shifted its focus globally to acquire a larger market for its products. In recognition of the dangers of tobacco, WHO (2014a) established the Framework Convention on Tobacco Control in June 2003 in Geneva, which was subsequently ratified and enforced in 2005. While efforts to reduce exposure to cigarette smoke have gained momentum in resource-rich countries, many resource-limited countries lag behind in public health efforts aimed at reducing the morbidity and mortality associated with smoking.

Occupational Injury as a Global Health Challenge

Occupational injuries are a major source of morbidity and mortality worldwide. Most workers face many challenges since resource-limited countries often do not have workplace protections similar to the U.S. Occupational Safety and Health Administration (OSHA). Musculoskeletal injuries are common and represent a global health urgency. Many occupations are inherently risky and attract less educated workers who have fewer employment options. These occupations—for example, manufacturing, mining, fishing, building, and agriculture—are linked to serious injuries, and workers place their health at great risk daily in their occupational settings. Similar to Nightingale's focus on environment and noise, in the following section we address noise as a global health threat.

Noise

Exposure to noise is a major health challenge worldwide and most often is related to occupational exposure or residing near worksites that control levels of noise poorly. Global regulations related to protection from occupational exposure vary widely and may not always be enforced even with the oversight of governmental agencies such as OSHA. OSHA (2002) suggests that noise (or unwanted sound) is a major public and occupational health problem that is often related to industrial processes; however, air and automobile traffic and wind turbines are other sources of noise. As OSHA (2002) describes:

> Exposure to high levels of noise causes hearing loss and may cause other harmful health effects as well. The extent of damage depends primarily on the intensity of the noise and the duration of the exposure. Noise-induced hearing loss can be temporary or permanent.

> Temporary hearing loss results from short-term exposures to noise, with normal hearing returning after [a] period of rest. Generally, prolonged exposure to high noise levels over a period of time gradually causes permanent damage. . . . Loud noise can also create physical and psychological stress, reduce productivity, interfere with communication and concentration, and contribute to workplace accidents and injuries by making it difficult to hear warning signals. Noise-induced hearing loss limits your ability to hear high frequency sounds, understand speech, and seriously impairs your ability to communicate. (p. 1)

In the United States and many other countries, there is an increased focus on reducing noise levels in hospitals. The Joint Commission on Accreditation of Healthcare Organizations (JCAHO) and Joint Commission International (JCI) have developed recommendations related to noise reduction in hospitals and other health care settings in recognition of the negative sequelae of noise and lack of adequate sleep. Increasingly, nurses in clinical practice and nurse researchers are focusing on improving sleep environments and sleep hygiene for patients.

ENVIRONMENTAL CONTAMINATION BY CHEMICALS

Chemical Exposure and the Potential Connection to Autism Spectrum Disorder and Cancer

Pesticide exposure is a health danger of enormous proportion. Pesticides pose a variety of health challenges due to their carcinogenic properties as well as the potential link to issues with proper brain development. Recently, a potential link between autism spectrum disorder (ASD) and maternal exposure to pesticides during pregnancy has been identified. Lyall, Schmidt, and Hertz-Picciotto (2014) examined prenatal maternal health and nutrition, substance use, and exposure to environmental agents and the prevalence of ASD in children. The interplay of genetics and environment is an area of intense research, particularly since the worldwide incidence of ASD has risen dramatically since 1990 (IOM, 2011).

Childhood vaccinations have also been implicated as a contributing factor in the development of ASD. However, the role of vaccines (particularly vaccines with thimerosal) and their link to ASD were investigated and culminated in the IOM (2011) report that found no causal link between vaccines and ASD. More recently, Maglione et al. (2014) published a systematic review that further validates the earlier IOM report. These researchers conducted a systematic review of the evidence published since the 2011 IOM report and found that the evidence was strongly related to the safety of vaccines for adults, adolescents, and children. Specifically, the investigation found that for children under the age of 6 years, vaccines including DTaP (diphtheria, tetanus, and acellular pertussis), hepatitis A, hepatitis B, influenza, meningococcal, MMR (measles, mumps, and rubella), and varicella were safe. The authors also reviewed the evidence on several childhood vaccines

(*Haemophilus influenzae* type b [Hib], pneumococcal, rotavirus, and inactivated poliovirus vaccines), which were not studied in the original 2011 IOM report, and concluded that the strength of the evidence suggests that MMR is not associated with autism and that MMR, DTaP, Td (tetanus), Hib, and hepatitis B vaccines are not associated with childhood leukemia (Maglione et al., 2014). The authors did report an association with vaccines and some serious adverse events, such as intus-susceptions after rotavirus vaccine, but these are exceedingly rare. The American Academy of Pediatrics (2014) noted that this new report emphasized the safety of vaccines for adults, adolescents, and children.

The role of pesticide exposure in carcinogenesis is another area of study that focuses on both those who apply pesticide as well as those who are bystanders to the application. The damaging effects of pesticide exposure and cancer are being studied in prostate cancer, non-Hodgkin's lymphoma, leukemia, multiple myeloma, breast cancer, and other cancers. In their review, Alavanja, Ross, and Bonner (2013) suggest that several studies support the role of pesticides used in agricultural, commercial, and home and garden applications and their association with excess cancer risk. It is also known that exposure to neonicotinoid pesticides may be harmful to bee populations even in lower concentrations, and these pesticides may have health consequences for humans (Larson, Redmond, & Potter, 2013).

Hydraulic Fracturing and Directional Drilling of Oil and Natural Gas (Fracking)

Health threats associated with the extraction of natural resources such as oil and natural gas, which involves deep drilling, is an emerging area of investigation. The process of fracking involves drilling thousands of feet deep into permeable rock, such as shale, to access natural gas. Weaknesses or fractures in the rock are opened in the process and large amounts of water mixed with sand and hazardous and nonhazardous chemicals are injected (Finkel & Law, 2011). Many of the chemicals are associated with respiratory, gastrointestinal, and nervous system disorders. McDermott-Levy, Kaktins, and Sattler (2013) report that the potential health consequences of fracking may begin at the onset of drilling, and those exposed may experience negative consequences for long periods after drilling ceases. Several researchers have identified outcomes of fracking that are linked to negative health consequences, including water and air contamination, elevated noise levels, increased intensity of diesel track traffic volume, occupational hazards, and stress and illness in rural communities located near fracking sites (Burton & Stretesky, 2014).

Methane leaks and exposure to silica dust are known hazards. Howarth Santoro, and Ingraffea (2011) suggest that fracking is believed to result in a 30% increase in methane escaping into the environment compared with conventional methods of gas extraction, thus threatening the health of the neighboring population. In addition to the human toll, the ecological damage must be addressed. Drinking water sources, including surface water, reservoirs, and wells, are at risk of contamination by methane and other chemicals, resulting in measurable levels of benzene in the blood—a known human carcinogen (McDermott-Levy et al., 2013). Because of the potential association with negative health effects, several countries have banned fracking.

Lead Poisoning

The prevalence of lead poisoning in children has decreased dramatically in many resource-rich countries due to governmental efforts aimed at limiting childhood exposure to lead. However, in some poorer countries and communities, exposure to lead may still be high. There are many emerging economies in the midst of rural and industrial development that have not enacted safeguards to mitigate negative consequences such as industrial pollution, which leads to contamination of water, soil, and air (Cohen & Amon, 2012). Lead poisoning is particularly toxic for children since they are more susceptible to the damage that lead can cause in the brain, liver, kidney, and nerves, as well as anemias and other serious outcomes including comas, convulsions, and death (UNICEF and United Nations Children's Program, 1997). The CDC (2014d) indicates that there is no acceptable level of blood lead concentration that is safe and that even concentrations less than 10 mcg of lead per deciliter of blood are associated with cognitive problems. In 2012, the CDC revised their earlier recommendations that suggested that if a child's blood lead level is elevated between 10 and 15 mcg, then the nutritional or environmental source be addressed (CDC, 2014d). The CDC (2014d) now uses a reference level of 5 mcg per deciliter to identify children with blood lead levels that are much higher than most children's levels. If the source is related to a contaminated environment, then people should be moved away to avoid exposure.

China is an example of a country that is in the midst of enormous rural and industrial development and is grappling with the environmental price that widespread industrial pollution has yielded—contaminated water, soil, and air due to lack of environmental protection regulations. As a result, lead poisoning in children has become a major health threat with the resulting problems of reduced IQ and attention span, reading and learning problems, behavioral problems, hearing loss, and problems with vision and motor functioning (UNICEF and United Nations Children's Program, 1997). The health concerns and global nursing efforts for the population of children in China require an urgent response.

Poor Countries and Communities as Recipients of Toxic Waste

Breivik et al. (2011) report on recent studies that suggest that polychlorinated biphenyl (PCB) air concentrations are high in parts of Africa and Asia, which are regions where PCBs were never extensively used and the levels are considered dangerous. Many countries of Africa and Asia are known to be recipients of obsolete products and wastes containing PCBs and other industrial contaminants.

This is a long-standing pattern both in the United States and globally whereby resource-rich communities tend to discard waste—often toxic waste—in communities and other poor countries to avoid having toxic material located in their home communities and countries. There is an urgent need to address the health challenges related to exposure to toxic waste and trash. In the United States, poorer communities often have greater numbers of waste disposal areas and have higher rates of asthma and chronic respiratory disease; these health consequences are also related to poor housing and environmental pollution from disposal and trash sites.

NATURAL DISASTERS AND NURSING'S ROLE GLOBALLY

Disasters are associated with emergent health consequences that require a nursing response. Humanitarian disasters like flooding, hurricanes, typhoons, tsunamis, earthquakes, and tornadoes, as well as infectious disease outbreaks, often exact a human toll on health. The Association of Public Health Nurses (APHN) developed a position paper titled *The Role of Public Health Nurses in Emergency and Disaster Preparedness, Response, and Recovery* in 2013. The APHN's vision for emergency and disaster preparedness is that "public health nurses understand their disaster roles in light of the scope of practice. . . . [to] be ready for practice across the disaster cycle, advocating for and working beside the whole community" (p. 4). APHN (2013) identifies four principles related to the role of nurses in disasters: that public health nursing roles are consistent with the scope of public health nursing practice; that the components of the nursing process align with the stages of preparedness (prevention, protection, and mitigation), response, and recovery; competencies and standards of practice are critical elements in addressing the disaster cycle; and the role of public health nurses is to bring leadership, policy, planning, and practice expertise. In the immediate aftermath of a disaster response, the need for expertise of nurses in fields other than public health may be urgent. For example, after the 2010 earthquake in Haiti, nurses with perioperative and orthopedic experience were key aspects to the effectiveness of the disaster response.

CONCLUSION

This chapter sought to provide an overview of some of the more pressing contemporary issues affecting health. Both the challenges that surround climate change and the environmental factors that impact health are extensive. Climate change and climate justice provide a new framework for examining consequences for human health. As described at the beginning of this chapter, nurses have and will continue to play a role at the individual, community, and population levels in addressing the climate-related and environmental health challenges of the 21st century.

REFERENCES

Ahlgren, I., Yamada, S., & Wong, A. (2014). Rising oceans, climate change, food aid, and human rights in the Marshall Islands. *Health and Human Rights, 16*, 69–80.

Alavanja, M. C., Ross, M. K., & Bonner, M. R. (2013). Increased cancer burden among pesticide applicators and others due to pesticide exposure. *CA: A Cancer Journal for Clinicians, 63*, 120–142.

American Academy of Pediatrics. (2014). *Systematic review of vaccine safety may allay parents' concerns.* Retrieved from http://www.aap.org/en-us/about-the-aap/aap-press-room/Pages/Systematic-Review-of-Vaccine-Safety-May-Allay-.aspx

American Nurses Association. (2001). *Code of ethics.* Washington, DC: Author.

Association of Public Health Nurses. (2013). *The role of public health nurses in emergency and disaster preparedness, response, and recovery.* Retrieved from http://www.apha.org/NR/rdonlyres/5B42E252-FA95-4AED-AD0C-2C878633A842/0/APHN_RoleofPHNinDisasterPRR_FINALJan14.pdf

Breivik, K., Gioia, R., Chakraboty, P., Zhang, G., & Jones, K. C. (2011). Are reductions in industrial organic contaminants emissions in rich countries achieved partly by export of toxic wastes? *Environmental Science and Technology, 45*, 9154–9160.

Bruce, N., Perez-Padilla, R., & Albalak, R. (2000). Indoor air pollution in developing countries: a major environmental and public health challenge. *Bulletin of the World Health Organization, 78*, 1078–1092.

Burton, L., & Stretesky, P. (2014). Wrong side of the tracks: The neglected human costs of transporting oil and gas. *Health and Human Rights, 16*, 82–92.

Cameron, E., Bevins, W., & Shine, T. (2013). *Climate justice.* Washington, DC: World Resources Institute. Retrieved from http://www.wri.org/publication/climate-justice-equity-and-justice-informing-new-climate-agreement

Centers for Disease Control and Prevention. (2014a). *Chikungunya in the Caribbean.* Retrieved from http://wwwnc.cdc.gov/travel/notices/watch/chikungunya-saint-martin

Centers for Disease Control and Prevention. (2014b). *Cholera in Haiti.* Retrieved from http://wwwnc.cdc.gov/travel/notices/watch/haiti-cholera

Centers for Disease Control and Prevention. (2014c). *Ebola hemorrhagic fever.* Retrieved from http://www.cdc.gov/vhf/ebola/index.html

Centers for Disease Control and Prevention. (2014d). *What do parents need to know to protect their children?* Retrieved from http://www.cdc.gov/nceh/lead/ACCLPP/blood_lead_levels.htm

Chang, A. Y., Fuller, D. O., Carrasquillo, O., & Beier, J. C. (2014). Social justice, climate change, and dengue. *Health and Human Rights, 16*, 93–104.

Cohen, J. E., & Amon, J. J. (2012). Lead poisoning in China: A health and human rights crisis. *Health and Human Rights, 14*, 74–86.

Finkel, M. L., & Law, A. (2011). The rush to drill for natural gas: A public health cautionary tale. *American Journal of Public Health, 101*(5), 784–785.

Gillis, J. (2014). *U.N. Draft report lists unchecked emissions' risks.* Retrieved from http://www.nytimes.com/2014/08/27/science/earth/greenhouse-gas-emissions-are-growing-and-growing-more-dangerous-draft-of-un-report-says.html?hp&action=click&pgtype=Homepage&version=HpSum&module=first-column-region&region=top-news&WT.nav=top-news&_r=4

Howarth, R. W., Santoro, R., & Ingraffea, A. (2011). Methane and the greenhouse-gas footprint of natural gas from shale formations. *Climatic Change, 106*, 679–690.

Institute of Medicine. (2011). *Safety of vaccines*. Washington, DC: The National Academies Press. Retrieved from http://www.iom.edu/Reports/2011/Adverse-Effects-of-Vaccines-Evidence-and-Causality.aspx

Institute of Medicine. (2014). *The influence of global environmental change on infectious disease dynamics*. Washington, DC: The National Academies Press.

Intergovernmental Panel on Climate Change. (2014). *Climate Change Report 2014: Summary for policy makers*. Retrieved from http://ipcc-wg2.gov/AR5/images/uploads/WG2AR5_SPM_FINAL.pdf

International Council of Nurses. (2006). *The ICN code of ethics for nurses*. Geneva, Switzerland: Author.

Larson, J. L., Redmond, C. T., & Potter, D. A. (2013). Assessing insecticide hazard to bumble bees foraging on flowering weeds in treated lawns. *PLoS One, 8*, e66375. doi:10.1371/journal.pone.0066375

Lemery, J., Williams, C., & Farmer, P. (2014). Editorial: The great procrastination. *Health and Human Rights, 16*(1), 1–3.

Levy, B. S., & Sidel, V. W. (2014). Collective violence caused by climate change and how it threatens health and human rights. *Health and Human Rights, 16*, 32–40.

Lyall, K., Schmidt, R. J., & Hertz-Picciotto, I. (2014). Maternal lifestyle and environmental risk factors for autism spectrum disorders. *International Journal of Epidemiology, 43*, 443–464.

Maglione, M. A., Lopamudra Das, L. R., Smith, A., Chari, R., Newberry, S., Shanman, R., . . . Gidengil, C. (2014). Safety of vaccines used for routine immunization of US children: A systematic review. *Pediatrics*. Retrieved from http://pediatrics.aappublications.org/content/early/2014/06/26/peds.2014–1079.abstract

McDermott-Levy, R., Kaktins, N., & Sattler, B. (2013). Fracking, the environment, and health. *American Journal of Nursing, 113*, 45–51.

Meason, B., & Paterson, R. (2014). Chikungunya, climate change, and human rights. *Health and Human Rights, 16*, 105–112.

Nightingale, F. (1860). *Notes on nursing: What it is and what it is not*. New York, NY: Appleton.

Occupational Safety and Health Administration. (2002). *Hearing conservation*. Washington, DC: U.S. Department of Labor.

Robinson, M. (2014). Foreword on climate change. *Health and Human Rights, 16*, 4–7.

Shaw, J. (2014). Time to tax carbon. *Harvard Magazine, 117*(1), 52–56.

UNICEF and United Nations Children's Program. (1997). *Childhood lead poisoning: Information for advocacy and action*. Retrieved from http://www.unicef.org/spanish/wash/files/lead_en.pdf

United Nations. (2014). *United Nations framework convention on climate change*. Retrieved from http://unfccc.int/kyoto_protocol/items/2830.php

United Nations International Children's Emergency Fund. (2014). *Water, sanitation, and hygiene*. Retrieved from http://www.unicef.org/wash

Varma, M. K., Satterthwaite, M. L., Klasing, A. M., Shoranick, T., Jean, J., Barry, D., . . . Lyon, E. (2008). Woch nan Soley: The denial of the right to water in Haiti. *Health and Human Rights, 10*, 67–89.

World Health Organization/UNICEF Joint Monitoring Program (JMP) for Water Supply and Sanitation. (2014). *Progress on drinking water and sanitation: 2014 Update*. Retrieved from http://www.wssinfo.org/fileadmin/user_upload/resources/JMP_report_2014_webEng.pdf

World Health Organization. (2013). *World malaria report 2013*. Retrieved from http://www.who.int/malaria/publications/world_malaria_report_2013/en

World Health Organization. (2014a). *Framework convention on tobacco control*. Retrieved from http://www.who.int/fctc/about/en

World Health Organization. (2014b). *Global alert and response ebola*. Retrieved from http://www.who.int/csr/disease/ebola/en

World Health Organization. (2014c). *Household (indoor) air pollution*. Retrieved from http://www.who.int/indoorair/en

CHAPTER 3

A Foundation for Global Health, *The Lancet Report on Health Professionals for a New Century:* An Interview With Dean Julio Frenk

Patrice K. Nicholas

D r. Julio Frenk is the dean of the faculty, Harvard T. H. Chan School of Public Health, and the T&G Angelopoulos professor of Public Health and International Development, a joint appointment with the Harvard Kennedy School of Government. He served as Mexico's minister of health from 2000 through 2006, notably instituting a national health insurance program to minimize social inequality in access to health care. Dr. Frenk also served as the founding director-general of the National Institute of Public Health in Mexico, the World Health Organization (WHO) executive director in charge of Evidence and Information Policy, and a senior fellow at the Gates Foundation's global health program. He holds a medical degree from the National University of Mexico, a master's of public health degree, and joint doctorate in Medical Care Organization and Sociology from the University of Michigan. Dr. Frenk is a member of the U.S. Institute of Medicine, the American Academy of Arts and Sciences, and the National Academy of Medicine in Mexico. He is the recipient of three honorary doctorates. In September 2008, Dr. Frenk received the Clinton Global Citizens Award. The questions that follow are based on *The Lancet* report. Dr. Frenk is the first author of *The Lancet Report on Health Professionals for a New Century*, published in 2010 to commemorate the 100th anniversary of the Flexner, Welch-Rose, and Goldmark reports.

PKN: Dean Frenk, thank you for joining us for this interview regarding your important work on transforming education to strengthen health systems in an interdependent world.

In the executive summary, you discuss the groundbreaking reforms in the education of health professionals that occurred nearly 100 years ago and culminated in the 1910 Flexner Report, as well as the subsequent reports: the Welch-Rose and Goldmark reports. You note that these reforms "equipped health professionals with the knowledge that contributed to the doubling of life span in the

20th century." Could you comment on how the Commission developed the shared vision and common strategy for education in the disciplines of medicine, nursing, and public health?

JF: The report was born out of a realization that 100 years had passed since the publication of that series of landmark reports, and that it was time for a fresh look at everything that had changed in this intervening 100 years. Something happened at the turn of the 19th to the 20th century, in that the way we educate health professionals became a matter of enormous interest, and that is what led to all of the series of reports—the Flexner Report on medical education, the Welch-Rose Report on public health education, the Goldmark Report on nursing education—and then the Gies Report a little bit later on dental education. The emergence of the scientific basis for the health professions spurred this great interest initially; subsequently, a number of foundations, including the Rockefeller and Carnegie Foundations . . . became involved and this is what led to this series of reports.

What occurred with *The Lancet* Commission was that we brought together a group of very distinguished thinkers and educators, and that is how the Commission came about, with the idea of not focusing on a single profession, but across all health professions.

PKN: You discuss the three generations of educational reforms that characterized progress over the past 100 years. The first generation was the focus on a science-based curriculum. The second generation introduced problem-based instructional innovations. The third generation is proposed as a systems-based approach to improve the performance of health systems by adapting core professional competencies to specific contexts. One of the most important statements in the Commission's report is that "realization of this vision will require a series of instructional and institutional reforms, which should be guided by two proposed outcomes: transformative learning and interdependence in education." As noted in the report, informative learning is about acquiring knowledge and skills and its purpose is to produce experts; formative learning is about socializing students around values and its purpose is to produce professionals; transformative learning is about developing leadership. Can you share your views on "moving from informative to formative to transformative learning?"

JF: We think of these as three successive levels–where all of the levels are required. We do need good informative learning, because we want people to be experts in their respective professions, but we say that's not enough. Educating experts is not enough. We need to take the second step, which is building on that basis of expertise to then socialize students into a series of values and a code of ethical behavior, which is mostly the ethic of service; this is what distinguishes the professions from other occupations. It is a fact that the members of a profession have been socialized into an ethic of service to others. One would say that it is the defining attribute of a professional. So that is the second level. This process occurs both through explicit parts of the curriculum, but also through the so-called *hidden curriculum*, the set of activities that happen in the course of education that are not necessarily codified in a formal curriculum or a formal syllabus. What we add to that analysis is that even formative learning is not enough, and it is what we call transformative learning, the third level. This is where the competencies that are developed are competencies related to leadership. This process produces an expert and a professional, but you also have a change agent—someone who is keenly aware of the social circumstances that surround his or her practice as a professional, and who then decides to be transformative in the sense of improving those circumstances. This is the specific meaning of a change agent. It doesn't mean that we are changing others' fields. It is very specific to the idea of professionals who understand the context in which they develop their practice and have a critical understanding through leadership competencies to possess the capacity to improve those circumstances.

PKN: The report also suggests that "opportunities are opening for a new round of reforms to craft professional education for the 21st century, spurred by mutual learning due to health interdependence, changes in educational pedagogy, the public prominence of health, and the growing recognition of the imperative for change." Can you talk about the vision for interprofessional education and what this might look like in the future for medicine, nursing, and other disciplines?

JF: Part of proposing a competency-based approach is that you develop those competencies that are required for professionals to function effectively in the health system, and also to serve as change agents in the health system. One of the attributes of the health care system is that because of its growing complexity, it requires teamwork. Yet in the more conventional forms of educating professionals—which are usually in silos and in isolation from one another—there is nothing in their educational experience that prepares them for teamwork. The goal of interprofessional education is exactly to change that and build into the education of health professionals the competencies to work effectively as teams. This report added its voice to a number of reports that have emerged at the 100th anniversary of the earlier reports. And most of those reports call on the importance of interprofessional education. We also added the notion of trans-professional education, by which we mean the competencies to work not just across professions, but also with the nonprofessional members of the health workforce. And this is particularly important in developing countries—focusing on the global perspective—because in many countries the vast majority of health workers are not professionals. These are community health workers, nursing assistants, and technicians. The idea of trans-professional education is exactly to extend the competencies of professionals—of interprofessionals—to the nonprofessional part of the workforce. What we suggest is that this is an explicit set of competencies—teamwork is an explicit set of competencies—that need to be developed purposefully as part of education.

PKN: Educational reform in the health professions is a key element of the report. You and your colleagues note that there is an "explosive increase not only in the total volume of health information, but also in ease of access to it." Can you share your vision of how the health professions will evolve globally as a result of this increase in information? How is public health as a discipline specifically influenced by this?

JF: That is a very good question. It again goes back to the point of competency-based education, and the idea here is that for most of history, you went to a school, to a university, to gain access to information. In a sense, if you looked at universities and other institutions of higher learning, what they controlled was access to a library where you would find the books and access to the professors who embodied the knowledge that you were seeking. In our era of the revolution in information and communication technology, it is not access to information that matters, it is the capacity to discriminate and then make use of that information that is really the competency that needs to be developed. And that is what we meant by stating that the competency set changes with technological improvements. I think developing those generic cross-cutting competencies that cross all of the health professions is a big part of interprofessional education. And one of them is the capacity to access, but more importantly, discriminate the validity of information, and then be able to utilize that information as evidence to guide decision making.

PKN: Dean Frenk, you note that "health security is being challenged by new infectious, environmental, and behavioral threats superimposed upon rapid demographic and epidemiological transitions" and that health systems are struggling to keep up. The emerging challenges to health systems are complex. How would you envision a future for health professionals in strengthening health systems in our interdependent world?

JF: The motivation to develop this report stemmed from the observation that the 100 years that have passed since the original report was published at the beginning of the 20th century are not just any 100 years. They are *the* 100 years of the most intense transformation in health conditions around the world. During these 100 years, we have witnessed unprecedented changes, not only in increased life expectancy, but in the radical shift in patterns of health and disease toward more chronic conditions. We see the emergence of the idea that access to information and the technological revolution have really expanded the array of effective interventions we have at our disposal, as well as the emergence of an ethical framework that says that access to those technologies is a right, and not a merchandise or a privilege. If you combine that with the large and rapid extent of professional differentiation, and the emergence in the 20th century of many new categories of health professionals, all of those forces are putting unprecedented pressures on health systems. The whole idea of the third level of transformative learning is a response to this growing complexity. For health professionals to be effective today, there is a need for them not just to be competent in their own practice, but to be cognizant of this unprecedented set of pressures that affect the performance of health systems, and to be a constructive element for improving that performance.

PKN: A major contribution of the report is the focus on all of the health professions and their contributions to the health of the world's people. The report discusses educational reforms in the 20th century and their roots in social movements. In particular, you note that "in the mid-1800s, Florence Nightingale campaigned that good nursing care saved lives, and good nursing care depended on educated nurses." The first nursing education program began in London in 1859, as 2-year, hospital-based training that soon spread quickly in the United Kingdom, the United States, Germany, and Scandinavian countries. The roots of modern medicine and public health go back similarly to the mid-1800s, propelled by discoveries that proved the germ theory. If you could envision the future of the health professions and their contributions in our interdependent world, what would you see in our future?

JF: Probably the most radical explanation of the report is the notion that, in an ideal world, the differentiation among the different health professions ought to be based on competencies, on a rational design of competencies, and then on a division of labor that emerges from those competencies. Instead, what we see is that health professions emerge, and then create their specific domain for practice. I think the most radical recommendation is that the division of labor among professions needs to be driven by competencies. Instead of that [process], what we have is that historically, the different professional groups emerged, and then the boundaries of their respective domains of practice have been very often driven by political clashes. We see this [phenomenon occurring frequently] in the boundary between elements of nursing and medicine. Why do nurses in the United Kingdom, especially in midwifery, have much larger spans of practice, or in some other countries have prescription privileges that you don't see in others? I think that as we're pointing toward the future with a higher sense of team-based health care, maybe it will be competencies that determine the division of labor, rather than historical turfs that have been established through other, mostly political, processes.

PKN: One compelling point addressed in the report is the following: "Like never before, the public prominence of health in general and global health in particular has generated an environment that is propitious for change. Health affects the most pressing global issues of our time: socioeconomic development, national and human security, and the global movement for human rights. We now understand that good health is not only a result of, but also a condition for development, security, and rights. At the same time, access to high-quality health care with financial protection for all has become one of the major domestic political priorities worldwide." How do you envision the future of health and health care nationally and internationally?

JF: I think the biggest change that has happened is that health has stopped being solely the concern of domain experts: physicians, nurses, public health professionals. Instead, it has really now become a key part of main themes in the national and global agenda—questions on economic growth and development, or national and global security, or the protection and promotion of human rights. So it is this idea that health is not just what health professionals care about, but that it is now a concern for everyone. And conversely, health promotion requires the mobilization of policy tools that may be outside of the health domain. For an issue like smoking, tax policy becomes a very powerful instrument. This is the idea of thinking about health not just as a sector, but as a social objective, to which many other areas of policy contribute. And my point in the [recent] opinion editorial in the *Boston Globe*, which is also reflected in the quote you mentioned, is that the way we manage health policy has now become one of the key political issues. We see this [occurring] in the United States. This is *the* dominant element of domestic politics in the United States. If we think of health as an objective, and not just a sector, then you need to mobilize policies in many other domains. This is true especially when you extend access to insurance and to health care; it is also important to set in motion upstream policy interventions that will stop people from getting sick in the first place. My opinion editorial was very much saying that one of the great aspects of the Affordable Care Act is that it actually has a whole chapter on health promotion and disease prevention. That [aspect] is critical. If you only extend insurance which is, of course, very important, but don't implement upstream interventions, then the system becomes unsustainable because you have a huge increase in demand without the necessary preventive and health promotion interventions. The idea is that health has become this hugely important social objective to which every other field of public policy has a contribution to make.

PKN: Yes. It was quite striking to see in the opinion editorial piece, that three percent of health care spending is focused on prevention and public health, and 75% on preventable conditions.

JF: Yes. By the way, when I talk about interprofessional education, I include, of course, the education among the health professionals, but I also include the introduction of health competencies for non-health professionals. For example, I don't think you can now be a lawyer if you do not understand elements of health. I do not think you can be an economist if you ignore that health care is the largest sector of the economy. Interprofessional education also includes the development of health-related competencies for non-health professionals.

PKN: The report also addresses recommendations for reform and enabling actions. Can you comment on how public health can engage in these reforms and how the discipline of nursing can embrace these reforms?

JF: Public health provides a population perspective that greatly complements the perspective centered on individual care that other health professionals bring.

But it is the population perspective, the idea of understanding not just the individual who shows up at a health care facility, but the population from which that individual comes, and the members of that population who may not have access—that, I think, distinguishes public health. And I believe that in interprofessional education, public health is a key ingredient in providing that population perspective. Most of what we have been seeing under the rubric of interprofessional education is education among the clinical professions. But we also need the public health perspective that addresses the needs of entire populations. And, by the way, with the Affordable Care Act, where there is a very specific objective of combining excellent care of individuals with taking care of whole populations, I think that combination is going to be more needed than ever. Also, public health offers a natural bridge to professions that are not health professions, but that influence other policy arenas—the attorneys, the economists, the anthropologists, etc. Public health then offers a natural bridge between the health professions and the non-health professions and this has a huge effect on health outcomes. Those are the two crucial roles that we play: we bring the population perspective of non-health professionals, and we serve as a bridge between health and non-health professionals in thinking about promoting health as a social objective.

PKN: Thank you for joining us for this very enlightening interview and sharing your wisdom on the report, *Health Professionals for a New Century: Transforming Education to Strengthen Health Systems in an Interdependent World.*

COMMENTARY ON INTERVIEW WITH JULIO FRENK, MD, MPH, PhD

Shira Winter, Holly Fulmer, Suellen Breakey, and Patrice K. Nicholas

Dr. Frenk's words predict how future health-professional education must evolve to meet current global health needs. Not only must health professionals be educated in their own field, but they must be able to lead health care initiatives with a lens of their own profession as well as an interprofessional view. For instance, global nursing education must incorporate clinical reasoning, skill, and ethos, as well as educating new nurses on how to work across disciplines for better health outcomes. Nurses will be tasked with leading and contributing to such interdisciplinary teams.

Dr. Frenk's creative view of the *hidden curriculum* is particularly relevant in nursing since a recent publication also addressed professional and interprofessional development. In the recent publication, *Educating Nurses: A Call for Radical Transformation* (Benner, Sutphen, Leonard, & Day, 2009), commissioned by the Carnegie Foundation for Advancement in Teaching, there is a significant focus on the development of professional identity, interprofessional roles, and team-focused efforts of nurses. Dr. Frenk stresses the importance of three levels that should build upon each other in the curricula of medical, nursing, and public health schools. He addresses the importance of informative learning to produce experts in the professions; socialization within a framework of values and ethics to distinguish the professions from occupations, and culminating in an ethic of service; and finally, transformative learning that focuses on the development of leadership and change agency in the professions. His views are in alignment with those of Benner et al. (2009) who note the importance of developing one's professional identity in the curriculum in nursing education and developing ethical comportment for leadership in one's career.

Another key professional shift that Dr. Frenk brings to the fore is the need for health professionals to collaborate with non-health professionals. He embraces the notion that more progress can be made if we harness the individual strengths of experts from diverse fields to alter the environment, circumstances, and systems in which health professionals provide care. In addition, the need for nurses to be skilled in interprofessional teamwork is particularly critical in global health settings where nurses comprise the majority of health professionals and work alongside physician colleagues as well as community health workers. In many resource-limited settings, nurses are the drivers of the entire health care system from rural clinics to district and urban centers.

REFERENCE

Benner, P. A., Sutphen, M., Leonard, V., & Day, L. (2009). *Educating nurses: A call for radical transformation.* San Francisco, CA: Jossey Bass.

CHAPTER 4

Global Health Ethics

Suellen Breakey and Linda A. Evans

WHAT IS GLOBAL HEALTH?

Global health has been defined as "an area for study, research, and practice that places a priority on improving health and achieving equity in health for all people worldwide" (Koplan et al., 2008, p. 1995). Working toward these goals is a challenging endeavor. Progress is slowly being made, but the factors that constrain these efforts are complex and extend beyond the limits of health care into economic, social, and political spheres. Millum and Emanuel (2012) observe that only recently have bioethicists begun to shift from a domestic to a global focus. They also point out that the complexity of the issues surrounding global health necessitates that ethicists expand their areas of concern from the traditional (issues that occur within patient–provider relationships, for example) to other areas such as health policy, as well as political and economic theory (Millum & Emanuel, 2012). In this chapter, we examine the effects that social determinants and economic globalization have had on the health of the world's people, particularly in low- and middle-income countries. We also explore the concept of global health ethics and how it is distinct from traditional ethics. Finally, we discuss frameworks that can be used to examine the complex global issues at the population health level.

INFLUENCE OF GLOBALIZATION ON GLOBAL HEALTH

According to Parekh and Wilcox (2014), globalization is the "economic, social, cultural, and political processes of integration that result from the expansion of transnational economic production, migration, communications, and technologies" (para 1). This definition implies that these processes are being integrated and shared equally. Sen (1999) contends that the process of integration has been unequal and that globalization has led to increased Westernization of the world as opposed to a more equal diffusion of these processes. One potential consequence of an increasingly Westernized world is the potential for Western values and beliefs to become the dominant view at the expense of local cultural values, beliefs, and traditions.

The current global political economy is based on neoliberal ideology. The policies derived from neoliberal thought support trade liberalization; deregulation; privatization of public assets, including natural resources such as minerals and forests; elimination of social welfare programs; and restrictions on immigration (Parekh & Wilcox, 2014). Specifically, economic integration, removing regulatory constraints such as tariffs and restrictions on investments, leads to freer movement of goods and, thus, economic growth (Shah, 2010). Proponents of the current global economy argue that the effects of these policies have created employment opportunities for people worldwide, particularly in developing countries, moving them out of poverty, while opponents disagree.

In addition to enhanced economic growth *for some*, the benefits of globalization include rapid advances in scientific and technological innovation, improved health and life expectancy *for some*, and expanded access to communication. These advances have increased our ability to generate new knowledge and to share knowledge among a larger global audience, which has led to what Roland Robertson refers to as the "compression of the world." As Benatar, Gill, and Bakker (2011) point out, the minority who benefit in the current global political economy are large investors and transnational corporations, resulting in a widening gap between the wealthy and the poor both between and within countries. For instance, in order to satisfy the conditions of World Bank or International Monetary Fund loans, some countries must prioritize profit-making over the interest and well-being of its citizens (Falk-Rafael, 2006).

For the sick living in poor countries, or to borrow Paul Farmer's term, "the destitute sick," economic integration has an even more direct effect on health. Tighter intellectual property rights protection, for example, which maximizes profits for wealthy companies by granting them exclusive rights, keeps the prices of goods high, which disadvantages poor countries (Haynes et al., 2013). In the case of pharmaceutical companies, such arrangements limit access to essential lifesaving medications that may be cost prohibitive for either governments in poor countries or individuals to purchase. Although globalization was predicted to be "the rising tide that would lift all boats" (WHO, 2012a, p. vii), low- and middle-income countries continue to bear a significant burden of poverty and, as a result, disease.

Extreme Poverty and the Global Burden of Disease

The total number of people living in extreme poverty may be decreasing, but the numbers are still devastatingly high. The gap between the wealthy and the poor continues to widen. More than 3 billion people live on less than US$2.50 per day (Shah, 2013), and the relationship between poverty and health is clear. When it comes to health, World Health Organization (WHO) statistics from 2012 indicate that people living in low- and middle-income countries fare far worse than those in high-income countries (WHO, 2014). Case in point: In 2012, the overall global life expectancy at birth was 70 years. When aggregated and compared according to level of income, however, the disparities become evident; those in high-income countries had a life expectancy of 79 years versus a life expectancy of 62 years for those living in low-income countries (WHO, 2014). This trend was similar for infant mortality and mortality by the age of 5. Likewise, when comparing the incidence and prevalence of infectious diseases, both the incidence and prevalence of disease (malaria, HIV/AIDS, and tuberculosis, for example) were consistently higher in low-income countries than the global measure and much lower than the global measure in high-income countries (WHO, 2014). African countries, in particular, fare worse in all areas compared to low-income countries on the whole (WHO, 2014; Table 4.1). In addition to the economic strain placed on poor countries as a result of a disproportionate amount of disease—both from the loss of productivity and the cost of illness—individuals and families are also directly affected financially, leading to further expansion of the wealth–poverty gap.

The conditions that contribute to poor health and premature death of individuals worldwide, and in poor countries in particular, are preventable. The most basic resources, such as access to clean water and sanitation, are critical for survival and freedom from preventable disease, yet 780 million people lack access to clean water. Moreover, greater than 3.4 million deaths each year, 99% of which occur in the developing world, are water, sanitation, and hygiene related (Prüss-Üstün, Bos, Gore, & Bartram, 2008). In many cases, the reason for lack of access to these most basic resources is not a lack of availability of the actual resource, for example, water. Instead, it is an economic issue either at the individual level, the government level, or both. Poor countries may lack the financial resources needed to create effective infrastructures that will protect its citizens, such as systems to provide access to clean water or health care systems to treat water-borne diseases. Even when appropriate infrastructures exist within low- or middle-income countries, many individuals are too poor to access these services and die a preventable death as a result.

The widening gap between the wealthy and the poor is a moral issue. Pogge (2010) identifies three facts that support the contention that global poverty is

TABLE 4.1 Impact of Wealth on the Occurrence of Selected Health Indicators (2012 data)

	GLOBAL	HIGH INCOME	LOW INCOME	AFRICAN
Life expectancy at birth (years)	70	79	62	58
Infant mortality by age 1 (1/1000)	35	5	56	63
Mortality by age 5 (1/1000)	48	6	82	95
Malaria (incidence per 100,000)	3,752	0	11,165	18,579
HIV/AIDS (incidence per 100,000)	33	16	89	176
HIV/AIDS (prevalence per 100,000)	511	265	1,788	3,203
Tuberculosis (incidence per 100,000)	122	23	246	255
Tuberculosis (prevalence per 100,000)	169	31	352	303

Source: WHO (2014).

morally troubling. First, the growing disparity occurs in the face of unprecedented global affluence. He estimates that a 2% shift in global household income would be sufficient to eradicate severe poverty. Second, global poverty continues to increase, and finally, as stated previously, the world is shaped by international interactions, including the development of treaties, conventions, and economic policies that disproportionately benefit the wealthy. Therefore, those who contribute to global economic inequality, the severe poverty it perpetuates, and the resultant detriments to health are morally implicated (Pogge, 2010).

Social Determinants of Health

Social determinants of health are the conditions into which people are born and live and are shaped by the distribution of power, money, and resources (WHO, 2008). Examples of such conditions include level of education, occupation, income, gender, ethnicity, and race. In all countries, regardless of income, health and illness follow a social gradient—the lower one's socioeconomic status, the poorer one's health (WHO, 2008). Further, much of the global burden of disease is in fact avoidable and is a result of a "toxic combination of poor social policies and programmes, unfair economic arrangements, and bad politics" (WHO, 2008, p. 1). As such, many have contended that working to improve social determinants cannot be successful within the health sector alone (WHO, 2012a). It follows, then, that if health is in part socially constructed, it is necessary to protect and promote not only the civil and political rights of all people but also economic, social, and cultural rights.

Human Rights and Health

> In short, we live in a world where inequalities in health and economic development continue to pervade our development trajectory and where exclusion from social systems remains the most fundamental obstacle to realizing human potential worldwide. (London, 2008, p. 66)

Forman and Nixon (2013) contend that human rights, in and of themselves, are also determinants of health. Human rights are those basic rights to which all persons are entitled; they are considered indivisible, interrelated, and interdependent. The Universal Declaration of Human Rights (UDHR) was adopted by the United Nations (UN) General Assembly in December 1948 following the atrocities of World War II and is considered to be the foundation for international human rights law. The purpose of the document is to make explicit those inalienable rights that are necessary for freedom, justice, and peace. Subsequently, the International Covenant for Civil and Political Rights (ICCPR) and the International Covenant for Social, Economic, and Cultural Rights (ICSECR) were derived from the UDHR and adopted in 1976. These International Covenants serve as a means to hold those member states who ratify them accountable under the law for promoting and observing the rights of their people. Together, these documents are known as the International Bill of Human Rights.

Article 25 (1) of the UDHR specifically addresses the right to health in the context of an adequate standard of living:

> Everyone has the right to a standard of living adequate for the health and well-being of himself and of his family, including food, clothing, housing, and medical care and necessary social services, and the right to security in the event of unemployment, sickness, disability, widowhood, old age or other lack of livelihood in circumstances beyond his control. (UN General Assembly, 1948)

In addition, Article 12 (1) of the ICSECR states that, "The States Parties to the present Covenant recognize the right of everyone to the enjoyment of the highest attainable standard of physical and mental health" (UN General Assembly, 1976). This treaty has been ratified by many member states of the UN. However, the United States has yet to ratify the ICSECR. Finally, the Declaration of Alma-Ata, developed at the International Conference on Primary Health Care in 1978, elaborated on the notion that health is a fundamental human right by recognizing that health inequalities exist between those in developed and developing countries and that attainment of health is a "world-wide social goal whose realization requires the action of many other social and economic sectors in addition to the health sector" (WHO, 1978).

Jonathan Mann, who some have characterized as the founder of the health and human rights movement, and his colleagues (1994) were the first to describe a provisional framework connecting health and human rights. Their framework is based on the following assumptions: Health policies impact human rights; human rights violations impact physical, mental, and social well-being; and human rights and health are fundamentally and inextricably linked (Mann et al., 1994). The link between human rights and health is exemplified in the following ways. First, certain human rights violations have a direct negative effect on health, such as in the case of torture or slavery. Second, violations that impact economic, social, and cultural rights—for instance, the right to education, food and nutrition, and water—lead to an increased vulnerability to illness. And finally, the development of programs that either do not consider individuals' rights or violate those rights altogether may be discriminatory or violate a person or group's right to privacy (WHO, n.d.).

Mann and colleagues argued that using public health research methodology, education, and field work expertise could not only advance our understanding of the health impacts resulting from human rights violations but also "give voice" to and possibly expedite actions to address these issues (Mann et al., 1994). While the links between human rights and health are complex, over the past 20 years their thesis has provided the basis for examining and understanding the effects that ignoring or violating certain human rights has had on health. Examples include violence against women, certain traditional practices within cultures such as female genital mutilation, and slavery.

CAN TRADITIONAL ETHICAL PRINCIPLES BE APPLIED TO GLOBAL HEALTH?

The challenges to promoting and defending human rights to achieve the highest standard of health and well-being and to eradicate inequities—in essence, creating a socially just society—are complex. The traditional ethical principles—autonomy, beneficence, nonmaleficence, and justice—are useful but not sufficient to examine global health issues. A global ethics framework is needed.

Respect for Autonomy

In the Western tradition, autonomy refers to one's right to self-determination, free from controlling influences or limitations (Beauchamp & Childress, 2012). Two general conditions must be met in order for a person to act autonomously: liberty and agency. *Liberty* refers to the ability to be free from controlling influences, and *agency* refers to the capacity for intentional action (Beauchamp & Childress, 2012). When we have full autonomy, that is, the ability to reason and to make choices based on our beliefs, values, and wishes, then one element necessary to achieve well-being has been satisfied.

Provision 1.4 of the American Nurses Association (ANA) *Code of Ethics for Nurses With Interpretive Statements* (2015) addresses the nurse's ethical responsibility to respect individual autonomy and the right to self-determination. From a traditional Western bioethical perspective, respect for autonomy is regarded as the ethical principle that underlies the concept of informed consent, the patient's right to make decisions based on accurate information regarding the nature of the treatment as well as the risks, benefits, and alternatives to that treatment. The International Council of Nurses (ICN) *Code of Ethics* (2006) addresses the nurse's duty to respect autonomy from a broader perspective, stating that, "In providing care, the nurse promotes an environment in which the human rights, values, customs and spiritual beliefs of the individual, family and community are respected" (p. 2).

Autonomy in social and political philosophy is used as the ideal against which unjust, or oppressive, social conditions are critiqued (Christman, 2009). To acknowledge an individual as an autonomous agent is to recognize and respect the right of that individual to have personal values and beliefs as well as her or his right to make choices and act on her or his values and beliefs. Conditions that interfere with an individual's or group's ability to exercise autonomy are considered oppressive.

Threats to Autonomy From a Global Ethics Perspective

As the ANA *Code of Ethics for Nurses* (2015) suggests, nurses working in wealthy countries often consider the principle of autonomy from the perspective of an individual's right to self-determination in decision making and care. In clinical settings, a nurse's role in protecting and respecting autonomy is often related to the patient's decision-making capacity and the extent to which it is affected by illness or the presence of comorbid conditions. In this way, the concern is often one of agency, the capacity to make informed decisions, and, to a lesser extent, liberty, or the freedom from forces that constrain decision making. On the other hand, from a global ethics perspective, a focus on liberty and on efforts to remove constraining forces—for example, poverty, lack of access to clean water and sanitation, or gender inequality—is often the central moral issue impacting health.

Crigger (2008) refers to autonomy as "the ethics of affluence" (p. 22). She argues that our Westernized view of autonomy, which places great importance on personal autonomy and individual rights, is not transferrable to all settings, particularly resource-challenged settings where poverty and a lack of material resources have a devastating impact on health (Crigger, 2008). These settings often differ in many ways from Western culture. Often, the social and economic welfare of the family is reliant on the joint efforts of each family member. Because of this dependency, family members are often key stakeholders in the decision-making process, and less emphasis is placed on the individual. Autonomy, then, would be understood differently in settings where this is true. Therefore, understanding relevant cultural values, beliefs, and norms that may shape one's definition of autonomy is essential. Using a global ethics perspective to understand threats to autonomy in global health necessitates a broader, deeper view, one that incorporates knowledge of the social, economic, and political constraints to achieving health and well-being and knowledge of the specific culture.

To illustrate the distinction between a traditional and a global ethics framework, consider the concept of informed consent. In order to ensure informed consent in a global health setting, one must first acknowledge that despite the social circumstances of an individual (e.g., poverty, illiteracy), the obligation to engage in the process of informed consent remains. In the case of HIV testing, an issue where people are particularly vulnerable to stigmatization and discrimination, the WHO (2012b) made explicit the steps to ensure basic human rights protections and optimal treatment of people living with HIV. Informed consent is a central concern as well as maintaining confidentiality, offering counseling, ensuring correct results, and connection to care.

However, results from Madhivanan et al. (2014) study in India to understand women's experiences and perceptions of HIV testing during antenatal care illustrate instances where these steps are violated. They found that informed consent was not obtained for either the antenatal care the women received or for HIV testing. Moreover, the participants' respect for privacy and confidentiality were routinely violated during visits when the women were informed of their positive test results. And while told they needed to be on medication, they were not given any further information and were not referred for counseling; clearly, the WHO guidelines were not practiced. In fact, although these private providers had the necessary resources to continue to care for these HIV-positive women, the women's care was transferred to either government facilities or nongovernmental organizations (NGOs; Madhivanan et al., 2014). Within a Western framework, autonomy was clearly violated. Informed consent was not obtained and the participants' right to privacy and confidentiality were violated. Solutions based on this analysis would be primarily based in the health care setting and include such things as educating providers on the elements and significance of informed consent, restructuring practices to adhere to WHO guidelines, and holding individual providers accountable for their breaches in practice.

Examination of the study from a broader global ethics perspective uncovers morally significant sociopolitical factors—poverty and gender inequality—that must be factored into an ethical solution to the problem. The moral issue, then, of violating individual women's rights to autonomy by disregarding the process of informed consent is raised to a societal level, taking into account the constraining effects of poverty and women's inequality on autonomy. Considering the issue this way takes into account not only actors at the local level (the physicians and nurses) but also the government and other institutions that permit or perpetuate these practices and fail to protect their citizens, in this case poor women. Therefore, the focus shifts from violations of informed consent and threats to individual autonomy to violations rooted in social inequity, thereby necessitating examination from a perspective of justice.

Beneficence

The principle of beneficence refers to a moral obligation *to act* for the good of others to help further their interests, often by preventing or removing harms (Beauchamp, 2013). Some have argued that this *positive obligation* to act for the good of others is too demanding, an ideal rather than an obligation, and that we are not morally obligated to benefit others even if we are so able. Anderson et al. (2009) point to a lack of concern for "distant and different others" (p. 282) and Wolff (2012) discusses a diffusion of responsibility as possible reasons why individuals disregard a humanitarian duty to assist those in need. But some, notably Singer (2009) and Pogge (2010), as discussed previously, dispute the contention that beneficence is an ideal and argue that individuals living in wealthy countries have a duty to assist those living in poverty.

Singer (2009) uses a hypothetical situation to state his case. He begins by first begging the question: If you were walking to work, wearing expensive shoes, and encountered a girl drowning in a shallow pond, would you save her? He asserts that people would choose to wade into the pond to save the girl because the girl's life is more important than the loss of the expensive shoes and the resulting inconveniences of getting wet, such as having to go home to change, or being late for work, for example. However, most people do not feel the same moral obligation to save the lives of poor children in Africa, even though we could through charitable giving. His analogy provides support for Anderson et al. (2009) notion that we feel more of a moral obligation to those in close proximity than for the distant and different other. Further, Singer (2009) argues that we do indeed have a duty to help the thousands of children whom we know are dying from poverty-related, preventable diseases daily, and this duty is as morally significant as our duty to save the drowning girl from a preventable death. He proposes that individuals give 1% of their income to the poor as a means to promote a culture of giving (Singer, 2009).

Yet, while there may be a wide consensus that those in middle income or poor countries are entitled to basic human rights that are essential for health and well-being, a consensus has not been reached on whether humans have a positive right to assistance or to what extent we are obligated to assist. Beauchamp (2013) suggests that beneficence exists on a continuum, starting with strict obligation (core norms of beneficence in ordinary morality) and ending with high-level supererogatory, or heroic, acts of self-sacrifice. As Beauchamp (2013) points out, the debate lies in where obligation ends and supererogation begins. While our individual duties to act for the good of others remain unclear, our professional responsibilities are well-articulated; Provision 8 of the *Code of Ethics for Nurses* (2001) states that the nurse has a responsibility to promote health at the community, national, and international level. Provision 8 also informs nurses of the responsibility to be aware of the "broader health concerns such as world hunger, environmental pollution, lack of access to health care, violation of human rights, and inequitable distribution of nursing and health care resources" (p. 13).

Nonmaleficence

Simply put, nonmaleficence refers to our moral obligation to not inflict harm on others. Whereas *beneficence* requires an action to promote good, *nonmaleficence* requires that we intentionally refrain from actions that cause harm to another (Beauchamp & Childress, 2012). Harms may take the form of physical or mental injury or danger, but may also include setbacks to other interests held by an individual or party (Beauchamp & Childress, 2001). Examples of moral rules that are supported by this principle include do not kill, do not incapacitate, and do not deprive others of the goods of life (Beauchamp & Childress, 2001).

To view this principle from a global ethics perspective, refer back to the earlier example related to intellectual property rights protections. International laws and agreements that favor pharmaceutical companies and the protection of their right to intellectual property could be considered a violation of the principle of nonmaleficence since the link between poor health and poverty is well-established. If a company is allowed to continue to hold exclusive rights to a drug that could save lives, it prohibits manufacturing and distribution of generic drugs that would be cheaper and more accessible to the poor. Such policies or arrangements that knowingly perpetuate a lack of access to lifesaving resources in order to financially benefit a large wealthy company inflict harm on the potential beneficiaries whose lives could be saved and violate the principle of nonmaleficence. While violations of nonmaleficence do occur, it should also be noted that many pharmaceutical companies include statements of social responsibility in their mission and contribute to humanitarian efforts. For example, in 2013, Janssen Pharmaceuticals, a pharmaceutical company of Johnson & Johnson in the United States, developed a drug donation program for HIV treatment-experienced children who are in need of new treatment options (Johnson & Johnson, 2013).

Threat of Doing More Harm Than Good

An increasing number of nurses are interested in engaging in global health work, either by providing direct care or by partnering with NGOs or governments to provide and develop education or to assist in developing programs to address specific health issues. In fact, nurses are perfectly suited to undertake this work, but need a broader global ethics view to enhance their understanding of how autonomy may be viewed differently depending on needs, priorities, and traditions in the setting in which one is working. It is equally as important to view the principles of beneficence and nonmaleficence from a global ethics perspective in order to avoid unintentionally doing more harm than good.

Fuller (2012) describes cultural imperialism as providing care or services in such a way that it forces potential recipients of those services to choose between accessing the care being offered that would be unavailable otherwise but that violates traditional norms and practices, or not receiving assistance (Fuller, 2012). Clearly, those who work in global health settings do not set out to cause harm. However, the recipient of care may be harmed if the care or assistance being offered does not cohere with the norms, values, or traditions that are important to the individual and community. The end result may be that the potential beneficiary of the assistance is forced to make the difficult decision to abandon those values and opt for the care from which she or he may benefit that, under normal circumstances, would not be available. This decision may have devastating social implications for the individual and her or his family. One important aspect in preventing such harm is the provision of culturally competent care, or what some call cultural humility. The recently published document, "Guidelines for Implementing Culturally Competent Nursing Care" (Douglas et al., 2014), which was endorsed by the ICN, provides recommendations that can assist nurses working globally. These provisions are listed in Box 4.1.

Anderson et al. (2009), along with Douglas et al. (2014), recommend that nurses working in global health settings should engage in critical self-reflection. Critical self-reflection takes into account not only the economic, cultural, and political context in which health inequities exist, but also the potential consequences of the power differentials behind the inequities. For instance, those providing assistance are often from wealthy countries while recipients of care live in poverty. Critical self-reflection can lessen the risk of nurses' objectifying the experience of those who are disadvantaged and marginalized, which can lead unintentionally to feelings of moral superiority or knowing "what's best"(Anderson et al., 2009). As Crigger (2008) points out, the risk of doing more harm than good may be realized if the focus of global health efforts does not match the needs and goals of the beneficiaries of the assistance. Moreover, when decisions to do "what's best" are made without regard for the local culture, traditions, or insights from stakeholders living in the local setting, the end result is paternalism.

Using a global ethics lens to design care, education, or assistance programs can mitigate this potential for harm. Fuller (2012) offers the following suggestions that, in addition to critical self-reflection, are particularly useful for global health nurses. The recommendations include engaging key local stakeholders in the work,

BOX 4.1 GUIDELINES FOR IMPLEMENTING CULTURALLY COMPETENT NURSING CARE

GUIDELINE	DESCRIPTION
1. Knowledge of cultures	Nurses shall gain an understanding of the perspectives, traditions, values, practices, and family systems of culturally diverse individuals, families, communities, and populations they care for, as well as knowledge of the complex variables that affect the achievement of health and well-being.
2. Education and training in culturally competent care	Nurses shall be educationally prepared to provide culturally congruent health care. Knowledge and skills necessary for assuring that nursing care is culturally congruent shall be included in global health care agendas that mandate formal education and clinical training, as well as required ongoing, continuing education for all practicing nurses.
3. Critical reflection	Nurses shall engage in critical reflection of their own values, beliefs, and cultural heritage in order to have an awareness of how these qualities and issues can impact culturally congruent nursing care.
4. Cross-cultural communication	Nurses shall use culturally competent verbal and nonverbal communication skills to identify client's values, beliefs, practices, perceptions, and unique health care needs.
5. Culturally competent practice	Nurses shall utilize cross-cultural knowledge and culturally sensitive skills in implementing culturally congruent nursing care.
6. Cultural competence in health care systems and organizations	Health care organizations should provide the structure and resources necessary to evaluate and meet the cultural and language needs of their diverse clients.
7. Patient advocacy and empowerment	Nurses shall recognize the effect of health care policies, delivery systems, and resources on their patient populations, and shall empower and advocate for their patients as indicated. Nurses shall advocate for the inclusion of their patient's cultural beliefs and practices in all dimensions of their health care.
8. Multicultural workforce	Nurses shall actively engage in the effort to ensure a multicultural workforce in health care settings. One measure to achieve a multicultural workforce is through strengthening of recruitment and retention efforts in the hospitals, clinics, and academic settings.

(continued)

BOX 4.1 GUIDELINES FOR IMPLEMENTING CULTURALLY
COMPETENT NURSING CARE (*CONTINUED*)

GUIDELINE	DESCRIPTION
9. Cross-cultural leadership	Nurses shall have the ability to influence individuals, groups, and systems to achieve outcomes of culturally competent care for diverse populations. Nurses shall have the knowledge and skills to work with public and private organizations, professional associations, and communities to establish policies and guidelines for comprehensive implementation and evaluation of culturally competent care.
10. Evidence-based practice and research	Nurses shall base their practice on interventions that have been systematically tested and shown to be the most effective for the culturally diverse populations that they serve. In areas where there is a lack of evidence of efficacy, nurse researchers shall investigate and test interventions that may be the most effective in reducing the dispanties in health outcomes.

From Douglas et al. (2014). Reprinted with permission from Sage Publishing Company.

focusing care or development efforts on the needs that are identified by the local experts, ensuring that the assistance being provided does not violate moral or religious beliefs that are central to those who live in the setting, and having a good understanding of the local cultural practices and incorporating them appropriately into the assistance being provided. Similarly, Murphy et al. (2013) outline elements of successful global health research partnerships. Although they discuss these in the context of international research, the elements they discuss can be applied to all types of global partnerships—whether aimed at capacity development, health programs and policies, clinical services, or education partnerships. Included are the importance of mutual trust and respect among global partners, shared decision making, and national ownership (Murphy et al., 2013); the presence of these characteristics indicates a true partnership rather than a paternalistic relationship.

Justice

The principle of justice is a fundamental consideration when examining possible solutions to address the inequities that impact global health. Theories of justice are complex; bioethicists as well as social and political philosophers have been and continue to be engaged in extensive discussions about the nature and scope of this concept. The overview of justice presented here provides a basic understanding of its importance in global health discussions.

Distributive justice refers to fair, equitable, and appropriate distribution of material goods and services such as income, wealth, health care, and jobs

(Lamont & Favor, 2013). The concept of distributive justice is very closely linked to the economic framework of each society, since it is that framework, comprised of its laws, policies, and institutions, that influences how both economic benefits and burdens are distributed to individuals (Lamont & Favor, 2013). In other words, who will reap the benefits, and who will be placed at an economic, political, or social disadvantage? Institutions refer to "a significant practice, relationship, or organization in a society or culture" (*Merriam-Webster*, n.d.). Examples of institutions include health care, religion, industry, law and the legal system, and the military. Principles of justice provide societies with a moral framework to determine the political processes and structures that affect the distribution of economic benefits and burdens (Lamont & Favor, 2013). Beauchamp and Childress (2001) define specific material principles of justice as those principles that specify the characteristics of equal treatment and help to guide distribution of resources.

1. To each person an equal share
2. To each person according to need
3. To each person according to effort
4. To each person according to contribution
5. To each person according to merit
6. To each person according to free-market exchanges (p. 228)

Principles of justice, therefore, have the potential for practical application if used to help shape the laws and policies that govern the distribution of economic benefits and burdens. There is, however, an ongoing discussion and a lack of consensus regarding the nature of equality—what goods and resources are we obligated to share equally? An equal need for certain resources does not necessarily exist universally, but consideration should be given to fair distribution. It is clear that there may be inherent conflicts of interest that would influence the determination of how resources ought to be distributed fairly. Realistically, there is no one pure theory; rather, a host of principles help shape decision making and attempt to address the questions: How do we distribute burdens and benefits fairly? and How do we define "fair or equal?" The four traditional theories of justice are egalitarianism, utilitarianism, libertarianism, and communitarianism (Beauchamp & Childress, 2012). What follows is a general description of each.

Theories of Justice

The belief that people are created as equals and have equal moral status underlies *egalitarian* theories of justice. Egalitarians, therefore, hold the belief that all people should be treated equally (Beauchamp & Childress, 2012). In this way, equality is central to justice, and there exist certain absolute humanitarian principles such as autonomy, freedom, and human dignity (Gordon, 2006). John Rawls's (1971) theory of justice as fairness has significantly shaped, informed, and influenced discussions related to justice. In his account, individuals are free and possess equal basic rights; the principal task of government is "to distribute fairly the liberties and economic resources individuals need to lead freely chosen lives" (Bell, 2012, para 1).

Utilitarians believe that the morally right action in a situation is that action that produces the most good or maximizes value (Driver, 2009). Utilitarianism falls into the category of consequentialism. Broadly, consequentialists believe that determination of whether an act is morally right depends only on the consequences of that act (Sinnott-Armstrong, 2011). As such, all other morally relevant factors are disregarded since it is the consequence or outcome that is morally significant.

Libertarian theories place significant emphasis on individual rights as opposed to social or economic liberty (Beauchamp & Childress, 2012). In this view, individuals have full self-ownership; a just society provides protection for individual rights, for example, property and liberty (Vallentyne & van der Vossen, 2014). All persons should have the freedom to improve their circumstances on their own initiative (Beauchamp & Childress, 2012). Determination of just acts from a libertarian viewpoint centers on whether people have been justly treated and whether their individual rights have been respected and not on the outcome or consequences of that act (Vallentyne & van der Vossen, 2014).

Unlike libertarianism, *communitarian* theories of justice define conceptions of good as those that are created in moral communities, and dismiss theories of justice based on individual rights (Beauchamp & Childress, 2012). Communities can take on several forms. They may be based on geographical location—for example, the place where one calls home; they may be based on memory—strangers who share a morally significant history; or they may be psychological communities—for example, families (Bell, 2012).

The Scope of Justice: Cosmopolitanism Versus Statism

Another question that is asked when issues of justice are examined is, "How far do our responsibilities extend?" How ethicists and political philosophers answer this question depends on whether they take a cosmopolitan or statist view. A cosmopolitan view suggests that all human beings are citizens of one community and that our collective duties to each other extend beyond national borders (Kleingeld & Brown, 2013). As Emanuel (2012) contends, where a person is born or lives is arbitrary from a moral perspective and should not factor in the determination of entitlement to basic rights, opportunities, or resources. In other words, regardless of how far we live from those who lack access to basic resources—for example, food, water, and health care—we have a collective duty to assist. This duty is based on the idea that those suffering from these burdens, many of whom live in low-income countries, have the same right to health as those living in wealthy countries. Singer's (2009) argument related to our individual duties to the poor is based not only on our obligation of beneficence, but also on a cosmopolitan view of justice.

On the other hand, the statist view, primarily put forth by Rawls, is concerned not with the well-being of individuals, but with creating just institutions within a society (Emanuel, 2012). Statists acknowledge the existence of states that experience abject poverty, but the primary concern lies not in the existence of economic insecurity, but with the inability of those nation-states to develop and establish just social and political institutions. There is, therefore, a duty to assist these states to allow them to reach a minimal level of economic security so just institutions may be established, but there is no ongoing obligation of justice (Emanuel, 2012). As one can see, justice as a duty to others and what we owe to others who have less than we have is complicated and influenced deeply by not only our individual values and beliefs but also by the moral and social norms that shape our communities and nations.

Emerging Theories of Justice: The Capability Approach

One responsibility of the society in which we live is to provide a social minimum, defined by White (2004) as, "the bundle of resources that a person needs in order to lead a minimally decent life in their society" (para 2). However, the fairness of this definition has been challenged since the idea of a minimally decent life will look different depending on one's circumstances. One born into deprivation may have different expectations and adapt to a lack of resources that will in turn affect her or his definition of a "minimally decent life" (White, 2004). Therefore, the bundle of resources will be different depending on whether you live in a poor or wealthy country. For the poor, a minimally decent life may mean access to food, water, or education. For those living in wealthy countries, a minimally decent life will extend beyond these basic needs; some have argued that the social minimum in wealthy societies is more costly (White, 2004).

A set of theories of justice, *capability theory*, has emerged over the past few decades that represents a departure from the traditional theories of justice and is particularly promising to address global issues, such as health inequities that have arisen from globalization. A capability approach may in some ways also address the inconsistencies with the social minimum. This approach was first developed by Sen (1999) as a means of making cross-cultural judgments regarding quality of life and was further explicated by Nussbaum (2000) and others. Capability theory is more normative than explanatory and takes into consideration what people are able to realistically be and do (Kleist, 2010). Beings and doings described by Sen (1992),

> can vary from such elementary things as being adequately nourished, being in good health, avoiding escapable morbidity and premature mortality, etc., to more complex achievements such as being happy, having self-respect, taking part in the life of the community, and so on. (p. 39, as cited in White, 2004)

Within this approach, poverty is not merely the lack of material resources required for survival, but is viewed as deprivation of the capability to live a good life, the quality of which is defined by the individual. As such, capability theory extends beyond traditional theories of justice; while basic needs are required for good health and well-being, the goal is to achieve human flourishing, or optimal well-being.

One of the difficulties with this theory is determining universally what capabilities are absolutely necessary to allow one to flourish since conceptions will surely be influenced by what is culturally accepted within a particular society.

However, there are some basic needs that ought to be considered urgent moral and political priorities—capabilities that most would agree are required; for example, education, nutrition, shelter and, importantly, health. Development and the distribution of resources, therefore, are focused on expanding capabilities (Wells, 2012).

Sen and Nussbaum have differing accounts of capability theory. For instance, Sen's account emphasizes freedom while an important aspect of Nussbaum's theory is the concept that human dignity is necessary for human flourishing (Wells, 2012). But the central tenet of the theories is similar—certain capabilities, those that are realistic and not unreachable possibilities—and forms of freedom are essential for a flourishing life, the kind of life we have reason to value (Beauchamp & Childress, 2012).

While Sen is reticent to make a list of essential capabilities (Wells, 2012), Nussbaum (2000) has identified 10 capabilities that are necessary for a full life. They are life; bodily health; bodily integrity; senses, imagination, and thought; emotions; practical reason; affiliation; relationship with other species; play; and control over one's environment (both political and material; Nussbaum, 2000). Nussbaum emphasizes two of the 10 capabilities that constitute a truly human pursuit, one that is self-constructed and where one is not just following or being shaped by others. The first practical reason is the ability to form a conception of and critically reflect on the notion of the good. The second is affiliation, which focuses on the ability to live with and show concern for others and the ability to have self-respect and be treated with dignity and self-worth (Kleist, 2010). Moreover, the capabilities approach shows promise for use in assessing individual well-being, evaluating and assessing social arrangements, and designing policies related to addressing inequities (Robeyns, 2011).

FRAMEWORKS FOR THE APPLICATION OF A GLOBAL HEALTH ETHIC TO ISSUES IN GLOBAL HEALTH

Examining the four traditional ethical principles—autonomy, beneficence, nonmaleficence, and justice—with respect to global health and reconceptualizing them through a global ethics lens serves as a guide for individuals to understand global health inequities and for ethical practice in global health. In addition, global health experts are engaged in serious discussions centered on developing viable population level scale solutions to address the global health crisis. Three frameworks that have particular merit are advanced here: Ford's Global Health Advocacy framework, a rights-based framework, and the more recently proposed Framework Convention on Global Health (FCGH).

An Ethical Framework for the Common Good: Global Health Advocacy

Ford (2013) describes global health advocacy as "people in one part of the world advocating for the improved health of people in another part of the world" (p. 136), clearly a cosmopolitan view of justice. This term and Ford's definition of it suggest an approach to global health that is rooted in normative ethics—what ought to be done. However, Ford (2013) also acknowledges that global health has a political context and, therefore, should have a political solution. His framework is useful for addressing global health issues affecting large numbers of people as a result of health inequities. He also notes that, while policy change is not a linear process, it is useful to have clear, logical, stepwise process to ensure a comprehensive approach to the issue at hand. The steps of his global health advocacy framework are outlined here.

- *Define the problem* and determine if it is important to overcome
- *Gather the evidence* in a way that ensures all aspects of the health problem—sociopolitical, cultural, and economic—are being addressed. This step may include, for example, gathering epidemiologic data, information on current effective standards of care related to the health issue being addressed, relevant health policy information, and any existing financial barriers to prevention or treatment.
- *Formulate and propose a possible solution*
- *Build alliances* with people who have expertise related to all aspects of the issue to strengthen the case
- *Challenge the status quo*
- *Seize opportunities* that may arise that will strengthen or increase public awareness of the global health issue
- *Build consensus*
- *Support implementation* (Ford, 2013)

This framework is particularly useful for addressing specific global health problems. Box 4.2 provides an illustration of the application of his framework to a global health issue, access to antiretroviral (ARV) medications for people living with HIV in Africa.

A Rights-Based Framework to Global Health

A tension exists between advances in science and technology and the ability of current social policies to meet the basic needs of the world's people such that technological innovation adds to health inequities since expensive technologies are not available to those unable to pay for them (Crigger, 2008; London, 2008). Crigger (2008) also notes that the ethical issues created from these cutting-edge technologies—for instance, ethical issues related to genetic mapping, face transplantation, or the development of an artificial heart—seem more relevant or interesting to some than issues such as dire poverty and lack of access to clean water and sanitation, all of which impact health negatively. To those living in wealthy countries, this second set of problems seems far removed from our everyday lives—or as Anderson et al. (2009) would suggest, problems of the distant and different others. Yet, at the core of all of these issues is the basic right to health.

Since the right to health is protected under international law through the International Bill of Human Rights, governments who have ratified the ICSECR owe a duty to promote and protect the health of their citizens, and this duty is legally binding (Forman & Nixon, 2013). This requirement applies mainly to governments, however, and much less so to the duties of organizations or transnational

BOX 4.2 EXAMINING ACCESS TO ARV MEDICATION USING FORD'S GLOBAL HEALTH ADVOCACY FRAMEWORK

Defining the problem	Lack of access to treatment for people living with HIV in Africa
	Concerns included: cost, ability of health care infrastructure in Africa to support care, concerns about adherence and drug resistance
Gathering the evidence	Included: epidemiological data, drug pricing data, treatment efficacy data
Championing a solution	In 2001, a company in India developed the capability to manufacture generic ARV drugs at a price that would allow access to those living with HIV in Africa
	This development could be used to pressure drug companies to lower cost
Building alliances	Stakeholders included intellectual property experts, clinicians, researchers to examine adherence and drug resistance, economists
Challenging the status quo	Global patent laws influenced pricing and, therefore, Africa's access to the drugs from Indian manufacturers.
	The challenge: The needs of patients living with HIV in developing countries ought to be placed over large pharmaceutical companies' profits
Seizing opportunities	A consortium of 36 pharmaceutical companies sue the South African government to try to stop the import of lower cost ARV medications; this led to global public attention and support for improving access to HIV treatment
Building consensus	Important for all stakeholders to agree to not only the nature of the problem, but also the solution
	Outcome: Over 90% of people receiving ARV medication in developing countries are receiving generic medication
Supporting implementation	Stakeholders involved (advocacy groups, national government, clinicians) were committed to the solution (increasing access to generic medication)
	Stakeholder support is necessary for sustainability

Source: Ford (2013).

corporations to uphold the right to health (Forman & Nixon, 2013). Further, while forward progress toward achieving a right to health is occurring, particularly through the work of the UN-appointed rapporteur, a more robust attempt to hold nation-state and nonstate actors accountable to their legal and ethical duties presents a challenge, particularly to economically disadvantaged countries where achievement of the right to health will be difficult (Forman & Nixon, 2013).

Civil and political rights are indivisible from economic, social, and political rights. Therefore, health and social policies need to be developed that address obligations to fulfill the human right to health (London, 2008). Integrating a human-rights approach into health and social policies can offer new opportunities for addressing global health challenges. In addition to providing standards for states' conduct, as emphasized by Forman and Nixon (2013), policies being developed should incorporate the voice and perspectives of those who suffer from human rights violations, firsthand. London (2008) specifically addresses the responsibilities of health workers in working to advance health as a human right by proposing that professional codes of conduct use stronger human rights language to make them a more effective means for self-regulation. Reliance on ethical frameworks, he argues, to guide professional behavior have limited effect. London admits that a human rights framework may not be successful in achieving the right to health but, at the very least, will mobilize civil society to action, which he believes is necessary for social change. *Social mobilization*, increasing society's awareness of the government's legal obligation to facilitate the right to health, will empower rights holders, particularly those whose rights to health are being violated, to make rights-based claims to health (Friedman, Gostin, & Buse, 2013; Haynes et al., 2013; London, 2008).

Framework Convention on Global Health (FCGH)

More recently, Gostin et al. (2013) have advanced a more formalized concept of a rights-based approach to health that they believe will increase accountability at both the domestic and international level. They point out that since the concept of a right to health is vague, it has had limited use in efforts to hold responsible parties accountable (Gostin et al., 2013). They propose a FCGH that will "dramatically reduce the health disadvantages experienced by the marginalized and the poor, both within countries and between them, while reducing health injustices across the socioeconomic gradient" (Gostin et al., 2013, p. 790). The authors of this proposal note that, while progress toward global health has been made through the implementation of the UN Millennium Development Goals (MDG), the health gap still exists; they contend that this is in part due to the lack of existing health and social policies that are equally as robust as current international trade and investment policies (Gostin et al., 2013). Therefore, to achieve global justice, the focus must extend beyond achieving health to include achieving equity (Gostin et al., 2013). The FCGH as proposed provides strategies for action to achieve equity by including interventions focused in the economic, social, and political domains. Specifically, the FCGH would ensure three conditions essential for a healthy life: well-functioning health systems that have the ability to provide quality care; a full range of public services such as the access to nutritious food, clean water, and healthy environments; and access to economic and social determinants for good health such as employment, housing, income support, and gender equality (Gostin et al., 2013). These conditions would be met through a global governance structure and new international law that would establish a health financing network with clear obligations and lines of accountability in addition to standards for monitoring and enforcement (Haynes et al., 2013).

The FCGH would also include actions against what they call "drivers" of health disparities, such as intellectual property rules, migration policies that encourage health worker migration, and policies that fail to address the harmful health effects of climate change and environmental hazards (Friedman et al., 2013; Gostin et al., 2013). Social mobilization underlies the proposed FCGH by not only promoting awareness among individuals regarding the right to health, but enlisting others engaged in global health, such as women's rights organizations, human rights groups, and environmental advocacy groups (Gostin et al., 2013). While some criticisms to the FCGH exist, the answers to which warrant further consideration, (Hoffman & Rottingen, 2013), it is a promising practical approach to advancing global health.

CONCLUSION

Globalization has benefitted civil society in many ways. Yet with those benefits have come great consequences that have been experienced disproportionately by the poor. The profession of nursing has a long history of attending to and advocating for the world's most vulnerable. Our work continues in this effort, and new problems continue to arise. Grootjans and Newman (2013) identify three essential attributes for nursing practice in a globalized world that complement the global ethics perspective presented in this chapter. First, the nurse must understand the environment, including environmental determinants as well as physical and socially constructed determinants of health; second, the nurse must make health promotion a priority where promotion of health is taken to mean not just the absence of disease but the promotion of well-being; and finally, the nurse practicing in a globalized world must consider how actions at the local level impact the health of others on a global level (Grootjans & Newman, 2013). These recommendations cohere with the notion that incorporating a global ethics perspective, one that leads us to examine the larger societal factors and their impact on an individual's potential to realize optimal health and well-being, can serve as a guide for action as we continue our important role in helping the world's people to flourish.

"Addressing injustice and enhancing global health is a matter of practical action. It requires careful thinking, initiative and a willingness to experiment with new approaches. Most importantly, it requires that we think ethically and then act ethically" (Orbinski, 2013, p. x).

REFERENCES

American Nurses Association. (2015). *Code of ethics for nurses with interpretive statements.* Retrieved from http://www.nursingworld.org/MainMenuCategories/EthicsStandards/CodeofEthicsforNurses/Code-of-Ethics.pdf

Anderson, J. M., Rodney, P., Reimer-Kirkham, S., Browne, A. J., Khan, K. B., & Lynam, M. J. (2009). Inequities in health and healthcare viewed through the ethical lens of critical social justice: A contextual knowledge for the global priorities ahead. *Advances in Nursing Science, 32*(4), 282–294.

Beauchamp, T. (2013). The principle of beneficence in applied ethics. *Stanford encyclopedia of philosophy.* Retrieved from http://plato.stanford.edu/entries/principle-beneficence

Beauchamp, T., & Childress, J. F. (2001). *Principles of biomedical ethics.* New York, NY: Oxford University Press.

Beauchamp, T., & Childress, J. F. (2012). *Principles of biomedical ethics* (7th ed.). New York, NY: Oxford University Press.

Bell, D. (2012). Communitarianism. *Stanford encyclopedia of philosophy.* Retrieved from http://plato.stanford.edu/entries/communitarianism

Benatar, S. R., Gill, S., & Bakker, L. (2011). Global health and the global economic crisis. *American Journal of Public Health, 101*(4), 646–653.

Christman, J. (2009). Autonomy in moral and political philosophy. *Stanford encyclopedia of philosophy.* Retrieved from http://plato.stanford.edu/entries/autonomy-moral

Crigger, N. J. (2008). Toward a viable and just global nursing ethics. *Nursing Ethics, 15*(1), 17–27.

Douglas, M. K., Rosenkoetter, M., Pacquiao, D. F., Clark Callister, L., Hattar-Pollara, M., Lauderdale, J., . . . Purnell, L. (2014). Guidelines for implementing culturally competent nursing care. *Journal of Transcultural Nursing, 25*(2), 109–121.

Driver, J. (2009). The history of utilitarianism. *Stanford encyclopedia of philosophy.* Retrieved from http://plato.stanford.edu/entries/utilitarianism-history

Emanuel, E. J. (2012). Global justice and the "standard of care" debates. In E. Emanuel & J. Millum (Eds.), *Global justice and bioethics.* New York, NY: Oxford University Press.

Falk-Rafael, A. (2006). Globalization and global health: Toward nursing praxis in the global community. *Advances in Nursing Science, 29*(1), 2–14.

Ford, N. (2013). The political context of global health and advocacy. In A. D. Pinto, & R. E. G. Upsher (Eds.), *An introduction to global health ethics* (pp. 136–147). New York, NY: Routledge.

Forman, L., & Nixon, S. (2013). Human rights discourse within global health ethics. In A. D. Pinto & R. E. G. Upsher (Eds.), *An introduction to global health ethics* (pp. 47–57). New York, NY: Routledge.

Friedman, E. A., Gostin, L. O., & Buse, K. (2013). Advancing the right to health through global organizations: The potential role of a framework convention on global health. *Health and Human Rights, 15* (1), 71–86.

Fuller, L. (2012). International NGO health programs in a non-ideal world: Imperialism, respect, and procedural justice. In E. Emanuel & J. Millum (Eds.), *Global justice and bioethics* (pp. 213–240). New York, NY: Oxford University Press.

Gordon, G. S. (2006). Moral egalitarianism. *Internet encyclopedia of philosophy.* Retrieved from http://www.iep.utm.edu/moral-eg

Gostin, L. O., Friedman, E. A., Buse, K., Waris, A., Mulumba, M., Joel, M., . . . Sridhar, D. (2013). Toward a framework convention on global health. *Bulletin of the World Health Organization, 91,* 790–793.

Grootjans, J., & Newman, S. (2013). The relevance of globalization to nursing: A concept analysis. *International Nursing Review, 60,* 78–85.

Haynes, L., Legge, D., London, L., McCoy, D., Sanders, D., & Schuftan, C. (2013). Will the struggle for health equity and social justice be best served by a Framework Convention on Global Health? *Health and Human Rights, 15*(1), 111–116.

Hoffman, S. J., & Rottingen, J. (2013). Dark sides of the proposed framework convention on global health's many virtues: A systematic review and critical analysis. *Health and Human Rights, 15*(1), 117–134.

International Council of Nurses. (2006). *The ICN code of ethics for nurses.* Geneva, Switzerland: Author.

Johnson & Johnson. (2013). *Janssen, the pharmaceutical companies of Johnson & Johnson, announces first-of-its-kind drug donation program for HIV treatment-experienced children.* Retrieved from http://www.jnj.com/news/all/Janssen-the-Pharmaceutical-Companies-of-Johnson-Johnson-Announces-First-of-its-Kind-Drug-Donation-Program-for-HIV-Treatment-Experienced-Children

Kleingeld, P., & Brown, E. (2013). Cosmopolitanism. *Stanford encyclopedia of philosophy.* Retrieved from http://plato.stanford.edu/search/searcher.py?query=cosmopolitanism

Kleist, C. (2010). Global ethics: Capabilities approach. *Internet encyclopedia of philosophy.* Retrieved from www.ep.utm.edu/ge-capab

Koplan, J. P., Bond, T. C., Merson, M. H., Reddy, K. S., Rodriguez, M. H., Sewankambo, N. K., & Wasserheit, J. N. (2008). Toward a definition of global health. *Lancet, 373,* 1993–1995.

Lamont, K., & Favor, C. (2013). Distributive justice. *Stanford encyclopedia of philosophy.* Retrieved from http://plato.stanford.edu/entries/justice-distributive

London, L. (2008). What is a human rights-based approach to health and does it matter? *Health and Human Rights Journal, 10*(1), 65–80.

Madhivanan, P., Krupp, K., Kulkarni, V., Kulkarni, S., Vaidya, N., Shaheen, R., . . . Fisher, C. (2014). HIV testing among pregnant women living with HIV in India: Are private healthcare providers routinely violating women's human rights? *BMC International Health and Human Rights, 24,* 7. Retrieved from http://www.biomedcentral.com/1472-698X/14/7

Mann, J., Gostin, L., Gruskin, S., Brennan, T., Lazzarini, Z., & Fineberg, H. V. (1994). Health and human rights. *Health and Human Rights, 1*(1), 7–23.

Merriam-Webster Dictionary Online. Retrieved from http://www.merriam-webster.com/dictionary/institution

Millum, J., & Emanuel, E. J. (2012). Introduction: Global justice and bioethics. In J. Millum & E. J. Emanuel (Eds.), *Global justice and bioethics* (pp. 1–14). New York, NY: Oxford University Press.

Murphy, J., Neufeld, V. R., Habte, D., Asseffa, A., Afsana, K., Kumar, A., . . . Hatfield, J. (2013). Ethical considerations of global health partnerships. In A. D. Pinto & R. E. G. Upsher (Eds.), *An introduction to global health ethics* (pp. 117–128). New York, NY: Routledge.

Nussbaum, M. (2000). *Women and human development: The capabilities approach.* Cambridge, MA: Cambridge University Press.

Orbkinski, J. (2013). Foreword. In A. D. Pinto & R. E. G. Upshur (Eds.), *An introduction to global health ethics* (p. x). New York, NY: Routledge.

Parekh, S., & Wilcox, S. (2014). Feminist perspectives on globalization. *Stanford encyclopedia of philosophy.* Retrieved from http://plato.stanford.edu/entries/feminism-globalization/

Pogge, T. W. (2010). *Politics as usual: What lies behind the pro-poor rhetoric.* Cambridge, UK: Polity Press.

Prüss-Üstün, A., Bos, R., Gore, F., & Bartram, J. (2008). *Safer water, better health: Costs, benefits, and sustainability of interventions to protect and promote health.* Geneva, Switzerland: World Health Organization.

Rawls, J. (1971). *A theory of justice.* Cambridge, MA: Harvard University Press.

Robeyns, I. (2011). The capability approach. *Stanford encyclopedia of philosophy.* Retrieved from http://plato.stanford.edu/entries/capability-approach

Sen, A. (1992). *Inequality reexamined.* Oxford, UK: Blackwell.

Sen, A. (1999). *Development as freedom.* New York, NY: Anchor Books.

Shah, A. (2010). A primer on neoliberalism. *Global Issues.* Retrieved from http://www.globalissues.org/article/39/a-primer-on-neoliberalism

Shah, A. (2013). Poverty facts and stats. *Global Issues.* Retrieved from http://www.globalissues.org/article/26/poverty-facts-and-stats

Singer, P. (2009). *The life you can save: Acting now to end world poverty.* New York, NY: Random House.

Sinnott-Armstrong, W. (2011). Consequentialism. *Stanford encyclopedia of philosophy.* Retrieved from www.plato.stanford.edu/entries/consequentialism

UN General Assembly. (1948). *Universal Declaration of Human Rights.* Retrieved from http://www.un.org/en/documents/udhr/index.shtml

UN General Assembly. (1976). *International Covenant on Economic, Social, and Cultural Rights.* Retrieved from http://www.ohchr.org/EN/ProfessionalInterest/Pages/CESCR.aspx

Vallentyne, P., & van der Vossen, B. (2014). Libertarianism. *Stanford encyclopedia of philosophy.* Retrieved from http://plato.stanford.edu/entries/libertarianism

Wells, T. (2012). Sen's capability approach. *Internet encyclopedia of philosophy.* Retrieved from www.iep.utm.edu/sen-cap

White, S. (2004). Social minimum. *Stanford encyclopedia of philosophy.* Retrieved from http://plato.stanford.edu/entries/social-minimum

Wolff, J. (2012). Global justice and health: The basis of the global health duty. In E. Emanuel & J. Millum (Eds.), *Global justice and bioethics* (pp. 78–101). New York, NY: Oxford University Press.

World Health Organization. (n.d.). *Linkages between health and human rights.* Retrieved from http://www.who.int/hhr/HHR%20linkages.pdf?ua=1

World Health Organization. (1978). *Declaration of Alma-Ata.* Retrieved from http://www.euro.who.int/__data/assets/pdf_file/0009/113877/E93944.pdf?ua=1

World Health Organization. (2008). *Closing the gap in a generation: Health equity through action on the social determinants of health.* Geneva, Switzerland: Author.

World Health Organization. (2012a). *All for equity: World conference on social determinants of health.* Geneva, Switzerland: Author.

World Health Organization. (2012b). *Service delivery approaches to HIV testing and counseling (HTC): A service policy framework.* Geneva, Switzerland: Author.

World Health Organization. (2014). *World health statistic 2014.* Geneva, Switzerland: Author.

CHAPTER 5

Health, Human Rights, and Social Justice: An Interview With Paul Farmer and Sheila Davis

Patrice K. Nicholas

Dr. Paul Farmer, physician and anthropologist, is chief strategist and cofounder of Partners In Health (PIH), Kolokotrones University Professor, and chair of the Department of Global Health and Social Medicine at Harvard Medical School, as well as chief of the Division of Global Health Equity at Brigham and Women's Hospital in Boston. He also serves as UN special adviser to the secretary-general on Community-Based Medicine and Lessons from Haiti. Dr. Farmer has written extensively on health, human rights, and the consequences of social inequality. His most recent books are *In the Company of the Poor: Conversations With Dr. Paul Farmer and Fr. Gustavo Gutiérrez, Reimagining Global Health: An Introduction,* and *To Repair the World: Paul Farmer Speaks to the Next Generation* (retrieved from www.pih.org).

Dr. Sheila Davis is the chief nursing officer at PIH, a global nongovernmental organization (NGO). She works in many of PIH's 12 countries on nursing-related programs in education, nursing practice and leadership, health care delivery programs, and health capacity building. She is an adult nurse practitioner specializing in HIV/AIDS and infectious diseases and had an active clinical practice in the Massachusetts General Hospital infectious diseases outpatient clinic for over 25 years. Dr. Davis is an internationally renowned nurse leader and a frequent national and international speaker on global health and the role of nursing in human rights. Dr. Davis was named one of the first 20 national Carl Wilkens Fellows from the Genocide Intervention Network in 2009.

PKN: Drs. Farmer and Davis, thank you for joining us for this interview regarding your important work on health, human rights, and social justice. Your work is so compelling in these areas. Dr. Farmer, can you share how you first became engaged in the work of human rights and social justice?

PF: Thank you, Patrice. I think it depends on what we term "involvement." I was certainly enchanted with the notion of health and social justice by the time I was an undergraduate and was lucky enough to spend time examining the mechanisms by which race, class, gender, and insurance status influenced care seeking at a university emergency room. But the moment this engagement became irrevocable for me was definitely in 1983 when I went to central Haiti for the first time.

PKN: Dr. Davis, can you share your insights on how global nursing has evolved over the past 20 years and what you anticipate in the future? Also, your doctoral work focused on your passion for social justice; can you share your wisdom and ideas on the ethics of global nursing with us.

SD: Thanks so much, Patrice. I don't think there is consensus on what "global health" is, let alone "global nursing." My definition of global nursing is less geographic and more focused on a health equity agenda that is patient centered and illuminates the critical role nurses and midwives (35 million of us) play in health care delivery. Global nursing is a dynamic field that has really taken off; before the infusion of HIV funding to non–United States settings, I don't think we heard much about global nursing as a specialty area. Global nursing has its roots in public health nursing, where social justice is a core component of practice. My first global nurse hero was Lillian Wald, who started the Henry Street Settlement in the Lower East Side of New York in 1893. What an amazing woman. She was committed to providing care for the poorest of the poor and I am so lucky to work with many amazing nurses today at the PIH sites around the world who also have this commitment.

Bringing it back to this century, my hope is that global nursing will become less about "helping" and more about partnership and bidirectionality. There is significant momentum in global health delivery and we have to make sure that we are front and center in this arena and provide vision and strategy to these efforts.

The ethical components of global nursing are important and multifactorial. There are the ethical dilemmas inherent in providing care in settings where there are too few resources and too few educated providers. Sadly, I think we will be faced with this for a long time. Ensuring that we insist that our global work be directed by those who are the beneficiaries of the effort is imperative. It is not acceptable that students and nurses who are not trained, licensed, or appropriate to give care feel empowered and allowed to do so in low resource settings. Sending inexperienced nurses or students to "teach" experienced seasoned professionals in Haiti, Rwanda, Lesotho, or beyond is unethical and must be halted. Responding to identified needs by the local community can be accomplished in a way that first benefits the nurses, students, and patients in the setting while still providing a valuable learning experience for well-intended visiting nurses and students. Nurses have a responsibility to provide fair and just care for our patients. I hope we can challenge each other to think beyond our borders and advocate for all of our patients.

PKN: Dr. Farmer, you wrote recently: "Poverty is arguably the greatest risk factor for acquiring and succumbing to disease worldwide, yet historically received less attention from the medical community than genetic or environmental risk factors. Several factors likely contributed to this oversight: first, being poor is not considered a disruption of normal physiologic function. Physicians and basic scientists viewed themselves as ill-equipped to understand or manipulate an individual's socioeconomic status. Second, unlike the largesse dedicated to finding technical solutions for population health problems, funding for research dedicated to understanding and alleviating poverty was sparse. Third, although some acknowledged that poverty plays a pivotal role in determining disease vulnerability and outcomes, the resultant solutions aimed at redressing poverty were often wrongheaded." Can you elaborate on your thoughts regarding your quote and link the solutions to your journey with PIH?

PF: First, it's not only basic scientists who are ill-equipped to understand links between deprivation and disease; so, too, are most clinicians—including doctors and nurses. At least, this is my view after three decades working with health care providers in settings from Boston to rural Haiti and Rwanda. That is, we clinicians are not trained to understand how poverty gets in the body. Second, it is not just a question of understanding these social determinants of disease—how poverty gets in the body—but also, and more critically for our professions, knowing how and having the capacity to get it out of the body. That is, we know that poverty determines, in significant measure, the incidence of pathologies ranging from measles and diabetes to AIDS and tuberculosis. But understanding social determinants is not the same as practicing social justice medicine (and as I stress in all of my writing, when I say "medicine," I include all of the health professions). This has as its goal the eradication or palliation of illness among the poor and otherwise marginalized. For example, if you were to say that poverty and gender inequality were risks for HIV infection—and few would dispute this now—it's not the same as saying, "how do we bring high-quality services (for prevention or care) to women living in poverty?" What Dr. Alsan, our colleagues, and I were trying to say in this article, and in so many others, is that it's one thing to understand how poverty gets in the body, and quite another to understand how to get it out—and to deliver on a commitment to do so (Alsan, Westerhaus, Herce, Nakashima, & Farmer, 2011).

PKN: Dr. Davis, can you share your thoughts on global nursing and the intersection of health and human rights?

SD: Viewing health as a human right provides a solid foundation for global nursing. As global nurses we are faced with so many challenging situations and it is hard—every day. In my early days working in global health, I was working in South Africa, where we had only a very limited supply of antiretroviral medications. It was impossible to make the decision who got the chance to receive the medications, literally life and death decisions. It was heart wrenching and sitting around that small table while this was being discussed will forever be imprinted in my mind. It felt like the lifeboat game in freshman psychology where you have to choose who gets tossed off the boat. Globally, where does nursing fit into this? If we truly see health as a human right, then part of our time and energy needs to be directed to fighting the realities that make that table scenario happen. It is unfathomable that we had to make those decisions when there were effective anti-retrovirals available in other countries.

Paul talks about being "socialized for scarcity." I had never heard this phrase before I came to PIH but once I heard it, it completely made sense. He describes it as accepting lower standards for poor people because that is the way things are (Farmer, Saussy, & Kidder, 2010). The entire world had been socialized for scarcity and thought that there was no way we could treat all of the millions of people with HIV from poor countries—hence that barbaric lifeboat game. Thankfully the world rallied and now many more people have access to antiretrovirals, but there are still millions who don't.

PKN: Dr. Farmer, you wrote the following in a recent article in *Global Public Health*. Can you share your thoughts on sustainability and its intersection with social justice and human rights?

"'Sustainability' has become a central criterion used by funders—including foundations, governmental agencies and international agencies—in evaluating public health programmes. The criterion became important as a result of frustration with discontinuities in the provision of care. As a result of its application, projects that involve building infrastructure, training or relatively narrow objectives tend to receive support. In this article, we argue for a reconceptualisation of sustainability criteria in light of the idea that health is an investment that is itself sustaining and sustainable, and for the abandonment of conceptualisations of sustainability that focus on the consumable medical interventions required to achieve health. The implication is a tailoring of the time horizon for creating value that reflects the challenges of achieving health in a community. We also argue that funders and coordinating bodies, rather than the specialised health providers that they support, are best positioned to develop integrated programmes of medical interventions to achieve truly sustainable health outcomes" (Yang, Farmer, & McGahan, 2010).

PF: I apologize if this excerpt sounds as though I argue that "group A should determine policies rather than group B." I think health care providers, like doctors and nurses, have a lot to contribute to policy, and need mostly to look beyond their own professional interests to focus on good outcomes for patients (which is what we mean by the term "value"). As for "sustainability," the notion is very often used as a blunt instrument—or even a weapon—in the context of settings of poverty, in part because there is a lack of conviction that the provision of high-quality health care services for poor people is possible, or even that it does constitute value. At least, such is my experience over the last 30 years, even if this claim is not always made explicitly. So as far as the notion of sustainability goes, in our work, it is always important to focus our efforts on sustaining high-quality, health-promoting efforts for those who might benefit most from them. That's what value means. And that simple shift—from asking, "Is this sustainable?" to asking, "How do we sustain this?"—makes all the difference. In recent years, I've written more about how this and other notions lead to the "House of No," meaning: If something is judged as "not cost-effective" or "not sustainable," especially when it concerns populations living in poverty, then it is unlikely to receive financing not only from the public sector, but also from influential foundations and funding agencies.

PKN: Dr. Davis, you recently had a widely read contribution to the *Huffington Post*. Can you share with us your views from that publication?

SD: It has been great to see the response from my *Huffington Post* blogs. I think there is a desire for more about the nursing profession in the media and it has been inspiring and humbling to hear from many nursing students and nurses who have connected with something I have written. In the Finding Our Compass blog from May 2, 2014, I really wanted to start the conversation about global nursing being focused on patient-centered care and less just nurse-centric dialogue. It will always be important to advocate and raise the visibility of nurses and nursing in all settings, but that has to be done in the landscape of providing quality care to patients, families, and communities. It does take a village to provide health care and in that village are nurses, doctors, families, community health workers, and so many others. At the center of that village is the patient. I hope that nurses can take up the charge for global patient-centered care and have that be our rallying call (Davis, 2014).

PKN: Dr. Farmer, you address the role that medical education has in addressing health as a human right, the growing disparities between the wealthy and poor, and the issues of brain drain from the poorer countries of Asia, Latin America, and Africa. You note that: "The burden of disease is growing disproportionately in precisely those regions most commonly afflicted by 'the brain drain.' From Africa and the poorer regions of Asia and Latin America, doctors and nurses who cannot make living wages flee rural areas for cities, then make their way to industrialized countries" (Farmer, Furin, & Katz, 2004, p. 1832).

PF: Reflecting on these claims 10 years later, I don't see any fundamental error in our analysis. But we weren't trying to win an argument so much as to address the so-called "human resources for health crisis." Over the past decade, we've launched a novel training program in global health equity for young physicians at Brigham and Women's Hospital and we've launched many more for physicians, nurses, and health managers in Haiti, Rwanda, and other settings in which PIH and its partners work. The main take-home message, in my view, is that there are two ways to address the brain drain. One includes addressing "pull forces," and the other "push." For example, pushing professionals not to emigrate by erecting barriers to their mobility is neither, in my opinion, a human rights approach nor a reasonable one in terms of understanding how the global political economy works. As for the pull forces that PIH has focused on, these include not only improved salaries, but also better working conditions and a chance for young health professionals to pursue the kind of advanced training that they often do in affluent countries. Trying to stop the brain drain by arguing that Malawian nurses, say, should not emigrate to the United Kingdom, doesn't strike me as particularly fruitful. But making their working conditions in Malawi better and even attractive does strike me as promising. And that approach always involves staff, stuff, and training (Farmer, Furin, & Katz, 2004).

PKN: Dr. Davis, your work in global nursing has been strongly influenced by your work in HIV nursing. Can you talk about the issues of health and human rights related to care of those with HIV as an exemplar of the inequalities in health that exist in resource-limited countries and those that PIH serves?

SD: The HIV epidemic illuminated the haves and have-nots of society unlike any other disease, virus, or public health pandemic in modern times. In the United States and other resource-rich countries, the virus preferentially invaded the most marginalized communities—first gay men and injection drug users. This made it "acceptable" for the government to ignore this fast-moving virus and the resulting devastating impact that occurred. As a new nurse in the early days of HIV, I did not understand why this was happening—this intersection of politics, stigma, and discrimination with public health was certainly eye-opening. I grew up in rural Maine and immersing myself in the gay and injection drug–using communities was a bit of a culture shock. But I, like many others, jumped in and we are richer because of it. My parents instilled the values of social justice and equality for all as I was growing up and this provided the foundation for the framework of health as a human right.

PIH's impact on HIV treatment for resource-limited settings was catalytic for the global AIDS movement. I was working at the Massachusetts General Hospital infectious diseases clinic at that time in Boston and heard about what was happening in rural Haiti when PIH launched its HIV Equity Initiative in rural Haiti in 1998. We were struggling to provide good care here in Boston and it was amazing to hear about this small NGO working with the poorest of the poor and making it happen. This was one of the first programs in the world to provide free, comprehensive HIV/AIDS treatment to the poor. This was a game-changer for global HIV treatment and funding.

PIH colleagues (Rich et al., 2012) from PIH's partner organization in Rwanda, Inshuti Mu Buzima, showed an amazing 92% retention rate of over 1,000 HIV patients 2 years after starting antiretroviral treatment. This retention rate far exceeds the average of 70% reported in a review by Mills of 39 published studies that looked at a combined 225,000 HIV patients across sub-Saharan Africa. Surprising to many, the retention rates in North America were even lower, with the average just 55% (Mills et al., 2006). This is such important information to get out there—withholding care and treatment for poor people because it will "not work" or the even more morally intolerable excuse of it being "wasted" is moot.

Now PIH provides antiretroviral treatment and care in Haiti, Rwanda, Lesotho, and Malawi to over 23,000 people and is involved in comprehensive health care to over 3 million people. Addressing the social determinants of health is part of what we do—providing and connecting our patients to food, water, transportation, and housing is a big part of our care. Team-based care is definitely in vogue now in the health care delivery literature; PIH has always exemplified team-based care including the key element of our success—community health workers.

PKN: Dr. Farmer and Dr. Davis, could each of you share what you view as the top three to five priorities in global health for the next 5 years, the next decade, and beyond?

PF: This is a perplexing question for all of us who seek to do the best we can with the limited resources that we have succeeded in marshaling. I'm certainly not saying that these conditions are fixed; it's just that we haven't succeeded in bringing even a fraction of the resources needed to bear on these problems. The best way to set priorities, in my view, is to understand burden and gap. By burden, I mean burden of disease, which is not always easy to assess. You can look at mortality, but it's also important to look at disability and suffering of all types—what's ailing the poor. The second interpretive grid we'd recommend is gap: What kinds of problems are being ignored because they're "too expensive," "not cost-effective," or "not sustainable"? Just thinking about these two interpretive grids—burden and gap—in many of the places that we're working leads me to underline the importance of improving cancer care and surgical services. Mental health receives whatever is the opposite of the lion's share (is that a lamb's share?) of resources. Finally, all of these vertical approaches can be useful, and often have been—the impact of PEPFAR [the President's Emergency Plan for AIDS Relief] on AIDS mortality across the world has been profound and inspiring—but most people involved in global health understand that we have to avoid pitting prevention against care and one disease against another, or one professional group against another. The goals of building strong health systems and looking toward universal health coverage will also come to dominate the global health agenda in the coming years.

SD: The priorities of global health delivery are best based on building strong health systems of care with the public sector. We don't know what the next big thing will be that we have to address in global health. Cholera is an example of where we had to deal with an emergency that required providing care to hundreds of people to save their lives in October 2010. The tragedy of cholera happened in Haiti postearthquake when the poor public infrastructure had already been devastated. Although many were worried about cholera or other opportunistic entities hitting postearthquake, 10 months later we thought we were out of the woods. It is impossible to anticipate all possible iterations of a global health crisis that may come our way, and the only way to be able to ride those storms is to have a system that can withstand the assaults. This does not just mean health care systems, but also public infrastructure for clean water, electricity, and an educated workforce.

The second priority has to include provisions for quality care delivery. This encompasses so much—a good supply chain for medications and goods, clinics and hospitals that are functional and provide a safe working environment, and most importantly educated nurses, doctors, pharmacists, and community health workers. Education is definitely the key to quality, and University Hospital in Mirebalais, Haiti, is a great example of a national teaching hospital that has physician residencies, nursing school rotations, and specialty education for nurses. Nurses are gaining expertise in leadership, critical care/emergency, oncology, and neonatal intensive care. The quality of care has improved as our clinicians develop expertise and are given the tools they need to provide that care.

Setting the expectation of compassionate care delivery has to be another priority for global health moving forward. In many ways, this is the most important, and if we don't treat our patients with dignity and respect, we have already failed. By focusing on patient-centered care, where the patient is the most important part of the team, we will shift care that is "tolerable" to care that is comprehensive and dignified. To accomplish this goal, we must invest in clinical providers and all members of the team to provide them with the support they need to continue to work in very challenging settings. Compassion begins with each other and the more we stand in active solidarity with our global colleagues, then our patients will benefit.

PKN: Please feel free to offer a closing observation about your views on global health, global health equity, and global medicine and nursing in the 21st century.

SD: We are at a crossroad today in global health delivery and we can either continue to limp along and accept our "socialization for scarcity" or we can be the catalyst for a global health equity movement. Focusing on team-based care that is inclusive and values all members of the team including, most importantly, patients and families will enable us to provide better care to those who need it most. It should not matter where you are born or live, if you have HIV, cancer, mental illness, or if you want to have a safe delivery and healthy child—I refuse to believe that we don't have the global resources to provide high-quality and dignified health care for all.

This is an exciting time for global nursing. If we can insist on the foundation of bidirectionality within our global nursing community then we will all win, especially our patients. Nurses are increasingly being recognized as the global health experts that we are and it is imperative that we continue our advocacy to ensure inclusion and recognition—all the while still focusing on the patient. As the United States health system is being reformed, lessons from health delivery in resource-limited settings are extremely valuable. Shifting the emphasis from tertiary care centers to community-based care that is less expensive creates better access and provides quality care, and positive health outcomes should be our goal. Mobilizing the like-minded, converting the skeptical by showing data and honing our messaging, and not settling for "less than" care will move us toward the path of global health equity.

PF: After decades of penury, there have finally been some timid advances in what we're now calling global health, and this is true whether we look at service delivery, training, or commitment to the development of new diagnostics, therapeutics, and deliverables. There are a host of foundations turning their attention and resources toward global health, and certainly more and more young people across the world are engaging in the movement. The biggest problem I'd signal right now is an absurd competition for resources, though not between those promoting global health equity and those in, let's say, the financial sector. Instead, we see absurd and dispiriting competition between various groups and causes that should all be subsumed under the rubric of global health equity. Not only is this dispiriting for obvious reasons—why should we pit better care for mental illnesses against better care for AIDS any more than we should pit prevention against care?—but also because problems run together. The synergies that would result from better coordination and fewer competitive, vertical programs would speed up our attempts to build stronger health systems. Without stronger health systems, there's no chance of universal health care, even in a modest form, and therefore no chance of removing catastrophic illness from the top of the list of causes of destitution. These are, admittedly, complex matters and rooted in place and time. Therefore, global health equity is always a moving target. But the good news is that there is a renewed interest among young people in these very topics, and this is a development that we should all welcome. I'm confident that the up-and-coming generation will be able to sort out these complexities and avoid the balkanization of medicine and public health that have, along with grotesque underfunding, slowed down progress and delayed the achievement of global health equity.

PKN: Thank you for joining us for this fascinating interview and sharing your wisdom on the issues of health, human rights, and social justice.

COMMENTARY ON INTERVIEW WITH PAUL FARMER, MD, PhD, AND SHEILA DAVIS, DNP, RN, FAAN

Suellen Breakey, Patrice K. Nicholas, Shira Winter, Nancy L. Meedzan, and Inge B. Corless

Health, human rights, and social justice are values long held by Drs. Farmer and Davis. Dr. Farmer addresses the social determinants of disease—how poverty produces changes *in* the body—and the importance of the health professions to get the effects of poverty *out* of the body. Dr. Davis further addresses the social determinants of disease in viewing health as a human right, which in turn can provide a solid foundation for global nursing. The concept of health professionals being *socialized for scarcity*—that is, accepting lower standards for poorer people because that is the status quo—is completely upended by the groundbreaking work that Drs. Farmer and Davis accomplish with colleagues at PIH. Dr. Farmer shifts the paradigm whereby lack of resources translates into lack of services by changing the question from "Is this sustainable?" to "How do we sustain this?" Dr. Davis points to the HIV epidemic as a complex challenge that marginalized populations face; PIH had a catalytic effect on the problem of resource scarcity in moving the discussion and care of marginalized populations to the fore.

Global nursing is now fully engaged in addressing human rights and integrating social justice in caring for individuals, communities, and populations. Our charge is not only to participate in caring for people, but our responsibility is also to engage in the amelioration of the root causes of poor health. This mandate is evident in our professional codes including Provision 9.4 of the American Nurses Association (ANA, 2015) *Code of Ethics for Nurses*, which states:

> Health is understood as being broader than delivery and reimbursement systems, but extending to health-related, sociocultural issues such as violation of human rights, homelessness, hunger, violence, and the stigma of illness. (p. 13)

The next steps are to engage in a global effort to address this through action.

Similarly, the International Council of Nurses (ICN) *Code of Ethics for Nurses*, most recently revised in 2012, is a guide for action for nurses worldwide. The Code has served as the standard for nurses worldwide since it was first adopted in 1953. From the preamble of the ICN *Code of Ethics*: "Inherent in nursing is a respect for human rights, including cultural rights, the right to life and choice, to dignity, and to be treated with respect" (p. 1). But respect, while necessary, is not sufficient. As the ICN states further:

> The nurse shares with society the responsibility for initiating and supporting action to meet the health and social needs of the public, in particular those of vulnerable populations. . . . [and] advocates for equity and social justice in resource allocation, access to health care, and other social and economic services.

The discipline of nursing has had a long history of advocating for the sick and vulnerable that positions us to play a pivotal role in advancing the health of the world's people through social justice efforts.

REFERENCES

Alsan, M. M., Westerhaus, M., Herce, M., Nakashima, K., & Farmer, P. (2011). Poverty, global health and infectious disease: Lessons from Haiti and Rwanda. *Infectious Disease Clinics of North America, 25*(3), 611–622.

American Nurses Association. (2015). *Code of ethics for nurses with interpretive statements.* Retrieved from http://www.nursingworld.org/MainMenuCategories/EthicsStandards/CodeofEthicsforNurses/Code-of-Ethics.pdf

Davis, S. (2014, May 2). Finding our compass. *Huffington Post.* Retrieved from http://www.huffingtonpost.com/sheila-davis-dnp-anpbc-faan/finding-our-compass-nurses_b_5242603.html

Farmer, P., Saussy, H., & Kidder, T. (2010). *Partner to the poor: A Paul Farmer reader.* Berkeley, CA: University of California Press.

Farmer, P. E., Furin, J. J., & Katz, J. T. (2004). Global health equity. *The Lancet, 363*(9423), 1832.

International Council of Nurses. (2006). *The ICN code of ethics for nurses.* Geneva, Switzerland: Author.

Mills, E. J., Nachega, J. B., Buchan, I., Orbinski, J., Attaran, A., Singh, S., . . . Bangsberg D. R. (2006). Adherence to antiretroviral therapy in sub-Saharan Africa and North America: A meta-analysis. *Journal of the American Medical Association, 296,* 679–690.

Rich, M., Miller, A. C., Niyigena, P., Franke, M. F., Niyonzima, J. B., Socci, A., . . . Binagwaho, A. (2012). Excellent clinical outcomes and high retention in care among adults in a community-based HIV treatment program in rural Rwanda. *Journal of Acquired Immune Deficiency Syndrome, 59,* e35–e42.

Yang, A., Farmer, P. E., & McGahan, A. M. (2010). "Sustainability" in global health. *Global Public Health, 5*(2), 129–135. doi:10.1080/17441690903418977

CHAPTER 6

The Intersection of Global Health and Community/Public Health Nursing

Karen Anne Wolf

Health is created and lived by people within the settings of their everyday life; where they learn, work, play, and love.

—*The Ottawa Charter (1986)*

The boundaries of community expand and blur as the speed of globalization intensifies the impact of worldwide interconnectedness (Held, McGrew, Goldblatt, & Perraton, 1999). This is evident as growing numbers of organizations take up the challenge of global health and changing health status and patterns of disease. Further, the myriad patterns of population migration, due to climatic, sociopolitical, or economic factors are identified as key determinants of health (Macpherson, Gushalak, & MacDonald, 2007). There is a growing awareness of the negative results of globalization as major shifts in economic markets, environmental degradation, and growing health disparities emerge. The problems of structural violence and social suffering have become more visible, unveiled by social media and the facility of travel (Hanna & Kleinman, 2013). As a response, the expenditures for global health have more than quadrupled from 1990 to 2007 as both public and private organizations have been directed at health problems such as infectious diseases in an effort to stabilize nation-states, economies, and trade (Ravishankar, Leach-Kemon, & Murray, 2011). Global health is now a multisector concern and "due to its links to security, sustainable environment, and good governance, global health is occupying an increasingly visible space in the international agenda" (Frenk, Gomez-Dantes, & Chacon, 2008, p. 16).

Globalization has made possible new exchanges of information and technology and new possibilities for action. Responding to the health challenge posed by globalization requires a multilevel and multisectorial strategy. This chapter discusses this multilevel approach and addresses the role of nursing action at the level of community. A basic premise is that global nursing requires a community framework. The first section of this chapter provides a context for the community framework and elaborates key concepts and principles of a globally responsive community health framework. The second section discusses competencies and potential frameworks to support global community nursing practice. The final section identifies opportunities and challenges that nursing faces in a global community health practice.

A RETURN TO COMMUNITY HEALTH

A health care provider caring for patients in a community health center in many U.S. cities can figuratively "travel around the world," providing care to patients from multiple continents. The provider singularly focused on a diabetic person's infected foot may fail to see the major health determinants of immigrant status, poverty, and homelessness. Thousands of miles away, another health care provider working as part of a medical mission in a rural village, caring for families beset with diarrheal disease, may treat the diarrhea but fail to appreciate the community's difficulty in securing clean water. In each situation, the health care provider confronts inequities shaped by a community context. In order for their efforts to be effective, nurses must shift their perspective of community from the background into the foreground. Whether the provider is working in New York or a rural village in Burundi or Nepal, to make real and lasting positive population health outcomes the programs of care must move away from the individual in isolation and engage the community.

Global health action begins and ends in a community context. From assessment of community needs to partnering with communities to improve health outcomes, community is the central focus of action. Community health is the collective expression of the health of individuals and groups within a defined community and is determined by the personal and family characteristics, the social, cultural, eco-environmental factors, as well as health systems services and the influence of societal, political factors, and globalization (Gofin & Gofin, 2011).

In this chapter, the term *community health*, or *community/public health*, is purposely used. These terms are often used interchangeably as they overlap and share common goals, knowledge, skills, and perspectives that are directed toward the improvement of population health outcomes. The rationale for this distinction is twofold; first, it is intended to recognize that much of community health occurs outside of formal public health structures. This is the case in the United States, where health care is largely privatized. While other nations have centralized national health systems, these vary in their alignment with public health. Second, but primary reason for this distinction is to underscore the centrality of community in the effort to improve population health.

The concept of population health has gained prominence over the past decade (Kindig & Stoffart, 2003). The concept readily applies to communities, as it describes the patterns of health status and health outcomes of an aggregated group of people. Population health has evolved in response to accountability for health care outcomes of individuals and the aggregate or group covered by a given health system, reimbursement, or financing mechanism. The focus of action of population health is more often individuals, and the action is not necessarily tied to an organized identity or locality (Kindig & Stoffart, 2003; Modeste & Tamayose, 2004).

By contrast, community health is inherently tied to identity or locale. Action to promote health is directed at the level of the community as the major influence on health.

Health is embodied in the community as a whole. Community is defined in the American Nurses Association's (ANA) *Public Health Nursing: Scope and Standards of Practice* as "a set of people in interaction, who may or may not share a place or belonging; and who act intentionally for a common purpose" (2013, p. 3). The community may be defined by a location, cultural or demographic characteristic, or actual or potential health problem. Community health, according to the World Health Organization (WHO, 2004), builds on a combination of sciences, skills, and beliefs directed toward the maintenance and improvement of the health of all people through collective or social action.

Prevention of disease or improving the health of the community as a whole is the goal of health programs, services, and institutions. The community health activities may change with changing technology and social values, but the goals remain the same. From assessment of community needs to partnering with community to improve health outcomes, action is focused on the community. For example, if we return to the example of childhood diarrheal disease, the improvement of health outcomes requires more than the availability of treatment, but changing practices in sanitation, water use, and childhood nutrition.

The health of a community is the result of intersecting contextual factors or social determinants. Social determinants are described by the WHO as the conditions in which people are born, grow, live, work, and eat, noting that they are the "causes of causes" of health inequities and outcomes (WHO, n.d.). The WHO Commission on the Social Determinants (WHO, 2008a) offers three overarching recommendations:

1. Improve daily living conditions
2. Tackle the inequitable distribution of power, money, and resources
3. Measure and understand the problem and assess the impact of action

The link between social determinants and population health outcomes has contributed to reorienting public health. Over the past decade, community health is increasingly viewed as part of the redefined public health. According to Porta (2008), this reflects the rhetorical shift away from expert-driven and top-down approaches in policy making and program development. Instead, there is greater emphasis on collective and social action organized by society to protect, promote, and restore the peoples' health (p. 188). The most recent edition of the ANA *Public Health Nursing: Scope and Standards of Practice* integrates a dominant population perspective with a focus on community:

> Public health nursing practice focuses on population health through continuous surveillance and assessment of the multiple determinants of health with the intent to promote health and wellness, prevent disease, disability and premature death, and improve neighborhood quality of life. (2013, p. 2)

Public health knowledge evolved over the past 200 years and nursing practice has taken a more formalized approach, most commonly by government with the intent to protect the public's health. Such formal government-sponsored approaches have been subject to changing leadership, variability of funding, and inadequate infrastructure and resources in many countries. The variability and unpredictability of public health services has led nongovernmental organizations (NGOs) to take up the mantle of public health action in many countries, alongside private nonprofit providers. The rise of actual or potential epidemics such as AIDS, hepatitis C, or avian influenza, as well as maternal child mortality, has led to overlapping and, too often, disjointed systems of health promotion, prevention, and health services delivery (Unger, De Paepe, Sen, & Soors, 2010). Nurses have an obligation to do more than stand witness to this system dysfunction. Their contribution to community health, whether at home or abroad, rests on public health competencies employed within a community-nursing framework.

COMMUNITY/PUBLIC HEALTH NURSING COMPETENCIES

From the early days of Florence Nightingale, nursing has viewed health within a global context. For more than 40 years, Nightingale worked to improve the public health of India (Vallée, 2006). The concept of public health was still nascent, and Nightingale used her knowledge and skills to advocate for the improvement of health conditions. Nurses in the United States followed the call to community, with leadership from nursing education and nursing activists such as Lillian Wald. From the outset, their efforts were directed to the prevention of diseases and the promotion of health. Some 50 years later, WHO (1961) noted that the need for community and public health nurses was expanding worldwide and that nurses were critical providers in communicable disease control, health education, and maternal–child health services.

Despite this need, a shortage of public health nurses persisted. Under medical dominance, hospital-based health care systems grew in numbers and size. In the United States and other countries, funding and attention shifted away from public health. The higher status and remuneration for hospital work refocused nursing education and practice toward hospital care of the sick. This left nurses ill-prepared in community/public health nursing. Esther Lucille Brown observed that "insufficient attention has been given to the progressively larger role that nursing has come to play and apparently must play if the current world-wide expansion of health services is not to be checked "(p. 10).

Nursing roles have grown globally with specialization and expansion of educational opportunities. As nursing organizations have moved to standardize and evaluate competencies within the profession, so too has the field of public/community health nursing. Since the initial publication of the ANA *Public Health Nursing: Scope and Standards of Practice* in 1986, there has been an ongoing dialogue about the evolving role of nurses in community and/or public health settings. As public and private health systems were grappling with infectious diseases such as AIDS and malaria and social conditions such as homelessness and forced migration, national and international attention was redirected toward the need for competent and strong public health services. The 1988 *The Future of Public Health* was the catalyst for strengthening and redefining the scope of community/public health nursing (IOM, 1988). This report outlined the key public health functions as: assessment, assurance, and policy development. In 1994, a joint statement on Essential Public Health Services followed, drafted by representatives from several national organizations and governmental agencies (Public Health Foundation, 1994).

The *Essential Public Health Services* document provided a framework for the development of principles of public health nursing (Centers for Disease Control and Prevention [CDC], n.d.; Table 6.1). The principles reflect a commitment toward the population or community, whether or not the nurse provides care to individuals, families, or groups. The authors emphasized the nurse's dominant responsibility is to the population or community as a whole. Collaboration with the client as equal partner is an essential principle. A focus on prevention is an essential principle that includes primary prevention strategies that incorporate the following to support a thriving population: healthy, environmental, social, and economic conditions. A public health nurse is expected to be proactive in active case-finding and outreach and use organized approaches to plan and provide effective, evidence-based care. Leadership in collaboration with other professionals, community groups, and organizations is viewed as essential to promote and protect the health of the community.

The ethics of community health, once rooted in the idea of *the greatest good for the greatest number of people*, are increasingly complex. This complexity has led to a more narrowed focus on protection of the public in the face of health threats such as infectious diseases and has led to the neglect of personal health services. An integrated ethical approach to community health requires investment in primary health care services, as well as improvements in basic preventative services such as sanitation and potable, clean water.

The global movement toward a competency-based education and practice in the health professions is rooted in the drive for educational and health system

TABLE 6.1 Essential Public Health Services

The 10 essential public health services describe the public health activities that all communities should undertake and serve as the framework for the National Public Health Performance Standards (NPHPS) instruments. Public health systems should:

1. Monitor health status to identify and solve community health problems
2. Diagnose and investigate health problems and health hazards in the community
3. Inform, educate, and empower people about health issues
4. Mobilize community partnerships and action to identify and solve health problems
5. Develop policies and plans that support individual and community health efforts
6. Enforce laws and regulations that protect health and ensure safety
7. Link people to needed personal health services and assure the provision of health care when otherwise unavailable
8. Assure competent public and personal health care workforce
9. Evaluate effectiveness, accessibility, and quality of personal and population-based health services
10. Research for new insights and innovative solutions to health problems

Source: CDC (2010).

accountability. The competency approach offers a more efficient and effective means of achieving defined outcomes of the educational process and defined roles of the health practitioner. Gruppen, Mangrulkar, and Kolars (2012) argue that competencies offer a flexibility that can be adapted to address contextual differences in educational settings as well as the differences in learners. One such competency approach in community/public health nursing is the ANA *Public Health Nursing: Scope and Standards of Practice* that was first developed in 1986. This document serves as a model for other nations for public health nursing. Revised in 2007 and again in 2013, the document aligns with the document on the ANA *Scope and Standards of Nursing Practice* (2010) as well as with the *Public Health Nursing Core Competencies* (Quad Council, 2011; Table 6.2).

The most current version of the ANA *Scope and Standards of Practice* includes 17 standards for practice, and each standard is correlated with a set of competencies. The first six standards address public health nursing practice; standards 7 through 17 address professional performance in public health nursing. The document has served as a resource as other nations develop similar documents to guide community or public health nursing. The global movement toward competency-based education and workforce development offers an opportunity to identify core knowledge, skills, and attitudes of community/public health nurses. However, the adaptation of this core set of standards and competencies to the unique context of nations poses a socioeconomic and political challenge. While such documents are useful to outline the role and functions of nurses working in community/public health, they form only a partial framework for action.

TABLE 6.2 *Public Health Nursing: Scope and Standards of Practice* **(Revised 2013)**

These standards were developed by a Public Health Nursing Scope and Standards Working Group in conjunction with American Nurses Association (ANA) staff. Each of the standards of public health nursing are aligned with the ANA Standards of Nursing Practice. The standards are further elaborated with a set of expected competencies. The entirety of the report on *Public Health Nursing: Scope and Standards of Pracitce* is available from the American Nurses Association/Nurses Books.org.

STANDARDS OF PUBLIC HEALTH NURSING PRACTICE

Standard 1. Assessment
The public health nurse collects comprehensive data pertinent to the health status of population.

Standard 2. Population Diagnosis and Priorities
The health nurse analyses the assessment data to determine the population diagnoses and priorities.

Standard 3. Outcomes Identification
The public health nurse identifies expected outcomes for a plan specific to the population or situation.

Standard 4. Planning
The public health nurse develops a plan that prescribes strategies and alternatives to attain expected outcomes.

(continued)

TABLE 6.2 *Public Health Nursing: Scope and Standards of Practice* (Revised 2013) (*continued*)

Standard 5. Implementation The public health nurse implements the identified plan.
Standard 5A. Coordination The public health nurse coordinates care delivery.
Standard 5B. Health Education and Health Promotion The public health nurse employs multiple strategies to promote health and a safe environment.
Standard 5C. Consultation The public health nurse provides consultation to influence the identified plan, enhance the abilities of others, and effect change.
Standard 5D. Prescriptive Authority Not applicable.
Standard 5E. Regulatory Activities The public health nurse participates in the application of public health laws, regulations, and policies.
Standard 6. Evaluation

Source: ANA (2013). ANA NurseBooks, with permission.

FRAMEWORKS FOR COMMUNITY HEALTH NURSING ACTION

The purpose of frameworks for community/public health nursing in global health is to guide the practice and the evaluation of practice. A distillation of the principles, standards, and competencies of community/public health nursing identifies key themes that guide effective practice. These are both translatable and scalable to global nursing practice. The intersection of themes forges powerful models for effective community/public health nursing practice in a global context and examples of these are demonstrated throughout this text. The themes are organized categorically into ethical, sociocultural, political, community, eco-epidemiological, and intersectorial/interdisciplinary collaboration; however, it is the synergistic interplay of these that matters in practice.

Ethical Stance: Communitarian and Social Justice

The first theme is the community health nursing ethical stance, which recognizes the humanity and uniqueness of individuals, families, and communities as foundational for community and public health. While Western bioethical traditions express the regard for individual rights, including the right to health, the community/public health perspective also embraces the communitarian tradition. This tradition purports that individuals are interreliant and part of a greater social and political network. According to Callahan (2003), "human beings are social animals... whose lives are lived out within deeply penetrating social, political, and cultural institutions and practices. It also assumes that no sharp distinction can be drawn between the public and private sphere. It is important that there be a private and protected sphere, but what counts as private will be a societal decision, not something inherent in the human condition" (p. 4). This analytical perspective grounds the work of community/public health nursing. Nursing action emanates from the moral commitment to provide for the relief of suffering of the individual, but also community-focused disease and injury prevention and the promotion of health. The communitarian tradition furthers the commitment to social justice and calls for attention to private suffering as a public responsibility. This shifts attention to the community as a whole, and the efforts to support the basic human needs for the community, as well as the individuals within it.

The "right to health" is often stated as a goal that is not guaranteed or readily attainable. The goal extends the health care provider's gaze to look beyond health problems to the social determinants of health, such as poverty, access to education, and the health of the environment. There are a variety of ethical theories that may be applied to health care. Harrowing et al. (2010) argue that western biomedical ethics reflect a narrow paternalistic perspective. The concept of social justice and an associated call to action and advocacy transcends this perspective as discussed by Drs. Farmer and Davis in Chapter 5.

Political Perspective: From Empowerment to Building Community Capacity

The second theme is the importance of power sharing through partnerships and empowerment of clients (individuals, families, and communities). This political perspective builds on the communitarian ethical commitment and on the principle of social justice. A foundational concept for global health is empowerment. Based on the work of Brazilian educator Paolo Freire (1970), empowerment is described as the process of conscientization and involves critical reflection, questioning, and dialogue within the community. The process is intended to guide the community in recognizing and analyzing the situation of the community. This may include inequities, causal chains, and root causes that impede health and wellness within the community. Community members gain power as they build the capacity to self-identify problems and solutions. Empowerment has replaced the top-down strategies in the public health approaches of the 1960s and 1970s and is now the dominant paradigm for community/public health development. This approach was advanced in nursing as the Community as Partner model, described by Anderson and McFarlane (2008) and first published in 1988. According to Racher and Annis (2008), the health of a community derives from the functioning of that community. This central characteristic embodies the extent to which the community is empowered to build or effectively use the community's assets "for the life of community members and the community as a whole within the context of the environment" (Racher & Annis, p. 182).

The processes of empowerment and partnership development share a heritage in community organizing and community building. The movement to build community capacity is grounded in community development models as well as in community building models. McKnight and Kretzman (2012), proponents of community building, argue that there is a need to shift the focus away from deficits to one of assets and community capacities. A reality of community building and partnerships is that they must transcend a rhetorical call for participation and integrate participation through the process of community-focused action. Wallerstein (2006) observes that "participatory processes are at the base of empowerment. Participation alone is insufficient if strategies don't also build capacity to challenge non-responsive or oppressive institutions and to redress power imbalances" (p. 6). Community building is essential to address the underlying determinants of health that confront the community on a daily basis. But, community building is also essential to the well-being and resiliency of a community. Resiliency is considered to be a critical characteristic, required for a community to manage adversity such as a disaster or other trauma (Kulig, 2000). Planning for the health of a community requires building networks of support and aid in advance.

Ecosocial Perspectives: Toward a Multilevel Perspective

A third theme is the use of an ecosocial epidemiological perspective as a means to understand and address the complexity of the interconnected relationship between populations of animals (including humans), plants, and the natural environment. This perspective allows the community/public health nurse to appreciate that there are multiple factors or determinants of health. Krieger (2001), a primary proponent of this model, argues that the ecosocial offers a multilevel framework to integrate social and biological reasoning for a dynamic analysis. As an analytical framework, it takes into account the historical and current ecological perspective to formulate new insights into determinants of population distributions of disease and social inequalities in health.

An ecosocial perspective holds that policies and public health care actions should be driven by sustainability. Sustainability, as defined by the United Nations, is "the ability to meet the needs of the present without compromising the needs of the future" and requires the reconciliation of environmental, social, and economic demands (United Nations General Assembly, 2005). "Sustainability creates and maintains the conditions under which humans and nature can exist in productive harmony that permit fulfilling the social, economic and other requirements of present and future generations." In the case of public health, other sector policies such as food production, the built environment, and/or transportation, may impact health in a ripple effect, creating changes in both the physical environment and in human and animal health behaviors. Recognition of the interaction has led to a growing "One Health" movement, bringing together interprofessional teams to collaborate in an integrated approach to addressing global issues such as feeding the world population, zoonosis and emerging infectious diseases, human-animal bonds, and many others (CDC, n.d.).

Building Collaboration: Intersectoral and Interdisciplinary

Collaboration is a central theme across community/public health nursing and an essential element of assessment, planning, implementation, and evaluation at both the macro-system level and the microlevel of service delivery. At the macro level, the responsibility for the health of the population is necessarily shared across a complexity of sociopolitical, economic, and health care systems. The ability to effectively collaborate poses a challenge. An outspoken complaint is that the silo mentality in governmental and nursing organizations obscures the big picture. This narrowed perspective, and the subsequent lack of collaboration, impedes the development of effective solutions. A recent approach to public policy development is the concept of *health in all policies*. This approach calls for health, equity, and sustainability to be placed at the center of decision-making processes of governments, engaging all sectors in collaboration with key stakeholders (Rudolph, Caplan, Mitchell, Ben Moshe, & Dillon, 2013). This intersectional approach requires that community/public health nurses engage with policy makers to consider the potential impact of policies on health as well as the determinants of health. This approach builds on the previous themes of communitarian ethics, empowerment, and the ecosocial perspective.

A second major focus of collaboration is the move to greater interprofessional and/or interdisciplinary teamwork in education and practice. The call for interprofessional collaboration reflects a growing twofold concern. First is the drive to improve the quality and safety of health care, which has been impeded by the lack of effective communication and teamwork. Second is the belief that interprofessional teamwork can be a means to increase flexibility and adaptability and expand worker potential in health care services. Interprofessional teamwork in public health is viewed as a primary means to build capacity and "scale up" programs (Reeves, Lewin, Espin, & Zwarnsetein, 2010). Capacity-building interventions in the community include the expansion of nursing roles in areas of physician shortage as well as the integration of community health workers or lay health workers as part of the health care team. Underfunded and underresourced, there continues to be a nursing shortage in many communities. While building nursing workforce capacity is critical, the integration of community health/lay health workers can help extend the reach of nursing work, expand culturally appropriate health education, and increase outreach as well as direct care. The community or lay health workers' relationships with the community can help bridge community support for and acceptability of health programs. The development of community workers also facilitates the flow of workers into the pipeline of nursing and health careers. Community health nurses play a critical role in the training and ongoing supervision of lay health workers. This includes formal and informal training of community health workers to provide effective health outreach and intervention in communities.

While policies and programs for health are established at international, national, or regional levels, it is increasingly understood that implementation of policies requires a multilevel strategy, rooted in the community. In a review of major reports and programs, Trickett and Beehler (2013) highlight the importance of adapting a social ecological model to frame multilevel actions directed at reducing social inequities. They further suggest:

• The formation of collaborative and empowering partnerships with communities
• The development of community capacity goals as well as individual goals

- The use of interprofessional and/transdisciplinary intervention teams
- The application of a sustaining commitment to programs
- The application of theory and evidence to support community change (p. 1231)

CHALLENGES FOR THE FUTURE OF GLOBAL NURSING

The nursing profession is part of a global community united by history and a commitment to advance the quality of nursing practice. Despite our common history, there continue to be different opportunities for nursing with disparities in opportunities, reflecting social, economic, and political realities of nation-states. Nursing leadership is needed to address issues both internal to nursing, such as workforce development goals, and external to nursing, such as the social determinants and the health needs of populations for whom nurses provide care. Effective leadership is required to develop new forms of collaboration across disciplines and sectors, as well as across nursing organizations.

Leadership in Support of Global Community Nursing

Leadership development is a major priority for global nursing. Leadership is needed on multiple levels to influence policy regarding funding, regulating health care and health programs, and developing nursing and health care labor forces. While there have been centralized approaches to leadership through groups such as the International Council on Nursing (ICN) and the Honor Society of Nursing, Sigma Theta Tau International (STTI), leadership at the community-program level will be most successful if it can grow from and be rooted in the nursing community. The establishment of a network of leaders is needed to advocate for health-promoting policies and maximizing the potential of nursing practice. A variety of governmental and NGOs are working globally to build nursing workforce capacity and leadership (Mulvihill & Debas, 2008). One example is the work of Partners In Health (PIH), which brings resources to impoverished communities and works in partnership with the communities to build sustainable programs and the capacity to address serious health problems and promote health (see Chapter 5). Other nursing organizations, such as the Nightingale Initiative for Global Health (NIGH), are building networks of support for advocacy (Beck, Dossey, & Rushton, 2013).

Nursing leadership is challenged to address the development of a strong global public health nursing workforce, creating the knowledge and research base to support effective practice. Priority areas for nursing leadership and action include:

- Building integrative programs that build capacity for sustainable and holistic primary care as well as problem- or disease-specific services
- Expanding access to formal and continuing nurse education programs with curricula that support and enhance evidence-based practice for community/public health

- Compensating and recognizing nurses working in the community
- Understanding and addressing the complexity of the global migration in the nursing workforce
- Providing for safety in the workplace, including protections from violence as well as physical, biological, or psychological injuries of all types
- Advocating for funding and support of research- and evidence-based practice, including a focus on the evaluation of community/public health nursing programs, community-participatory research approaches and interdisciplinary approaches that render nursing, and community health workers visible

Expanding Access and Knowledge for Global Nursing Practice

Global nursing practice includes a variety of nursing roles and addresses a variety of health care needs. Global nursing practice, based on best evidence, is challenged by lack of a well-developed knowledge base in community/public health practice. Too often, problems of funding persist as the imperative to implement direct care projects takes precedence over project evaluation. For those projects that do integrate an evaluation component, the push to publish is impaired by resource limitations, as well as the small project sample sizes. Potential strategies to overcome barriers include partnering with academic partnerships through such formal structures as the ICN Nursing Education Network (ICN, n.d.) or academic institutional partnerships in sustained partnerships that build capacity for knowledge development, as well as generate or translate knowledge.

The globalization of knowledge through a process of quality systematic review reshapes the perception of what is possible. The Cochrane Collaborative sets a standard for the development and dissemination of systematic reviews of best practices and has been particularly effective in advancing the practice in global HIV/AIDS care (Wall, 2014). There is also the potential to aggregate the results of smaller projects. One resource for the aggregation and review of results is the launching of the Joanna Briggs Institute (JBI), which became affiliated with the Cochrane Collaborative in 2006. The JBI is a system similar to Cochrane, and is directed to a global nursing audience. Similar to the Cochrane Collaborative process, researchers aggregate, extract, and critique research to build evidence in support of nursing practice. The JBI training in the conduct of systematic reviews is slowly gaining momentum globally; however, in some areas of the world, the cost of training may be prohibitive. The JBI, however, has purposely established centers in a variety of underserved regions with training subsidies.

The Honor Society of Nursing, STTI (n.d), offers members access to evidence-based information through publications in the Henderson Library. As with the JBI, affordability remains a problem in many settings. An alternative is the expansion of open access resources. These usually depend on Internet access and include a variety of resources, often governmental, such as the WHO and the CDC, as well as NGOs such as social media sites and listserves.

One example is the Open Courseware Consortium (OCWC), which offers courses, webinars, and access to textbooks from a number of universities in an open access format. This site focuses on solving real problems. Another successful example is the Internet site Supercourse, a repository of lectures on global health and prevention (Shishani et al., 2012). The Supercourse networks scientists and academics in over 174 countries who offer free lectures in over 24 different languages. A third example is Unite for Sight University, which evolved from a program directed at improving vision health to a wide array of courses and programs that support global health action. Technology is making possible the sharing of knowledge and best practices. There is a growing need for nurses to become astute consumers through not only information and health literacy, but also epidemiology and evidence-based practice development.

Building Networks of Support

An important resource for global health practitioners is their shared experience and expertise. As noted in the previous discussion on knowledge resources, there are some key areas of shared knowledge in global health, but also some very specialized areas such as management of HIV infection in prenatal patients. Building support networks for health care practitioners offers the potential to aid in knowledge development as well as to provide guidance in managing issues related to program implementation and day-to-day practice. Support networks also assist practitioners to address power struggles in the field. Social media offers one approach to network support. One example is the Global Health Delivery Project at Harvard University, which offers online courses and topical community forums on global health issues. This is one approach to strengthening support networks to improve the delivery of health care.

Support for Respectful Collaborative Interprofessional Practice

Interprofessional collaborative practice is viewed as an essential element to meet the needs of community and global health in the future. Interprofessional collaboration and team-based health care offer an opportunity to strengthen systems of care and improve population outcomes. The interprofessional team approach offers a flexibility and adaptability necessary to respond to changing situations in global health care. Building effective teamwork requires a culture change in both the education of health care providers and the organizational culture in which they work. In addition, there may be a need to improve clarity in institutional or governmental regulations as well as in practice settings. The WHO (2012) highlighted this in the 2012 *Report on Strategic Directions for Strengthening Nursing and Midwifery Services*, calling for each health profession to establish standards and appropriate regulations that support high-quality evidence-based practice. The implementation of such strategies must therefore take into account the realities, priorities, and needs of each country. Two significant challenges must be faced in developing interprofessional models for global health practice. First, as Holzemer (2013) argues, there must be sufficient nursing resources, as well as the opportunities for interprofessonal education and practice collaboration, if interprofessional models are to be developed. Second, task shifting in the health professions is typically met with ambivalence and resistance by many in nursing (Holzemer, 2008). There is also a reluctance to acknowledge and compensate for task shifting in the cases where nurses are similarly taking on medical tasks (WHO, 2008b).

CONCLUSION

As nurses and other health care professionals heed the call to global health, it is important to recognize that *global is local*. Policies and action toward improved population health must be anchored within a community context. Community/public health nursing provides an essential set of competencies and services to address the health of the community. Community/public health nursing actions are guided by intersecting frameworks of ethics, partnership models, and eco-social epidemiology. These serve as a strong base for attending to social determinants of health and forging strong partnerships within the community. There is a need for nursing leadership and advocacy to address the growing challenges of global health at home and abroad. Building support for the nursing workforce is critical to ensure that nurses are visible and available to build capacity for healthy communities. As emphasized in the WHO Ottawa Charter (1986), the promotion of health is "a process of enabling people to increase control over and to improve their health" (p. 1).

Nurses and other health care providers must embrace the reality that public health is global. Nursing will be challenged to develop innovative population health strategies that respect, engage, and partner with communities. Nurses working within a community framework have an essential role in the forging of community partnerships grounded in trust and evidence-based practice. Through nurses' efforts, communities may be empowered to become more resilient and healthy.

REFERENCES

American Nurses Association. (1986). *Public health nursing: Scope and standards of practice.* Silver Spring, MD: American Nurses Association/Nurse Books.

American Nurses Association. (2010). *Public health nursing: Scope and standards of practice* (2nd ed.). Silver Spring, MD: American Nurses Association/Nurse Books.

American Nurses Association. (2013). *Public health nursing: Scope and standards of practice* (3rd ed.). Silver Spring, MD: American Nurses Association/Nurse Books.

Anderson, E. T., & McFarlane, J. (2008). *Community as partner: Theory and practice in nursing.* Philadelphia, PA: Lippincott, Williams, & Wilkins.

Beck, D. M., Dossey, B., & Rushton, C. (2013). Building the Nightingale initiative for global health—NIGH: Can we engage and empower the public voices of nurses worldwide? *Nursing Science Quarterly, 26*(4), 366–371.

Brown, E. L. (1948). *Nursing for the future*. New York, NY: Russell Sage Foundation.

Callahan, D. (2003). Principlism and communitarianism. *Journal of Medical Ethics, 29*(5), 287–291. doi:10.1136/jme.29.5.287

Centers for Disease Control and Health Promotion. (n.d.). *Office of one health*. Retrieved from http://www.cdc.gov/onehealth

Centers for Disease Control and Health Promotion. (2010). *The public health system and the 10 essential public health services*. Retrieved from http://www.cdc.gov/nphpsp/essentialservices.html

Freire, P. (1970). *Pedagogy of the oppressed*. New York, NY: Continuum.

Frenk, J., Gomez-Dantes, O., & Chacon, F. (2008). Global health in transition. In R. Parkers & M. Sommer (Eds.), *Routledge handbook of global public health* (pp. 11–18). New York, NY: Routledge.

Gofin, J., & Gofin, R. (2011). *Essentials of global community health*. Sudbury, MA: Jones and Bartlett.

Gruppen, L. D., Mangrulkar, R. S., & Kolars, J. C. (2012). The promise of competency-based education in the health professions for improving global health. *Human Resources for Health, 10*(1), 10–43. doi:10.1186/1478-4491-10-43

Hanna, B., & Kleinman, A. (2013). Unpacking global health, theory and critique. In P. Farmer, J. M. Kim, A. Kleinman, & M. Basilico (Eds.)., *Reimaging global health* (pp. 30–31). Berkeley, CA: University of California Press.

Harrowing, J. N., Mill, J., Spiers, J., Kulig, J., & Kipp, W. (2010). Culture, context, and community: Ethics consideration for global nursing research. *International Nursing Review, 57*, 70–77. doi:10.1111/j.1466-7657.2009.00766.x

Held, D., McGrew, A., Goldblatt, D., & Perraton, J. (1999). *Global transformations: Politics economics and culture*. Cambridge, UK: Polity Press.

Holzemer, W. (2008). Building a qualified global nursing workforce. *International Nursing Review, 55*(3), 241–242. doi:10.1111/j.1466-7657.2008.00675.x

Holzemer, W. (2013). Nursing and health policy perspective-global interprofessional education: Is the time now? *International Nursing Review, 60*(2), 145–146. doi:10.1111/inr.12029

Institute of Medicine. (1988). *The future of public health*. Washington, DC: The National Academies Press.

Institute of Medicine. (2003). *The future of the public's health in the 21st century*. Washington, DC: The National Academies Press.

International Council of Nurses Nursing Education Network. (n.d.). Retrieved from http://www.icn.ch/networks/nursing-education-network

Joanna Briggs Institute. (n.d.). Retrieved from http://joannabriggs.org

Kindig, D., & Stoffart, G., (2003). What is population health? *American Journal of Public Health, 93*(3), 380–383.

Krieger, N. (2001). Theories for social epidemiology in the 21st century: An ecosocial perspective. *International Journal of Epidemiology, 30*, 668–677. doi:10.1093/ije/30.4.668

Kulig, J. (2000). Community resiliency: The potential for community health theory development. *Public Health Nursing, 17*(5), 374–385.

Macpherson, D., Gushalak, B., & MacDonald, L. (2007). Health and foreign policy: Influences on migration and population mobility. *Bulletin of the World Health Organization, 85*(3), 200–206.

McKnight, J., & Kretzman, J. P. (2012). Mapping community capacity. In M. Minkler (Ed.), *Community organizing and community building for health and welfare* (3rd ed.). New Brunswick, NJ: Rutgers Press.

Modeste, N. N., & Tamayose, T. S. (2004). *Dictionary of public health promotion and education* (p. 97). San Francisco, CA: Jossey-Bass.

Mulvihill, J. D., & Debas, H. T. (2008). Long-term academic partnerships in capacity building in health developing countries. In R. Parkers & M. Sommer (Eds.), *Routledge handbook in global health* (pp. 506–515). New York, NY: Routledge.

Open Courseware Consortium. (n.d). Retrieved from http://www.ocwconsortium.org

Partners In Health. (2014, March 23). Retrieved from http://www.pih.org

Porta, M. (2008). *A dictionary of epidemiology*. New York, NY: Oxford University Press.

Public Health Foundation. (1994). *Core public health functions expenditures*. Washington, DC: Author.

Quad Council. (2011). *Quad council competencies for public health nurses*. Retrieved from http://quadcouncilphn.org

Racher, F., & Annis, R. (2008). The Community Health Action model: Health promotion by the community. *Research and Theory for Nursing Practice: An International Journal, 22*(3), 181–192. doi:10.1891/0889-7182.22.3.182

Ravishankar, N., Leach-Kemon, K., & Murray, C. J. L. (2011). Tracking development assistance for health, 1990–2007. In R. Parker & M. Sommer (Eds.), *Routledge handbook of global public health* (pp. 329–345). New York, NY: Routledge.

Reeves, S., Lewin, S., Espin, S., & Zwarnsetein, M. (2010). *Interprofessional teamwork for health and social care*. Hoboken, NJ: Wiley.

Rudolph, L., Caplan, J., Mitchell, C., Ben Moshe, K., & Dillon, L. (2013). *Health in all policies: Improving health through intersectoral collaboration, a discussion paper*. Washington, DC: Institute of Medicine (IOM)/National Academies Press.

Shishani, K., Allen, C., Shubkinkov, E., Salman, K., Laporte, R. L., & Linkov, F. (2012). Nurse educators establishing new venues in global nursing education. *Journal of Professional Nursing, 28*(2), 132–134. doi:10.1016/j.profnurs.2011.11.008

Trickett, E. J., & Beehler, S. (2013). The ecology of multi-level interventions to reduce social inequalities in health. *American Behavioral Scientist, 57*(8), 1227–1246. doi:10.1177/0002764213487342

Unger, J. P., De Paepe, P., Sen, K., & Soors, W. (2010). *International aid policies, a need for alternatives*. Cambridge, UK: Cambridge University Press.

United Nations. (1987). *United Nations World Commission on Environment and Development, 1987*. Retrieved from http://www.un-documents.net/ocf-01.htm#I

United Nations General Assembly. (2005). *The World Summit on Sustainable Development: Reaffirming the centrality of health*. Retrieved from http://www.globalizationandhealth.com/content/1/1/8

Vallée, G. (2006). *Florence Nightingale on health in India: Collected works of Florence Nightingale, (Vol. 9)*. Waterloo, ON: Wilfrid Laurier University Press.

Wall, D. (2014). The Cochrane Collaboration and evidence-based practice: Where the art and science of HIV nursing meet. *Journal of the Association of Nursing in AIDS Care, 25*(1), 4–6. doi:10.1016/j.jana.2013.09.003

Wallerstein, N. (2006, February). *What is the evidence on effectiveness of empowerment to improve health?* WHO Regional Office for Europe's Health Evidence Network (HEN) February 2006. Retrieved from http://www.euro.who.int/__data/assets/pdf_file/0010/74656/E88086.pdf

World Health Organization. (1961). *Aspects of public health nursing*. Geneva, Switzerland: Author.

World Health Organization. (1986). *The Ottawa Charter for Health Promotion First International Conference on Health Promotion*, Ottawa, November 21, 1986. Retrieved from http://www.who.int/healthpromotion/conferences/previous/ottawa/en

World Health Organization (WHO). (2004). *A glossary of terms for community health care and services for older persons*. Retrieved from http://www.who.int/kobe_centre/ageing/ahp_vol5_glossary.pdf

World Health Organization. (2008a). *Commission on the Social Determinants of Health closing the gap in a generation: Health equity through action on the social determinants of health*. Geneva, Switzerland: Author. Retrieved from http://www.who.int/social_determinants/thecommission/finalreport/en/index.html

World Health Organization. (2008b). *Task shifting: Rational redistribution of tasks among health workforce teams: Global recommendations and guidelines*. Geneva, Switzerland: Author.

World Health Organization. (2012). *2012 Report on strategic directions for strengthening nursing and midwifery services*. Retrieved from http://www.who.int/hrh/resources/nmsd/en

ADDITIONAL READING AND RESOURCES

Buhler-Wilkerson, K. (1993). Bringing care to the people: Lillian Wald's legacy to public health nursing. *American Journal of Public Health, 83*(12), 1778–1786.

Cochrane Nursing Care Field. (2014). Retrieved from http://ccnf.cochrane.org

Community Health Nurses of Canada. (2008). *Canadian community health nursing standards of practice*. Toronto, Canada: Community Health Nurses Association of Canada.

Gostin, L. (Ed.). (2002). *Public health law and ethics*. Berkeley, CA: University of California Press.

Hoffman, S. J., & Frenk, J. (2012). Producing and translating health evidence for improved global health. *Journal of Interprofessional Care, 26*, 4–5.

Horrocks, S., Anderson, E., & Salisbury, C. (2002). Systematic review of where nurse practitioners working in primary care can provide equivalent care to doctors. *British Medical Journal, 324*, 819–823.

Institute of Medicine (IOM). (2006). *Promoting health: Intervention strategies for social and behavior sciences*. Washington, DC: The National Academies Press.

International Council of Nurses (ICN). (2008). *Nursing care continuum–framework and competencies*. Geneva, Switzerland: Author.

Interprofessional Education Collaborative Expert Panel. (2011). *Core competencies for interprofessional collaborative practice: Report of an expert panel*. Washington, DC: Interprofessional Education Collaborative.

Kingma, M. (2005). *Nurses on the move: Migration and the global health care economy*. Ithaca, NY: Cornell University Press.

Lewin, S. A., Dick, J., Pond, P., Zwarenstein, M., Aja, G., van Wyk, B., . . . Scheel, I. B. (2005). Lay health workers in primary and community health care. *Cochrane Database of Systematic Reviews, 1*. doi:10.1002/14651858.CD004015

McMichael, A. J. (1995). The health of persons, populations, and planets. Epidemiology comes full circle. *Epidemiology, 6*(6), 633–636.

OpenCourseWare Consortium. (2014). Retrieved from http://www.ocwconsortium.org

World Health Organization (WHO) (2004). *A glossary of terms for community health care and services for older persons*. Retrieved from http://www.who.int/kobe_centre/ageing/ahp_vol5_glossary.pdf

World Health Organization. (2012). *Strategic directions for strengthening nursing and midwifery services 2011–2015*. Retrieved from http://www.who.int/hrh/resources/nmsd/en

World Health Organization. (n.d). *Social determinants of health*. Retrieved from http://www.who.int/social_determinants/en

CHAPTER 7

Global Health Partnerships

Anne Sliney

*F*or nurses and nursing students new to the global health sphere, there may be a hazy notion of what it means to work in global health. The images that often come to mind may be somewhat romantic notions of providing care and treatment to people without access, relieving pain and suffering with the nurse's own two hands, and using nursing knowledge and skill to teach people who are sorely lacking in those skills. While some of that might actually happen, the vast majority of programs in which nurses participate are complex initiatives with political, financial, cultural, and ethical components. Governments, donors, academic institutions, clinical sites, churches, and civil society all influence and help define how global health programs work. It is important for nurses to understand the complexities of global health initiatives as they plan and carry out their programs. In order to think about effective partnerships in global health, it is critical that we understand the recent evolution of global aid and approaches to addressing the most serious health issues in low-income countries.

A HISTORICAL PERSPECTIVE: THE IMPLEMENTATION OF GLOBAL HIV/AIDS INITIATIVES

The world has seen dramatic change in the way global health programs are designed, funded, and carried out since the early part of the 21st century. Complex health issues have been tackled across multiple countries, requiring unprecedented levels of funding. The global HIV pandemic presented the world with the opportunity to confront a seemingly overwhelming problem from multiple vantage points. In fact, many people believed that treatment of HIV on a wide scale was not possible in low-income countries. Barriers to care included the cost of antiretroviral (ARV) medications, poor supply chain and pharmacy systems, weak laboratory systems, and health professionals without the knowledge or experience to provide care and treatment. Surely challenges of this magnitude would require coordinated planning and implementation of programs.

Out of the challenge that arose from the AIDS pandemic came two huge global funders—the Global Fund to Fight AIDS, Tuberculosis, and Malaria; and the U.S. President's Emergency Plan for AIDS Relief (PEPFAR). The Clinton HIV/AIDS

Initiative took the lead in negotiating with generic drug companies to dramatically reduce the prices of generic ARVs, making them affordable for governments, nongovernmental organizations (NGOs), faith-based organizations, and others to purchase and provide at very low cost or no cost. Other bilateral donors developed their own funding plans to support the scale-up of diagnosis and treatment. From 2003 to 2005, almost every high-prevalence country developed multisectoral AIDS coordinating bodies, national strategic plans, and national treatment guidelines.

Many of the initially funded programs led to a flood of foreign clinical experts who actually provided direct care and treatment by setting up systems that were parallel to the existing government systems. This "emergency" strategy certainly saved many lives, but has been criticized for not increasing the capacity of the public health care systems from the start. Nurses initially were not fully included in the global response to the HIV pandemic, since diagnosis and treatment of HIV was seen as a very specialized area of medicine. Treatment programs were often established at the main referral hospitals in large cities and utilized infectious disease physicians and other doctors with specialized training. Physicians with expertise in HIV from the United States and other high-income countries were recruited and funded to provide technical advising, training, and consultation to physicians in virtually every high-prevalence country, but the demand for nursing expertise lagged behind.

Once the first cohorts of patients were successfully initiated on ARVs (with astoundingly positive results), national plans for providing access to treatment were developed that mandated that comprehensive HIV care be made available in more rural settings. It became apparent that the vast need for care and treatment could not be met by specialized physicians, or even general physicians. In most sub-Saharan countries, the majority of health facilities are staffed by nurses and midwives only. If treatment was to be made available to the large number of patients requiring it, nurses had to be an integral part of the plan. This led PEPFAR and other donors to acknowledge the need for nursing expertise in their funded programs. Experts in HIV nursing in high-income countries set out to form the partnerships necessary to work in foreign countries and to support their colleagues in taking on the monumental task of providing comprehensive care and treatment to their clients.

WHAT IS A PARTNERSHIP?

Many relationships in global health have been called *partnerships*. This term can cover a wide range of organizational structures and institutional relationships. The word "partner" is used in everyday language to describe everything from a life partner to a tennis partner. Clearly there is a vast difference between the two. Calling something a global health partnership does not make it so.

The Merriam-Webster's Dictionary Online defines partnership as "a legal relationship existing between two or more persons contractually associated as joint principles in a business . . . usually involving close cooperation between parties having specified and joint rights and responsibilities" (*Merriam-Webster*, n.d.). Clearly this is the strictest interpretation of the word and would pertain to personal partnerships, such as marriage, and business partnerships. An example of a legal partnership in global health might be a government contracting with a pharmaceuticals supplier. The supplier delivers the products at an agreed upon price according to a set timeline, and the government commits to payment for the products. The terms of the contract are clearly defined, and there are clear consequences for violating the contract.

The World Health Organization (WHO, 2009) states that, "Partnership can be defined as a collaborative relationship between two or more parties based on trust, equality, and mutual understanding for the achievement of a specified goal" (p. 2). Partnerships involve risks as well as benefits, making shared accountability critical. True partnerships lend a sense of mutual respect and responsibility to a program, a seriousness of purpose that is written in black and white and publicly agreed to by the parties involved in the partnership. Partners must share the same goal and consider each other capable and trustworthy.

Partnership Versus Collaboration

Global health programs may use the word "partnership" when they actually mean "collaboration." To collaborate is to work with another person or group in order to achieve or do something (*Merriam-Webster*, n.d.). It implies joint planning and joint implementation, but does not indicate that the parties have the same legal responsibilities to each other as they would in a partnership. For example, a U.S. school of nursing may collaborate with a private African school of nursing to develop a preservice curriculum on care of the patient infected with HIV. They would plan and implement the project together, but would not have contractual obligations to each other. They would not share a funding source. If the U.S. institution does not fully understand the role of nursing in HIV care in that particular country, the scope of nursing practice, the available medications, the positions of the nursing council, or the national HIV strategy, they may design a curriculum that does not make sense for those nursing students. It may actually have a negative impact by preparing nurses to practice in a way that is not approved by the regulatory bodies. The curriculum may not be sufficient for the expanded role that nurses will have in rural areas. Even more concerning is the potential for multiple curricula that are not coordinated or approved by nursing educators and leaders in the country.

If the foreign institution does not require that local nurses define and lead a particular program, the potential for major missteps is quite real. Well-meaning foreigners have developed training programs and curricula that, at worst, are at odds with each other and the national plan, and are often duplicative. In the past, institutions in the target country, whether NGOs, faith-based organizations, health facilities, or academic institutions, may have been reluctant to decline a suggested project from a donor or to redirect that work to better meet their needs. While both parties may state that they are collaborating, there is a danger that the foreign-funded party may actually wield most of the power in the relationship.

Cooperation

The softest of the terms used in global health relationships is *cooperation*. Virtually all foreign global health leaders state that they cooperate with someone in-country. For some, it is strictly having permission to be there. An example of this kind of cooperation might be a church in the United States recruiting nurses with knowledge and skill in HIV nursing and sending them to train nurses at one of its hospitals in a low-income country. They may ask the receiving hospital if it is all right to send these people, but, once again, it is difficult for the receiving institution to say no or request a different kind of support. As pointed out in the previous example, the training developed by these church members may not meet the needs of the nurses, may not be consistent with national guidelines, and may duplicate or interfere with the national plan for training HIV nurses. Similarly, a group may say that it is cooperating with the nursing council, but really have no ongoing relationship with those nursing leaders. They may have met with the council once, described their project, and, not hearing any objections, assumed approval. This kind of relationship is quite far from collaboration, and is definitely not a partnership.

Consensus on the Need for Partnerships

Most of the major global health organizations include partnerships as part of their mission or values statements. They are acutely aware that the issues being addressed in global health today are increasingly complex, requiring expertise across multiple fields. Many funders require organizations to work together to avoid duplication of work and waste of resources. Most importantly, in order to achieve any success or contribute to sustainable change, engagement with local government, academic, and health care institutions and the private sector within target countries is required. Three of the major global health funders attest to their commitment to supporting partnerships. The Bill and Melinda Gates Foundation (n.d.) "How We Work" statement says,

> The problems we seek to solve demand the coordination and focus of leaders, governments, private sector resources, communities, and individuals. *We believe in the power of partnership.* We bring together the best and the brightest people in the world to envision change and build the path to get there. Together, we work for a world where all can thrive.

Similarly, PEPFAR, which has provided billions of dollars to support the scale-up of treatment to people infected with HIV around the world, is built on a model of partnership with the governments of countries receiving its aid. Its partnership framework requires cooperation among the host government, the U.S. government, and the agencies receiving funds to carry out the work. Established as a partnership in global health, the Global Fund to Fight AIDS, Tuberculosis, and Malaria (n.d.), which has to date disbursed close to $23 billion, works closely with a wide diversity of partners—implementing governments, donors, civil society, international development organizations, the private sector, and communities living with and affected by the diseases. This partnership model actively supports country-owned approaches that develop and implement effective, evidence-based programs to respond to AIDS, tuberculosis, and malaria.

As these giants in global health declare their commitment to public and private partnerships, the smaller players in global health have also moved in that direction. Smaller organizations and academic institutions have demonstrated increased levels of awareness of the inappropriateness of programs that are designed by foreigners and dropped into their country of choice. The colonial approach of "knowing what's best" for another country is increasingly looked upon with disdain. Deb Goldman, a long-time global health nurse, describes her first venture into an international project and how she views it in retrospect (Box 7.1).

BOX 7.1 THE PITFALLS OF A COLONIAL APPROACH TO GLOBAL HEALTH

There is an NGO with which I did a 2-week volunteer trip to sub-Saharan Africa a few years ago. A doctor from the United States set up a clinic in a very rural town. The doctor was still in residency in the United States, and organized groups of providers—doctors, nurses and others—to go two or three times a year to provide direct medical care to the people in the village and surrounding villages. People came from surrounding villages when these providers were in the clinic. It was an incredible experience for me, but I felt it was not a sustainable program and was more like a "Band-Aid" effect and an imperialistic way of coming in to "save" the people. It cost nine of us about $2,500 each to go. Multiply that by two or three times per year, and the total is more than $65,000. The money could have been better used, in my opinion, to send someone from the village to medical or nursing school or partner with a medical/nursing school in the city to come and do internships, and so forth.

There appeared to be little assessment of the needs of the people. For example, we saw many men, women, and children daily in the clinic for a myriad of problems, but we never saw any pregnant women. No one from the organization knew anything about the childbirth practices in the village, and the women did not seem to want to share. Another public health nurse and I wanted to do an informal focus group while we were there to at least meet the women in the village and start a dialogue, but the organizers felt the need to see patients was greater.

Another example: They brought hundreds of toothbrushes to give out and went to the local school to demonstrate how to use them and found when they returned that no one used them. A third example: The organizers, who came to visit the first year the clinic opened, saw the women from the village who were cooks for the medical brigades squatting on the ground to cook. They decided to build picnic tables and benches for them to use to cook without really asking them if they would use them. The medical brigades used them but the cooks never did. You can see by these examples that their intentions were good but misguided by not doing appropriate needs assessments of the people in the villages.

Deb Goldman, personal communication, February 26, 2014.

The Rwanda Human Resources for Health Program involves multiple partners in a large and complex initiative aimed at dramatically improving the quality of education of health professionals; increasing the number of highly trained doctors, nurses, midwives, dentists, and health managers; and developing specialty training in specific areas of medicine and nursing. The program also aims to produce sufficient numbers of qualified faculty members for future education of health professionals. The primary partnership is between the Ministry of Health (MoH) and each of 25 U.S. academic institutions. These institutions have signed memoranda of understanding (MOU) with the government that ensures their commitment to recruiting and deploying a specified number of faculty members to teach in the University of Rwanda's College of Medicine and Health Sciences and its teaching hospitals. The institutions also agree to abide by the rules of engagement established by the government of Rwanda. The program is governed by a steering committee, chaired by the permanent secretary of the MoH, and made up of the deans of the University of Rwanda's School of Medicine, School of Nursing, School of Public Health, and other health care leaders in Rwanda.

A secondary level of partnership exists among the U.S. universities engaged in the recruitment of faculty in a clinical specialty. Six U.S. schools of nursing work closely with each other to respond to the needs of the Rwandan nursing leaders and educators. They have displayed a remarkable degree of collaboration. As of February 2014, these institutions had placed 75 full-time nursing and midwifery faculty in Rwanda, each of them committed to a minimum of 1 year. Each foreign faculty member is paired with at least one Rwandan nurse/midwife or faculty member in an effort to improve the educational experience of nursing and midwifery students. These faculty members also focus on curriculum development, simulation education, e-learning, professional and educational standards, and faculty development under the direction of Rwandan nursing leadership. The HRH program is an illustration of an effective global health partnership. Effective partnerships create opportunities for programs to stand the best chance of success and benefit all of the parties. On the other hand, there are common pitfalls that result in partnerships that are not beneficial to all parties and fail to reach their goals (Box 7.2).

HOW TO BUILD AN EFFECTIVE PARTNERSHIP

Global health partnerships in nursing should begin with the identification of the needs of one's own institution, hospital, MoH, nursing workforce, students, faculty, or other entity. It does not begin with identifying someone else's need. For example, a U.S. NGO should not respond to a high newborn mortality rate in a sub-Saharan African country by designing a program to train midwives on infant resuscitation and then offering that program to those midwives. That need should be identified by the MoH, midwifery leaders or educators, midwives themselves, or other in-country leaders who are responsible for improving infant survival. The problem may not be midwifery education or practice at all. If the lack of training is determined to be one of the contributing factors to newborn

BOX 7.2 EFFECTIVE AND INEFFECTIVE PARTNERSHIPS

ELEMENTS OF EFFECTIVE PARTNERSHIPS	COMMON PITFALLS OF INEFFECTIVE PARTNERSHIPS
• Clearly defined reasons for the partnership • Trust • Shared vision • Shared goals • Clearly articulated roles and responsibilities • In-country leadership • Joint planning • Equity • Accountability • Shared evaluation process • Recognition of the particular strengths and weaknesses of each partner • Sustainability as a key value for all parties	• Priorities driven by the donor agency • Imbalance in commitment to the project • Partners not fulfilling their commitments • Lack of transparency related to finances • Cultural misunderstandings or insensitivity • Poor planning for sustainability

mortality, and the government has not been able to address the gap in midwifery education with its available resources, there could be an opportunity for a partnership. This step is tremendously important, and it may seem unrealistic at first glance, but it demonstrates respect for the sovereignty of the country in which you plan to work. It acknowledges that the nursing, midwifery, and public health leaders in-country are the rightful authorities in determining priorities and needs. If the country does not own its problem and the proposed solution, the problem will not be resolved, no matter how much money and good intent is poured into it. This first step is also the key to sustainability of any new interventions.

Not every country will have a strong MoH, nursing council, or other official body, but every country has highly qualified leaders in education, health care, and public policy with whom foreign institutions can work. It is the responsibility of the foreign institution to assist the official bodies to increase their capacity for leadership and to seek out other recognized leaders for collaboration. It may be that in-country leaders will request technical assistance on getting to the root of a problem, or they may ask for advice on potential paths to overcoming public health challenges. That could also be a good beginning of a partnership, but they are ultimately the decision makers.

The United States, or other high-income country institutions, can simultaneously identify its own needs. Perhaps they need opportunities for students to study abroad, or they need research sites. They may be developing courses or programs in global health, and they need those global partnerships in order to attract faculty and students. An NGO may have a mandate from a donor that they work to reduce infant mortality, or a church may have a mission to serve those in need in other countries. Being honest about what the U.S. institution needs from the partnership is the next major step.

Once there is agreement on the benefits of a partnership, the hard work begins. Agreeing on the vision, goals, and program design requires trust, respect, and transparency. Acknowledging the strengths and weaknesses of partners, seeking out others with expertise that is needed, agreeing on decision-making processes, and confirming the ultimate leadership of the in-country partners are essential components of an effective partnership. The partnership should be formalized to the extent possible. MOU that clearly lay out the roles and responsibilities, the timeline, the evaluation process, and the financial obligations should be carefully constructed and signed. There is something very sobering about signing on the dotted line. It binds the partners together in a common purpose, with clear consequences for not delivering on promises made. Each partner must respect and abide by the laws of the countries involved, including scrupulous attention to visa requirements and licensing and registration of health professionals working in a foreign country.

Neither partner should assume that there is one right model of care, nor one acceptable model of nursing practice. There are many paths to becoming a professional nurse or midwife. No one system can be deemed to be the "correct" path. Open-mindedness to alternative experiences and ways of doing things will benefit all partners.

Every public health issue has political, financial, and cultural implications. This is true in every country on earth, no more so in African or Asian countries than it is in the United States. Those who work in foreign countries will always be guests. They will never understand the politics and culture as well as someone who has lived her or his whole life there, speaks the language, and is part of the culture. Acknowledging those facts and being always sensitive to the very real political and cultural landscape is a must.

HOW HAVE GLOBAL NURSING PARTNERSHIPS EVOLVED?

With the growing recognition that efforts to address global health issues must be built on mutual goal-setting and respect and be formalized relationships, global health partnerships are beginning to put more control in the hands of the local experts, government entities responsible for health and education systems, and professional bodies. Donors are beginning to require country ownership and real partnerships.

Nursing leaders in global health have seen the evolution of nursing partnerships. Two nursing leaders share their thoughts on global health nursing partnerships. Dorothy Powell, associate dean, Office of Global and Community Health Initiatives at the Duke University School of Nursing, observes:

> Partnerships are generally more egalitarian with more attention
> to principles of community engagement, as mutual visioning and
> planning are more likely to occur. At least the perceived dominant
> partner is less likely to be as ethno-centric as they were previously and
> [we are] beginning to recognize the rights of targeted underserved

communities to self-determination. Negotiation is emerging as more prevalent than silent receptivity. Control is also becoming more centered in the community of need versus the "more advanced" partner. (personal communication, January 27, 2014)

Mi Ja Kim, professor and dean emerita, executive director, Global Health Leadership Office at the University of Illinois at Chicago College of Nursing, echoes these thoughts:

> Global partnerships previously tended to be one-sided (i.e., U.S. leading developing countries); I note that this is changing to make it bi-directional or multi-directional in recent years. Hence, the product/outcome of the global work now reflects the input from all involved. (personal communication, January 30, 2014)

In conclusion, whether global health programs achieve their goals, provide donors with successful returns on investment, create country-specific solutions, and effect sustainable change will ultimately depend on the strength and quality of the partnerships created.

REFERENCES

Bill and Melinda Gates Foundation. (n.d.). *How we work.* Retrieved from http://www.gatesfoundation.org/How-We-Work

Collaborate. (n.d.). In *Merriam-Webster's online dictionary.* Retrieved from http://www.merriam-webster.com/dictionary/collaborate

Global Fund to Fight AIDS, Tuberculosis, and Malaria. (n.d.). *Partners.* Retrieved from http://www.theglobalfund.org/en/partners

Merriam-Webster's Dictionary Online. (n.d.). Partnership. Retrieved from http://www.merriam-webster.com/dictionary/partnership

World Health Organization. (2009). *Building a working definition of partnership.* Geneva, Switzerland: Author.

UNIT II

Issues in Global Health

Nancy L. Meedzan

Global health issues have sociopolitical, economic, ethical, and cultural implications. Nurses, by the very nature of their work, have direct experience caring for vulnerable populations worldwide and are in a unique position to offer expertise in global health. Unit II presents a range of contemporary global health issues impacting our world. The authors highlight and share their perspectives on specific global health issues from their work in Haiti, India, Brazil, South Africa, Democratic Republic of the Congo, Mozambique, and the United States.

The section begins with one of the most pressing issues—if not *the* most pressing issue—in global health; access to clean water. Access to water, proper sanitation, and hygiene are inextricably linked to the health of the world's people. In Chapter 8, Prevost and Dye provide an in-depth overview of the myriad issues of water scarcity and water contamination. Water access and sanitation are discussed in Chapter 9 in an interview with Gary White, chief executive officer and founder of Water.org. In addition to describing the issues around water and sanitation, he also discusses successful strategies for increasing access to clean water.

In Chapter 10, Bhengu and Ncama, academic nurse leaders in South Africa, add their views of the HIV/AIDS epidemic as it has unfolded with a lens on the roles of nurse leaders in addressing the challenges that have emerged. In Chapter 11, Dawson-Rose and Wishner present the ethical issues in HIV care that may impact vulnerable populations, particularly women, through a series of vignettes. Chapter 12 focuses on George's views on the issues that nurses, midwives, and women confront related to maternal health and maternal mortality in resource limited settings. A framework utilizing Millennium Development Goal 5 was developed. Lewis O'Connor, Conley, and Breakey describe the trends in violence against women and its negative impact on health in Chapter 13. In Chapter 14, de Chesnay explores the problem of sex trafficking, offers clinical exemplars that highlight the potential role of nursing, and proposes an innovative intervention model. In Chapter 15, Makosky highlights the health issues—both physical and mental—that occur in conflict areas. Additionally, she provides essential information for nurses preparing for global health experiences. In Chapter 16, Nadeau, Nicholas, and Stevens address the issues of mental health in the growing number of asylum seekers in the United States. Hazel, Ladd, and Begre use the UNICEF Conceptual Framework for Undernutrition to describe the state of childhood malnutrition in India. Case studies are used to highlight the impact of malnutrition on growth. Finally, Corless, Limbo, Syzlet, and Rochon offer the global health context in hospice and palliative care with case examples from Brazil and South Africa. This unit develops the reader's understanding of the many issues that affect global health and a context for framing solutions to achieve global health, which is the focus of Unit III.

CHAPTER 8

The Importance of Water for Global Nursing

Suzanne S. Prevost and Tabatha Dye

For over a century, nurses have acknowledged the relationship between cleanliness and health. Accessible and potable water and sanitation facilities are fundamental elements supporting that relationship. Without safe water, health promotion and health care delivery interventions are futile. In highly developed countries, nurses use massive amounts of water to care for their patients. From hydration to patient hygiene to hand washing, clean water flows freely; and nurses rarely stop to contemplate the importance of it until a natural disaster or other unplanned emergency threatens the safe water supply. Yet in underdeveloped countries, safe water access is one of the most obvious determinants of the health of individuals and populations. In those areas, basic nursing interventions may include advocating for citizens in partnership with governmental or nongovernmental organizations to secure the infrastructure for safe water and sanitation facilities.

Various agencies within the United Nations (UN), including the United Nations Children's Fund (UNICEF) and the World Health Organization (WHO), have combined forces to affirm the importance of, and promote access to, safe drinking water and sanitation. The UN Millennium Development Goals (MDGs) include a specific goal (Goal 7.C) to decrease by half the proportion of people without access to safe drinking water and basic sanitation by the year 2015 (UN, 2013). Furthermore, the UN Human Rights Council has published annual resolutions, including one in 2013, reaffirming the human right to safe drinking water and sanitation (United Nations Human Rights Council, 2013).

The WHO/UNICEF Joint Monitoring Programme (JMP) for Water Supply and Sanitation publishes an annual progress report on various indicators related to Goal 7.C. The baseline rate for safe drinking water access was 76% of the global population in 1990. The portion of the population without safe drinking water decreased by over half from 24% in 1990 to 11% in 2012, thus achieving the first part of Goal 7C. However, the sanitation goal is unlikely to be met by 2015 (UNICEF, WHO, 2014).

Water Scarcity

The two major global problems linking water and health are water scarcity and water contamination. Water scarcity is quantified by the relationship between population and available water supply. Water stress is experienced when the annual water supply is less than 1,700 m³ per person (World Water Assessment Programme [WWAP], 2012). Regions with less than 1,000 m³ per person experience water scarcity (WWAP, 2012). About 20% of the world's population currently experiences physical water scarcity, and many more experience water shortages due to lack of infrastructure or funding to effectively access and distribute water from rivers or aquifers (Molden, 2007).

The map in Figure 8.1 illustrates regions of the world experiencing physical water scarcity and economic water scarcity. While water scarcity affects all regions, including North America, the sub-Saharan Africa region has the broadest and most significant problem. If recent climate changes continue, the UN predicts that about half the world's population will be experiencing water stress by 2030 (UN, 2009).

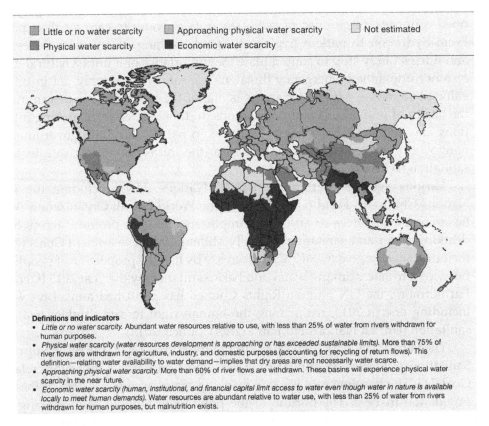

Little or no water scarcity   Approaching physical water scarcity   Not estimated

Physical water scarcity   Economic water scarcity

Definitions and indicators
- *Little or no water scarcity.* Abundant water resources relative to use, with less than 25% of water from rivers withdrawn for human purposes.
- *Physical water scarcity (water resources development is approaching or has exceeded sustainable limits).* More than 75% of river flows are withdrawn for agriculture, industry, and domestic purposes (accounting for recycling of return flows). This definition—relating water availability to water demand—implies that dry areas are not necessarily water scarce.
- *Approaching physical water scarcity.* More than 60% of river flows are withdrawn. These basins will experience physical water scarcity in the near future.
- *Economic water scarcity (human, institutional, and financial capital limit access to water even though water in nature is available locally to meet human demands).* Water resources are abundant relative to water use, with less than 25% of water from rivers withdrawn for human purposes, but malnutrition exists.

FIGURE 8.1 Areas of physical and economic water scarcity.

Adapted from International Water Management Institute (2007). Copyright 2007. Adapted with permission.

While sub-Saharan Africa has the largest population without safe drinking water, several other underdeveloped regions are affected as well. The following list illustrates the scope of the problem in terms of the number of people (in millions) without safe water access in each area: Southern Asia (149), (mostly in India [92]); Eastern Asia (114), mostly in China (112); Southeastern Asia (67); Latin America and Caribbean (36); Western Asia (20); Northern Africa (13); Caucasus and Central Asia (11); developed regions (9); and Oceania (5) (UNICEF, WHO, 2014).

Water Contamination

In regions of extreme water scarcity, inhabitants often access the most readily available water sources, with a high likelihood that those sources are contaminated. The two basic types of water contaminants are biological and chemical, which can be further categorized as pathogens, wastes, inorganic pollutants, nutrients, organic pollutants, suspended sediment, and radioactive pollutants (Lenntech, 2014). Both major categories can affect the health of the communities with contaminated water.

In 2008, 39% of diseases contributing to the water, sanitation, and hygiene-related disease burden were diarrheal diseases (Prüss-Üstün, Bos, Gore, & Bartram, 2008). In water treatment, pathogens that cause these diseases are monitored through the measurement of coliforms (New York State Department of Health: Center for Environmental Health, 2011). Coliforms are naturally present in soil and surface water, but are also present in the digestive system and feces of warm-blooded animals. Coliforms can enter a drinking water system through well maintenance deficiencies and flooding. Most coliforms are harmless, but some strains of *Escherichia coli* (*E. coli* O157: H7) can cause serious illness (New York State Department of Health: Center for Environmental Health, 2011).

Cryptosporidium, Giardia lamblia, *Legionella*, and enteroviruses are the pathogens that coliforms represent (U.S. Environmental Protection Agency [EPA], 2013). Despite advances in public health and technology in the United States, outbreaks of these diseases continue to occur (see Figure 8.2). The number of etiologic agents in outbreaks associated with U.S. drinking water from 1971 to 2010 has declined but not diminished (Centers for Disease Control and Prevention [CDC], 2013).

In recent years, *Legionella* outbreaks have been easier to identify, as noted in CDC surveillance reports, and is seemingly a bigger issue than previously thought (CDC, 2013). From 2009 to 2010, *Legionella* accounted for 58% of the U.S. drinking water outbreaks and 7% of resulting illnesses. When the outbreaks occurred 58% of them were caused by deficiencies in plumbing systems, 23% were caused by untreated ground water, and 12% were caused by deficiencies in the distribution system (CDC, 2013). These outbreaks can occur in developed countries with drinking water regulations and sanitary facilities; however, these outbreaks are far more lethal for less developed countries (Pontius, 2008).

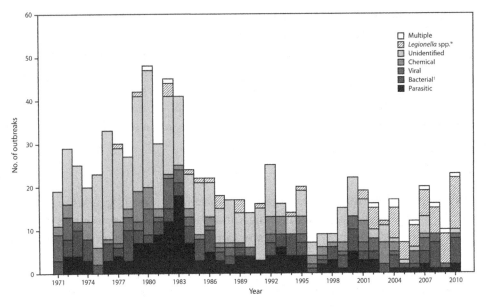

FIGURE 8.2 Number of waterborne disease outbreaks from 1971 to 2010. Adapted from the CDC (2013).

SANITATION AND CONTAMINATION

In 2012, 2.5 billion people were without improved sanitation worldwide. Even though many agencies are working together to address this problem, the prediction for 2015 remains at 2.4 billion people without sanitation access (UNICEF, WHO, 2014). More than half of the 2.5 billion people without improved sanitation live in India (UNICEF, WHO, 2014).

Globally, improved access to drinking water is more frequently financially and politically supported than sanitation access (UN-Water, 2008). Sanitation is perceived to be distasteful; despite that, sanitation access is necessary to maintain drinking water safety. Water from latrines or pits often infiltrates rivers and streams that are used as agricultural or drinking water sources. Up to 90% of human excreta ends up in rivers of the worst environments in developing nations (UN-Water, 2008). As of 2012, in the least developed countries 9% of the people drink surface water and 23% openly defecate (UNICEF, WHO, 2009). Poor sanitation does not only contaminate water and deliver diseases, but also affects the skin and lungs of those exposed to waste.

Although biological contamination is the biggest threat to developing nations, chemical contamination can also cause dangerous health problems. There are several sources of chemical contamination in drinking water: naturally occurring, agricultural, residential, industrial, and water treatment (Thompson et al., 2007). Of the chemicals that contaminate drinking water, the following list includes the chemicals that most often cause adverse effects in humans: fluoride, arsenic, selenium, nitrate, phosphorus, pesticides, petroleum, fuel oils, chlorinated solvents, industry-specific chemicals, heavy metals, mineral-processing chemicals (cyanide), disinfection byproducts, and chemicals from corroding pipes (copper or lead) (Thompson et al., 2007). Fortunately, chemical outbreaks do not occur as frequently as other types of outbreaks. These chemical and biological outbreaks lead to short- and long-term effects on individuals and entire communities afflicted with unsafe water.

HEALTH AND MORTALITY IMPLICATIONS

Water and sanitation-related diseases are among the most common causes of disability and death in underdeveloped countries. These problems create both direct (exposure to disease) and indirect (economic and lifestyle) negative health outcomes. Most water-related deaths are due to three infectious types of diseases: diarrheal diseases (2.2 million deaths per year); schistosomiasis (200,000 deaths per year); and intestinal helminths (100,000 deaths per year; Tarrass & Benjelloon, 2012). Diarrheal diseases are the seventh leading cause of death worldwide, and the third leading cause of death in low-income countries (WHO, 2013). Globally, 88% of diarrheal deaths are attributed to unsafe water, poor sanitation, and hygiene (UNICEF, WHO, 2009).

Infants and children are at significantly greater risk for water and sanitation-related diseases and deaths. Each year, between 1.5 and 2 million children die from illnesses related to water and sanitation (Tarrass & Benjelloon, 2012). In 2009, diarrheal diseases were the second highest killer of children worldwide (UN, 2009),

Health and well-being are indirectly affected by the constant search and retrieval of water that is often miles from home. Women and children are often forced to walk significant distances each day, crossing unpaved surfaces, in excessive heat, with minimal clothing or foot cover; and then to carry heavy water containers that can contribute to musculoskeletal pain and deformities. The search also limits time available for other healthier activities such as income-producing work and school attendance.

Nursing Implications

Clearly, clean, safe water and sanitation facilities are a basic requirement for promoting health and wellness around the world. Considering that the adult human body is composed of 55% to 60% water and children's bodies are 65% to 78% water (United States Geological Survey [USGS], 2014), water is essential for normal, healthy physiological functioning, not to mention disease prevention. In addition to providing for this physical need, nurses have a moral and ethical obligation to support and advocate for patients, families, and communities in their pursuits to access safe water and sanitation.

Under the Nursing Practice, Chemical Exposures and Right to Know policy in 2006, the American Nurses Association (ANA) advocated for increased research on the relationship between health and the environment, and the integration of environmental health policy into nursing education, practice, research, advocacy, and public policy (ANA, 2007). The ANA developed 10 principles of environmental health that advocate for the inclusion of environmental health concepts in nursing practice. The principles focus on nursing participation in assessing the quality of the environment in which they live and work, nursing participation in research for best practices for a safe and healthy environment, and support for nurses to advocate and implement environmental health principles (ANA, 2007). Further, in today's cost-conscious health care environments, health care savings are estimated at 7 billion U.S. dollars a year for health agencies by investing in drinking water and sanitation (Prüss-Üstün et al., 2008)

Partnerships to Increase Safe Water Access

Nurses are collaborating with other health care providers, engineers and environmentalists, policy makers, government and nongovernmental agencies, and community leaders around the world to respond to the global water and sanitation crisis. A recent example is Nurse Rise, which is a social media advocacy group dedicated to raising public awareness of dangers to clean water supplies. Members of this organization share a specific interest in the process of hydraulic fracturing, or "fracking," a relatively new and controversial approach to obtaining deep natural gas supplies that can violate clean water supplies in affected areas (Nurse Rise–Nurses for Safe Water, 2014).

The Alliance of Nurses for Healthy Environments (ANHE) is an international network of nurses who focus on the linkages between environmental issues and health. This organization promotes the incorporation of environmental health and sustainability practices and related content into nursing education and health care delivery institutions. Nurses have also partnered with Physicians for Social Responsibility (PSR), which has been organized for over 50 years. PSR advocates for a variety of issues, including the adverse effects of climate change and the environmental and health impact of toxic waste.

In the interview with Gary White, he focuses on global efforts to increase access to water, such as microfinancing, as well as policy and legislation to address the challenges of access to water. One can argue that those living in developed countries have a moral obligation to assist in the efforts to provide access to clean water and sanitation. For instance, several local chapters of Sigma Theta Tau, International (STTI) Nursing Honor Society, have partnered with nonprofit organizations, such as Water.Org, to raise funds and promote the development of improved water sources for underserved communities throughout the world. The commitment of STTI and other organizations is an example of nursing's professional commitment to continue the legacy of Florence Nightingale's focus on the environment in the 21st century.

REFERENCES

American Nurses Association (ANA). (2007). *ANA's principles of environmental health for nursing practice with implementation strategies.* Silver Spring, MD: Author.

Centers for Disease Control and Prevention (CDC). (2013, September 6). Surveillance for waterborne disease outbreaks associated with drinking water and other nonrecreational water—United States, 2009–2010. *Morbidity and Mortality Weekly Report (MMWR), 62*(35), 714–720.

International Water Management Institute. (2007). *Water for food, water for life: A comprehensive assessment of water management in agriculture.* London, UK: Earthscan.

Institute of Medicine (IOM). (2009). Panel discussion: Coordination and prioritization of water needs. In *Global rnvironmental health: Research gaps and barriers for providing sustainable water, sanitation, and hygiene services: Workshop summary* (pp. 43–49). Washington, DC: The National Acadamies Press.

Lenntech, B. V. (2014). *Water pollution FAQ (frequently asked questions).* Retrieved from http://www.lenntech.com/water-pollution-faq.htm

Molden, D. (Ed.). (2007). *Water for food, water for life: Comprehensive assessment of water management in agriculture.* London, UK: Earthscan.

New York State Department of Health: Center for Environmental Health. (2011, June). *Coliform bacteria in drinking water supplies.* Retrieved from http://www.health.ny.gov/environmental/water/drinking/coliform_bacteria.htm

Nurse Rise–Nurses for Safe Water. (2014). Retrieved from https://www.facebook.com/NurseRiseNursesforSafeWater/info

Pontius, N. L. (2008, October 31). *U.S. health agency provides expertise in dealing with cholera outbreaks.* Retrieved from Team Fights Waterborne Diseases in Developing Countries: iipdigital.usembassy.gov/st/english/article/2008/10/20081030171124abretnuh0.6893122.html

Prüss-Üstün, A., Bos, R., Gore, F., & Bartram, J. (2008). *Safer water, better health: Costs, benefits and sustainability of interventions to protect and promote health.* Geneva, Switzerland: World Health Organization.

Tarrass, F., & Benjelloun, M. (2012). The effects of water shortages on health and human development. *Perspectives in Public Health, 132* (5), 240–244.

Thompson, T., Fawell, J., Kunikane, S., Jackson, D., Appleyard, S., Callan, P., . . . Kingston, P. (2007). *Chemical safety of drinking-water: Assessing priorities for risk management.* Geneva, Switzerland: World Health Organization.

United Nations. (2009). *World water development report 3.* Paris, France: United Nations Educational, Scientific, and Cultural Organization.

United Nations. (2013). *The Millenium Development Goals report.* New York, NY: Author.

United Nations Children's Fund (UNICEF), World Health Organization (WHO). (2009). *Diarrhea: Why children are still dying and what can be done.* New York, NY: UNICEF Division of Communication/WHO.

United Nations Children's Fund, World Health Organization (WHO). (2012). *Progress on drinking water and sanitation 2012 update.* UNICEF/WHO Joint Monitoring Programme (JMP) for Water Supply and Sanitation. Geneva, Switzerland: World Health Organization Press.

United Nations Children's Fund, World Health Organization (WHO). (2014). *Progress on drinking water and sanitation 2014 update.* UNICEF/WHO Joint Monitoring Programme (JMP) for Water Supply and Sanitation. Geneva, Switzerland: World Health Organization Press.

United Nations Human Rights Council. (2013). The human right to safe drinking water and sanitation. *Human Rights Council Twenty-fourth Session* (p. 1). Geneva, Switzerland: World Health Organization Press.

United States Environmental Protection Agency (EPA). (2013, December 13). *Basic information about pathogens and indicators in drinking water.* Retrieved from http://water.epa.gov/drink/contaminants/basicinformation/pathogens.cfm

United States Geological Survey (USGS). (2014, March 17). *The water in you.* Retrieved from http://water.usgs.gov/edu/propertyyou.html

UN-Water. (2008). *Tackling a global crisis: International year of sanitation 2008.* UN-Water. Retrieved from http://esa.un.org/iys/docs/IYS_flagship_web_small.pdf

World Health Organization (WHO). (2013). *The top 10 causes of death.* Retrieved from Media Centre: http://www.who.int/mediacentre/factsheets/fs310/en

World Water Assessment Programme (WWAP). (2012). *The United Nations World Water Development Report 4: Managing water under uncertainty and risk.* Paris, France: United Nations Educational, Scientific and Cultural Organization (UNESCO).

CHAPTER 9

Access to Clean Water and the Impact on Global Health: An Interview With Gary White, CEO and Cofounder, Water.org

Nancy L. Meedzan, Patrice K. Nicholas, Suellen Breakey, and Inge B. Corless

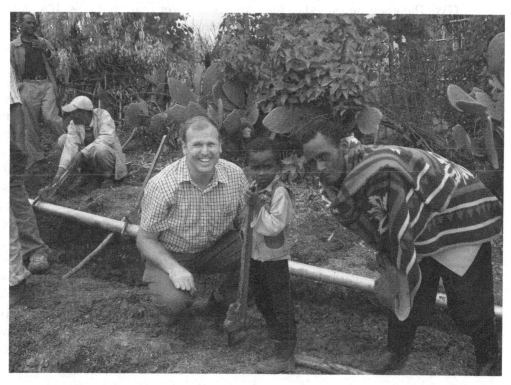

Gary White at the pipeline construction site (Ethiopia). Photo courtesy of water.org Flickr site.

NLM: Would you share with us the history of your organization, Water.org, and its role in the global movement for addressing the issues of access to water?

GW: Sure. All I've ever done since I was an undergraduate was to focus on water supply in developing countries. I cofounded an organization called Water Partners

International in 1990. Water Partners International was very much about working directly with local partners on the ground to implement infrastructure through water projects and sanitation. Matt [Damon] had started H2O Africa in 2006. In 2008, Matt and I crossed paths. At that point, Water Partners International had become one of the implementing partners for H2O Africa, and eventually we became the exclusive implementing partner helping them find local nongovernmental organizations (NGOs) on the ground in the developing world. They found that we were doing solid work in getting programs implemented and in doing the oversight, monitoring, and evaluation as well. That went really well. So, as Matt and I got to know each other better we thought: Why not just merge the organizations? In 2009, we merged and formed Water.org with Matt and me as the cofounders.

NLM: Your organization has focused on the fact that one billion people lack access to safe water. How did you mobilize your efforts to address this problem and are there successes that you would like to highlight?

GW: The good news is that the number is lower than that now. It's more in the neighborhood of 780 million people lacking access to water, which doesn't sound like a huge gain except for the fact that the global population [requiring access to water] has gone up dramatically in the last couple of decades. The good news is that from 1990 to 2010, about 2 billion people received water access for the first time. From Water.org's perspective, we absolutely believe this is a solvable problem. Our "philosophical drivers" around this and what solutions are needed focus on issues such as access to capital for those at the base of the economic pyramid. How do you help people living in poverty get access to the capital that they need so they can find their own water and sanitation solutions? What we've done is focus on something we call *WaterCredit*. WaterCredit starts off with the assumption, or throws off the assumption I guess you could say, that all the poor who lack water and sanitation are too poor to provide it from their own resources. Our belief is that there is a huge segment of people that, if they had access to small loans as little as $100 to $150, would then be able to get a water connection to the utility, or buy a water filter to treat the water in their home, or build a toilet. They could then repay that loan over about 2 years, and they would be much better off. Subsequently, there would be more funds available to reach more people. We believe that one of the fundamental solutions to this is not just top-down charity; it is using charity catalytically to spur more and more loans to people living in poverty.

NLM: You also note that the economics of access to water are inequitable worldwide. For example, in countries where there is less money, the cost of water tends to be much higher than in wealthier countries. Can you comment on successful water management projects and how they affect the costs of access to water and have influenced the health of the people?

GW: There is such a wealth of data and research out there that points to the fundamental importance of water, proper sanitation, and hygiene to health. And for me, being in the sector, I just tend to take that for granted. It may seem obvious that getting global access to water and sanitation for everyone—that this is going to pay tremendous health dividends. The challenge is the cost of access to water. Everyone supports the idea of access to safe water and sanitation; everybody's in favor of it. But the challenge is in actually paying for the infrastructure and these services. That becomes a real stumbling block. This is because it is a pretty expensive proposition, particularly when we start talking about urban infrastructure and getting people in slums connected to the utilities. A double challenge is that even though it may cost more to supply water, the water tariffs that the people pay to connect to the water utility are ridiculously low in developing countries; ridiculously low in terms of needing to recover the cost to maintain that infrastructure or to expand it. Water becomes this political tool where no one really wants to raise the water rate high enough to be able to actually pay to operate and maintain the infrastructure. This is where the great disparity comes in for people who are too poor. Because if you are so poor that you can't connect to the utility, you can't capture the subsidy that comes through the utility. Thus, if you are poor and you can't afford to get connected, you are forced to pay these water vendors—these private water vendors—who sell often-times contaminated water in your slum for about 10 to 15 times the cost per liter than the water that is coming from the tap if you could get connected to the utility. The whole system is built on a house of cards of a financial model because the infrastructure cannot be kept up. On top of that, even as distorted as that system is, the people who are really poor cannot even get into the system and take advantage of those lower tariffs. That is really part of what we are trying to do: to level that playing field for some of the poor who want to get connected to the utility but cannot afford the connection fee. They receive the loan through the WaterCredit program to afford the connection fee and become a paying customer and then can capture the subsidy. It is a way that we see the whole lower economic strata capturing more health benefits by getting connected to the utility and having a reliable source of water.

NLM: In addressing the health of the world's people, you note that improved health for women and girls is largely dependent on access to water and that safe water can reduce child and maternal mortality. You state that there are "billions of hours of unproductive time that is used to fetch water that rule out income-generating activities and education which could occur if clean water were closer to home." Can you address your WaterCredit initiatives and how water credit can impact women's and girls' lives?

GW: When you look at WaterCredit, it can do two things: It can free up time on the part of women and girls who would otherwise be scavenging for water, and it can save the family cash outlays that they would otherwise be spending on water and sanitation. Either of these has the potential to boost family income, the latter because you're not spending as much on the water vendors, and the former because of the time saving. You have women and girls scavenging for water in urban areas and they don't know where they will be going to get their water on any given day. They may walk several kilometers to a public standpost and find that there is no water there because it is only turned on erratically. The women and girls spend a huge amount of time just trying to secure water every day due to its unpredictability. They cannot really turn that time into a paying job. Once they get the connection at their home, however, then they do have daily access to water. They can then turn their time into a paying job, which happens quite a bit if the individual has access to the labor market in an urban area, for example. In terms of saving money and boosting family income, it is significant. Just last August, I was in the slums of Bangalore, and I met a woman who was paying 20 rupees every day to obtain water for her family from the water vendor. They were also paying 20 rupees a day to use the public toilet in their slum. She was spending 40 rupees a day for her family. If you add that up over the course of a year, it is a tremendous cost. She took out a WaterCredit loan to build a toilet in her home and to obtain a water connection and her monthly payments on that loan are 1,200 rupees

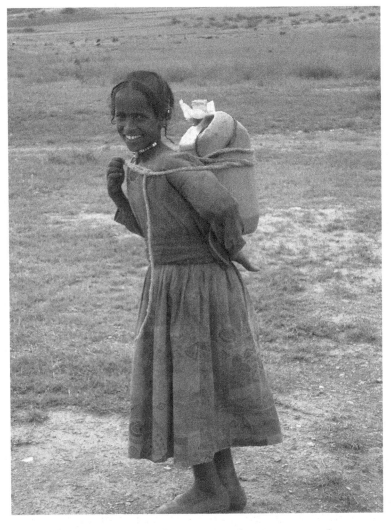

Young girl carrying water-collecting jug. Photo courtesy of water.org Flickr site.

per month, exactly 40 rupees a day. Over the next 2 years, the 1,200 rupees she is paying on her loan will go away and her income will increase by that amount with the exception of the water tariff that she will have to pay to the utility. What we find is that WaterCredit is boosting family income and boosting how much time women have. It does not take too much to draw a line from this to the fact that women are able to invest more in other family health issues.

NLM: Would you comment on the physical issues associated with carrying water that affect women and girls?

GW: Of course. I don't have any medical expertise myself but I have seen the problems that exist in rural areas where people—almost always women and girls—spend up to six hours a day walking incredible distances while carrying jerry cans on their backs. Sometimes they have straps wrapped around their forehead, while other times they just wrap them around their shoulders. They often times have a baby wrapped on their back or on their chest as well. Being hunched over, fetching water, day after day for their whole lives, has a huge impact in terms of musculoskeletal issues and other health issues. I also think the bacteriologically contaminated water people are drinking has a huge impact on health. And then you also get into areas of fluorosis, where you actually have too much fluoride and arsenic contamination in the drinking water, particularly in Asia. There's just a whole host of these issues beyond just the carrying of water and the physical aspects associated with that.

NLM: Safety issues exist for women and girls to obtain access to water. Are there successful programs that you can share that have reduced the dangers associated with obtaining water?

GW: We hear a lot anecdotally about women and girls not defecating during the day because of privacy issues and instead waiting until the cover of darkness to go out to defecate. When they do go out, they face the dangers of sexual assault. In India, I know that women also fear snakes that are out in the darkness when they go out in the evening to defecate. Some of the experiences we have to back that up, actually, when we look at some areas where we support WaterCredit—which is a bit of a misnomer because it also provides loans equally for construction of toilets—there is actually a greater demand for toilet loans than there is for water connection. You can see the financial or economic payoff for the family with the water loan. And to a certain degree, if they are in urban areas, they are not paying to use a toilet anymore. But even in rural areas, in small villages, we will see a stronger demand for toilets than water, even though there is not the financial benefit associated with that. What I'm reading into that is because 93% of the borrowers are women, they see an intrinsic value in having that privacy of the toilet at home as opposed to open defecation. They value that so much that they are willing to take out these loans in order to build those private toilets. It is a strong indicator of how much women value that security of having a toilet in their home.

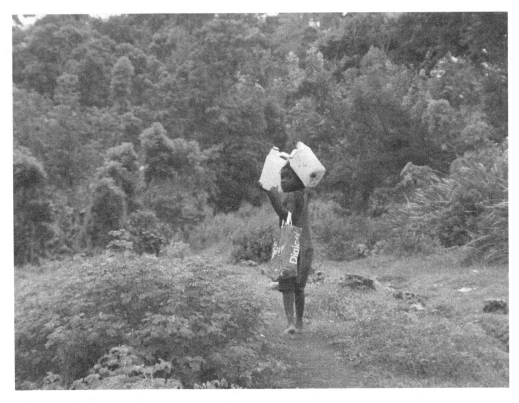

Young girl walking to gather water. Photo courtesy of water.org Flickr site.

NLM: You've noted that "every 21 seconds, a child dies due to waterborne illness." Has progress been made in addressing this issue?

GW: I don't know the exact statistics to date, but certainly when I first started in this, it was much more often than that. I have been involved in this work for a long time and in the 1990s the number of deaths was closer to 6 million each year. Now it is down to about 3.5 million, however, the majority of those are younger than age 5. During my time in this sector, the number of kids dying from water-related disease per year has definitely decreased.

NLM: In our work in global nursing efforts worldwide, we have seen firsthand that diarrheal disease is the leading cause of illness and death due to lack of access to safe drinking water and sanitation, as well as poorer overall health, hygiene, and nutrition. In our work globally, we've seen the impact that this has had for people living with HIV who have limited access to safe water and who have symptoms like diarrhea which can be life threatening. Do you envision any major projects that can alleviate the challenges that we face in caring for those with diarrhea and other water-borne illnesses?

GW: For me it has always been an incredible irony. The average cost per person for an antiretroviral (ARV) is about $1,000 per person per year. The cost of getting safe water to a whole village can be less than $10,000 for a permanent solution. It is so unfortunate that you might have a lot of people around the world taking ARVs with contaminated water, when the cost of getting them access to safe water is so low. The dangers of contaminated water, especially in an immunocompromised individual, are overwhelming. It just doesn't seem to make sense from a resource allocation perspective. The short answer to the question is: We just need to get safe water access to more people. Access to water will have a cascading effect on better health for the world's people. It is easier said than done, obviously, since we still have so many people without access to water. The more people you serve, the more important it is to continue the efforts to serve the next person or population. I think it will take continued emphasis on the capital side of this as well as trying to understand who out there doesn't have water that could be helped simply by a loan. Knowing that there is still going to be a segment of the population that is so poor; this strategy wouldn't suffice. Then you start to turn to something else that we think is also very important, which is accountability and transparency on the part of governments whose mandate it is to provide safe water to communities. We need to focus on assisting people in these countries and in these situations to find ways and tools to help them hold their government and their utilities more accountable for providing affordable water as well as for cross-subsidizing water. That is another big tool that we can take advantage of for those in extreme poverty. Maybe the first couple of cubic meters of water per month to them are free, or incredibly subsidized, and the more cubic meters per month that a household is consuming, the higher per-cubic-meter price. This way you are basically able to cross-subsidize those who are just barely surviving with the fees that are paid by people who are filling their swimming pools. I think we can do a lot more from a policy, financial, and accountability perspective than we can from a straight technology and engineering perspective. And I say that as someone with three engineering degrees. The engineering of it is important, but I think often that we place too much emphasis on finding that silver bullet technology that is going to get everybody safe water when we need to pay a lot more attention to accountability, transparency, and finance.

Suellen Breakey (SB): I'm just wondering, are you, or is Water.org, involved in any efforts at the policy level in any country that you're working in now?

GW: We've been very involved at the policy level in the United States in terms of getting the Water for the Poor Act passed and also in continuing to pursue the Water for the World Act. The Water for the World Act mandated that the executive branch of the government, particularly the U.S. Agency for International Development (USAID) and the U.S. State Department, make access to water supply in other countries part of our foreign policy for the first time ever. That has been, I think, incredibly successful at turning around the almost decimation of water supply funding coming out of the U.S. government for other countries. It really went down dramatically for years, for decades actually, and we've been able to get that number back up to $315 million a year that the U.S. government is focusing toward water access. That has been really good. Also, that focus has been on ensuring that the funds are invested in the countries with the greatest need oftentimes instead of our strategic allies. For example, we invested about $100 million in Jordan for some water treatment facilities there during a period of time when all of sub-Saharan Africa was getting about $8 million a year due to the politics of the region. Those policy issues are improving, but there is still plenty of room to make strategy even better. We have not focused so much on trying to impact policy at the country level in developing countries as we feel like that is just too big for us to fight at this point. It is not that it doesn't need to be done, but that different towns hold different sets of expertise needed to effect change. We have been working with partners in financial institutions within countries around the world to try to further us in that direction. We are also not a huge organization. A part of our philosophy is that it is better to light a candle than to curse in the darkness. By that I mean we could always be hitting the policy issues and saying, "There should be more money; there should be more money. " Or we can say, "You know what, there is already a system out there, and the poor are already paying huge amounts of money to these vendors. There exists a system out there in the form of microfinance infrastructure." We know that in the past people have said that they only earned 25% interest for loan charge so they could get toilets or water connection. That is because the microfinance institutions wouldn't lend for water and sanitation until we nudged them. Instead of trying to get all of the policy issues accomplished and obtaining more money, we are focusing on helping the poor take advantage of the system already in place to introduce them to the microfinance institutions so they can get loans. We want to get them connected to the public water infrastructure where the subsidies already exist. Water.org has been much more about trying to work within the present system as it exists and tilting it more in favor of the poor, as opposed to eliminating the entire existing system and starting from scratch.

NLM: Since this book is for nurses and other health professionals, what should their role be in addressing the water problem?

GW: Well, I think it is looking at water as the most basic *medicine*. I think nurses have really made incredible strides over the decades in terms of not just curing health problems, but also helping people to think about their lifestyle, their diet, their exercise, and so on, to head off those problems. The more that nurses, particularly in developing countries, view water as a medical intervention and sanitation as a medical intervention the more proactive nurses will be in addressing some of these waterborne diseases. I believe this view has already taken root in the global nursing community. I think that part of the problem is that it is still outside of the domain of the medical profession to a certain degree, to address access to water. It was Hippocrates who said water adds much to health. The fact that *The Lancet* declared that sanitation, proper sanitation, as the biggest lifesaving invention in the history of mankind is noteworthy. These issues clearly contribute to health, but they are constantly placed as part of the engineering and public sector domains. I propose that, perhaps, it should also be in the health sector domain. So I am struggling with the question. I turn to the medical profession and the nursing profession in particular to lobby and educate so that the facts and the connection between the water that people are drinking and the health impact on them and their children are being circulated and understood. There is probably a great underlying truth right there: helping people understand the connection between contaminated water, disease, and health. Beyond that, nurses make the case to support those efforts that are in the public policy arena to assist countries to expand access to water and sanitation.

NLM: Why did you select the issue of water, when there are so many worthy causes globally in which you could engage?

GW: I was drawn to issues of access to water because of my background in engineering. I also had this thirst for social justice instilled in me from an early age. When you look at the intersection of engineering and social justice, you do not have to go much further than water and sanitation to find an area where you can have a huge impact. I knew this at an intellectual level when I was an undergraduate but then in college I traveled to Guatemala to volunteer. I think that kind of experience where I was volunteering and was able to take a side trip to the slums in Guatemala City was when the issues became apparent. I was struck by the realization that within this short distance from the United States, there were kids drinking incredibly contaminated water that was provided to them from barrels. Then to see the sewage in the street; that just had a tremendous impact on me. Having learned about this type of thing on an intellectual level and then seeing it firsthand, it just seemed like an incredible injustice. I have heard it said that your life should be about finding the intersection of your greatest passion and the world's greatest need. I had a passion for engineering and then I saw this huge need. I felt I couldn't not do something about it.

NLM: What is the future of Water.org?

GW: Well, at one level, what we really want to do is continue working with philanthropists and philanthropic organizations and corporations. We have been very successful with support from the PepsiCo Foundation, Caterpillar, IKEA, Cartier, and a number of other corporate foundations. On one hand, we really want to continue to use that philanthropy to reach more people directly through programs like WaterCredit. We have reached 1.5 million people now with WaterCredit alone. I did not mention before, but the loans are being repaid at a rate of 99%. We feel that we have a tremendous initiative that we have pioneered and if we can get the principles rolled out to other organizations that are doing work in the water sector that can have even more of an impact. One of the things we want to do more of is what we call global advocacy, which is taking the experience base that we have today—the programming around WaterCredit—and pushing it out to more organizations so that they can use the philosophy and expand tools and learning platforms that people can use in order to replicate it. This is where we feel we are going to have the most impact—by advocating for this issue, but also and of equal importance, advocating for a solution that works. We will also be moving into the accountability space a bit more. For example, how can we help the poor get access to the tools they need to hold their governments and utilities more accountable for supplying water? That is a very new area for us, and we are just starting to explore it, but I think it is something that we really need to do so that we can help a certain segment of the population with WaterCredit. As you go down to those in absolute poverty, we ask the question: "How can we help them tap into what I see as their intrinsic power as citizens to hold their governments accountable?"

Inge Corless (IC): Patrice Nicholas and I, in particular, have spent time over the years in South Africa and there what we see is, in the urban areas, no problem in terms of toilets and running water. In the rural areas, there is the village tap and there may also be some latrines. I also went out last June with a hospice group and palliative care and down through the brush where there is the village tap for people to collect their water. You go into the homes that were previously shacks and are now concrete. You see in the kitchen this big basin, but then when you look, it is not connected to anything. The problem is there is no pipe connection to the homes for water. There is a real disconnect here, where you do need engineering and you also need the government to recognize this is an important thing to be done for their countrymen.

GW: Yes, it does vary. The situations vary tremendously from country to country and the lack of water as a resource is critical. In arid regions, they are already water stressed or water critical. South Africa has actually done better than most in terms of getting better water access, particularly among some of the poorer communities there. But at the same time, it can be a very expensive proposition to find that next water resource because common sense dictates that you have already exploited water resources that are the cheapest to develop and that are closer to where the populations are; however, that next incremental development of the water resource is going to naturally be farther away, harder to access, more expensive to pump, and so on. I think this must occur at the policy level, in order to ensure that the resources are allocated for this. And equally important, making sure that they are allocated equitably so you do have the things like cross-subsidy tariffs—which actually South Africa has done a great job on—and these other mechanisms in place. It is important to make sure that when the public treasure is expended to develop these resources, that it is not all the middle class and the wealthy neighborhoods and the five-star hotels that capture all the subsidy, but that they are properly targeted to those most in need as well.

SB: I just have two quick questions; one may be a little bit repetitive. I am curious as to how you came to partner with the countries that you have partnered with, and I am also curious as to what about the future of Water.org excites you most?

GW: In the countries that we selected, it is kind of a combination. When I first started in this business, it was basically Central America, because there was no money for travel. So I was paying that out of my own pocket, or more appropriately, my wife was paying it for me to subsidize my volunteer efforts. So we really focused on Central America because it was much more affordable to travel there. And there was obviously a critical need, particularly at a time when, in Central America, the war was starting to wind down. There was plenty of dislocation and poverty, particularly in the rural areas, so we began with Honduras and Guatemala. As we refined our approach to selecting partners, we began looking at other countries through the lens of evaluating the presence of strong NGOs that were addressing access to water. We asked the question: "Was there either a high absolute number of people who lacked water and sanitation or a high percentage of people who lacked these resources?" In Africa, you do not have large absolute populations, but you have high percentages of people who do not have access to those services. In India, 90% of the population has access to an improved water supply, but that still means more than 100 million people do not have access. We were looking at whether there were strong NGOs there that we could partner with, and now it is also whether there are strong microfinance institutions that we can partner with. We look at the microfinance ecosystem in the countries where we want to work and if there are large amounts of people without access to water. We are not an emergency relief organization, so we do look for political stability in the countries where we work together. And finally, what we look for is an overlap with funders. If we meet all those other criteria, then we will also try to work with funders where they want to work. For example, this occurred in both India and even Indonesia, where all of those criteria were met for us. For the Caterpillar Foundation, these were some of the countries of interest for them; so we looked at launching work there. What am I most excited about the future of Water.org? It really is WaterCredit. The accountability for this work that we will be doing in the future is growing and really important. It is so nascent that I do not want to expect too much quite yet. So, for me it is WaterCredit and how it can expand beyond microfinance institutions. To ask the question: "How can we help small entrepreneurs push out more water access in rural areas where you would possibly need a small business to help make that happen, or somebody is putting in a well to help provide water to a community at low cost?" Now, we can help them cover their startup costs. By working more directly with utilities so that they may possibly waive the connection fee or help people pay that connection fee over more time, then we do not have to be involved as much.

One of the things that we just launched was a debt fund. We really believe that, for the first time, we can actually raise debt capital in the United States and generate a financial return to investors. This may be very modest, I would say 2%, and then we can take those funds and lend them to our microfinance partners to fund their loan portfolios. Then they, in turn, use those funds to loan to poor people so that they can get these water connections and the WaterCredit loans. We are seeing that, right now in India, alone, our partner network has about $55 million in demand for capital; and right now they're having to pay 15% interest to source that from commercial banks there. What if we could help them drive down that

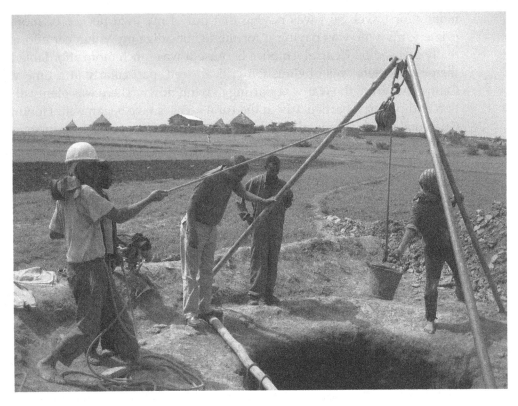

Digging the new well. Photo courtesy of water.org Flickr site.

cost of capital? And then when they make that final loan to an individual woman, the price of that loan can come down and expand even further. We already have $3 million in commitments for the first loan fund and if we can do that, it then becomes inherently scalable in terms of funding more and more of these loan portfolios. I am really excited about the potential of using more of these market forces to help drive water and sanitation to the poor, because if you can make that happen, again, it is infinitely scalable.

NLM: Thank you so much for this fascinating interview, Mr. White. Safe travels.

COMMENTARY BY NANCY L. MEEDZAN, SUELLEN BREAKEY, PATRICE K. NICHOLAS, SHIRA WINTER, AND INGE B. CORLESS

Access to clean water and sanitation is necessary to ensure freedom from preventable disease. As Matt Damon suggests:

> Looking ahead, I think access to water will be one of the most critical challenges of our time. There are a lot of ways to tackle it but for me, ensuring that every human being has access to safe drinking water and the dignity of a toilet—two incredibly basic and inextricably linked requirements for survival—is one of the most urgent and pressing

causes in the world today. The good news is that there are solutions that work. I'm convinced that we can overcome the global water crisis in our lifetime.

—Matt Damon, cofounder, Water.org

In his interview, Mr. White discusses two key pieces of legislation: The Senator Paul Simon Water for the Poor Act of 2005 (WfP) (H.R. 1973, 2005) and the Senator Paul Simon Water for the World Act (H.R. 2901, 2013). The first bill, sponsored by Representative Earl Blumenauer (Democrat, Oregon), was enacted into law on December 1, 2005. WfP required the government, in collaboration with USAID and other governmental agencies, to develop and implement a strategy to assist developing countries to make access to clean water and sanitation equitable and affordable. Reports are published annually detailing progress in this area and any changes to U.S. strategy. In 2012, "more than three million people gained access to drinking water, and one million people gained access to improved sanitation" (Office of Conservation and Water, 2013, p. 2).

The Senator Paul Simon Water for the World Act of 2013 (H.R. 2901, 2013) is a bipartisan bill sponsored by Representative Earl Blumenauer (Democrat, Oregon) and Representative Ted Poe (Republican, Texas). As its full title suggests, this bill would strengthen the implementation of the WfP by improving capacity of the U.S. government to implement, leverage, and monitor and evaluate programs to provide first-time or improved access to safe drinking water, sanitation, and hygiene to the world's poorest (H.R. 2901, 2013). This bill was introduced on August 1, 2013, and was referred to the House Committee on Foreign Affairs.

The following story, which appeared in the news soon after our interview with Gary White, illustrates the complex nature of lack of access to toilets and how the legislation may improve the lives of people globally. In the Uttar Pradesh state in northern India, two young girls were gang-raped and murdered, and hung from a tree near their village. The press noted that the two girls, cousins from an impoverished family with no toilets in their home, had disappeared at night after going into a field to seek privacy in toileting. As Mr. White notes, women and girls are often at risk of sexual violence and lack of safety when access to toilets and water are not available. This story underscores how incredibly important a global human rights issue it is, particularly for women and girls to have access to safe latrines and sources of water (British Broadcasting Company [BBC], 2014).

Another example of the importance of access to clean water for global health is evident in a recent film, *A Walk to Beautiful*. This is a poignant story about the incidence of obstetric fistula in women of Ethiopia and the devastation this condition causes in the lives of young girls. Although many circumstances contribute to the development of obstetrical fistula, lack of access to clean water is a major contributing factor because cleanliness requires water. Florence Nightingale would certainly concur.

As Mr. White points out in this interview, young girls and women spend many hours walking long distances to find water and then carrying that very heavy water back to their family. This difficult manual work consumes many of the calories that young girls take in for nourishment and thus they do not grow at the

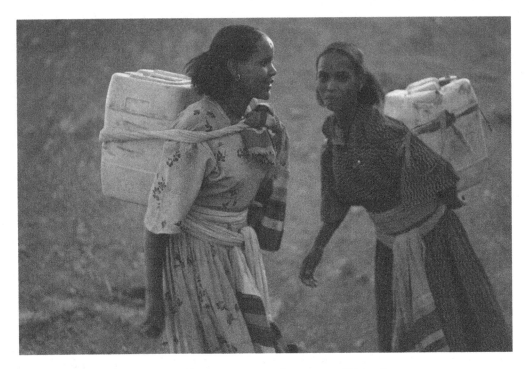

Ethiopian girls carrying water. Photo courtesy of water.org Flickr site.

rate of girls in resource-rich countries. This smaller development can be seen in the development of a small pelvis, which can lead to obstructed labor. In addition to stunted pelvic growth, is the fact that poor girls in the countryside often marry and become pregnant at ages as young as 14 years old. Because a doctor does not attend most births, many young girls labor for many hours, even days, and have resulting trauma to the bladder and/or bowel during labor that results in a fistula—and quite often a stillbirth. A woman's life with a fistula is one of total isolation, discrimination, and devastation. What is tragic is that the condition and the stigma associated with this condition could decrease in many countries around the world.

REFERENCES

British Broadcasting Company (BBC). (2014). *Two India girls gang raped and hanged in Uttar Pradesh*. Retrieved from http://www.bbc.com/news/world-asia-india-27615590

Office of Conservation and Water. (2013). *Report to Congress on strategy for safe water and sanitation: Senator Paul Simon Water for the Poor Act*. P.L. 109–121.

Senator Paul Simon Water for the Poor Act of 2005. H.R. 1973-109th Congress. (2005). In www.GovTrack.us. Retrieved from http://www.govtrack.us/congress/bills/109/hr1973

Senator Paul Simon Water for the World Act of 2013. H.R. 2901-113th Congress. (2013). In www.GovTrack.us. Retrieved from http://www.govtrack.us/congress/bills/113/hr2901

CHAPTER 10

The Impact of HIV/AIDS on the Nursing Profession in Sub-Saharan Africa

Busisiwe Rosemary Bhengu and Busisiwe P. Ncama

The HIV/AIDS epidemic has been one of the greatest challenges in public health for more than three decades. While reports indicate a decline in transmission of HIV/AIDS in some populations, particularly mother-to-child transmission, there has been a profound impact on the nursing profession. Nurses form the majority of health care workers in sub-Saharan Africa. For instance, 85% of the health care workers in Botswana are nurses (Phaladze, 2003). Ehlers (2006) maintains that the increasing number of HIV-positive persons in a country increases the possibility of the health care workers in that country contracting the disease, thus posing both a personal risk for health care workers and a potential loss for the health care workforce. Indeed, it has been reported that between 11.5% and 15.7% of health care workers in South Africa were reported as HIV/AIDS positive early in the advent of the disease (Britz, as cited in Ehlers, 2006; Connelly et al., 2007; Shisana, Hall, Maluleke, Chaveau, & Schwabe, 2004). Nursing, which is primarily a female-dominated profession, and a marginalized group in many countries of southern Africa, has an added burden in the HIV/AIDS epidemic in caring for those who are sick or dying from the disease.

Interestingly, out of the tragedy of the HIV/AIDS epidemic, great strides were made in the advancement and development of the nursing and midwifery professions in southern Africa because HIV/AIDS necessitated new ways of thinking. Such advancements are evident in nursing and midwifery practice, research, education, and community service. This chapter examines the impact of HIV/AIDS on the nursing profession, with a focus on advancements and developments in practice, education, regulation, policy, and research.

MAGNITUDE OF THE PROBLEM

Since the identification of the first case of HIV in San Francisco, California, in 1981, the world has confronted an epidemic that not only caused the death of large numbers of people, but also had a substantial impact on socioeconomic capacities, especially in developing countries (UNAIDS, 2012). Sub-Saharan Africa carried most of the disease burden and impact, with an estimated 2.1 million people dying from the disease in 2011 alone (AVERT, 2013).

UNAIDS (2013) states that worldwide approximately 35.3 (32.2 to 38.8) million people were living with HIV in 2012. The increase from previous years is largely due to the exponential increase in global access to lifesaving antiretroviral therapy (ART). There was also a 33% decline in the number of new infections since 2001. At the same time the number of AIDS deaths worldwide was also declining, with an estimated 1.6 million AIDS deaths in 2012, down from 2.3 million in 2000. Over the first decade of the 21st century, African states have also made substantial strides in reducing adult (ages 15 to 49) prevalence rates. Thirty of 42 sub-Saharan African states have seen their adult HIV prevalence rates decline between 2001 and 2009, and the region's overall prevalence rate went down by nearly one sixth (UNAIDS, 2010, p. 181).

Of the estimated 35.3 million people living with HIV/AIDS worldwide (UNAIDS, 2012), only about 9.7 million have access to ART. The World Health Organization (WHO) has set a target of 15 million people receiving ART by 2015 (WHO, 2013). Access to ART services has been influenced by factors such as urban–rural areas, age, gender, and other sociodemographic differentials across and within nations (UNAIDS, 2012; WHO, 2013). People living in rural areas, female gender, people with low economic status, and migrants have an increased risk of HIV and benefit less from HIV/AIDS prevention and control services (Agadjanian, 2005; Heckman, Somlai, Kelly, Stevenson, & Galdabini, 1996; Reid, 2006; Reif, Golin, & Smith, 2005). Sub-Saharan Africa consists of about 10% of the world's population, with more than two thirds of HIV-infected individuals but where more than three quarters of HIV-related deaths occurred in 2007. The southern Africa region is the most affected, with more than 35% of the world's HIV-infected people, half of whom live in South Africa.

IMPACT OF HIV/AIDS ON NURSING PRACTICE

HIV/AIDS has impacted the profession of nursing in the areas of increased workload, fear among nurses of contracting HIV/AIDS, stigma attached to HIV/AIDS, ethical issues surrounding HIV/AIDS in practice, and support to HIV-infected/affected employees.

Increased Workload

The impact of HIV/AIDS on the health workforce and health systems is an added burden to the already fragile health systems in developing countries, which are characterized by poor infrastructure, depleted health workforce, lack of drugs and commodities, and frequently poor management. The burden of disease has quadrupled in South Africa and other sub-Saharan African countries yet the available number of RNs in these areas to care for those with HIV/AIDS has decreased due to emigration (brain drain). According to Hall (2004), 80% of remaining nurses report heavier workloads while 22.8% felt that caring for AIDS patients was in itself demanding and time consuming due to longer recovery times and lack of support from families of patients. Moreover, nurses found caring for the terminally ill as emotionally challenging and demoralizing with the knowledge that the patient likely would not recover (Hall, 2004).

Fear Among Health Workers on the Possibility of Contracting the Disease

While nurses are overwhelmed with HIV/AIDS workload, the possibility of becoming infected with HIV has been a major concern, especially in the early period of the HIV epidemic (Fusilier, Manning, Santini Villar, & Rodriguez, 1998; Horsman & Sheeran, 1995; Loewenbrück, 2000). These authors maintain that the fear of contracting HIV/AIDS is far greater than the actual risk of infection. Nurses perceive the risk of contracting HIV infection after exposure to be much higher than the risk of contracting other infectious diseases such as the hepatitis B virus (Hall, 2004). This fear is fueled by the amount of contact with HIV patients at work (which is greatest among nurses); the prevalence rates in a particular country (e.g., South Africa), region (e.g., sub-Saharan Africa), or area of work (e.g., trauma unit); confidentiality surrounding patient's medical information preventing nurses from knowing the HIV status of their patients; and finally lack of government-enforced precautions. These fears may not be unfounded. Nurses seem to be at particularly higher risk for contracting HIV/AIDS—and at higher risk than physicians and medical students in care provision for those with HIV. A study by Shisana et al. (2004) found that HIV prevalence was higher among student nurses (13.8%) and nurses (13.7%) than among physicians (2%). It should be noted that very few physicians volunteered to participate in this study. Furthermore, in a study by Hall (2004), 46.4% of nurses feared infecting their partners and children at home because of exposure at work while 25% of their partners, in turn, were concerned about being in close contact with patients who suffered from infectious diseases such as HIV/AIDS. The fear of contracting HIV/AIDS was attributed to inadequate implementation of universal precautions, lack of reliable infection control programs, and lack of availability of sterilizing equipment in some areas. This fear was so serious that 16.2% of the nurses who participated in the study reported considering alternative employment and 7.7% reported considering another profession (Hall, 2004).

Needlestick injuries from administration of injections, suturing, and cuts from scalpel blades in cutting incisions like episiotomies add to the risk of contracting HIV/AIDS for nurses and midwives. These types of situations warrant wearing protective gear, which is cumbersome, expensive, time consuming to put on, often unavailable, and extremely hot in a region like sub-Saharan Africa that has limited air-conditioned facilities. There are also medical–legal issues associated with the delay in care in emergency situations while seeking and applying protective gear. Vengeance theory, which states that patients driven by anger may intentionally cause an injury in which a health care worker would contract HIV/AIDS, is another area of concern for nurses. Nurses who unfortunately have needlestick injuries in the clinical setting are offered post-exposure prophylaxis (PEP) drugs; however, other issues, such as the potential for drug resistance with repeated exposures, inaccessibility to the drugs, and supervisor control to access such drugs are complex. Some hospital nurses viewed protective measures, including PEP, primarily as a means for the hospital to protect itself against liability rather than for worker protection. Furthermore, workplace exposure policies were presumed by hospital nurses to protect the patient's rights to confidentiality ahead of protecting nurse's rights and health on the job (Zelnick & O'Donnell, 2005). Often when a nurse is exposed, stigma occurs in the clinical setting regarding the nurse's HIV status (Ehlers, 2006).

One initiative aimed at addressing stigma was aimed at developing a supportive work environment for HIV-affected staff following the death of four staff members over 4 months in one hospital in KwaZulu-Natal. Unfortunately, the program was met with denial, fear, hopelessness, and an unwillingness to be tested or treated. After improving communication aimed at decreasing stigma, the hospital succeeded in establishing a trusted and well-used diagnostic and treatment program for its staff (Uebel, Friedland, Pawinski, & Holst, 2004).

Stigma Attached to HIV/AIDS

Sources of stigma include fear of illness, fear of contagion, and fear of death among health workers, coworkers, and caregivers, as well as the general population (Brown, Macintyre, & Trujillo, 2003). Stigma was also identified as occurring in clinical settings by 49.2% of nurses, who believed that HIV/AIDS patients were treated differently from other patients. The secrecy surrounding the disease due to lack of understanding has also fueled stigma. It appears that family members often leave patients in the hospital for fear of being stigmatized themselves and for lack of alternative types of care; this was noted during the denialist period in South Africa (Hall, 2004). However, a qualitative study by Orner, Cooper, and Palmer (2011) has revealed that stigma toward HIV has lessened among many communities, though it may not have completely disappeared. Many of those who are living with it remain in denial or fearful of disclosing their HIV status. Although treatment is widely available, many nurses are reluctant to receive care in the institution in which they work because of the stigma (Guberski, 2007).

The HIV status of patients is often unknown due to policies related to voluntary disclosure. A policy was therefore developed in African countries that health care workers must plan care based on the assumption that every patient may be HIV positive. In the United States, this policy is known as universal precautions. A study completed in the United States suggests that nurses increased their use of protection if they knew their patients were HIV positive (Young, Forti, & Preston, 1996). However, if nurses believed that their patients were HIV positive or if they did not know their patients' HIV status, they did not always use adequate protection (Young et al., 1996, p. 249).

ETHICAL ISSUES RELATED TO HIV/AIDS IN PRACTICE

Nurses in the sub-Saharan region also faced ethical issues related to sending mixed messages. For example, recommending voluntary counseling and testing (VCT) without offering options such as ART and options for pregnant women to choose caesarian section delivery occurred during the period of denial in South Africa. Discouraging breastfeeding if the mother was HIV positive after a long-standing impetus to support breastfeeding in the population was a difficult health message. Breastfeeding offered advantages, particularly related to affordability, accessibility, and avoiding illness due to contaminated water in underresourced countries; with the HIV epidemic, educating mothers about shifting to bottle feeding placed nurses and midwives in a dilemma. Providing ART during pregnancy brought about the controversy of resistance in future treatment. Bottle feeding was accompanied by stigma because the message in the community was that this signified that the mother was positive (Ehlers, 2006).

Often nurses are the sole decision makers in addressing immunization and opportunistic infections related to HIV/AIDS. Confidentiality or secrecy surrounding the status of patients with HIV/AIDS was a complex issue for nurses regarding how to involve families in the care of patients. In addition, educating patients and their families on measures to protect themselves from contracting HIV created a widespread ethical dilemma. Furthermore, many myths and misconceptions regarding HIV/AIDS in relation to its origin and its presentation existed in South Africa, specifically. For example, politics dominated the political system both during apartheid and postapartheid. Under apartheid in South Africa, many people were marginalized, which fueled suspicion and paranoia. Patients living with HIV often presented with opportunistic infections such as tuberculosis (TB), pneumonia, and meningitis; in addition to providing care, nurses needed to offer sexual education for prevention of the spread of HIV, as well as other interventions. However, the predominantly illiterate population in rural communities in sub-Saharan Africa could not grasp the relationship between HIV, opportunistic infections, and the need for sexual education to prevent the spread of the epidemic (Ehlers, 2006).

SUPPORT OF HEALTH WORKERS INFECTED/AFFECTED WITH HIV/AIDS

Hall (2004) addressed the engagement of companies with HIV/AIDS in terms of policies on HIV/AIDS and individual support of workers. A 2003 survey on the economic impact of HIV/AIDS on business in South Africa, conducted by the Bureau for Economic Research (BER) and the South African Business Coalition on HIV and AIDS (SABCOHA), suggested that only 25% of the 1,006 participating companies had an HIV/AIDS policy (BER, 2003). Another study focused on large companies reported that only 60% of the 25 largest companies in South Africa had HIV/AIDS policies or programs (Bendell, 2003). This could be related to companies not seeing the impact of HIV/AIDS on their companies. For example, a survey by Deloite & Touche, LLP (2003) found that most employers envisaged that HIV/AIDS would have either little or no more than a moderate impact on their companies. The denialist stance in the country could also be the reason not to engage with HIV/AIDS policies in these companies. The BER and SABCOHA survey showed that only 14% of companies (most of them larger companies) had conducted research to assess the impact of HIV on the labor force, whereas 9% of survey participants indicated that the disease had already had a "significant adverse impact" on their business and another 34% foresaw a "significant negative" effect within 5 years (BER, 2003). The impact manifested in things such as increased worker absenteeism, higher labor turnover, and higher employee benefit costs (Hall, 2004). The lack of support from employers was also found in the health services substudy, where only 42.4% of health facilities indicated the existence of an official HIV/AIDS policy to guide health workers in the management of HIV/AIDS. In fact, in this later study more than a third of the nurses surveyed (37.7%) did not know if an official HIV/AIDS workplace policy was in place in the health facilities where they worked (Hall, 2004). Less than half of the respondents (48.8%) had access to any form of official support such as counseling for work-related stress in the earlier period of the HIV/AIDS epidemic (Hall, 2004). A similar trend was found among hospital-based health workers in Uganda, who also perceived infection control equipment and HIV counseling facilities to be inadequate (Mungherera et al., 1997).

However, recently numerous government policies and legislation were developed related to workplace protection from needlestick injuries, compensation, and human resource management of HIV/AIDS infected/affected nurses. These policies and precepts are scattered in several government documents so that an average nurse or even a nurse manager may find it difficult to access. The human resource departments in hospitals where a qualitative study was done were not helpful either in providing such information (Kerr, Brysiewicz, & Bhengu, 2014).

NURSING RESPONSE TO HIV/AIDS EPIDEMIC

HIV/AIDS led to the redesigning of the scope and responsibilities of nursing practice, especially in the areas of task shifting and relevant education to accommodate the changing environment.

Redesigning Practice

Escalating opportunistic infections and terminal illness from AIDS led to overcrowding in health facilities, necessitating early discharge of patients for care at home (home-based care) or community services (community-based care). Most of these home-based facilities and services are solely managed by nurses in sub-Saharan Africa. The HIV/AIDS epidemic necessitated greater preventive health education input from health workers, including basic care of those in the late stages of HIV/AIDS. Nurses played a pivotal role in implementing and maintaining effective health education in a variety of settings, including schools, youth centers, colleges and universities, clinics, and hospitals. Nurses are also familiar with the cultural traditions and taboos of specific communities and can convey health education messages in culturally congruent terms. Later, nurses were faced with the need to diagnose HIV/AIDS through rapid testing that was performed in both the fixed clinics and through campaigns within communities. However, most of these community-based health facilities where nurses perform their functions and services do not have laboratories or pharmacies to address the important care needs that arise. Prior to the HIV/AIDS epidemic, primary health care (PHC) nurses in South Africa were authorized to prescribe and administer medications according to section 38 of the old Nursing Act (Act no. 50 of 1978), as amended, and now section 56 of the South Africa Nursing Act (Act no. 33 of 2005). These roles are similar to primary care nurse practitioners in international terms. In the absence and/or shortage of doctors, pressure grew for RNs to take over the function of initially diagnosing, initiating ART, and maintaining patients on ART in nurse-led health facilities. One proposed solution to the increasing demand for care in Uganda was the shifting of HIV/AIDS care, including ART, to nonphysician providers. Nonphysician providers include clinical officers whose education is similar to physician assistants and nurses (Guberski, 2007). This role was embraced by nurses and nursing academics in South Africa through the initiative, nurse-initiated and managed ART (NIMART). After a recent major study indicated that circumcision played a role in prevention of HIV/AIDS, RNs were given the authority to perform circumcisions. All of this built on task shifting and task sharing that WHO recommended to member countries due to shortages of qualified/specialized health care workers. The HIV epidemic led to an increase in task shifting of medical tasks to RNs and of moving RNs' tasks to other health care workers. New cadres of workers were also created, such as predominantly voluntary HIV/AIDS counselors.

Task Shifting and Requirements

Task shifting is a process of delegation whereby tasks are moved, where appropriate, to less specialized health care workers. This makes more efficient use of the available human resources (WHO, 2007). The Streamlining Tasks and Roles to Expand Treatment and Care for HIV (STRETCH) implementation and testing were conducted to determine the difference in outcomes of patients treated by nurses and doctors (Uebel et al., 2011). The study found that there were similar outcomes in terms of viral load suppression; however, there was no improvement in survival. There was also no difference in the percentage started on ART. The study suggested that there was improvement in the numbers of patients with higher CD4 counts. (Fairall, 2012). Sanne et al. (2010) suggested that management of patients on ART by a nurse had similar outcomes to physician care.

Task shifting can cascade further down from the level of qualified nurses to community workers to free the time of qualified nurses to attend to their expanded role of prescribing and dispensing. However, the Practical Approach to Lung Health in South Africa (PALSA PLUS) program, which provides guidelines and training for PHC nurses in the management of adult lung diseases and HIV/AIDS, was later introduced based on the fact that South Africa has the highest coinfection rate of HIV and TB in the world. Since TB is the leading cause of death among HIV-infected South Africans, it made clinical sense to combine a lung health-training program with the additional training on ART. A study evaluating this program found that PALSA PLUS training successfully engaged all PHC nurses in a comprehensive approach to a range of illnesses affecting both HIV-positive and HIV-negative patients (Stein et al., 2008). Community workers, for example, could perform home-based care that may include a wide range of activities such as basic nursing care, health education, and counseling, to name a few (Fairall, 2012). One nurse, however, in the STRETCH study indicated that while they embraced task shifting they were overburdened: "Nurses can do everyone's job, but no one can do the nurse's job, that's the problem, we are overloaded. We are really exhausted" (Fairall, 2012).

Advancing Nursing Education to Meet the HIV/AIDS Challenges

In *The Lancet* Commission Report (Frenk et al., 2010) on transforming education to strengthen health systems in an interdependent world, a recommendation was that education and training be aligned with competencies to support the dynamic environment and changing contexts. This has great relevance for the clinical care of those with HIV/AIDS in southern Africa and South Africa. *The Lancet* Commission further recommended a systems approach to accommodate PHC that would support professional interdependence, including nursing roles in HIV care and ART delivery. The challenges of HIV/AIDS should urge nurses to engage in responsive, context driven, and lifelong education for nurses (Frenk et al., 2010). Nurses must possess the necessary knowledge to address health education, prescribing and administering ART, circumcision, and end-of-life care. Continued global support of African countries is urgently needed—financially, scientifically, and technologically—to address the epidemic. One example is the U.S. initiative, the President's Emergency Plan for AIDS Relief (PEPFAR), that was initiated to address the urgent need for ART in Africa.

Nursing Preregistration Curriculum

The nursing curricula at various levels was critical to review in order to meet the compelling country imperative of the HIV/AIDS epidemic in South Africa and other countries in Africa, as well as short-term and long-term solutions to address

BOX 10.1 INTEGRATION OF HIV/AIDS

1st year: Basic nursing care and infection control

2nd year: Community-based care including health education and counseling

3rd year: HIV/AIDS disease and management including pharmacology

4th year: Issues on HIV/AIDS care, including nurse-initiated and managed antiretroviral treatment (NIMART) and the prevention of mother-to-child transmission (PMTCT); circumcision, which came later, could be added to fourth year

the epidemic. The comprehensive 4-year degree and diploma nursing education programs had to incorporate or integrate HIV/AIDS content. Workshops were held with international partners, including Johns Hopkins University, and South African nurse managers, clinicians, and educators were invited to add expertise and to explore ways of integrating HIV/AIDS content into these curricula. The rationale was that African countries could not afford to wait for specialization in an area like HIV/AIDS, and that basic nurses at 1 year needed to acquire the knowledge to protect themselves from infection and offer basic care to those patients who were already streaming into the health facilities. One example for integration of HIV/AIDS is illustrated in Box 10.1.

POSTREGISTRATION CURRICULA

Specialization courses were also expected to incorporate HIV/AIDS content according to relevance in their areas. For example, the critical care nursing curriculum placed an emphasis on complications of HIV/AIDS disease and ART such as metabolic acidosis, dyslipidemia, acute myocardial infarction, and acute infections. The family nurse practitioner course focused on NIMART as it involves prescribing, dispensing, administrating, and monitoring of patients on ART. The advanced midwifery course focused on prevention of mother-to-child transmission (PMTCT), treatment, and ART during pregnancy, as well as breastfeeding issues.

Short Courses

Short courses were developed by the local and global community and offered widely in South Africa. The local municipalities and the provincial departments of health ran short courses to meet the immediate needs of the health facilities. The global community offered funds to support short courses and multidisciplinary teams. There were also individual RNs who, after obtaining university qualifications, ran private courses in HIV/AIDS and serviced some of the large companies and their health workforces. The focus of these courses was mainly

HIV/AIDS counseling. Often, the short courses were not well coordinated. However, Guberski (2007) described a curriculum in Uganda that includes an overview of HIV pathogenesis and transmission, PMTCT, triage, symptom evaluation and management, ART, drug side effects and adverse effects, common opportunistic infections, and adherence. Many universities offered various modules and courses. The medical school in KwaZulu-Natal, in collaboration with the Department of Health and the Global Fund to Fight AIDS, Tuberculosis, and Malaria, began a graduate diploma program in HIV and AIDS Management in which students could accrue credits toward a formal master's degree. This diploma became very popular with nurses, especially those nurses who manned the health facilities and initiated courses in educational institutions. The psychology department at the University of KwaZulu-Natal, South Africa, introduced a decentralized module on HIV/AIDS counseling that became compulsory for all RNs pursuing a bachelor's degree for advanced practice. This is a bridging degree for RNs who completed their basic education and training at a nursing college to enable them to access graduate studies. Although this degree was a redress for the diploma nurses from colleges, it also provided for specialization with several streams, for example, advanced midwifery, advanced psychiatry, critical care nursing, oncological nursing and palliative care, community health nursing, primary care (family practice nursing), nursing education, and nursing management. After some time, a stream on HIV/AIDS was created within the bachelor's degree advanced practice. This stream included four modules: Fundamentals of HIV/AIDS; HIV/AIDS Nursing Management; Issues Related to HIV/AIDS; and HIV/AIDS Care in Pregnancy, Labor, and Puerperium. In graduate studies at the master's degree level, similar modules were added; however, these were independent modules rather than specialization.

HIV/AIDS in South Africa became an emerging and complex epidemic for which solutions to address care were urgently needed; hence, the need to quickly develop HIV/AIDS content to incorporate into existing courses. Education and training for HIV/AIDS was not fully incorporated into a specific advanced practice nursing category. Since African countries are resource limited in health and health professions education, it was necessary to weigh the option of educating and training specialist nurses against providing basic, predominantly preventive care for the large number of infected and affected people with HIV/AIDS. In South Africa, postregistration courses are also regulated within the South African Nursing Council. Debates surrounding the accreditation of HIV/AIDS as a specialization resulted in controversy among nursing professionals. Some suggested that HIV/AIDS could be accommodated in oncological nursing and palliative care because HIV/AIDS patients had flooded the hospice care facilities to an extent that these facilities became overcrowded and decentralization of this service was needed. NIMART prompted the creation of nurse practitioner specialization in HIV/AIDS. However, primary care nurse practitioners remained in the forefront of care provision.

REGULATION TO ACCOMMODATE TASK SHIFTING

There is wide agreement in the global health community that, in order to be sustainable, workforce strategies such as preservice strengthening and task shifting should be incorporated into nationally endorsed health professional regulatory frameworks. Health professional regulation ensures the safety and quality of health professional practice and education. Many countries in sub-Saharan Africa have a professional regulatory body, such as a nursing and midwifery council, that issues the national regulations and standards for nursing and midwifery education and practice in their country. Eleven of the 13 registrars indicated that task shifting occurs. Of the 11 countries in which task shifting is taking place, only Tanzania indicated that current regulations for nurses and midwives could allow for task shifting. Eight countries updated their scope of practice within the past 5 years to accommodate recent changes (McCarthy et al., 2013). Training and licensing nurses for prescription of ART and management of HIV/AIDS patients has been implemented in some East, Central, and Southern Africa (ECSA) countries, most notably Botswana, South Africa, and Zambia. These countries could offer an effective method of expanding nurse-initiated HIV treatment and delivery of vital health services across sub-Saharan Africa if support and authorization could be secured from nursing and midwifery councils. Sanne et al. (2010) conclude by suggesting that health system decisions require dedicated planning and a responsive regulatory environment, believing that regulatory bodies limit the scope of practice of practitioners. Furthermore, Phaladze (2003, p. 22) maintains that there is limited involvement of nurses in formulating policies and in allocating resources, which could cause policy implementation problems and compromise the quality of services rendered in Africa. Therefore, this author proposes greater inputs into policy formulation processes by nurses. Edwards and Roelofs (2007) support this claim by arguing that nurses are at the forefront of HIV prevention and AIDS care in these countries but have limited involvement in related policy decisions. These authors therefore engaged in a participatory action research to address the contributions of sub-Saharan and Caribbean nurses to health policy development and health systems reform in order to improve the effectiveness of HIV and AIDS policies and practices.

IMPACT OF HIV AND AIDS IN DEVELOPING AND ADVANCING RESEARCH IN NURSING AND MIDWIFERY

The Influence of International Nursing Organizations

The development of the WHO Collaborating Centers (CC) in Africa and the formation of Sigma Theta Tau International Honor Society of Nursing, African Chapter, contributed substantially to the development of scholarship among nurses in southern Africa. Currently, there are four WHO CCs for nursing and midwifery in Africa; two are in South Africa at the University of KwaZulu-Natal (UKZN) and University of South Africa (UNISA). The other WHO CC is at Botswana University, and recently Kamuzu College of Nursing in Malawi joined. Research and scholarship are critical to the mission of the WHO CCs. The WHO CCs were instrumental in producing PhD-credentialed nurses that eventually engaged in leadership positions in Africa, as well as research activities in the whole of the WHO Regional Office for Africa (AFRO). PhD graduates contributed to the pool of leaders in nursing and midwifery in countries such as Rwanda, Namibia, Nigeria, Ethiopia, Malawi, South Africa, Swaziland, Uganda, Liberia, Sierra Leone, Zambia, and many other countries (UKZN WHO CC, 2013).

The WHO CC activities also brought countries together in conducting research activities. For example, the UKZN WHO CC collaborated with the UNISA and Botswana WHO CCs in writing evidence-based policy briefs. Professor Busisiwe Bhengu presented to the Minister of Health, the Honorable Dr. Aaron Motsoaledi, and to the South African Nursing Council on the policy brief written regarding Human Resources for Health. Another policy brief on task shifting is still being finalized (UKZN WHO CC, 2013). A number of publications and systematic reviews were published in journals as part of the terms of reference of the WHO CC. For example, UKZN CC published several systematic reviews on e-learning and tele-health in southern Africa (UKZN WHO CC, 2013).

The Joanna Briggs Institute as a Driver of Evidence-Based Research in Southern Africa

The affiliation of UKZN, University of the Witwatersrand (Wits), and Ethiopia with the Joanna Briggs Institute (JBI) in Australia has encouraged the development and growth of evidence-based research in southern Africa. The JBI conducted initial training for staff in these centers to qualify them to conduct and publish evidence-based systematic reviews. Mcinerney and Brysiewicz (2009) conducted a systematic review on experiences of caregivers in providing home-based care to persons with HIV/AIDS in Africa. Graduate students and academic staff were also trained on conducting systematic reviews with the aim of advancing nursing research in southern Africa. UKZN WHO CC's core group of trainers in systematic reviews were further trained by WHO Geneva and the WHO AFRO in the compilation of evidence-based policy briefs; subsequently, two policy briefs were developed.

Research Conducted by Nurses on HIV and AIDS in Southern Africa/Sub-Saharan Africa

The emergence of HIV/AIDS was instrumental in advancing nursing research related to the epidemic. Many nursing research studies have been conducted by researchers, educators, and practitioners, and in the community at large. Nursing advancement in research, education, practice, and community service flourished amid the complex and tragic landscape of HIV disease. The research trajectory followed the same course as the HIV/AIDS educational interventions and this was largely driven by the course of the epidemic and the response to it. The Southern African Nursing Research group also benefited from collaborations with international partners and organizations involved in HIV/AIDS care and research.

Prevention Research

Behavior Change Research as Part of Communication, Information, and Education Strategies Implemented

Initially, the research focused on knowledge, attitudes, practices, and behaviors (KAPB) relating to HIV/AIDS, homophobia levels, willingness to care for people with AIDS, and their approach to possible sexual risk behaviors. Prevention messages included behavior modification and communication strategies and there was evaluation of the effectiveness of the behavior messages, especially the ABC message (Abstinence, Be Faithful, and Condomize). Uganda, Botswana, Swaziland, Senegal, and a number of countries in Africa actively promoted the ABC approach to prevention, and Uganda promoted VCT through nongovernment organizations (NGOs) such as the AIDS Support Organization (TASO; AVERT, 2013).

The uptake of intervention and condom use became a large focus both in terms of effectiveness and of efficiency of usage. Consistent use of condoms was proven to be effective and efficient (up to 99%) with correct use. According to a meta-analysis conducted by Herbst et al. (2005), interpersonal skills training was a successful intervention in reducing risky sexual behavior of men who have sex with men. This interpersonal skills training incorporated several delivery methods and was offered over multiple sessions spanning a minimum of 3 weeks.

Intervention research has also been conducted in the following areas:

- Male and female condoms
- Male circumcision
- Voluntary counselling and testing
- Testing and treatment of sexually transmitted infections (STIs)
- Needle exchange programs (NEP)
- Opioid substitution treatment (OST)
- Universal health care precautions
- Blood screening
- Antiretroviral (ARV) drugs for PMTCT; preexposure prophylaxis (PrEP); PEP; and treatment as prevention (TasP)
- Microbicides
- Vaccines

Research on structural approaches to HIV/AIDS prevention was highlighted in a *Lancet* paper (Gupta, Parkhurst, Ogden, Aggleton, & Maha, 2008).

Structural factors were defined as physical, social, cultural, organizational, community, economic, legal, or policy aspects of the environment that impede or facilitate efforts to avoid HIV infection (Sumartojo, Doll, Holtgrave, Gayle, & Merson, 2000).

Research on Migration

The research conducted on migration revealed that migration has fueled the HIV/AIDS epidemic in southern Africa. During that era, denialism had engulfed the South African government and there was widespread denial that HIV/AIDS was an epidemic under the leadership of Dr. Mantombazana Tshabalala. Denialism led to a rapid increase in the numbers of people living with HIV, continued the stigmatization of the disease, and led to late entry to treatment. The issues of migration are complex in South Africa and are linked with apartheid since men often left their rural villages to work in cities, particularly in mining and manufacturing. Migrants frequently lived in hostels where sex work was common due to poverty of women, thus fueling the HIV epidemic further. Often migrant men would then return home and infect their partners in rural villages.

Research on Fear of Contracting HIV/AIDS

During the earlier days of the HIV/AIDS epidemic, fear of contracting the disease was studied among nurses. The study was necessitated by the fear surrounding the mode of spread of the disease and the fact that the disease was ill understood at the time. Not only were nurses fearful of contracting HIV, but even spouses and family members were fearful of being infected through their contact with the nurses after their care of patients with AIDS (Greeff & Phetlhu, 2007; Ullah, 2011).

Research on Prevention of Mother-to-Child Transmission

The Treatment Action Campaign (TAC) group focused heavily on research related to PMTCT. In fact, TAC brought suit against the South African government and forced the South African government to offer nevirapine to pregnant women to prevent the spread of HIV from mothers to unborn children.

Microbicide Studies

Subsequent research focused on the microbicides as a method of HIV prevention. One study was conducted by the Center for the AIDS Program of Research in South Africa (CAPRISA), specifically the 004 Tenofovir Gel trial. Studies are continuing in the area of microbicides. Although nurses are not lead researchers in the microbicides studies, frequently they are involved as members of the research team in fieldwork, recruitment of participants, and management of patients in the studies. Condom usage messages and monitoring of condom use also became a significant part of the nurses' work as well as tracing of participants who were lost to follow-up.

Circumcision

Nurses were involved in conducting research on circumcision, initially on traditional circumcision, then later on circumcision as a prevention tool against HIV/AIDS. The uptake of circumcision as a tool was evaluated and nurses also became involved in conducting circumcision as a task-shifting element of care.

Research on HIV/AIDS Treatment and Care

A substantial amount of research was conducted on community home-based care. The South Coast Hospice initiated an integrated community home-based care model for HIV/AIDS care; as such, research was conducted on the evaluation of the model and its usefulness in caring for people with AIDS. Professor Leanna Uys conducted a number of studies on community home-based care. This occurred during the time that ART was not available and the focus of research was on palliative care and how best it should be delivered. The University of Botswana became a WHO CC with a focus on community home-based care and, as such, also conducted substantial research on that topic. Research on community home-based care revealed that home care was a viable option for caring for those with HIV outside of hospital settings; the need for proper coordination and supervision by experienced staff was suggested, including having an available visiting medical doctor. Symptom control was the major focus of research conducted in home-based settings, as well as research associated with emotional well-being and effectiveness of interventions, such as counseling, social aspects of care, and spiritual care. Poverty was identified as a major issue confronted by home-based care volunteers. The transport and payment of home-based care volunteers was also identified as another impediment in the delivery of home-based care. The financial viability of home-based care remained a challenge in the absence of a proper funding model, and sustainability is a concern. Research on caring for the care provider is an important area of study since it is well established that caring for a patient with HIV/AIDS is emotionally and physically challenging.

Symptom Control and Self-Care Management Research

Another major focus of research conducted by nurses was related to symptom control. This type of research began prior to the availability of ART and grew upon the initiation of therapy. This research also incorporated symptom management in the treatment of HIV. The research was mainly stimulated by the work of the International Nursing Network for HIV/AIDS Research. A series of research studies were conducted across the sub-Saharan countries on symptom control and management. Strategies were identified for control of symptoms and a symptom management intervention was developed (Wantland et al., 2008). This symptom management manual was further evaluated in different settings in sub-Saharan Africa and found to be beneficial for people living with HIV/AIDS.

Stigma Research

Research on stigma and discrimination became another major thrust after funding support was provided by the U.S. National Institutes of Health (NIH) under the leadership of Dr. William Holzemer and Dr. Leana Uys in South Africa (Holzemer et al., 2007). The research was conducted in five African countries: Lesotho, Malawi, South Africa, Swaziland, and Tanzania. The research suggested that stigma associated with HIV/AIDS was a deterrent to people living with HIV in seeking care and disclosing their HIV status. Accessing care at VCT facilities was also hampered by stigmatization, and many people preferred not testing out of fear of being stigmatized. Stigma was also described as a violation of human rights in the settings where the research was conducted. From this research, both a conceptual model and a validated stigma measurement tool were developed (Holzemer et al., 2007).

ARV Treatment Research

Nurses became involved in research trials that tested specific ARV medications in southern Africa. In these trials, nurses served on research teams, primarily as recruiters of participants, field workers, phlebotomists, data collectors, and subsequently monitors of patients enrolled in the clinical trials. A significant amount of research was conducted on VCT, such as comparing the different models of testing and their effectiveness as well as the messages that encouraged people to come forward for testing.

Research on Support Groups

In the absence of ART, support groups played a major role in encouraging positive living among people living with HIV/AIDS (PLWHA). Research on usefulness of support groups, effectiveness, and efficiency were conducted. Support groups were identified as effective in encouraging PLWHA to accept and disclose their status, as well as encouraging PLWHA to live positively with the disease.

Research on Adherence to Treatment

Research on adherence to HIV/AIDS treatment became another important area for study in the early days of ART. Since adherence to therapy at a level of 95% or more is known to be necessary to achieve complete suppression of viral activity, adherence studies by nurses were critical to investigating this. Studies conducted in sub-Saharan Africa demonstrated high levels of adherence among the PLWHA who were on treatment (Corless et al., 2009; Weiser et al., 2010). Another study conducted in South Africa revealed that a supportive social environment is critical for those with HIV/AIDS (Ncama et al., 2008). Further studies compared adherence to ARV medications with adherence to TB medications. Corless et al. (2009) suggested that these studies may indicate the likely success to adherence to ARVs as access to these medications becomes more available.

Research on NIMART

Through the Global Fund to Fight AIDS, TB, and Malaria, ARV treatment became available, initially mainly in research sites, and was eventually rolled out throughout the sub-Saharan Africa countries. Due to the massive numbers of PLWHAs that needed to commence treatment, different systems of reaching large numbers had to be explored. Research on NIMART was conducted and found to be effective in reaching large numbers of PLWHA. Funding through institutions such as the Johns Hopkins Program for International Education in Gynecology and Obstetrics (JHPIEGO), an international, nonprofit health organization affiliated with Johns Hopkins University, were key to success. The Medical Education Partnership Initiative (MEPI) made it possible to further study the effectiveness of NIMART as part of the undergraduate curricula.

CONCLUSION

Despite the complex epidemic of HIV, the nursing profession has emerged successfully in addressing this urgent public health problem. Many advancements have occurred in nursing practice, education, research, and policy as a result of the need to engage in addressing the human toll on health that is caused by HIV disease. The successes in addressing HIV have led to a dramatic increase in those successfully treated and in gaining further understanding of the contributions of nursing to care across the continuum.

REFERENCES

Agadjanian, V. (2005). *War, migration and HIV/AIDS risk in Angola.* Poster presented at the XXV IUSSP International Population Conference, Tours, France.
AVERT. (2013). *AVERTing HIV and AIDS. HIV prevention strategies.* Retrieved from http://www.avert.org/worldwide-hiv-aids-statistics.htm

Bendell, J. (2003). *Waking up to risk. Corporate responses to HIV/AIDS in the workplace.* United Nations Research Institute for Social Development (UNRISD) UNAIDS. Retrieved from http://www.unaids.org/EN/other/functionalities/Search.asp

Brown, L., Macintyre, K., & Trujillo, L. (2003). Interventions to reduce HIV/AIDS stigma: What have we learned? *AIDS Education and Prevention, 15*(1), 49–69.

Bureau for Economic Research (BER). (2003). *The economic impact of HIV/AIDS on business in South Africa.* Retrieved from http://www.redribbon.co.za/business/default.asp

Connelly, D., Veriava, Y., Roberts, S., Tsotetsi, J., Jordan, A., DeSilva, E., . . . DeSilva, M. B. (2007). Prevalence of HIV infection and median CD4 counts among health care workers in South Africa. *South African Medical Journal, 97,* 115–120.

Corless, I. B., Wantland, D., Bhengu, B., McInerney, P., Ncama, B., Nicholas, P. K., . . . Davis, S. M. (2009). HIV and tuberculosis in Durban, South Africa: Adherence to two medication regimens. *AIDS Care, 21*(9), 1106–1113.

Deloitte & Touche. (2003). *AIDS in the workplace 2003.* Johannesburg, South Africa: Deloitte & Touche.

Edwards, N. C., & Roelofs, S. (2007). Strengthening nurses' capacity in HIV policy development in sub-Saharan Africa and the Caribbean: An international program of research and capacity building. *Canadian Journal of Nursing Research, 39*(3), 187–189.

Ehlers, V. J. (2006). Challenges nurses face in coping with the HIV/AIDS pandemic in Africa. *International Journal of Nursing Studies, 43,* 657–662.

Fairall, L. (2012, November). Does nurse initiation of ART improve access? SA Clinicians Society Conference, Cape Town, South Africa.

Frenk, J., Chen, l., Bhutta, Z., Cohen, J., Crisp, N., Evans, T., . . . Fineberg, H. (2010). Health professionals for a new century: Transforming education to strengthen health system in an interdependent world. *The Lancet Commission.* Retrieved from www.thelancet.com

Fusilier, M., Manning, M. R., Santini Villar, A. J., & Rodriguez, D. T. (1998). AIDS knowledge and attitudes of health-care workers in Mexico. *The Journal of Social Psychology, 138*(2), 203–210.

Greeff, M., & Phetlhu, R. (2007). The meaning and effect of HIV/AIDS stigma for people living with AIDS and nurses involved in their care in the North West Province, South Africa. *Curationis, 30*(2), 12–23.

Guberski, T. D. (2007). Nurse practitioners, HIV/AIDS, and nursing in resource-limited settings. *The Journal for Nurse Practitioners, 3*(10), 695–702.

Gupta, G., Parkhurst, J. O., Ogden, J. A., Aggleton, P., & Maha, A. (2008). Structural approaches to HIV prevention. *The Lancet, 372*(9640), 764–775.

Hall, E. (2004). Nursing attrition and the work environment in South African health facilities. *Curationis, 27*(4), 28–36.

Heckman, T., Somlai, A., Kelly, J. I., Stevenson, L., & Galdabini, K. (1996). Reducing barriers to care and improving quality of life for rural persons with HIV. *AIDS Patient Care and STDs, 11,* 37–43.

Herbst, J. H., Sherba, R. T., Crepaz, N., Deluca, J. B., Zohrabyan, L., Stall, R. D., & Lyles, C. M. (2005). A meta-analytic review of HIV behavioral interventions for reducing sexual risk behavior of men who have sex with men. *Journal of Acquired Immune Deficiency Syndromes (1999), 39*(2), 228–241.

Holzemer, W. L., Uys, L., Makoae, L., Stewart, A., Phetlhu, R., Dlamini, P. S., . . . Naidoo, J. (2007). A conceptual model of HIV/AIDS stigma from five African countries. *Journal of Advanced Nursing, 58*(6), 541–551.

Horsman, J., & Sheeran, P. (1995). Health care workers and HIV/AIDS: A critical review of the literature. *Social Science and Medicine, 41*(110), 1535–1567.

Kerr, J., Brysiewicz, P., & Bhengu, B. (2014). *An analysis of nurse managers' human resource management of HIV/AIDS affected/infected nurses in selected hospitals in KwaZulu-Natal*, (Unpublished doctoral thesis). University of KwaZulu-Natal, Durban.

Loewenbrück, K. (2000). *Impact of HIV/AIDS patients on hospitals: Hospital response and behavior*. Organization of Health Services Delivery (Unpublished report). World Health Organization, Geneva, Switzerland.

McCarthy, C. F., Voss, J., Verani, A., Vidot, P., Marla, E., Salmon, M. E., & Riley, P. L. (2013). Nursing and midwifery regulation and HIV scale-up: Establishing a baseline in east, central and southern Africa. *Journal of the International AIDS Society, 16*, 18051.

Mcinerney, P., & Brysiewicz, P. (2009). A systematic review of the experiences of caregivers in providing home-based care to persons with HIV/AIDS in Africa. *JBI Library of Systematic Reviews, 7*, 130–153.

Mungherera, M., Van der Straten, A., Hall, T. L., Faigeles, B., Fowler, G., & Mandel, S. (1997). HIV/AIDS-related attitudes and practices of hospital-based health workers in Kampala, Uganda. *AIDS, 11*(Suppl. 1), S79–S85.

Ncama, B., McInerney, P., Bhengu, B., Corless, I., Wantland, D., Nicholas, P., . . . Davis, S. (2008). Social support and medication adherence in HIV disease in KwaZulu-Natal, South Africa. *International Journal of Nursing Studies, 45*(12), 1757–1763. doi:10.1016/j.ijnurstu.2008.06.006

Orner, P., Cooper, D., & Palmer, N. (2011). *Investigation of health care workers' responses to HIV/AIDS care and treatment in South Africa*. Report funded by PEPFAR. Washington, DC: Anova Health Institute/PEPFAR.

Phaladze, N. A. (2003). The role of nurses in the human immunodeficiency virus/acquired immune deficiency syndrome policy process in Botswana. *International Nursing Reviewx, 50*, 22–33.

Reid, S. D. (2006). Poor educational attainment and sexually transmitted infections associated with positive HIV serostatus among female inpatient substance abusers in Trinidad and Tobago. *Drug and Alcohol Dependence, 82*(1), S81–S84.

Reif, J. C., Golin, C. E., & Smith, S. R. (2005). Barriers to accessing HIV/AIDS care in North Carolina: Rural and urban differences. *AIDS Care, 17*(5), 558–565.

Sanne, I., Orrell, C., Matthew, P., Fox, M. P., Conradie, F., Ive, P., . . . Wood, R. (2010). For the CIPRA-SA Study Team. Nurse versus doctor management of HIV-infected patients receiving antiretroviral therapy (CIPRA-SA): A randomized non-inferiority trial. *The Lancet, 376*, 33–40.

Shisana, O., Hall, E. J., Maluleke, R., Chauveau, J., & Schwabe, C. (2004). HIV prevalence among South African health workers. *South African Medical Journal, 94*, 846–850.

Stein, J., Lewin S., Fairall, L., Mayers, P., English, R., Bheekie, A., . . . Zwarenstein, M. (2008). Building capacity for antiretroviral delivery in South Africa: A qualitative evaluation of the PALSA PLUS nurse training program. *BMC Health Services Research, 8*, 240.

Sumartojo, E., Doll, D., Holtgrave, D., Gayle, H., & Merson, M. (2000), Enriching the mix: Incorporating structural factors into HIV prevention. *AIDS, 14*(Suppl. 1), s1–s2.

Uebel, K. E., Fairall, L. R., Dingie, H. C. J., van Rensburg, D. H., Mollentze, W. F., Bachmann, M. O., . . . Bateman, E. D. (2011). Task shifting and integration of HIV care into primary care in South Africa: The development and content of the streamlining tasks and roles to expand treatment and care for HIV (STRETCH) intervention. *Implementation Science, 6*, 86.

Uebel K. E., Friedland, G., Pawinski, R., & Holst, H. (2004). HAART for hospital health care workers—An innovative program. *South African Medical Journal, 94*, 423–427.

UKZN WHO CC. (2013). Annual Report 2013, University of KwaZulu-Natal World Health Organization Collaborating Center for Nursing and Midwifery Development (Unpublished document). University of KwaZulu-Natal, Durban, South Africa.

Ullah, A. A. (2011). HIV/AIDS-related stigma and discrimination: A study of health care providers in Bangladesh. *Journal of the International Association of Physicians in AIDS Care, 10*(2), 97–104.

UNAIDS. (2010). Combination HIV prevention: Tailoring and coordinating biomedical, behavioral and structural strategies to reduce new HIV infections: A UNAIDS discussion paper. Geneva, Switzerland: Author. Retrieved from http://www.unaids.org/en/media/unaids/contentassets/documents/unaidspublication/2011/20111110_JC2007_Combination_Prevention_paper_en.pdf

UNAIDS. (2012). *UNAIDS Report on the global AIDS epidemic.* Retrieved from http://www.unaids.org/en/media/unaids/contentassets/documents/epidemiology/2012/gr2012/20121120_UNAIDS_Global_Report_2012_with_annexes_en.pdf

UNAIDS. (2013). *UNAIDS Report on the global AIDS epidemic.* Retrieved from http://www.unaids.org/en/media/unaids/contentassets/documents/epidemiology/2013/gr201 3/unaids_global_report_2013_en.pdf

Wantland, D. J., Holzemer, W. L., Moezzi, S., Willard, S., Arudo, J., Kirksey, K. M., . . . Huang, E. (2008). A randomized controlled trial testing the efficacy of an HIV/AIDS symptom management manual. *Journal of Pain and Symptom Management, 36*(3), 235–246. doi:10.1016/j.jpainsymman.2007.10.011

Weiser, S. D., Tuller, D. M., Frongillo, E. A., Senkingu, J., Mukiibi, N., & Bangsberg, D. R. (2010). Food insecurity as a barrier to sustained antiretroviral therapy adherence in Uganda. *PLoS One, 5*(4), e10340.

World Health Organization (WHO). (2007). *Treat train retain. Task shifting: Global recommendations and guidelines.* Geneva, Switzerland: Author. Retrieved from http://www.who.int/healthsystems/task_shifting/en

World Health Organization (WHO). (2013). *Research for universal health coverage.* Geneva, Switzerland: Author. Retrieved from http://apps.who.int/iris/bitstream/10665/85761/2/9789240690837_eng.pdf

Young, E. W., Forti, E., & Preston, D. B. (1996). Rural nurses' use of universal precautions in relation to perceived knowledge of patient's HIV status. *International Journal of Nursing Studies, 33*(3), 249–258.

Zelnick, J., & O'Donnell, M. (2005). The impact of the HIV/AIDS epidemic on hospital nurses in KwaZulu Natal, South Africa: Nurses' perspectives and implications for health policy. *Journal of Public Health Policy, 26*(2), 163–185.

CHAPTER 11

Vulnerable Populations: Ethical Issues in HIV Care

Carol Dawson-Rose and Denise Kelsey Wishner

Nurses must seek approaches toward caregiving that demonstrate ethical behavior when practicing in a system that has been contaminated by colonialism and patriarchy
—Batiste, 2008, p. 497

What does it mean to be vulnerable? The *Merriam-Webster* definition of *vulnerable* is the following: [one who is] easily hurt or harmed physically, mentally, or emotionally; [or is] open to attack, harm, or damage (*Merriam-Webster*, n.d.). From the everyday practice of nurses, globally, vulnerability can be seen in nearly every shape, size, and color of humanity. Many describe the vulnerable populations living among us as the children, the frail elderly, the homeless, the poor, the mentally ill, substance abusers (including injection drug users), prisoners, migrants, lesbian/gay/bisexual/transgender, and those who are forced into occupations that put them at constant risk for violence and disease acquisition, such as sex workers. Regardless of age, universally, women (at least 50% of the population) rank as the gender that experiences the highest degree of vulnerability at some point during their life course (Macklin, 2012). Macklin (2012) states that women and girls are disadvantaged by discrimination that has its roots in their own social and cultural norms. It is because of these disadvantages that the World Health Organization (WHO, n.d.) states that women and girls are increasingly vulnerable to HIV/AIDS (Box 11.1). Because of the WHO emphasis and Dr. Carol Dawson-Rose's global research experiences, we focus this chapter on women, specifically women who are HIV positive, from a global perspective.

Before we proceed, we should clarify that we use Mozambique as the international backdrop, and San Francisco, California, as an example of a high-resource country, although these examples and situations can occur anywhere. We evaluate these issues through an ethical lens that can help guide the practice of the global health (GH) nurse.

For the purpose of this chapter, GH is defined as health concerns that affect people globally and that are not specific to one location or limited to countries outside of our borders.

BOX 11.1 SOCIOCULTURAL FACTORS THAT INCREASE RISK OF CONTRACTING HIV/AIDS IN WOMEN AND GIRLS

The WHO (n.d.) identifies some of the sociocultural factors that place women and girls at higher risk and prevents them from attaining the highest level of health possible (among their own country/culture); they include:

• Unequal power relationship between men and women
• Social norms that decrease education and paid employment opportunities
• An exclusive focus on women's reproductive roles
• Potential or actual experience of physical, sexual, and emotional violence

What do we mean when we think about ethics in the context of a global nursing practice? We are not thinking about the typical acute-care, end-of-life decision making, or the wrenching outpatient decision making related to an unwanted pregnancy. What we are thinking about are values. What does one value? Family, religion, the ability to work, free time, water, honesty, freedom of choice, health, friendship, books, long hugs, and feeling safe are some common values. Write your own values down and hold on to them. Got it? Now tuck them away, you won't need them for this chapter.

The values that a person possesses inform the nurse about what is important to that person (Carter, 2014). An ethical evaluation of a situation requires answering the question: What is the right thing to do, and what is the right reason for doing it? Frequently something that feels ethically or morally wrong brings about a visceral response—the proverbial "pit in the stomach" feeling. In essence, we must consider each ethical challenge through the lens of the other person's values and then help that person determine what is the right thing to do, and what is the justification for doing so? At times, there may be competing values between two people or, in GH, between person and country; this adds an additional valuation for consideration. This process is rarely easy, or quick, in any situation. But when one is immersed into an entirely new culture, it is complicated further, and often difficult to find a resolution that is satisfying to all. As we discuss the informational vignettes that follow we identify some ethically charged issues, situations, or dilemmas for discussion.

The topic of vulnerable populations is coming to the forefront of conversation, especially when we combine vulnerable populations with GH. Country and GH definitions of vulnerable populations range from specific groups of people who exhibit a higher burden of disease to people who are most at risk for acquiring the illnesses that are associated with vulnerability and the vulnerable. When we look at GH and transnational vulnerability, we can become overwhelmed by the global burden of disease and the litany of inequalities that exist in our world today.

In this chapter, we focus on women living with HIV. In so doing, we can illustrate more easily what makes groups of people, and in this case women, vulnerable and then consider vulnerability from a GH perspective using the chronic illness, HIV. The diagnosis of HIV in itself has a propensity for impacting the most vulnerable in any country or global region. We present some examples of situations that make women vulnerable to HIV and, once infected, vulnerable for life, and use a case-based approach to highlight women as a vulnerable population. Next, we turn our focus to identifying the real ethical issues that occurred with each case, which we anticipate will help prepare the new GH nurse for practice in the global environment.

MOZAMBIQUE VIGNETTE #1

The first time Dr. Dawson-Rose went to Mozambique, she spoke with a group of women who were visiting a community-based center where they went to receive the results of their HIV tests. The center was set up to conduct HIV counseling and testing but not HIV treatment or care, per se. There was no other place where these women could go where they felt comfortable discussing their HIV status, concern for their health, their children's health, or to ask about new information, or any new clinics where they could go for the anti-HIV medication that could save their lives. The year was 2006, 20 years since the availability of antiretroviral (ARV) medication to treat HIV in the United States. Thousands of HIV-positive men and women could access medication that would halt the damage HIV was doing to both their bodies and their health. The health care landscape of Mozambique in 2006 was barren compared with higher resource countries. Getting back to the story, the women were interviewed to discuss the program Dawson-Rose was interested in starting in three rural settings in Mozambique, to gauge interest and to see if the program made sense to them. The positive prevention (PP) project was about working with women living with HIV in communities and health care settings to address the prevention needs of those living with HIV (Box 11.2). Prevention refers to the "meaning of prevention needs" for those who are already living with HIV. It is about the concerns and strategies that people living with HIV use to keep from infecting others, their sexual partner, the people they use drugs with, and their children.

The first story is about Mare, a widow who was obviously in a lot of pain. We wanted to ask her the planned "key informant" questions but could not look past the pain she was experiencing. The grant afforded food to be given

BOX 11.2 MOZAMBIQUE PP PROJECT

In 2006, Dr. Dawson-Rose began collaborating with the Ministry of Health and the Centers for Disease Control Global AIDS Program in Mozambique, to adapt, pilot, and implement a national PP strategy to integrate evidence-based HIV behavioral interventions for prevention. Utilizing a U.S. clinic-based model (Dawson-Rose et al., 2010), they adapted the HIV Intervention for Providers for use in rural health centers (Dawson-Rose, Gutin, & Reyes, 2011).

to those who came to be interviewed as a token of gratitude, yet despite the pain Mare was in, she was willing to sustain the interview so she could get the food to feed her six children. She did not have the energy to work or farm. The nurse began asking assessment questions about whether Mare had been to a clinic, seen a medical doctor, or reported her pain to anyone. Mare had been to a clinic three times and had seen a doctor once who told her she had something wrong with her abdomen, but she had to wait for yet another month for an additional examination. Sitting with Mare and the translator, the nurse paused the interview and went searching through her purse to retrieve an over-the-counter (OTC) pain medication. She handed the bottle to Mare and began to give her instructions on how to take the medication. Then in haste, the translator took the bottle of pills away from Mare and told the nurse not to give out pills since patients there did not know how to take them. The GH nurse was stunned by this interaction. The nurse, acting as advocate, started to disagree with the translator and then thought better of it, and waited until Mare left with the food provided to her. Following the interview, a heated debate began with the translator (who, incidentally, was also the executive director for the community partnership) about the importance of honoring the patient's autonomy by allowing her to make her own treatment decisions. Suffice to say neither a happy nor harmonious agreement was reached about whether it was Mare's decision to determine if she was capable of taking the pills offered to her.

Ethics

As you read Vignette #1, were you able to identify anything that could be considered an ethical issue? Read on to see if you identified any of the ethical issues described.

In many resource-limited countries, such as Mozambique, food insecurity is a significant issue, so the token of food that the PP project was able to offer to its participants was extremely valuable; as such, Mare was willing to suffer in pain in order to fulfill her primary value of feeding her family. Resources, such as food and other materials, are sometimes lacking. As a result of diminished resources, women in Mozambique do not necessarily have control of when or with whom they have sexual relations. And when sexual relations occur, there may be condoms available, but that does not guarantee that they will be used, despite the woman's preference. Unfortunately, many women are driven to have sexual relations in exchange for needed resources that will satisfy their survival needs—for example, food or objects to sell in order to get food. This leads to the slippery slope of using sex work as one avenue to acquire vital material resources such as food. This trade-off is not unique to Mozambique, but it was a common story told by the women interviewed as part of this project. In this scenario, to whose value do you believe it was to use condoms? Could this represent an inherent conflict of the government's wanting to treat HIV but not having the resources to provide condoms to prevent HIV?

As you learned in Chapter 4, autonomy is the right to self-determination, which is a priority for most people in the United States. Wishner certainly believes that one would want to make her own medical decisions and maintain the right to accept or refuse treatment; however, what about Mare's lack of protest about not getting the OTC pain meds? The interference of the translator and the lack of protest from Mare, demonstrate (1) that patients in Mozambique are not used to having the luxury of health care self-determination, and (2) that her personal values were not aligned with self-care or self-determination. Mare's priority value in this situation was getting food to feed her family, at the expense of her own physical pain.

Resources That Influence Vulnerability

In Mozambique, in working with both HIV-positive women and health care providers (primarily nurses), we understand the need for HIV medical treatment. Treatment adherence is accepted as an important mechanism for improved health and reduced HIV transmission; however, both groups have repeatedly mentioned food insecurity as perhaps the greatest barrier that people living with HIV face (Cummings et al., 2014). Food insecurity is defined as "having uncertain or limited availability of nutritionally adequate or safe food or the inability to procure food in socially acceptable ways" (Weiser et al., 2009). Women living with HIV and health care staff speak of the link between lack of food and a patient's inability to adhere to ARV medication. The United Nations Development Programme estimates that the majority of individuals in Mozambique are living in poverty (Food and Agriculture Organization [FAO], 2011). Furthermore, the proportion of people in Mozambique who are estimated to be food insecure is over 60%, and is as high as 75% of the population in the southern region of the country (FAO, 2011). In prior research, food insecurity has been strongly associated with low ARV adherence (Kalichman et al., 2011; Weiser et al., 2009), lower viral load suppression, and earlier death from HIV/AIDS (Weiser et al., 2009).

As treatment access increases in Mozambique with government efforts to increase clinical sites, barriers to adherence may become more pronounced. Our data highlight the need for a more systematic effort to understand the role of food insecurity relative to other adherence barriers in this population and the need to examine various approaches to address this issue. Other countries that have documented food insecurity with HIV-positive individuals have implemented small interventions that focus on integrating food or agricultural programs with HIV/AIDS activities. This approach has been promoted by various international organizations including the WHO, the Joint United Nations Program on HIV/AIDS (UNAIDS), and the World Food Program (WFP; Kalichman et al., 2011; WFP, 2003).

Ethics

A final question that remains to be answered is, "Will improving food security improve HIV outcomes?" Given that many HIV-positive people think they cannot take their HIV medications without food, and that the adherence rate drops when they are without food, are we not ethically obligated to ensure that HIV-positive people obtain food to eat so they will adhere to their treatment regimen? So whose responsibility is it to provide adequate food? The United States provides funds to the government of Mozambique so that they can purchase ARV medications. From there on, the responsibility to subsidize food, baby formula, and any other essential needs falls to the government of Mozambique. The government of Mozambique, however, allocates their limited resources based on priorities that may not rank food before medicine at this time of the HIV/AIDS epidemic.

MOZAMBIQUE VIGNETTE #2

Another story from Dr. Dawson-Rose's first visit to Mozambique involves Nyeka, another young woman that was interviewed for the PP program who was pregnant and HIV positive. The interview began by talking to Nyeka about her HIV and her pregnancy and how she felt about having a child at this time in her life. She was excited. Her boyfriend had just started a coveted job working in a mine in South Africa, and they were looking forward to what his new employment would bring to their child. I asked Nyeka if she understood how she could prevent transmitting HIV to her child while she was pregnant. She spoke about the ARV medication she was being given as an enrollee in a program for pregnant women with HIV.

When I asked her about preventing HIV to the baby during and after birth, she said she knew that if she could formula feed the baby, the baby might not get HIV. Obviously, she had been educated that breastfeeding was a risk for HIV transmission. Then she proceeded to ask me if I knew where she could get infant formula, or if I could provide any formula for her baby. Formula was not readily available in Mozambique. Infant formula feeding is the international standardized recommendation for preventing mother-to-child transmission of HIV during the infant period (WHO, n.d.); however, in Mozambique formula was only available in the capital city. In any case, infant formula was too expensive to purchase, and it is rare that a poor HIV-positive women could purchase formula. What do you say to a question like that? With a pit in my stomach, I said the only thing I could, which was no; and then I assumed the nurse-as-educator role and taught her about the latest WHO guidelines on breastfeeding.

Ethics

The reader might find the ethical issue in Nyeka's story a bit more transparent than in the first vignette. The U.S. government sends researchers to Mozambique to learn how to prevent the transmission of HIV, and we know how to prevent transmission of HIV to infants (WHO, n.d.). However, despite the strong evidence that HIV transmission is eliminated if a baby is not breastfed, mothers in low-resource settings are often not given any other feeding option but to breastfeed. This is an example of the ethical conundrums that, in your GH nursing practice, you may encounter many times.

Let's break this down ethically using the principles taught in Chapter 4. Nyeka's value is that it would be beneficial for her child to receive formula to prevent acquisition of HIV through breast milk. The competing value comes from the government—there are limited financial resources, which limits the government's ability to supply both formula and ARV medications. So the government evaluates its resources and options and chooses the option that they believe will have the greatest benefit for the greatest number. The role of public health ethics is to determine which health inequalities are the most egregious and then to make decisions as to where the health care resource priorities should be focused (Macklin, 2012). In the previous example, the priority is supplying more people with ARV medications (including ARV meds for the prevention of vertical transmission of HIV to unborn children) over preventing infant transmission of HIV by supplying infant formula. There is one other competing value that we have yet to consider: There is a moral concern for the health of children as a helpless vulnerable population dependent on the decisions of others for their well-being (Macklin, 2012; Schouten et al., 2011). This becomes a social justice issue, perhaps an international justice issue, one beyond the scope of this chapter's discussion.

Mozambique Postscripts

Nyeka delivered a baby girl 3 months after our interview, and her child, Cibele, remains HIV uninfected. Mare's story did not end so happily. She died 6 weeks after the interview, without being seen at the clinic again. It was suspected that Mare's severe abdominal pain was caused by uterine cancer. Neighbors in Mare's village are now raising her six children.

During the subsequent 3 years that Dr. Dawson-Rose was working with the rural community groups of men and women with HIV in Mozambique, she ran into Nyeka, who appeared to be pregnant again. Nyeka had obtained a small cleaning job at the community center; because of her very thin body habitus, it was obvious that she was pregnant. When I asked her if she was expecting, she responded "yes" and immediately began apologizing, saying, "We could not always find condoms, and then the condoms didn't always work." Finally, she added, "I know I shouldn't have become pregnant again." My comments were meant to be congratulatory, as she had said she wanted more children, but instead she acted as if I were shaming her. We then spoke for a bit about her health related to HIV. What was most striking about this interaction was the shame Nyeka expressed for being pregnant and perhaps feeling that she was "going against nursing advice." The clinic "nurses" in Mozambique believe and preach that woman who are HIV positive should not be having sexual intercourse without condoms nor should they be having additional children. Nyeka's response was an example of feeling stigmatized for being pregnant while having HIV, as well as the result of the clinic nurses' shaming her. I suspect she had been prey to these judgments time and again from her health care providers who could not check their own personal values at the door. Recall the exercise we went through at the beginning of this chapter? As humans, we are fallible, and no one person has the right to impose her or his own values (judgment or shame) upon another just because she or he does agree with that person's decisions. In order to deliver beneficial care to our patients, we need to enlist their trust and provide a safe harbor in which our caring relationship and dialogue can grow. Having a good understanding of our personal values allows us to separate them from the values of those for whom we care, which facilitates a trusting relationship.

MOVING ON

The story of the HIV epidemic and how this disease is impacting the lives of women is currently being written. Women are the majority of people living with HIV globally, and the number continues to increase. This increase is occurring disproportionately in groups of vulnerable women, as the next story demonstrates.

The U.S. story we want to tell is about a study Dr. Dawson-Rose conducted with a group of HIV-positive women drug users who were living in a single room occupancy hotel in San Francisco, California. The hotel for this research study also provided on-site hospice/home care for HIV-positive individuals, including some of the women who participated in this study. The aim of this research study was to understand more about the women who were living and receiving HIV care or care for HIV-related conditions in this hotel (Adih, Campsmith, Williams, Hardnett, & Hughes, 2011). From my observations (CD-R), the women in the hotel were living with multiple stigmatized conditions: They were actively using drugs; they made money through sex work; they were poor; they had been homeless; and they were HIV positive. Considering all of these factors I felt sure that these women could provide narratives about how they had experienced health care for HIV-related conditions. Specifically, I wanted to know about any experiences with discrimination that they had encountered. I had witnessed some of this discrimination, so I believed their claims to be true. These disadvantaged women are frequently not believed, and further, they feel punished by their health care providers because of who they are and how they have to live.

Some of the literature on HIV and women has focused on the unique experiences of women—the victimization and vulnerability—without mention of the social and structural relationships that may contribute to the lived experience of women. Additionally, the positive aspects of living with HIV infection for women, specifically for poor or drug-addicted women, is not well described in the literature. The study discussed here was a qualitative study utilizing ethnographic methods. Through the stories from the interviews of seven women and from observations over a 5-month time period, I saw a broader picture emerge than I anticipated based on my initial questions. I learned about the hotel and what happened there, the relationships, the drug use, the money issues, the participants' former and current lives, experiences of loss, and the vulnerability of these women.

When I first started this study I took field notes on whatever I saw, for example, what the participants were wearing and whether or not they looked like they belonged in this hotel. In other words, I would try to discern whether I could tell this person lived there or whether this person was so put together that I would have never thought that she lived in the hotel; many of my descriptions of the hotel focused on the chaotic environment. Depending on the time of the month and who had money and who was around, I noticed the changing mood of the hotel and its wide swings toward chaos in one form or another. As I was encouraged to describe more than just the superficial chaos, I began focusing on the entire environment of the hotel.

The following paragraphs from my early field notes illustrate the chaos and disorder of the hotel.

On going down the stairs, two flights, I am trying to be more aware and vivid in my description of the environment. There is a man mopping the hallways with a strong smell of bleach mixed with urine. On the stairs there is a carpet, a very dirty carpet that used to have a flower pattern. Today I notice the cockroaches on the carpet. They are not even hiding just crawling everywhere your foot touches. On Friday, I wanted to see Julie, who was a woman I had asked to participate in the study, but when I went to her room down the hall, no one answered the door. Sam, the nurse, came in, and I told him I could not find Julie. [H]e said maybe she is at the clinic getting her methadone. He needed to call the hospital and see if they had taken her off the detox program and put her on methadone maintenance. Sam then went down to Julie's room, and when he came back, he said she wasn't there and gave me a passkey, so I knocked and then let myself into her room. He said there is a pile of [expletive] in her sink. I said what kind of [expletive]. He said literally a pile of [expletive]. He said there is a bedside commode in her room but the bucket was not in it. And Sam said, I thought her diarrhea was under control.

About a half hour later, Julie came by the nurse's office, and she was visibly happy. She said, "They put me back on methadone maintenance." The nurse congratulated her. Julie is a small woman and very emaciated; she is about 5'2"and looks like she weighs less than 90 pounds. She is White, has dark brown hair, and her skin color appears pale gray. She has on a sweatshirt, pants, and slippers. She is carrying a tray of food that she picked up in the office next door [part of the social services available at the hotel]. [S]he asks if she can get her pills. Sam asked her how her diarrhea was, and she said it was better. He said, "[W]ell, are you using the bedside commode?" [S]he said, "No, I am going down the hall to the bathroom." He tells her that he went down to her room, knocked and announced himself, and then let himself in with the passkey because he didn't know if she was all right. He asked her if she minded him doing this. She said no and asked if there was anyone in there when he went in. He said no.

She said, "[W]ell, there was a guy there that I let spend the night with me last night and I'm glad he is gone." Sam said he was gone and then said, "and he left you a present," and told her about the [expletive] in the sink. She said, "[O]h well, he wasn't that good of a friend, and I guess I won't be letting him stay anymore."

Another woman I had interviewed was named Sheila... whose husband had just died a few days prior. She was staying in his hotel room until the end of the month because the rent was paid. I walked up the flights of stairs to her door. I knocked on her door, and she opened it... part way. The room is very dark; a TV is on, and I can see the arm and leg of a man on the bed. Sheila is a young White woman with blonde hair pulled into a ponytail and has eyes that are off center on her face. She also has several missing front teeth. I tell her about the study. She starts talking and says this is not a good time, that she is trying to arrange the funeral and everything because her old man died three days ago. [S]he didn't know if I knew. I said I knew, and that I was sorry about him dying. She said, "[Y]eah, I have to get things straightened out, but I will talk to you sometime."

I went back downstairs, and Sam asked me what Sheila had to say. I told him that she had someone in her room. He asked who it was and I said I didn't know. I had just seen his arm and leg. He said, "Sheila is only 23 and we are trying to get her into a drug treatment program or something before she gets hooked up with another abusive dope fiend that beats the [expletive] out of her... that's why I wanted to know who was in her room." The other nurse tells me that she has actually been doing better since her husband was hospitalized 3 weeks before his death. And that she thought he had been injecting Sheila (with heroin), which Sheila could not do on her own or without his help, so now she is trying to stop using.

I asked another woman I interviewed about what the hotel meant to her, "I met Miss Bunny, and I stayed with her off and on for years. We was good friends like Miss Lola across the hall. We were good friends. Both of them died from AIDS. When Miss Bunny died I was out on the streets, real messed up, and I had full-blown AIDS. My friend Miss Rene found me and made me get cleaned up and tested for HIV. It took a while. I stayed out on the streets but finally I went home with her to try and get straightened around, and I got tested for HIV. When I got tested everything changed. I got a diagnosis, I got the paper work to get disability for having AIDS, and I got a place to live here at the hotel. I have been here one and a half years. I am trying to take care of my health, and I get a lot of services from the nurses...I have friends here. One of the things I get from them every day is food."

I hope from these field notes you can get a picture of what life was like for these HIV-positive women living in the hotel, the environment, and some of the conditions of the hotel, in general. I will tell you what I thought: Women live like this?

It is disgusting and unacceptable that women with HIV live in these conditions literally a block from one of the most exclusive areas of California and in a wealthy American city such as San Francisco.

Ethics

Justice is the ethical principle that comes to mind as I (DKW) read these excerpted field notes. Justice is about an equal distribution of scarce resources among equals. Given the living conditions previously described, do you feel that resources have been equally distributed among people living under these same circumstances? Justice can be examined on several levels: resources, social, materials. It seems these residents missed out on all of these three levels of justice.

Individual beneficence, the duty to do good for others, is demonstrated by the presence of the hotel, those who work there, and the benefits (food) provided to its residents. This beneficence allows the residents a certain level of autonomy that comes with having a secure place to stay, which may allow them the opportunity to make their own life choices, in essence allowing them some autonomy (self-determination).

WOMEN LIVING WITH HIV

According to UNAIDS (Joint UN Program on HIV/AIDS, 2013), 52% of people living with HIV/AIDS worldwide are women. In sub-Saharan Africa, women account for over 57 % of all the people living with HIV (Box 11.3). In other countries, such as the United States, the proportion of HIV cases affecting women, while still low when compared with other groups (e.g., men who have sex with men), is increasing (Centers for Disease Control and Prevention [CDC], 2014). Globally, women bear a disproportionate impact of HIV.

In Mozambique, similar to other countries with limited resources for health, there are an estimated 130,000 new HIV infections annually, and women are significantly impacted. The national prevalence of HIV is 11.5% among adults aged

---

BOX 11.3 FACTORS LEADING TO INCREASED VULNERABILITY IN WOMEN LIVING WITH HIV

Women living with HIV have a number of co-occurring conditions that lead to a considerable amount of suffering and increase their vulnerability. These conditions include high rates of stigma (Sengupta, Banks, Jonas, Miles, & Smith, 2011; Vanable, Carey, Blair, & Littlewood, 2006), social isolation (Machtinger, Wilson, Haberer, & Weiss, 2012), depression (Bing et al., 2001; Tsao, Dobalian, Moreau, & Dobalian, 2004), trauma and PTSD (Machtinger et al., 2012), and substance abuse (Bing et al., 2001; Machtinger et al., 2012). Increasingly, the term "syndemic" has been used to describe the high rates of co-occurring HIV, gender-based violence, substance abuse, and mental illness in this population (Meyer, Springer, & Altice, 2011).

15 to 49 years. In some of the hardest hit provinces, the group prevalence rates are as high as 25.1%. The government of Mozambique Ministry of Health (MoH) has done much to stem this epidemic, but the continued high prevalence rates demonstrate the need for additional prevention strategies to effectively reduce HIV transmission. The scale-up of HIV care and treatment in Mozambique has created an opportunity to give priority to people living with HIV by providing prevention interventions within HIV care and treatment settings.

In the United States, more than three quarters (79%) of U.S. women diagnosed with HIV/AIDS in 2010 were either African American or Latina (CDC, 2014); African American and Latina women represent approximately 30% of the U.S. population (United States Census Bureau [U.S. Census], 2014). And while often overlooked, Asian Pacific Islanders are also impacted. A recent study by Adih et al. (2011) demonstrated a statistically significant increase in the incidence of Asian Pacific Islanders diagnosed with HIV/AIDS.

Transgender women also represent a highly vulnerable group of women globally. The term *transgender women* refers to people whose current gender identity or expression is in discordance with their assigned gender at birth. Although data are lacking regarding the proportion of people who identify as transgender women globally, a conservative estimate of 0.3% of U.S. adults, approximately 1 million people, identify as transgender (Conway, 2002). Global estimates suggest that transgender women are 48% more likely to acquire HIV when compared to other women across racial and socioeconomic groups (Baral et al., 2013). As noted earlier, many issues place women in a vulnerable position to acquire HIV (Grown, Gupta, & Pande, 2005). Once infected, women living with HIV continue to be vulnerable in many other aspects of their lives.

CONCLUSIONS

It is certainly clear that most of us would find the examples described in this chapter to be situations in which we would not like to live. Furthermore, we certainly would never want to live in a country where the choice of whether we are receiving needed medicine or the food to keep us alive is not within our control. But these are the realities within which the people who make up the global vulnerable populations continue to exist. In order to prepare to be a GH nurse working in trying circumstances such as poverty, starvation, and rampant disease, it is important to understand your own values and separate them from those who you will serve as you begin this honorable path in your career. When working with patients from different cultures across the globe, it is important to understand and respect the values of the patient (and country) where you are working and to be able to place those values paramount to your own personal values during your work.

As this chapter has demonstrated by using an exemplar of HIV-positive women, vulnerable populations exist both within and outside the United States. Shifting our view to consider ethics when we approach new populations or groups of people provides us with the opportunity to consider not only what makes people vulnerable but also how we can help them while preserving their values. In both low-resource and high-resource countries worldwide, HIV-positive women are considered vulnerable. Reasons for vulnerability may include stigma, victimization, mental illness, migration, limited access to needed health care or food, or substance use (Meyer et al., 2011). Evidence suggests that mainstream systems of health care that currently deliver essential services to vulnerable populations in settings where there is a high prevalence of HIV need to increase their capacity to address ethical issues. Nurses and the discipline of nursing's interest in GH and international settings represent opportunities to integrate ethical concepts into the care we deliver in various settings and where we encounter vulnerable populations.

We hope we have provided opportunities for nurses to examine the situational ethics and to begin to adopt an ethical approach to the work done with vulnerable populations in GH. A grounding in ethical approaches to nursing care that are only U.S.-centric, together with constraints in resource-limited environments, can result in unintended adverse consequences for the people for whom we provide care. However, these same constraints allow us the opportunity as nurses to engage in our own values assessment when caring for vulnerable populations and to realign our nursing care with what is needed. Sometimes the results of a values assessment will mean putting our personal values in our pocket in order to deliver the individualized patient- and family-centered nursing care that is the bedrock of our profession.

By looking through an ethical lens, we are more able to understand and to try to make sense of the human rights violations of vulnerable populations that we believe to be morally wrong. As we stated earlier, vulnerable populations are more at risk for HIV acquisition and decreased access to care. As leaders in GH delivery and as nurses, we must always be mindful of what our role is in these situations.

REFERENCES

Adih, W. K., Campsmith, M., Willaims, C. L., Hardnett, F. P., & Hughes, D. (2011). Epidemiology of HIV among Asians and Pacific Islanders in the United States, 2001–2008. *Journal of the International Association of Physician in AIDS Care, 10*(3), 150–159. Retrieved from http://dx.doi.org/10.1177/1545109711399805

Baral, S. D., Poteat, T., Stromdahl, S., Wirtz, A. L., Guadamuz, T. E., & Beyrer, C. (2013). Worldwide burden of HIV in transgender women: A systemic review and meta-analysis. *Lancet, 13*(3), 214–222. Retrieved from http://dx.doi.org/10.1016/s1473-3099(12)70315-8

Batiste, M. (2008). Research ethics for protecting indigenous knowledge and heritage: Institutional and research responsibilities. In N. K. Denzin, Y. S. Lincoln, & L. Tuhiwai (Eds.), *Handbook of critical and indigenous methodologies* (pp. 497–510). London, UK: Sage.

Bing, E. G., Burnam, M. A., Longshore, D., Fleishman, J. A., Sherbourne, C. D., London, A. S., . . . Shapiro, M. (2001, August). Psychiatric disorders and drug use among human immunodeficiency virus-infected adults in the United States. *Archives of General Psychiatry, 58*, 721–728.

Carter, S. M. (2014, April). Health promotion: An ethical analysis. *Health Promotion Journal of Australia, 25,* 19–24.

Centers for Disease Control and Prevention. (2014). *HIV among women.* Retrieved from www.cdc.gov/hiv/risk/gender/women/facta/index/html

Conway, L. (2002). *How frequently does transsexualism occur?* Retrieved from http://www.conseil-lgbt.ca/wp-content/uploads/2013/12/How-Frequently-Does-Transsexualism-Occur.pdf

Cummings, B., Gutin, S. A., Jaiantilal, P., Correia, D., Malimane, I., & Dawson-Rose, C. S. (2014). The role of social support among people living with HIV in rural Mozambique. *AIDS Patient Care and STDs, 28*(11), 602-612.

Dawson-Rose, C. S., Courtenay-Quirk, C., Knight, K., Shade, S., Vittinghoff, E., Gomez, C., . . . Colfax, G. (2010, December). HIV intervention for providers study: A randomized controlled trial of a clinician-delivered HIV risk-reduction intervention for HIV-positive people. *Journal of Acquired Immune Deficiency Syndrome, 55,* 572–581.

Dawson-Rose, C. S., Gutin, S. A., & Reyes, M. (2011). Adapting positive prevention interventions for international settings: Applying U.S. evidence to epidemics in developing countries. *Journal of the Association of Nurses in AIDS Care, 22,* 38–52.

Food and Agriculture Organization (FAO). (2011). *Nutrition country profile: Republic of Mozambique.* Retrieved from http://www.fao.org/countryprofiles/index/en/?iso3=MOZ

Grown, C., Gupta, G. R., & Pande, R. (2005). Tak-ing action to improve women's health through gender equality and women's empowerment. *Lancet, 365,* 541–543.

Joint United Nations Program on HIV/AIDS (UNAIDS). (2013). *Global Report UNAIDS report on the global AIDS epidemic 2013.* Retrieved from http://www.unaids.org/en/media/unaids/contentassets/documents/epidemiology/2013/gr2013/UNAIDS_Global_Report_2013_en.pdf

Kalichman, S. C., Pellowski, J., Kalichman, M. O., Cherry, C., Deterio, M., Caliendo, A. M., & Schinazi, R. F. (2011). Food insufficiency and medication adherence among people living with HIV/AIDS in urban and peri-urban settings. *Prevention science: The Official Journal of the Society for Prevention Research, 12,* 324–332.

Machtinger, E. L., Wilson, T. C., Haberer, J. E., & Weiss, D. S. (2012, November). Psychological trauma and PTSD in HIV-positive women: A meta-analysis. *AIDS Behavior, 16*(8), 2091–2100. Retrieved from http://dx.doi.org/10.1007/s10461-011-0127-4

Macklin, R. (2012). *Ethics in global health: Research, policy, and practice.* New York, NY: Oxford.

Merriam-Webster Dictionary Online. (n.d.). Retrieved from http://www.merriam-webster.com/dictionary/vulnerable

Meyer, J. P., Springer, S. A., & Altice, F. L. (2011, July). Substance abuse, violence, and HIV in women: A literature review of the syndemic. *Journal of Women's Health, 20,* 991–1006. Retrieved from http://dx.doi.org/10.1089/jwh.2010.2328

Schouten, E. J., Jahn, A., Midiani, D., Makombe, S. D., Mnthambala, A., Chirwa, Z., . . . Chimbwandira, F. (2011). Prevention of mother-to-child transmission of HIV and the health-related Millennium Development Goals: Time for a public health approach. *The Lancet, 378,* 282–284.

Sengupta, S., Banks, B., Jonas, D., Miles, M. S., & Smith, G. C. (2011, August 15). HIV interventions to reduce HIV/AIDS stigma: A systematic review. *AIDS Behavior, 6,* 1075–1087.

Tsao, J. C., Dobalian, A., Moreau, C., & Dobalian, K. (2004, February). Stability of anxiety and depression in a national sample of adults with human immunodeficiency virus. *Journal of Nervous and Mental Disorders, 192,* 111–118.

United States Census Bureau. (2014). *Population estimates program*. Retrieved from http://quickfacts.census.gov/qfd/meta/long_PST045213.htm

Vanable, P. A., Carey, M. P., Blair, D. C., & Littlewood, R. A. (2006, September). Impact of HIV-related stigma on health behaviors and psychological adjustment among HIV-positive men and women. *AIDS Behavior, 10*, 473–482.

Weiser, S. D., Fernandes, K. A., Brandson, E. K., Lima, V. D., Anema, A., Bangsberg, D. R., . . . Hogg, R. S. (2009). The association between food insecurity and mortality among HIV-infected individuals on HAART. *Journal of Acquired Immune Deficiency Syndrome, 52*, 342–349.

World Food Program. (2003). *Programming in the era of AIDS: WFPs response to HIV/AIDS*. Geneva, Switzerland: Author.

World Health Organization. (n.d.). *Women's health*. Retrieved from http://www.who.int/topics/womens_health/en

The Role of Midwives and Nurses in Reducing Global Maternal Mortality Around the World and in Haiti

Erin George

*E*very year, hundreds of thousands of preventable deaths of women and girls during pregnancy and childbirth occur as the appalling result of limited access to health services and resources, especially in poor countries. Midwives and nurses are critical to the reduction of maternal mortality, providing crucial access to reproductive health services, often serving as the only health care workers serving marginalized communities. This chapter provides an overview of the current state of global maternal mortality rates and explores the causes of maternal mortality through a gender equity and women's rights perspective. It also offers a review of midwifery and nursing efforts to eliminate maternal mortality around the globe and a case study of midwifery, nursing, and maternal mortality in Haiti.

MATERNAL MORTALITY: AN OVERVIEW

The deaths of women and girls during pregnancy and childbirth disproportionately occur in resource-limited settings. In 2013, the World Health Organization (WHO, 2014) estimated 289,000 women died during pregnancy or childbirth. This number translates into a maternal mortality ratio (MMR), or number of maternal deaths per 100,000 live births, of 210 deaths per 100,000 live births (WHO, 2013b). Approximately 99% of these maternal deaths occur in developing countries (WHO, 2012). The MMR is far higher in low-income countries, where 410 women die as a result of pregnancy or childbirth per 100,000 live births. This ratio is highest in sub-Saharan Africa, a region that experienced 500 deaths per 100,000 live births (United Nations [UN], 2013). A country is considered to have a high MMR if the MMR is equal to or greater than 300 maternal deaths and an extremely high MMR if the MMR is equal to or greater than 1,000 maternal deaths per 100,000 live births. In 2013, WHO (2014) indicated that Sierra Leone had the highest MMR in the world: 1,100 maternal deaths per 100,000 live births. The two countries that accounted for one third of all maternal deaths were India and Nigeria; sub-Saharan Africa accounted for 62% of global maternal deaths (WHO, 2014).

In high-income countries, women and girls die at a rate of 14 deaths per 100,000 live births (WHO, 2013b). This figure is nearly 1/25th the average MMR present in low-income countries. The vastly lower MMR in high-income countries is directly related to the availability of functional and accessible health care services provided by well-trained health personnel. WHO attributes low maternal mortality rates to several advances: increased use of contraception to delay and limit childbearing, access to high-quality health care, and socioeconomic and political gains of women in areas such as political representation and higher education (WHO, 2009). These advances have slowed dramatically in low-income countries, where maternal deaths occur in tragically astronomical numbers. The most recent worldwide effort to reduce global maternal mortality and foster the political, social, and economic wills of countries to end such disparities in maternal deaths is the pursuit of the Millennium Development Goals (MDGs).

Monitoring Worldwide Progress on Reducing Maternal Mortality: MDG 5

In 2000, nearly 200 world leaders gathered at the UN Millennium Summit to discuss solutions to eradicate poverty and to address the inequities that cause deleterious health outcomes for people living in poor countries around the globe. From the summit came the MDGs, a set of eight goals that, if achieved, could significantly reduce illness and death in low- and middle-income countries (UN Millennium Development Project, 2006). Each MDG has target outcomes to attain by 2015 as a way of measuring time-bound progress toward the eight goals (see Table 12.1 for a complete list of MDGs and their targets).

The MDGs are lauded for guiding a straightforward global agenda that has galvanized political and economic support from donor nations, multilateral organizations, private foundations, and others for achieving their targets. They have also come under criticism for failing to include priorities of less politically and economically powerful countries in the articulation of the goals and to oversimplifying complex global problems (UN System Task Team on the Post-2015 Development Agenda, 2012). Despite the legitimate criticisms of the MDGs, the MDG agenda sparked a new age of attempting to align worldwide global health priorities across continents, governments, and communities. The MDGs have "helped generate support, in high-income countries as in many of those in which poverty and disruption make such goals a matter of urgency, for more ambitious agendas in global health and development" (Farmer et al., 2013). The MDG agenda endures as an unprecedented attempt to better the lives of millions of people living in poverty worldwide.

One of these goals, MDG 5, specifically seeks to improve global maternal health. MDG 5 has two chief aims to accomplish by 2015: to reduce worldwide maternal mortality by 75% and to provide universal access to reproductive health

TABLE 12.1 Official List of Millennium Development Goal (MDG) Indicators

GOALS AND TARGETS (FROM THE MILLENNIUM DECLARATION)	INDICATORS FOR MONITORING PROGRESS
Goal 1: Eradicate extreme poverty and hunger	
Target 1.A: Halve, between 1990 and 2015, the proportion of people whose income is less than $1 a day	1.1 Proportion of population below $1 (PPP) per day[1] 1.2 Poverty gap ratio 1.3 Share of poorest quintile in national consumption
Target 1.B: Achieve full and productive employment and decent work for all, including women and young people	1.4 Growth rate of GDP per person employed 1.5 Employment-to-population ratio 1.6 Proportion of employed people living below $1 (PPP) per day 1.7 Proportion of own-account and contributing family workers in total employment
Target 1.C: Halve, between 1990 and 2015, the proportion of people who suffer from hunger	1.8 Prevalence of underweight children younger than 5 years of age 1.9 Proportion of population below minimum level of dietary energy consumption
Goal 2: Achieve universal primary education	
Target 2.A: Ensure that, by 2015, children everywhere, boys and girls alike, will be able to complete a full course of primary schooling	2.1 Net enrollment ratio in primary education 2.2 Proportion of pupils starting grade 1 who reach last grade of primary 2.3 Literacy rate of 15- to 24-year-old women and men
Goal 3: Promote gender equality and empower women	
Target 3.A: Eliminate gender disparity in primary and secondary education, preferably by 2005, and in all levels of education no later than 2015	3.1 Ratios of girls to boys in primary, secondary, and tertiary education 3.2 Share of women in wage employment in the nonagricultural sector 3.3 Proportion of seats held by women in national parliament
Goal 4: Reduce child mortality	
Target 4.A: Reduce by two thirds, between 1990 and 2015, the under-5 mortality rate	4.1 Under-5 mortality rate 4.2 Infant mortality rate 4.3 Proportion of 1-year-old children immunized against measles
Goal 5: Improve maternal health	
Target 5.A: Reduce by three quarters, between 1990 and 2015, the MMR	5.1 Maternal mortality ratio 5.2 Proportion of births attended by skilled health personnel

(continued)

TABLE 12.1 Official List of Millennium Development Goal (MDG) Indicators (*continued*)

GOALS AND TARGETS (FROM THE MILLENNIUM DECLARATION)	INDICATORS FOR MONITORING PROGRESS
Target 5.B: Achieve, by 2015, universal access to reproductive health	5.3 Contraceptive prevalence rate 5.4 Adolescent birth rate 5.5 Antenatal care coverage (at least one visit and at least four visits) 5.6 Unmet need for family planning
Goal 6: Combat HIV/AIDS, malaria, and other diseases	
Target 6.A: Have halted by 2015 and begun to reverse the spread of HIV/AIDS	6.1 HIV prevalence among population aged 15 to 24 years 6.2 Condom use to avoid getting HIV during last high-risk sex 6.3 Proportion of population aged 15 to 24 years with comprehensive correct knowledge of HIV/AIDS 6.4 Ratio of school attendance of orphans to school attendance of nonorphans aged 10 to 14 years
Target 6.B: Achieve, by 2010, universal access to treatment for HIV/AIDS for all those who need it	6.5 Proportion of population with advanced HIV infection with access to antiretroviral drugs
Target 6.C: Have halted by 2015 and begun to reverse the incidence of malaria and other major diseases	6.6 Incidence and death rates associated with malaria 6.7 Proportion of children younger than 5 sleeping under insecticide-treated bednets 6.8 Proportion of children younger than 5 with fever who are treated with appropriate antimalarial drugs 6.9 Incidence, prevalence, and death rates associated with tuberculosis 6.10 Proportion of tuberculosis cases detected and cured under directly observed treatment short course
Goal 7: Ensure environmental sustainability	
Target 7.A: Integrate the principles of sustainable development into country policies and programs and reverse the loss of environmental resources	7.1 Proportion of land area covered by forest 7.2 CO_2 emissions, total, per capita and per $1 GDP (PPP)
Target 7.B: Reduce biodiversity loss, achieving, by 2010, a significant reduction in the rate of loss	7.3 Consumption of ozone-depleting substances 7.4 Proportion of fish stocks within safe biological limits 7.5 Proportion of total water resources used 7.6 Proportion of terrestrial and marine areas protected 7.7 Proportion of species threatened with extinction

TABLE 12.1 Official List of Millennium Development Goal (MDG) Indicators (*continued*)

GOALS AND TARGETS (FROM THE MILLENNIUM DECLARATION)	INDICATORS FOR MONITORING PROGRESS
Target 7.C: Halve, by 2015, the proportion of people without sustainable access to safe drinking water and basic sanitation	7.8 Proportion of population using an improved drinking water source 7.9 Proportion of population using an improved sanitation facility
Target 7.D: By 2020, to have achieved a significant improvement in the lives of at least 100 million slum dwellers	7.10 Proportion of urban population living in slums[2]
Goal 8: Develop a global partnership for development	
Target 8.A: Develop further an open, rule-based, predictable, nondiscriminatory trading and financial system Includes a commitment to good governance, development, and poverty reduction, both nationally and internationally	*Some of the indicators listed here are monitored separately for the least developed countries (LDCs), Africa, landlocked developing countries, and small island developing states.* Official development assistance (ODA)
Target 8.B: Address the special needs of the least-developed countries Includes tariff- and quota-free access for the least-developed countries' exports; enhanced program of debt relief for HIPC and cancellation of official bilateral debt; and more generous ODA for countries committed to poverty reduction	8.1 Net ODA, total and to the least-developed countries, as percentage of OECD/DAC donors' gross national income 8.2 Proportion of total bilateral, sector-allocable ODA of OECD/DAC donors to basic social services (basic education, primary health care, nutrition, safe water and sanitation) 8.3 Proportion of bilateral official development assistance of OECD/DAC donors that is untied
Target 8.C: Address the special needs of landlocked developing countries and small island developing states (through the Program of Action for the Sustainable Development of Small Island Developing States and the outcome of the 20-second special session of the General Assembly) Target 8.D: Deal comprehensively with the debt problems of developing countries through national and international measures in order to make debt sustainable in the long term	8.4 ODA received in landlocked developing countries as a proportion of their gross national incomes 8.5 ODA received in small island developing States as a proportion of their gross national incomes Market access 8.6 Proportion of total developed country imports (by value and excluding arms) from developing countries and least-developed countries admitted free of duty 8.7 Average tariffs imposed by developed countries on agricultural products and textiles and clothing from developing countries 8.8 Agricultural support estimate for OECD countries as a percentage of their gross domestic product 8.9 Proportion of ODA provided to help build trade capacity

(continued)

TABLE 12.1 Official List of Millennium Development Goal (MDG) Indicators (*continued*)

GOALS AND TARGETS (FROM THE MILLENNIUM DECLARATION)	INDICATORS FOR MONITORING PROGRESS
	Debt sustainability
	8.10 Total number of countries that have reached their HIPC decision points and number that have reached their HIPC completion points (cumulative)
	8.11 Debt relief committed under HIPC and MDRI Initiatives
	8.12 Debt service as a percentage of exports of goods and services
Target 8.E: In cooperation with pharmaceutical companies, provide access to affordable essential drugs in developing countries	8.13 Proportion of population with access to affordable essential drugs on a sustainable basis
Target 8.F: In cooperation with the private sector, make available the benefits of new technologies, especially information and communications	8.14 Fixed telephone lines per 100 inhabitants
	8.15 Mobile cellular subscriptions per 100 inhabitants
	8.16 Internet users per 100 inhabitants

DAC, development assistance committee; HIPC, heavily indebted poor countries; MDRI, Multilateral Debt Relief Initiative; MMR, maternal mortality ratio; ODA, official development assistance; OECD, Organization for Economic Cooperation and Development.

Notes: [1] For monitoring country poverty trends, indicators based on national poverty lines should be used, where available.

[2] The actual proportion of people living in slums is measured by a proxy, represented by the urban population living in households with at least one of the four characteristics: (a) lack of access to improved water supply; (b) lack of access to improved sanitation; (c) overcrowding (three or more persons per room); and (d) dwellings made of nondurable material.

services. There are six indicators used to monitor progress toward MDG 5, including the measurement of the MMR by country, the proportion of births attended by skilled health personnel, and the rate of contraceptive prevalence among women of reproductive age (see Table 12.1 for a complete list and description of the MDG 5 indicators). Since 1990, the world has experienced a 47% reduction in maternal deaths, a significant amount of progress toward the goal of decreasing the MMR by 75%. The proportion of births where a skilled birth attendant—defined by the United Nations as a nurse, midwife, or doctor with skills to care for women during pregnancy and childbirth—is present rose by 11% by 2011, to 66% of births worldwide (UN, 2013). In women of reproductive age (ages 15 to 49) 63% were using some form of contraception in 2010, compared with 54.8% in 1990 (Alkema, Kantorova, Menozzi, & Biddlecom, 2013).

While there is much progress to celebrate among the MDG 5 targets, the goals set forth in 2000 will not be met by 2015 across much of the globe. Several countries are on track to meet the MDG 5 goals, but most have many years or even decades before they will be within reach of achieving MDG 5 and beyond. In sub-Saharan

Africa, only Rwanda is on track to meet its MDG 5 goals. The poorest regions of the world are unlikely to meet MDG 5 until the year 2040 or later. In these regions, where women are burdened by the highest rates of maternal mortality, there exists the least amount of progress toward reducing the incidence of maternal mortality (WHO, 2012).

Why Women Die: Gender Equity, Women's Rights, and Maternal Mortality

To understand why women die in pregnancy and childbirth, it is first important to consider how the political, economic, and social standing of girls and women is inextricably linked to maternal survival. The countries where women experience the highest risk of dying in pregnancy and childbirth also struggle with equitable political representation, access to education, and fair-paying jobs for women (WHO, 2009). On average, only 20% of the members of the world's parliaments are women. Fewer girls attend primary school than boys, a gap that grows wider in secondary school and at university levels. Women hold 40% of wage-earning jobs, and continue to earn less on average than men for similar work (UN, 2013). When girls and women lack power and resources, they are less likely to be able to access and advocate for health care services necessary for safe pregnancy and childbirth (Paruzzolo, Mehra, Kes, & Ashbaugh, 2010). In resource-poor settings, where the provision of health care services is limited by chronic shortages of health care personnel, essential medicines, and medical equipment, women become exponentially more vulnerable to dying in pregnancy and childbirth (Mukherjee et al., 2011; WHO, 2009).

So critical is the plight of gender equality for women that there is a separate MDG devoted to monitoring global progress toward promoting gender equality and empowering women around the world, MDG 3 (see Table 12.1). Two direct consequences of poverty, inequity, and lack of power for women that impact their risk of dying during pregnancy and childbirth are child marriage and violence against women. Millions of girls around the world are married as children and teenagers, often as a way for their families to earn money. Child marriages dramatically contribute to the rates of adolescent pregnancy worldwide, where 95% of all adolescent pregnancies occur in developing countries and 19% of women in developing countries become pregnant before the age of 18. Pregnancy during adolescence comes with increased risks of complications that can cause maternal death, such as postpartum hemorrhage, hypertensive disorders, and obstructed labor (UN Population Fund [UNFPA], 2013a).

Violence against women is a universal phenomenon, blind to poverty and power. At least one third of all women have experienced violence during their lifetimes, in the richest and poorest corners of the world, among the most and least empowered (WHO, 2013a). While violence against women can occur indiscriminately anywhere in the world, the laws to criminalize acts of violence against women and the resources available to protect and support women who survive acts of violence vary widely. On the whole, poorer nations have more limited laws and resources to protect women from violence. Additionally, regions experiencing natural disasters, wars, and other periods of upheaval are less able to protect women against violence. Rape is one act of violence against women that contributes to rates of unintended pregnancy and abortion worldwide. In addition, rates of violence against women increase during pregnancy, leaving women more vulnerable to injury or death from violence (UNFPA, 2005).

The Risks of Pregnancy and Childbirth in Resource-Limited Settings

Similarly, the obstetric causes of maternal deaths around the world occur at the intersection of gender equity, women's rights, and poverty. Globally, postpartum hemorrhage is the leading cause of maternal mortality, followed by hypertensive disorders, sepsis, and unsafe abortion. Other causes can include, but are not limited to, obstructed labor, embolism, and HIV/AIDS. These causes vary widely by region. For instance, postpartum hemorrhage is the leading cause of maternal death in Africa and Asia, whereas hypertensive disorders are the leading cause of maternal death in Latin America and developed countries (Khan, Wojdyla, Say, Gulmezoglu, & Van Look, 2006). The HIV epidemic has contributed enormously to maternal mortality, most significantly in sub-Saharan Africa, the epicenter of the epidemic. An estimated 60,000 maternal deaths would be averted per year if the world had an HIV seroprevalence rate of zero. Even so, in regions where women living with HIV have access to high-quality health care and antiretroviral medications, the risk of dying from HIV during pregnancy and childbirth is extremely low (Hogan et al., 2010).

Women living in poverty are disproportionately impacted by the obstetric causes of maternal mortality for a number of reasons. First, women who are poor are less likely to have access to family planning, a critical component to the prevention of unintended pregnancy. In addition, effective contraception is crucial to limiting and spacing the number of pregnancies a woman experiences over her lifetime. It is believed that the number of maternal deaths around the world would be anywhere from one to eight times higher without the current prevalence of contraception use. Further, an estimated 104,000 maternal deaths could be prevented every year if the unmet need for contraception among women of reproductive age was addressed (Ahmed, Li, Liu, & Tsui, 2012).

Access to contraception is only part of the story. Women in poor countries also endure barriers to controlling their own fertility. These barriers include the ability to purchase available methods of contraception, the desire to have large families to ensure the survival of some children in areas where infant and child mortality rates are high, and the unwillingness of women's partners to use and engage in contraceptive methods (UNFPA, 2012; WHO, 2009). The highest fertility rates in the world largely occur in low-income countries, where barriers to contraception use are greatest. Women in low-income countries are frequently forced to resort to desperate measures to cope with unintended pregnancy, seeking unsafe, and often illegal, abortions. In 2012, an estimated 80 million unintended pregnancies occurred, with half of these pregnancies ending in abortion. Of the 80 million unintended births, 63 million occurred in developing countries. Nearly 50,000 women died from abortion, the vast majority occurring in resource-poor settings, accounting for the fourth leading cause of maternal death worldwide (Singh & Darroch, 2012).

The number of pregnancies that a woman experiences during her lifetime directly correlates to her risk of postpartum hemorrhage. Over 70% of postpartum hemorrhages occur as a result of uterine atony, or the inability of the uterus to involute once a baby is born. In women who have had five or more births, they have an increased chance of experiencing uterine atony due to precipitous or prolonged labors, both significant risk factors for uterine atony (Sosa, Althabe, Belizan, & Buekens, 2010). To treat postpartum hemorrhage and prevent maternal deaths, women must have access to uterotonics, blood transfusions, and surgical infrastructure, if necessary. Essential to emergency obstetrical care, the availability of uterotonics, blood transfusions, and surgery is the amount of financial support given to a health care institution to supply such measures (Prata, Bell, & Weidert, 2013).

Similarly, the prevention and treatment of hypertensive disorders in pregnancy, the second leading cause of maternal death around the world, are contingent upon the availability of antihypertensive medications; equipment to deliver intravenous routes of medications, if necessary; and the ability to perform cesarean sections when warranted for women in hypertensive crisis. Underlying the incidence of hypertensive disorders in pregnancy is poor nutrition of women before and during pregnancy. For instance, high sodium levels are associated with hypertensive disorders (Lo, Mission, & Caughey, 2013). Although high sodium intake is a public health issue across nations, diets high in salt are common in poor countries where salt is used as a food preservative in areas without refrigeration and concentrated in cheap, processed foods (Ibrahim & Damasceno, 2012).

The issues around gender equity and women's rights are further exacerbated in low-income countries, where chronic shortages of skilled health personnel (midwives, or nurses and doctors with midwifery skills) available to provide safe care during pregnancy and childbirth exist. In addition to possessing the background, knowledge, and skills to address issues such as postpartum hemorrhage and hypertensive disorders, skilled health personnel are key to the prevention of sepsis, the provision of safe abortion (where legal), and the delivery of emergency obstetrical care (UNFPA, 2011). Approximately 50 million babies are born each year without nurse, midwife, or doctor present at their births (UN, 2013). If women around the world had universal access to skilled health personnel, they would experience 74% fewer maternal deaths every year. A midwife or nurse attends the vast majority of births attended by skilled health personnel (UNFPA, 2011).

Overwhelmingly, midwives and nurses around the world are women, women who had the access to education and the resources to become skilled health personnel. In countries where women experience gender inequity and unequal rights, midwives and nurses confront barriers to providing health care, advocating for their patients, and acquiring much-needed health resources that are often related to their status as women (WHO, 2009). Despite these challenges, midwives and nurses serve as the frontline health care providers to millions of women around the world and represent professions uniquely poised to reduce maternal mortality around the globe (UNFPA, 2011).

Nurses and Midwives: Essential to Maternal Mortality Reduction

Integral to the midwifery and nursing professions is a deep commitment to health and human rights. The International Confederation of Midwives (ICM) and the International Council of Nurses (ICN) uphold the recognition of human rights and the importance of practicing midwifery and nursing from a human rights perspective with a focus on women's health in their governing documents. The ICM's "Bill of Rights for Women and Midwives" functions as a human rights framework through which governments can effect change in women's health. The Bill of Rights demands that governments recognize and provide midwifery care as a basic human right for all women and babies, and that women and midwives should be respected by governments and governmental institutions for health and education. Nationally, midwifery workforce planning is identified as key to ensuring sufficient numbers of midwives to meet the needs of society. Further, the ICM (2011) notes that:

> The issues for women around gender equity and access to education also extend to midwives as a woman-dominated profession. . . . Midwives and women have the right to a system of regulation that will ensure a safe, competent and autonomous midwifery workforce for women and their babies. . . .

Similarly, the ICN has a specific "Nurses and Human Rights" position statement that outlines its expectations for nurses, with a specific emphasis on serving vulnerable populations such as women and children. The ICN (2011) further notes that the nursing profession has an obligation to safeguard, respect, and promote society's health. The utilization of human rights principles and protections has a special emphasis on vulnerable groups, including women, children, the elderly, refugees, and stigmatized groups. There is additional emphasis on nurses' accountability for their own actions in safeguarding human rights and the role of national nurses associations (NNAs, 2011) in developing health and social policy legislation.

> Nurses individually and collectively through their national nurses associations have a duty to report and speak up when there are violations of human rights, particularly those related to access to essential health care, torture and inhumane, cruel and degrading treatment and/or patient safety.

Such dedication to health and human rights from the ICM and ICN also serve as the foundation for national midwifery and nursing organizations worldwide. In the United States, the American College of Nurse-Midwives (ACNM) and the American Nurses Association (ANA) both incorporate a call within their membership to practice with a commitment to human rights and gender equity (ACNM, 2013; ANA, 2001).

Midwifery and nursing scholars further explore this call to uphold human rights in treatises that discuss the responsibility of midwives and nurses to ameliorate poverty, gender inequity, and women's rights, recognizing the impact of these issues as the underlying causes of maternal mortality around the globe. In her sentinel article outlining a human rights framework for midwifery care, Thompson states, "Gender discrimination is a global concern for women and all those who provide health services to them. The link between health and the lack of basic, human right . . . is vivid throughout the life cycles of girls and women" (Thompson, 2004). Tyer-Viola and Cesario (2010) further expound on the global concern for women by stating:

> Nurses have direct knowledge of and experience with working with
> poor and vulnerable members of society. Nurses should use this
> knowledge to promote advocacy and partnerships to create
> anti-poverty measures within communities and work with
> organizations that will provide income opportunities and health
> related education for women. (p. 586)

Tyer-Viola and Cesario (2010) also note that the nursing profession is responsible for increasing the visibility of those most vulnerable, often the women of a community and particularly those living in poverty. In recognition of the commitment within the midwifery and nursing professions to human rights and the roles that midwives and nurses can play in addressing poverty and gender inequity, the UNFPA states that midwives and nurses with midwifery skills are not only critical to the reduction of maternal mortality around the world, but also "contribute to the advancement of gender equality and women's rights." One key component widely acknowledged as vital to the reduction of maternal deaths is the scaling up of the midwifery and nursing workforce around the world. In well-resourced health systems, midwifery-led care provides positive health outcomes for women, equal to or superior than physician-led models of care (Sandall, Soltani, Gates, Shennan, & Devane, 2013).

However, this model is contingent upon the availability of emergency obstetric services, particularly the availability of cesarean sections when necessary. In poor countries, it is common for midwives and nurses to function as the sole health personnel in health centers and often hospitals. Over two thirds of midwives and nurses providing care to women during pregnancy and childbirth in low-income countries do not have access to emergency obstetric services. Like all cadres of health care providers in resource-poor settings, midwives and nurses also grapple with a limited workforce available to high-quality and safe care. It is estimated that the optimal midwife-to-population ratio is six midwives for every 1,000 births, health care coverage that would significantly reduce maternal mortality. The midwifery workforce in resource-poor settings, including nurses with midwifery skills, is approximately 860,000, dismally inadequate for the tens of millions of births that occur annually worldwide. Over 110,000 more midwives are needed among the 38 countries with the largest shortages (UNFPA, 2011). Such low provider-to-population ratios stretch nursing and midwifery capacity to its limits, leaving nurses and midwives feeling dissatisfied in their work and patients vulnerable to inadequate care (ICN, 2006).

Many obstacles exist to scaling up the midwifery workforce in resource-poor settings. Chief among them are financing and gender equity. First, many would-be midwives and nurses with midwifery skills are unable to attain the education necessary to apply to midwifery and nursing schools, a direct result of inequitable education access for girls and women, particularly in low-income settings. Qualified, prospective students also require access to the funding necessary to complete their educations. If students are qualified and have the ability to pay for school, they then require access to a midwifery training program. In impoverished countries, there is scant availability of well-run midwifery programs with qualified faculty and well-resourced teaching facilities. If students are able to complete a midwifery training program, they then need fairly paid jobs through which they can provide their newly acquired skills. Low-income countries often struggle with their ability to fund the salaries of their health workforce. When funds are available, midwives and nurses are relegated to significantly lower pay scales than doctors, a reflection of the gender inequity of female dominant versus male dominant professions. This inequity is also reflected in the lack of midwives and nurses holding positions of power and authority in health care systems, eroding the opportunities for midwives and nurses to advocate for themselves and the women they serve (WHO, 2009, 2010).

In the face of such challenges and obstacles, midwives and nurses centrally figure in the major successes of reducing maternal mortality in resource poor settings. A few examples include the progress toward MDG 5 in Rwanda, Afghanistan, and Sri Lanka. Rwanda, home to the second highest gender equality index in the world, a female minister of health, and the only sub-Saharan African nation on track to meet its MDG 5 targets (UN Development Program, 2013), the strengthening of midwifery education and increasing its midwifery workforce are central to its progress (Maliqi & Mugabo, 2011). The MMR in Afghanistan, one of the highest in the world due to the ravages of war and gender inequality, dropped dramatically when the Afghani government was provided the funding to expand its midwifery workforce (Turkmani et al., 2013). In Sri Lanka, another country on target to meet its MDG 5 goals and home to universal education access for women and men, the government's commitment to its midwifery workforce is lauded as the main factor for reducing maternal mortality (Senanayake et al., 2011).

In observing the progress and challenges to the reduction of maternal mortality in countries that are not on track to meeting MDG 5, midwives and nurses also play a central role in plans for preventing maternal deaths. Using one country, Haiti, as a case study, efforts to expand the midwifery workforce, in conjunction with the need to increase gender equity and women's rights, illustrate the critical role of midwives and nurses in improving Haiti's MMR and meeting its MDG 5 targets.

GENDER INEQUITY AND WOMEN'S RIGHTS IN HAITI

Haiti, a small island nation of approximately 10.1 million people, has the highest MMR in the Western Hemisphere. In 2010, 350 women died for every 100,000 live births in Haiti, compared with just 12 maternal deaths that occurred in the United States for every 100,000 live births in the same year (WHO, 2013b). Not only is Haiti behind on its MDG 5 targets, the country is not on track to meet is MDG 5 targets for at least another three decades, given its current rate of progress (see Figure 7.2). As expected, given its high MMR, Haiti is also the poorest country in the Western Hemisphere. The average annual income per capita in Haiti is just $771. In the United States, an individual can expect to earn an average of $51,749 per year (World Bank, 2014).

In addition to its status as the poorest country in the Western Hemisphere, Haiti is still recovering from a catastrophic earthquake that struck the most populated part of the country, its capital, Port-au-Prince, on January 12, 2010. An estimated 220,000 people were killed, more than 300,000 were injured, and 1.5 million people lost their homes (Pan American Health Organization, 2011). The earthquake decimated Haiti's health care sector, as an estimated 10% of its entire health care workforce was killed during the earthquake or emigrated in the earthquake's aftermath. Over 60% of the country's total health facilities, largely concentrated in the Port-au-Prince area, were damaged or destroyed (Human Rights Watch, 2011). The earthquake was cruelly followed by a cholera outbreak in October 2010, the first outbreak of cholera in Haiti in its history. Over 6% of the Haitian population has experienced at least one bout of cholera since the outbreak began and over 8,000 people have died (Gelting, Bliss, Patrick, Lockhart, & Handzel, 2013).

Similar to other low-income countries, Haiti also has many gains to achieve in regards to gender equality and women's rights, which are critical to improving its MMR. It is one of only four countries in the world where not a single member of its parliament is a woman (UN, 2013). There are no laws that specifically protect women against domestic violence or prohibit sexual harassment in the workplace. Rape officially became an illegal act in 2005. As is the case in other countries that have experienced repressive rule, Haiti endured a spate of high rates of sexual violence against women during the Duvalier dictatorship and the decades of political upheaval that have followed since the dictatorship ended in 1986. Rates of sexual violence also soared after the catastrophic January 2010 earthquake that struck the nation on January 12, 2010 (Human Rights Watch, 2011).

Maternal Mortality in Haiti: Nursing and Midwifery Impact and Challenges

In part due to its dismal record on gender equity and women's rights, Haiti is home to a long-standing shortage of nurses and midwives. Haiti has the lowest nurse-to-population ratio in the Americas. The nationwide nurse-to-population ratio is 1.1 nurses for every 10,000 people, compared with 97.2 nurses per 10,000 people in the United States (Pan American Health Organization, 2005). The midwife-to-birth ratio in Haiti is even more dismal. Statistically, less than one midwife is available per 1,000 births, far lower than the recommended ratio of six midwives per 1,000 births (UNFPA, 2011). As of 2008, a mere 174 midwives worked in Haiti. Tragically, the shortage of nurses and midwives became even more severe following the January 2010 earthquake that caused the collapse of the public nursing and midwifery school in the Haitian capital of Port-au-Prince and killed 150 nursing and midwifery students (UNFPA, 2010).

Unlike most low-income countries, where doctors are often in even shorter supply than midwives and nurses, in Haiti, there exist three times as many physicians as midwives and nurses. It is estimated that Haiti is home to more than 200 obstetricians and an additional 373 general practitioners with midwifery skills. This imbalance is largely due to the relative ease for Haitian nurses and midwives to immigrate to wealthier nations and receive higher salaries for their work. Physicians usually have to repeat their medical residencies in other countries before being able to practice in their professions, whereas nurses and midwives generally have to pass licensure and competency exams, but not repeat their training (WHO, 2010). However, the relative abundance of physicians does not equate to access to skilled attendance during pregnancy and birth for women living in Haiti. Most doctors in Haiti remain concentrated in Port-au-Prince, leaving smaller cities and rural areas extremely underserved. In order to attain the MDG 5 goal of having 95% of all births attended by a midwife, or a doctor or nurse who has training and competency in care during pregnancy and birth, an additional 563 midwives, nurses, and doctors would be required in communities across Haiti. This estimate assumes that the existing and additional nurses, midwives, and doctors with such competencies were distributed equitably according to need across the country (UNFPA, 2011). The shortage of health care providers is a direct contributor to Haiti's high MMR. In addition, an estimated 37% of women of reproductive age have an unmet need for contraception and a mere 26% of all births are attended by a midwife, or a doctor or nurse with midwifery skills (WHO, 2013b).

Recent Efforts to Reduce Maternal Mortality in Haiti

To respond to the economic barriers most women in Haiti confront in seeking health care, the Haitian Ministry of Health launched a program in 2008 to reimburse a group of 63 hospitals and health centers for the cost of providing free maternal health care, largely delivered by nurses and midwives. With the support of the Pan American Health Organization, over the course of the 5-year program, the MMR in the population served by the program was 135 maternal deaths per 100,000 live births, nearly half the current MMR in Haiti, and the rate of prenatal visits increased by sixfold (Pan American Health Organization, 2012).

Like many low-income nations, a major barrier for women in accessing health care is the centralization of available health care services in urban areas. Most hospitals and health centers in Haiti serve the population of Port-au-Prince and smaller coastal cities, leaving the rural interior vulnerable to inadequate numbers of skilled health personnel and functional, well-resourced infrastructure. In an effort to decentralize health care services in Haiti and enhance the limited tertiary care available across the country, Partners In Health (PIH), a health and human rights organization headquartered in Boston, Massachusetts, led the efforts to build an 18,000 square foot, 300-bed tertiary-care academic medical center in Mirebalais, Haiti. PIH, in partnership with the Haitian Ministry of Health, opened Hôpital Universitaire de Mirebalais (HUM) in March 2013. The hallmark of HUM is women's health: one third of the entire hospital is devoted to providing comprehensive women's health services, including family planning, prenatal care, vaginal and operative births, postpartum care, and gynecology services. Most significantly for women in the Mirebalais region, HUM will serve as the referral center for women in the surrounding rural communities who require emergency obstetrical services, an option tragically limited to a few smaller, severely understaffed hospitals less centrally located than HUM. In addition to full-scope, lifesaving women's health services, HUM is only the second national teaching hospital to exist in Haiti. HUM will serve as a critical training ground for the midwives, nurses, and doctors of Haiti's future, which is urgently needed in a country that has suffered too long from the shortage of skilled health personnel available to serve its people (PIH, 2014).

One major success from the relief effort following the January 2010 earthquake in Haiti is the rebuilding of the public nursing and midwifery school in Port-au-Prince. In October 2013, the Haitian Ministry of Health, in partnership with the UNFPA, reopened the National Midwifery School. In its first year, 80 students enrolled, including 39 nurses who want to formally train to become midwives. Also, for the first time, the school is offering a 3-year, direct-entry program for high school graduates interested in becoming midwives. Prior to this option, students wishing to become midwives had to complete 6 years of schooling, becoming nurses first and then completing midwifery training. The direct-entry program will help build the desperately needed midwifery workforce more quickly and immediately in Haiti (UNFPA, 2013b).

THE END OF MATERNAL MORTALITY: SUPPORTING MIDWIVES AND NURSES, ACHIEVING GENDER EQUITY AND EQUAL RIGHTS FOR WOMEN

In Haiti and in other countries where women senselessly die during pregnancy and childbirth, the solutions to reducing maternal mortality are clear. By investing in midwives and nurses, by supporting health resources, and by ensuring women have more equitable power, access, and rights, the burden of maternal mortality decreases exponentially. However, huge changes must still occur in the political, social, and economic infrastructure of regions where the numbers of maternal deaths every year remain unacceptably high. These changes require enormous and sustained financial investments and political stability to endure, in addition to the political and social will to improve survival of girls and women during pregnancy and childbirth. As the year 2015 continues, it is vital to consider the progress of the MDGs and where to go once the deadline for each MDG target passes.

In the "post-2015" landscape of global health, one major consideration is to ensure broader access to financial resources for poor countries to fund midwifery and nursing positions and supply the medical and health equipment necessary to provide health care services. In addition, expanding the MDG 5 target of universal access to reproductive health services to universal access to reproductive health rights could help ensure a firmer commitment to gender equity and women's rights (Hill, Huntington, Dodd, & Buttsworth, 2013). Midwives and nurses have a specific duty to support women's health and to advocate for the resources necessary to reduce maternal mortality, increase access to family planning, and elevate the pursuit of gender equity and women's rights around the globe. Without the service and leadership of midwives and nurses, it will be impossible for the world to achieve MDG 5 and, ultimately, the elimination of maternal mortality.

REFERENCES

Ahmed, S., Li, Q., Liu, L., & Tsui, A. O. (2012). Maternal deaths averted by contraceptive use: An analysis of 172 countries. *The Lancet, 380,* 111–125.

Alkema, L., Kantorova, V., Menozzi, C., & Biddlecom, A. (2013). National, regional and global rates and trends in contraceptive prevalence and unmet need for family planning between 1990 and 2015: A systematic and comprehensive analysis. *The Lancet, 381,* 1642–1652.

American College of Nurse-Midwives (ACNM). (2013). *Code of ethics.* Retrieved from http://www.midwife.org/ACNM/files/ACNMLibraryData/UPLOADFILENAME/000000000048/Code-of-Ethics.pdf

American Nurses Association (ANA). (2001). *Code of ethics for nurses with interpretive statements.* Retrieved from http://www.nursingworld.org/MainMenuCategories/EthicsStandards/CodeofEthicsforNurses/Code-of-Ethics.pdf

Farmer, P., Basilico, M., Kerry, V., Ballard, M., Becker, A., Bukhman, G., . . . Yamamoto, A. (2013). Global health priorities for the early twenty-first century. In P. Farmer, J. Y. Kim, A., Kleinman, & M. Basilico (Eds.), *Reimagining global health: An introduction* (pp. 302–339). Berkeley, CA: University of California Press.

Gelting, R., Bliss, K., Patrick, M., Lockhart, G., & Handzel, T. (2013). Water, sanitation and hygiene in Haiti: Past, present and future. *American Journal of Tropical Medicine and Hygiene, 89,* 665–670.

Hill, P. S., Huntington, D., Dodd, R., & Buttsworth, M. (2013). From Millennium Development Goals to post-2015 sustainable development: Sexual and reproductive health and rights in an evolving aid environment. *Reproductive Health Matters, 21,* 113–124.

Hogan, M. C., Foreman, K. J., Naghavi, M., Ahn, S. Y., Wang, M., Makela, S. M., . . . Murray, C. J. L. (2010). Maternal mortality for 181 countries, 1980–2008: A systematic analysis of progress toward Millennium Development Goal 5. *The Lancet, 375,* 1609–1623.

Human Rights Watch. (2011). *"Nobody remembers us": Failure to protect women's and girls' rights to health and security in post-earthquake Haiti.* Retrieved from http://www.hrw.org/sites/default/files/reports/haiti0811webwcover.pdf

Ibrahim, M. M., & Damasceno, A. (2012). Hypertension in developing countries. *The Lancet, 380,* 611–619.

International Confederation of Midwives. (2011). *Bill of rights for women and midwives.* Retrieved from http://www.internationalmidwives.org/assets/uploads/documents/CoreDocuments/CD2011_002%20ENG%20Bill%20of%20Rights%20for%20Women%20and%20Midwives.pdf

International Council of Nurses (ICN). (2006). The global nursing shortage: Priority areas for intervention. Retrieved from http://www1.icn.ch/global/report2006.pdf

International Council of Nurses. (2011). Nurses and human rights. Retrieved from http://www.icn.ch/images/stories/documents/publications/position_statements/E10_Nurses_Human_Rights.pdf

Khan, K. S., Wojdyla, D., Say, L., Gulmezoglu, A. M., & Van Look, P. F. A. (2006). WHO analysis of causes of maternal death: A systematic review. *The Lancet, 367,* 1066–1074.

Lo, J. O., Mission, J. F., & Caughey, A. B. (2013). Hypertensive disease of pregnancy and maternal mortality. *Current Opinion in Obstetrics and Gynecology, 25,* 124–132.

Maliqi, B., & Mugabo, M. (2011). *The state of the world's midwifery 2011–Rwanda Summary.* Retrieved from http://www.unfpa.org/sowmy/resources/docs/country_info/short_summary/Rwanda_SoWMyShortSummary.pdf

Mukherjee, J. S., Barry, D. J., Satti, H., Raymonville, M., Marsh, S., & Smith-Fawzi, M. K. (2011). Structural violence: A barrier to achieving the Millennium Development Goals for women. *Journal of Women's Health, 20,* 593–597.

Pan American Health Organization (PAHO). (2005). *Overview of the nursing workforce in Latin America.* Retrieved from http://www1.icn.ch/global/Issue6LatinAmerica.pdf

Pan American Health Organization. (2011). *Earthquake in Haiti—One year later: PAHO/WHO report on the health situation.* Retrieved from http://www.who.int/hac/crises/hti/haiti_one_year_after_january2011.pdf

Pan American Health Organization. (2012). *Free obstetric care in Haiti.* Retrieved from http://www.paho.org/hq/index.php?option=com_docman&task=doc_view&gid=19673&Itemid=

Partners In Health. (2014). *Hôpital Universitaire de Mirebalais.* Retrieved from http://www.pih.org/pages/mirebalais

Paruzzolo, S., Mehra, R., Kes, A., & Ashbaugh, C. (2010). *Targeting poverty and gender inequality to improve maternal health.* Retrieved from http://www.womendeliver.org/assets/ICRW-Women_Deliver_FINAL.pdf

Prata, N., Bell, S., & Weidert, K. (2013). Prevention of postpartum hemorrhage in low-resource settings: Current perspectives. *International Journal of Women's Health, 5,* 737–752.

Sandall, J., Soltani, H., Gates, S., Shennan, A., & Devane, D. (2013). Midwife-led continuity models versus other models of care for childbearing women. *Cochrane Database of Systematic Reviews.*

Senanayake, H., Goonewardene, M., Ranatunga, A., Hattotuwa, R., Amarasekera, S., & Amarasinghe, I. (2011). Achieving Millennium Development Goals 4 and 5 in Sri Lanka. *BJOG: An International Journal of Obstetrics and Gynecology, 118,* 78–87.

Singh, S., & Darroch, J. (2012). Adding it up: *The costs and benefits of contraceptive services.* Retrieved from http://www.guttmacher.org/pubs/AIU-2012-estimates.pdf

Sosa, C. G., Althabe, F., Belizan, J. M., & Buekens, P. (2010). Risk factors for postpartum hemorrhage in vaginal deliveries in a Latin American population. *Obstetrics & Gynecology, 113,* 1313–1319.

Thompson, J. B. (2004). A human rights framework for midwifery care. *Journal of Midwifery and Women's Health, 49,* 175–181.

Turkmani, S., Currie, S., Mungia, J., Assefi, N., Rahmanzai, A. J., Azfar, P., & Bartlett, L. (2013). "Midwives are the backbone of our health care system": Lessons from Afghanistan to guide expansion of midwifery in challenging settings. *Midwifery, 29,* 1166–1172.

Tyer-Viola, L. A., & Cesario, S. K. (2010). Addressing poverty, education, and gender equality to improve the health of women worldwide. *Journal of Obstetric, Gynecologic and Neonatal Nursing, 39*, 580–589.

United Nations. (2013). *The Millennium Development Goals reports 2013.* Retrieved from http://www.un.org/millenniumgoals/pdf/report-2013/mdg-report-2013-english.pdf

United Nations Development Program. (2013). *Eight goals for 2015.* Retrieved from http://www.undp.org/content/undp/en/home/mdgoverview

United Nations Millennium Development Project. (2006). *About MDGs—What they are.* Retrieved from http://www.unmillenniumproject.org/goals/index.htm

United Nations Population Fund (UNFPA). (2005). *Combating gender-based violence: A key to achieving the Millennium Development Goals.* Retrieved from http://www.unfpa.org/webdav/site/global/shared/documents/publications/2005/combating_gbv_en.pdf

United Nations Population Fund (UNFPA). (2010). *Midwifery and nursing schools destroyed by Haiti earthquake.* Retrieved from http://www.unfpa.org/public/site/global/lang/en/pid/4756

United Nations Population Fund. (2011). *State of the world's midwifery 2011: Delivering health, saving lives.* Retrieved from http://www.unfpa.org/sowmy/resources/docs/main_report/en_SOWMR_Full.pdf

United Nations Population Fund. (2012). *By choice, not by chance: Family planning, human rights and development.* Retrieved from http://www.unfpa.org/webdav/site/global/shared/swp/2012/EN_SWOP2012_Report.pdf

United Nations Population Fund. (2013a). *Motherhood in childhood: Facing the challenges of adolescent pregnancy.* Retrieved from https://www.unfpa.org/webdav/site/global/shared/swp2013/EN-SWOP2013-final.pdf

United Nations Population Fund. (2013b). *A new midwifery school brings hope to Haitian mothers.* Retrieved from http://www.unfpa.org/public/home/news/pid/15524

United Nations System Task Team on the Post-2015 Development Agenda. (2012). *Review of the contributions of the MDG agenda to foster development: Lessons for the post-2015 agenda.* Retrieved from http://sustainabledevelopment.un.org/content/documents/843taskteam.pdf

United Nations Women. (2012). *Violence against women prevalence data: Surveys by country.* Retrieved from http://www.endvawnow.org/uploads/browser/files/vaw_prevalence_matrix_15april_2011.pdf

World Bank. (2014). *GDP per capita (current US$).* Retrieved from http://data.worldbank.org/indicator/NY.GDP.PCAP.CD

World Health Organization (WHO). (2009). *Women and health: Today's evidence, tomorrow's agenda.* Retrieved from http://whqlibdoc.who.int/publications/2009/9789241563857_eng.pdf?ua=1

World Health Organization. (2010). *A global survey monitoring progress in nursing and midwifery.* Retrieved from http://whqlibdoc.who.int/hq/2010/WHO_HRH_HPN_10.4_eng.pdf?ua=1

World Health Organization. (2012). *Trends in maternal mortality: 1990 to 2010.* Retrieved from http://www.unfpa.org/webdav/site/global/shared/documents/publications/2012/Trends_in_maternal_mortality_A4-1.pdf

World Health Organization. (2013a). *Global and regional estimates of violence against women: Prevalence and health effects of intimate partner violence and non-partner sexual violence.* Retrieved from http://apps.who.int/iris/bitstream/10665/85239/1/9789241564625_eng.pdf?ua=1

World Health Organization. (2013b). *World health statistics 2013.* Retrieved from http://
www.who.int/gho/publications/world_health_statistics/EN_WHS2013_Full.pdf

World Health Organization (2014). *Trends in maternal mortality: 1990-2013. Estimates
by WHO, UNICEF, UNFPA, the World Bank and the United Nations population division.* Geneva, Switzerland: Author. Retrieved from http://apps.who.int/iris/bitstr
eam/10665/112682/2/9789241507226_eng.pdf

CHAPTER 13

Violence Against Women

Annie Lewis O'Connor, Karen A. Conley, and Suellen Breakey

Violence is immoral because it thrives on hatred rather than love. Violence is impractical because it is a descending spiral ending in destruction for all. It is immoral because it seeks to humiliate the opponent rather than win his understanding; it seeks to annihilate rather than convert. Violence ends up defeating itself. It creates bitterness in the survivors and brutality in the destroyers.

—*Martin Luther King*

VIOLENCE AGAINST WOMEN: A GLOBAL PUBLIC HEALTH PROBLEM

In 1993, the United Nations Declaration on the Elimination of Violence Against Women was passed (United Nations [UN] General Assembly, 1993). Violence against women, also referred to as gender-based violence (GBV), can be physical, sexual, or psychological. The UN defines violence against women as

> any act of gender-based violence that results in, or is likely to result in, physical, sexual or mental harm or suffering to women, including threats of such acts, coercion or arbitrary deprivation of liberty, whether occurring in public or in private life. (UN General Assembly, 1993)

Examples of GBV include, but are not limited to, sexual harassment, rape, sexual violence during conflict, sexual slavery, and traditional practices such as female genital mutilation. It has been more than 20 years since the promulgation of the Declaration on the Elimination of Violence Against Women was passed and yet, worldwide, women and girls remain plagued by violence. Moreover, this violence has a direct impact on the health of women globally.

Intimate partner violence (IPV) is more narrowly defined as "any behavior within an intimate relationship that causes physical, psychological or sexual harm" (Heise & Garcia-Moreno, 2002, p. 89). While both men and women perpetrate IPV, women are three times more likely than men to sustain injuries from IPV (Black et al., 2011). Effects of IPV on mental health include depressive symptoms, posttraumatic stress disorder, and substance use (Beydoun, Beydoun, Kaufman, Lo, & Zonderman, 2012; Campbell, 2002; Coker, Smith, Bethea, King, & McKeown,

2000; Dillon, Hussain, Loxton, & Rahman, 2013); physical health concerns include lower levels of physical functioning as a result of injury and chronic conditions such as chronic pain and fatigue (Campbell, 2002; Campbell, Abrahams, & Martin, 2008; Coker et al., 2002; Dillon et al., 2013; Felitti et al., 1998). Reproductive and gynecological issues have been reported related to sexual violence such as pelvic inflammatory disease and unintended pregnancy (American College of Obstetricians and Gynecologists, 2012; Chamberlain & Levenson, 2012; Dillon et al., 2013; Miller et al., 2010). These adverse health effects are more severe in cases of more recent as well as prolonged exposure to violence (Bonomi et al., 2006).

In addition to these health effects, women who experience violence are more likely to acquire HIV (Joint United Nations Program on HIV/AIDS [UNAIDS], 2014a). Finally, the incidence of homicide, suicide, and AIDS-related deaths are higher in women who experience IPV (Heise & Garcia-Moreno, 2002). Globally, more than one third of female homicide is at the hands of an intimate partner (Stockl et al., 2013) It is clear from these disturbing statistics that women's basic human rights continue to be denied despite social justice efforts (UNAIDS, 2014b; Watts & Zimmerman, 2002).

The Incidence and Prevalence of Violence Against Women: Global Estimates

Population-level surveys provide the most accurate estimates of the prevalence of GBV in nonconflict settings. Heise, Ellsberg, and Gottemoeller (1999) reported in a review of 48 population-based surveys from around the world that the range of women who reported being physically assaulted by an intimate male partner at some point in their lives was 10% to 69%. Subsequently, in 2005, the World Health Organization (WHO), in collaboration with the London School of Hygiene and Tropical Medicine and the Program for Appropriate Technology in Health, published a multicountry study on women's health and domestic violence against women from culturally and geographically diverse settings (Garcia-Moreno, Jansen, Ellsberg, Heise, & Watts, 2005).

As part of the aims of the study, the researchers sought to obtain valid estimates of the prevalence and frequency of physical, sexual, and emotional violence against women and to assess the association between violence and health outcomes (Garcia-Moreno et al., 2005). More than 24,000 women, ages 15 to 49, from 15 sites in 10 developing countries were interviewed using a standardized survey. The following findings are representative of the overall results of the study and indicate the extent of GBV involving intimate partners as well as nonpartner violence from a global perspective. These data and the full report published by WHO emphasize the widespread incidence and prevalence of GBV globally.

- The range of lifetime prevalence of physical or sexual IPV, or both, was between 15% (Japan city) and 71% (Ethiopia province).
- The reported levels of violence by a nonintimate partner since age 15 ranged from less than 1% (Ethiopia, Bangladesh provinces) to between 10% and 12% (Peru, Samoa, United Republic of Tanzania city).

- Many participants reported that their first sexual experience was forced: 17% in rural Tanzania, 24% in rural Peru, and 30% in rural Bangladesh (Garcia-Moreno et al., 2005).

More recently, WHO (2013), in collaboration with the London School of Hygiene and Tropical Medicine and the South African Medical Research Council, published the results of a comprehensive systematic review and synthesis of the existing global data on the prevalence of violence against women and sexual violence by a nonpartner. The results underscore the fact that violence against women is a global health problem. Troubling statistics suggest the following:

- 35% of women worldwide have experienced either physical and/or sexual IPV or nonpartner sexual violence at some point in their lives.
- Almost one third (30%) of all women who have been in a relationship have experienced physical and/or sexual violence by their intimate partner, and in some regions of the world, this statistic is much higher.
- Globally, as many as 38% of all murders of women are committed by intimate partners (WHO, 2013).

U.S. Estimates of Violence Against Women

Prevalence estimates calculated from data collected in 2010 using the Centers for Disease Control and Prevention (CDC) National Intimate Partner and Sexual Violence Survey (NIPSVS) in the United States reveal that approximately 42 million women (36%) have experienced rape, physical violence, and/or stalking by an intimate partner at some point in their lifetime (Black et al., 2011). One in three women (33%) has experienced physical violence by an intimate partner, and nearly one in 10 has been raped by an intimate partner in her lifetime. Approximately 6% of the women in the United States—almost 7 million women—reported experiencing these forms of IPV in the past year (Black et al., 2011). Moreover, in the United States, 40% to 50% of all women murdered are killed by an intimate partner (Campbell et al., 2003). In 2010, IPV accounted for 10% of all homicides (CDC, 2014a). It is clear that violence against women is a major public health issue both in the United States and globally. While the problem is recognized widely, successful interventions lag behind, and the issue remains an epidemic.

THE IMPACT OF CULTURE AND SOCIOPOLITICAL FORCES ON VIOLENCE AGAINST WOMEN

Cultural and sociopolitical influences have a major impact on how we, as a global society, prevent and intervene in violence against women. In fact, GBV and IPV are solely products of social context (Jewkes, 2002). A social ecological model of violence, like that described by Dahlberg and Krug (2002), considers the complex interrelationships between individual, relationship (peers, partners, and family), community (schools, neighborhoods, and places of employment), and societal characteristics (e.g., cultural norms) that increase the likelihood of either being a victim or perpetrator of violence. They propose that this model can be used to not only explain but also to develop prevention and intervention strategies. Garcia-Moreno, Guedes, and Knerr (2012) use this framework to categorize risk factors for IPV (Table 13.1).

Cultural and social norms shape our behavior and contribute in various ways to the normalization of certain kinds of violence (WHO, 2009). Violence as a learned social behavior begets violence, and this is borne out in the research. For instance, sons of mothers who are beaten are more likely to beat their partners, and daughters of mothers who have been beaten are more likely to be victims of IPV (Jewkes, 2002). In some cultures, a man's honor is linked to a woman's sexual behavior; this relationship increases the perpetration of violence against women (Heise & Garcia-Moreno, 2002). For example, in India, Nigeria, and Ghana, men are considered superior and have the right to assert power over women; in South Africa and China, physical violence is an accepted way to resolve relationship conflicts; and in Pakistan, sex is a man's right within the marriage, and divorce is shameful (WHO, 2009). Events that trigger IPV include refusing sex, going out without the man's permission, arguing back, and not obeying a male partner (Heise & Garcia-Moreno, 2002).

IPV, however, occurs in all countries, irrespective of the social, economic, religious, or cultural groups to which one belongs. Although women can be violent in relationships with men, and violence also occurs in same-sex relationships, the overwhelming burden of IPV is borne by women at the hands of men (Black et al., 2011; Garcia-Moreno et al., 2005; Heise et al., 1999).

TABLE 13.1 Using an Ecological Model of Violence to Identify Risk Factors for Experiencing Intimate Partner Violence (IPV)

Individual factors	Low level of education Exposure to violence between parents Childhood sexual abuse Acceptance of violence
Relationship factors	Conflict in the relationship Male dominance in the family Economic stress Disparity in education where woman is more highly educated
Community and societal factors	Poverty Low socioeconomic status of women Social norms that accept gender inequities Weak legal and community sanctions against IPV Lack of women's civil rights Armed conflict Social acceptance of use of violence to resolve conflict

Source: Garcia-Moreno et al. (2012).

While large-scale studies have been useful to identify the nature and extent of violence against women worldwide as well as the prevalence of violence-related physical and mental health outcomes, qualitative research has proven useful to identify culturally, community-, or values-specific factors that relate to violence. The use of qualitative research offers rich descriptions of the experience of being abused as well as the impact that being a victim of violence has had on women. These data are critical to the development of effective strategies aimed at both intervention and prevention. The following narrative illustrates the complexity of IPV:

> My husband . . . used to beat me when I refused to sleep with him . . . .
> He wouldn't use a condom. . . . It's a wife's duty to have sex with her
> husband because that is the main reason you come together. . . . When
> I knew about his girlfriends, I feared that I would get infected with
> HIV. . . . I tried to insist on using a condom but he refused. So I gave in
> because I really feared [him]. (Karanja, 2003, p. 24)

Other examples of qualitative studies that have increased our understanding of the social context of violence include studies that described the relationships between women and their partners and family responses to IPV (Hatcher et al., 2013); the resources used by women who experience IPV and the barriers to accessing those resources (Odero et al., 2014); and health providers' experiences and practices related to prenatal screening for IPV (LoGuidice, 2014).

VIOLENCE AGAINST WOMEN: NATIONAL AND INTERNATIONAL POLICY IMPLICATIONS

In the United States, much attention has been given to federal legislation on violence against women. It is helpful to review the historical milestones that have led to progress in IPV prevention and intervention in order to understand the context in which efforts are occurring today. *Herstory of Domestic Violence: A Timeline of the Battered Women's Movement* (SafeNetwork, 1999) provides a timeline that describes the following notable events: In 1967, one of the first domestic violence shelters opened in Maine. Five years later, in 1972, the nation's first emergency rape crisis hotline was established in Washington, DC. In 1977, at the request of those working with women who were victims of domestic violence, Emerge was founded in Boston, Massachusetts, to provide counseling services for men who abused their partners. In 1985, almost 20 years after the establishment of the first domestic violence shelter, a seminal event in the history of violence against women occurred when U.S. Surgeon General C. Everett Koop identified domestic violence as not only a law enforcement issue but also a public health issue (SafeNetwork, 1999). Categorizing domestic violence in this way required a proactive response from law enforcement officials as well as the health care community.

The Violence Against Women Act of 1994

In 1994, Joseph Biden, then a U.S. senator from Delaware, introduced the first Violence Against Women Act (VAWA). This landmark piece of federal legislation changed the sociopolitical response to violence against women in the United States. With strong bipartisan support, the VAWA was signed into law. For the first time, the VAWA provided a comprehensive approach that included provisions that held perpetrators accountable and also provided necessary services for victims. To that end, the VAWA not only improved the criminal justice approach to violence but ensured that victims and their families had access to necessary services (Seghetti & Bjelopera, 2010). During the 113th Congress in 2013, the VAWA was renewed as the Violence Against Women Reauthorization Act of 2013, with new provisions that expanded protections and services to Native American women; immigrants; lesbian, gay, bisexual, and transgender (LGBT) persons; college students; and public housing residents.

Additionally, from 2011 to 2013 national policy recommendations underscored the central role of health care professionals in identifying and intervening in cases of intentional violence against women. In 2011, fueled by the accumulating evidence supporting the benefits of screening for IPV, the Institute of Medicine (IOM), in their publication, *Clinical Preventive Services for Women: Closing the Gaps*, recommended that IPV screening become part of routine preventive care for women of childbearing age (IOM, 2011). The passage of the Patient Protection and Affordable Care Act in 2010 codified these recommendations and required that insurance cover IPV screening and counseling as an essential health service to women at no additional cost to the patient.

In 2004, prior to the publication of these current recommendations, the U.S. Preventive Services Task Force (USPSTF) concluded that there was insufficient evidence to support screening women for IPV. However, in January 2013, based on a systematic review (Nelson, Bougatsos, & Blazina, 2012), the USPSTF upgraded their earlier recommendation on screening for IPV. Their suggestion for practice is that clinicians should not only screen all women of childbearing age for IPV but also provide or refer women who screen positive for intervention (USPSTF, 2013). These policies and recommendations strengthen the opportunities for providers to address the health of women exposed to IPV and sexual violence.

The International Violence Against Women Act (I-VAWA)

In 2005, I-VAWA was initiated with the support of more than 150 groups, including nongovernmental organizations (NGOs), UN agencies, and women's groups worldwide. The goal of this legislation was to respond to violence against women on a global level. In 2007, the proposed legislation was introduced into the 110th Congress, sponsored by then Senator Joseph Biden, among others. It has been reintroduced into the 111th and 112th Congresses without being successfully enacted into law. In November 2013, Representative Jan Schakowsky, on behalf of a group of sponsors, reintroduced the bill at the 113th Congress.

On November 21, 2013, the legislation was referred to the House Committee on Foreign Affairs. As of the printing of this book, there has been no further action.

If enacted into law, the I-VAWA of 2013 would for the first time create a comprehensive approach to combat violence against women and girls internationally and commit financial resources to the effort. Specifically, the legislation would direct the secretary of state to establish an Office of Global Women's Issues and appoint an ambassador-at-large to coordinate U.S. governmental efforts to address the status of women and girls in foreign policy efforts (Congress.Gov, 2013). Additionally, it would support the appointment of a senior coordinator for Gender Equality and Women's Empowerment within the U.S. Agency for International Development (USAID). Ultimately, the bill would authorize the U.S. secretary of state to provide assistance to prevent and respond to violence against women worldwide (Congress.Gov, 2013). Enactment of this legislation would signify a U.S. commitment to making violence against women and girls a diplomatic priority (Amnesty International, n.d.). Yet, despite bipartisan support, passing this legislation remains a goal rather than an achievement.

INTERSECTION OF VIOLENCE AND HEALTH: THE EXTENT OF THE PROBLEM

Health Effects of Violence on Women

It is now well established that nearly one third of the world's women have been victims of physical or sexual violence by an intimate partner in their lifetime (WHO, 2013). However, violence often takes many forms—such as psychological and sexual—compounding the challenges that women face. National and international data further illustrate the impact that exposure to violence has on different aspects of one's health that was discussed in the introduction to this chapter.

In the United States, there are approximately 2 million self-reported injuries to women related to IPV (National Center for Injury Prevention and Control, 2003). Further, we know that women who experience IPV are 70% more likely to be diagnosed with cardiac disease and asthma (60%), and are more likely to drink excessively (70%) compared with women who have not experienced IPV (CDC, 2008).

Moreover, a significant number of the women who participated in the NIPSVS in 2010 reported adverse emotional effects of IPV. Women reported feeling fearful (approximately 25%), concerned for their safety (22%), and had at least one symptom associated with posttraumatic stress disorder (22%) (Black et al., 2011). Adverse health outcomes reported with the most frequency included difficulty sleeping (37.7%), activity limitations (35%), chronic pain (29.8%), and frequent headaches (28.7%). In addition, the prevalence of adverse mental or physical health outcomes was significantly higher in women who reported a history of IPV compared with women with no report of IPV (Black et al., 2011).

These findings are similar to results published by Breiding, Black, and Ryan (2008) based on an earlier survey conducted in 2005. They found that women who experienced IPV victimization were more likely to report joint disease, activity limitation, and use of disability devices, most likely related to direct physical injury. Similarly, women who reported IPV were also more likely to report heart disease, stroke, current smoking, current asthma, HIV risk factors, and heavy or binge drinking (Breiding et al., 2008).

Health outcomes reported in the WHO multicountry study provide international results that are similar to U.S. data. The prevalence of injury in women who reported IPV ranged from 19% (Ethiopia province) to 55% (Peru) (Garcia-Moreno et al., 2005). In most settings where the study was conducted, women who had experienced IPV were more likely to report their health as poor or very poor (Garcia-Moreno et al., 2005). The impact on the mental health of women who report IPV is also significant. In all settings, women who reported IPV had significantly higher levels of emotional distress and were more likely to have considered or attempted suicide compared to woman who did not experience IPV (Garcia-Moreno et al., 2005). The authors also suggest that these health challenges may be more prevalent in developing countries (Garcia-Moreno et al., 2005). The prevalence of IPV and the health impacts that have been consistently reported across studies discussed here point to the devastating burden of violence.

Violence and Women's Sexual and Reproductive Health

Findings from research conducted over the last few decades have established that women are at significant risk for experiencing IPV, sustaining serious injury, and being killed at the hands of their partner. Sexual violence and sexual coercion, such as threats of force, forced noncondom use, and use of drugs or alcohol, limit women's decision making regarding their reproductive health and often their access to care (Chamberlain & Levenson, 2012). In the WHO multicountry study, Garcia-Moreno et al. (2005) found that the percentage of women who experienced sexual violence ranged from 10% to 50%. Further, in the majority of instances of sexual violence, forced sex was a result of physical force, not fear (Garcia-Moreno et al.).

In addition to increasing a woman's risk of sexually transmitted infections and HIV, sexual violence and coercion may also lead to unintended pregnancy. Pregnancy coercion is defined as "behaviors such as threats or acts of violence if she [the woman experiencing IPV] does not comply with her partner's wishes regarding the decision of whether to terminate or continue a pregnancy" (Chamberlain & Levenson, 2012, p. 7). To that end, women and teens who seek abortions are three times more likely to have experienced IPV in the past year than women who continue their pregnancies (Chamberlain & Levenson, 2012), and women in the WHO multicountry study who experienced IPV reported more induced abortions and more miscarriages than women who did not report violence (Garcia-Moreno et al., 2005).

Pregnancy may be a time that women are protected from violence, but this is not consistently reported (Garcia-Moreno et al., 2005). Coker, Sanderson, and Dong (2004) found that 14.7% of the 755 women surveyed experienced IPV while pregnant. Moreover, pregnancy outcomes differ between women who experience IPV during pregnancy and those who do not. In a systematic review examining the impact of IPV on women's reproductive health, Sarkar (2008) found that violence during pregnancy increased the risk for low-birth-weight infants, preterm deliveries, and neonatal death. Similar findings were reported by Coker et al. (2004).

Violence and Women's Exposure to HIV

Numerous studies worldwide have linked exposure to violence and lack of sexual autonomy to risk for HIV infection (Stockman, Lucea, & Campbell, 2013). Approximately 35.3 million people worldwide—half of whom are women—are living with HIV, and there are an estimated 6,300 new HIV infections per day (Joint UN Program on AIDS, 2013). Millions of those infected with HIV are young people aged 15 to 24 years who currently account for an estimated 37% of all new infections (Joint UN Program on AIDS, 2013). While 97% of those living with HIV/AIDS reside in low- and middle-income countries, sub-Saharan Africa has the highest HIV prevalence rates and bears the greatest global burden of HIV disease (Joint UN Program on AIDS, 2013). Women are 55% more likely to be HIV positive if they experience IPV (Joint UN Program on AIDS, 2014b).

Women who live with violent partners have little to say with regard to their reproductive health. The past two decades have brought a growing recognition that women's and girls' risk of and vulnerability to HIV infection is deep rooted in social and gender inequalities. The factors that place women who experience IPV at risk for HIV include fear of requesting condom use, fear of disclosing HIV status and seeking treatment, forced vaginal penetration, and risky sexual behavior stemming from instances of abuse (Joint UN Program on AIDS, 2014a). Additionally, women who are HIV positive suffer more frequent and severe abuse when compared with HIV-negative women in violent relationships (Chamberlain & Levenson, 2012).

The Impact of Childhood Exposure to Violence

Children exposed to the toxic stressors of violence and abuse during childhood are at significantly higher risk of experiencing medical and mental health issues in childhood and across their adult lives (CDC, 2014b; Felitti et al., 1998). The Adverse Childhood Experiences (ACE) study was conducted by the CDC in collaboration with Kaiser Permanente. During the initial phase of the study, approximately 17,000 adults were enrolled to examine the relationship between health and well-being later in life and exposure to adverse events during childhood (CDC, 2014b). While the ACE study was conducted in the United States, it is probable that similar findings would be discovered globally if this research were replicated. Findings from the ACE study indicate that the more a child is exposed to abuse, neglect, and other traumatic stressors, the more at risk they are for a host of health problems including but not limited to depression, illicit drug use, chronic obstructive pulmonary disease, ischemic heart disease, liver disease, and risk for IPV (CDC, 2014b). The evidence from the ACE study also suggests that childhood exposure to violence was also a risk for future IPV (CDC, 2014b; Felitti et al., 1998).

INTERVENTIONS TO PREVENT AND ADDRESS VIOLENCE AGAINST WOMEN

Over the past several decades, violence against women has received significant media and legislative attention. There is a growing openness to media coverage of violence against women worldwide. While we recognize this notable shift, we also know more efforts are needed. Globally, advertising campaigns help to raise public awareness and facilitate conversations that did not occur previously. Information can be found on television, on the radio, on the Internet, and in booklets. Communities have developed programs on prevention that seek to challenge gender norms while encouraging social justice and supporting women's human rights.

The social ecological model (Dahlberg & Krug, 2002) discussed earlier not only provides a framework to identify risk factors for IPV, but also provides a framework for prevention aimed at halting violence before it begins. This model represents an integration of individual, relationship, community, and societal factors that may limit the cycle of violence. Therefore, developing strategies to intervene at each level may result in a more comprehensive approach to violence.

WHO and CDC Recommendations

Violence against women is a major public health problem globally, but it can be prevented. Efforts to prevent violence against women should be comprehensive, addressing the myriad factors that place women at risk. Public recognition that violence in a relationship is not the norm is a necessary first step to preventing violence and addressing gender inequality.

Public health experts would agree that prevention strategies developed by community members offer the best opportunity for behavior change and sustainability. While it is true that efforts must occur at the local level, including community leaders, efforts are also necessary at the national and international levels, including both government and nongovernmental agencies (Garcia-Moreno et al., 2005). In 2005, WHO offered 15 recommendations in the following five domains: strengthening national commitment and action; promoting primary prevention; strengthening the health sector response; supporting women living with violence; and sensitizing criminal justice systems (Garcia-Moreno et al., 2005). Table 13.2 provides a sampling of these recommendations.

TABLE 13.2 Recommendations to Prevent and Address Intimate Partner Violence (IPV) Based on the Findings From the WHO Multicountry Study

STRENGTHENING NATIONAL COMMITMENT AND ACTION
1. Promote gender equality and women's human rights, and compliance with international agreements
2. Establish, implement, and monitor multisectoral action plans to address violence against women
3. Enlist social, political, religious, and other leaders in speaking out against violence against women
4. Enhance capacity for data collection to monitor violence against women, and the attitudes and beliefs that perpetuate it

(continued)

TABLE 13.2 Recommendations to Prevent and Address Intimate Partner Violence (IPV) Based on the Findings From the WHO Multicountry Study (*continued*)

PROMOTING PRIMARY PREVENTION
5. Develop, implement and evaluate programs aimed at primary prevention of intimate-partner violence
6. Prioritize the prevention of child sexual abuse
7. Integrate responses to violence against women into existing programs, such as for the prevention of HIV/AIDs and for the promotion of adolescent health
8. Make physical environments safer for women
9. Make schools safe for girls
STRENGTHENING THE HEALTH SECTOR RESPONSE
10. Develop a comprehensive health sector response to the various impacts of violence against women
11. Use the potential of reproductive health services as entry points for identifying women in abusive relationships, and for delivering referral and support services
SUPPORTING WOMEN LIVING WITH VIOLENCE
12. Strengthen formal and informal support systems for women living with violence
SENSITIZING CRIMINAL JUSTICE SYSTEMS
13. Sensitize legal and justice systems to the particular needs of women victims of violence
SUPPORTING RESEARCH AND COLLABORATION
14. Support research on the causes, consequences, and costs of violence against women and on effective prevention measures
15. Increase support to programs to reduce and respond to violence against women

Source: Garcia-Moreno et al. (2005).

TABLE 13.3 Recommendations for the Prevention of Intimate Partner and Sexual Violence Based on the CDC NIPSVS

IMPLEMENT PREVENTION APPROACHES
1. Promote healthy, respectful relationships among youth
2. Address beliefs, attitudes, and messages that condone, encourage, or facilitate sexual violence, stalking, or IPV
ENSURE APPROPRIATE RESPONSE
3. Provide survivors with coordinated services and develop a system of care to ensure healing and prevent the recurrence of victimization
4. Ensure access to services and resources
HOLD PERPETRATORS ACCOUNTABLE
5. Support efforts based on strong research data
6. Implement strong data systems for monitoring and evaluation
7. Identify ways to prevent first-time perpetration of sexual violence, stalking, and IPV

IPV, intimate partner violence; NIPSVS, National Intimate Partner and Sexual Violence Survey.
Source: Black et al. (2011).

Likewise, based on findings from the CDC's NIPSVS, Black et al. (2011) made six recommendations within four domains aimed at prevention, appropriate response, holding perpetrators accountable, and supporting the development of a strong research database (Table 13.3). Recommendations from both the WHO and the CDC underscore the importance health providers have in both addressing and preventing violence. They also support the notion that preventing and intervening with women who experience violence must occur on several levels.

Social Strategies

Worldwide, since 2008, there are 16 days of activism focused on the elimination of violence against women. These days of activism occur between November 25 and December 10. WHO, in coordination with international organizers, promotes a number of activities that highlight the intersection between violence against women and health. Advocacy messages and *Resource and Take Action Kits* are developed annually, and the events can be followed on Twitter and Facebook. For more information on this initiative, see www.who.int/gender/violence/sixteendays/en.

Finally, another evolving social strategy to increase violence awareness is the use of applications for mobile devices (apps) for victims of violence and their health care providers. Table 13.4 provides examples of available applications for mobile devices. This method is particularly useful for teens and young

TABLE 13.4 Apps for Intimate and Teen Dating Violence and Education for Providers

APPs	DESCRIPTION
The ASPIRE News App	ASPIRE News is a free application. Designed from When Georgia Smiled: Robin McGraw Foundation (and powered by Yahoo!). Able to reach out to trusted friends with your GPS location. Free. Target: Adults. For use with Androids and iPhones. https://www.whengeorgiasmiled.org/the-aspire-news-app
AURORA Australia	The Aurora domestic and family violence app is for people experiencing domestic and family violence or for those worried about their relationship. It is also a valuable resource for those worried that a friend or family member is experiencing domestic and family violence. Free. Target: Adults. Has GPS ability. For use with Androids and iPhones. http://www.women.nsw.gov.au/violence_prevention/domestic_and_family_violence_app
Circle of 6	This app can connect an individual with friends to stay close, stay safe, and prevent violence before it happens. Designed for college students, it is quick and easy to reach six friends you need help getting home? Need an interruption? Two touches let your circle know where you are and how they can help. It's the mobile way to look out for your friends on campus or when you're out for the night. Free. Target: Teens and college students. Has GPS ability. For use with Androids and iPhones. Winner of the White House/Health and Human Service Apps Against Abuse Technology Challenge. Winner of the IOM/Avon Foundation for Women Ending Violence @ home Challenge. http://www.circleof6app.com
Grace's Diary	This app can prevent dating violence through awareness, education, and advocacy (+video games) in memory of Jennifer Ann Crecente. Free. Target: Teens. For use with Androids. http://www.jenniferann.org

(continued)

TABLE 13.4 Apps for Intimate and Teen Dating Violence and Education for Providers (*continued*)

APPs	DESCRIPTION
Love Is Not Abuse	Launched in August 2011, the Love Is Not Abuse iPhone app is an educational resource for parents that demonstrates the dangers of digital dating abuse and provides much needed information on the growing problem of teen dating violence and abuse. Free. Target: Teens. For use with Androids and iPhones. http://www.breakthecycle.org/lina-app
One Love MyPlan App	Helps an individual determine if a relationship is unsafe and helps to create the best action plan by weighing an individual's unique characteristics and values. In partnership with LoveisRespect.org, the app provides access to trained advocate support 24/7 through an embedded live chat function. Free. Target: Teens and Young Adults. For use with Androids and iPhones. http://www.joinonelove.org/resources-help
One Love Danger Assessment App	Helps individuals to assess safety in their relationships and connect to resources. Danger Assessment has over 20 years of research. Free. Target: Teens and Adults. For use with Androids and iPhones. http://www.joinonelove.org/resources-help
R3 App	Recognize, respond, and refer. Created to educate medical professionals in hospitals, doctors' offices, and clinics to make appropriate assessments of domestic violence victims and refer them to resources that can help. Free. Target: Health care providers. For use with Androids and iPhones. http://www.harborhousefl.com/2012/01/r3-app-2
Safety Siren	This app was developed by the YMCA in Canada and is available in both English and French. Offers health and safety information for young women. Free. Target: Young Women and Adults. For use with Androids, iPhones, iPods, and BlackBerrys. http://ywcacanada.ca/en/pages/mall/apps
TD 411	Designed to bring awareness about teen dating violence and cyber awareness. This app provides an individual with information to avoid abuse and finding resources. Free. Target: Teens. For use with Androids and iPhones. http://www.td411.org

women at risk or who are experiencing violence victimization since smartphone technology is often appealing to individuals in this age group. While these mobile applications were developed in resource-rich countries, they provide a platform for the development of mobile technologies in resource-limited countries as well, since cell phones are often accessible in many countries worldwide.

Research: Opportunities and Challenges

Despite the advances made in the past decades in the field of IPV, there are many lingering questions and opportunities to close these gaps through nursing research. Much is known about the health-related outcomes of victims of IPV. However, global prevention programs, strategies, and initiatives have not been systematically reviewed or evaluated. Research has a central role in examining the effectiveness and impact of various global initiatives (Devries et al., 2013). Other

TABLE 13.5 Ethical and Safety Recommendations for Domestic Violence Research

- The safety of respondents and the research team is paramount, and should guide all project decisions.
- Prevalence studies need to be methodologically sound and to build upon current research experience about how to minimize the underreporting of violence.
- Protecting confidentiality is essential to ensure both women's safety and data quality.
- All research team members should be carefully selected and receive specialized training and ongoing support.
- The study design must include actions aimed at reducing any possible distress cause to the participants by the research.
- Fieldworkers should be trained to refer women requesting assistance to available local services and sources of support. Where few resources exist, it may be necessary for the study to create short-term support mechanisms.
- Researchers and donors have an ethical obligation to help ensure that their findings are properly interpreted and used to advance policy and intervention development.
- Violence questions should only be incorporated into surveys designed for other purposes when ethical and methodological requirements cannot be met.

Source: Watts et al. (1999).

areas for research include the effect of lifetime exposures to violence, effects of screening tools and screening approaches, management of health outcomes, ways to improve care for women living with IPV, and the evaluation of interventions in different countries (Guruge, 2012).

A major challenge in conducting research on women who are IPV victims is protecting their safety and ensuring that the studies conducted are ethical and sensitive to the participants. Understanding the need for research in this area and the challenges inherent in conducting research with this population, Watts, Heise, Ellsberg, and Garcia-Moreno (1999) developed a set of eight recommendations to guide research related to domestic violence (Table 13.5). These recommendations should serve as guiding principles for nurse researchers in the field.

IMPLICATIONS FOR NURSING PRACTICE

The prevalence of violence against women globally is staggering and is a concern for all health providers. Despite the high incidence of violence worldwide and the global challenges nurses face when caring for women, there are steps that can be taken in order to continue to identify and reduce violence. Nurses are in a position to impact this problem. Several nurse researchers, including Drs. Jacquelyn Campbell, Ann Burgess, Barbara Parker, Judith McFarlane, and Janice Humphreys, were pioneers in developing programs of research on violence against women.

Globally, investments have been made in the treatment of victims who have experienced GBV. Victims of GBV typically do not seek assistance from law enforcement, but rather turn to health care professionals (Chibber & Krishnan, 2011). Women's health services, particularly in developing countries, have expanded. Thus, access for women and opportunities for GBV-related care are becoming an essential aspect of the spectrum of services for screening and identification.

The expansion of women's health services has been supported by the UN and addressed in several of the Millennium Development Goals (MDGs). Notably, one MDG focuses specifically on gender inequality and improving the health of women and girls.

The health system, along with other sectors of governments worldwide, must take an active role in addressing the IPV global crisis. Nurses have a key role in addressing IPV. The nursing profession is well positioned to address the policy issues and develop programs and interventions that may result in a reduction in the incidence of IPV and associated adverse health outcomes. Mitigating the long-term negative health outcomes for victims of IPV is critical to achieving optimal health and addressing the toll on health care costs.

Moreover, nurses are well suited to designing IPV education programs to address women's reproductive health. The incidence and prevalence of IPV are influenced by cultural, societal, interpersonal, and situational factors, including gender inequality. Health promotion interventions focusing on overall awareness of the widespread occurrence of IPV, the importance of healthy relationships, and the effects of IPV on women's and children's health are specific areas that professional nurses must address. The involvement of men in IPV awareness and prevention is another key intervention. Promoting healthy relationships and engaging men in violence prevention may impact the incidence of IPV. Nurses must expand their prevention focus to include not only the individual, but also family, community, and societal influences that lead to IPV (Guruge, 2012). Additionally, developing educational programs that focus on violence prevention awareness and life skill development along with support programs for victims are critical for IPV prevention and breaking the cycle of violence (Guruge, 2012). When equipped with the proper skill, education, and material resources, nurses may be key drivers in social change regarding IPV.

Incorporating IPV assessment, identification, and intervention techniques into nursing curricula and interprofessional education are critical (Campbell, Abrahams, & Martin, 2008). Many nursing organizations worldwide have developed position statements that focus on the nurse's role related to GBV and IPV and serve as a guide for professional practice.

CONCLUSION

For the past three decades, IPV has been documented as an epidemic. The health risks and sequelae associated with violence have been well documented in the nursing and health care literature. Scientific research and professional moral and ethical obligations underscore the need for nurses to provide care and promote safety and well-being for individuals and families. Progress has been made, but further research and clinical work are needed to address the gaps. As Mahatma Gandhi stated:

> Woman is the companion of man, gifted with equal capacities. She has the right to participate in minutest details in the activities of man, and she has an equal right of freedom and liberty with him.

REFERENCES

American College of Obstetricians and Gynecologists. (2012). ACOG Committee opinion No. 518: Intimate partner violence. *Obstetrics and Gynecology, 119*, 412–417.

Amnesty International. (n.d.). *Violence against women.* Retrieved from http://www.amnestyusa.org/our-work/issues/women-s-rights/violence-against-women?id=1011012

Beydoun, H. A., Beydoun, M. A., Kaufman, J. S., Lo, B., & Zonderman, A. B. (2012). Intimate partner violence against adult women and its association with major depressive disorder, depressive symptoms and postpartum depression: A systematic review and meta-analysis. *Social Science and Medicine, 75*(6), 959–975.

Black, M. C., Basile, K. C., Breiding, M. J., Smith, S. G., Walters, M. L., Merrick, M. T., . . . Stevens, M. R. (2011). *The national intimate partner and sexual violence survey: 2010 Summary report.* Atlanta, GA: Centers for Disease Control and Prevention.

Bonomi, A. E., Thompson, R. S., Anderson, M., Reid, R. J., Carrell, D., Dimer, J. A., & Rivara, F. P. (2006). Intimate partner violence and women's physical, mental, and social functioning. *American Journal of Preventive Medicine, 30*, 458–466.

Breiding, M. J., Black, M. C., & Ryan, G. W. (2008). Prevalence and risk factors of intimate partner violence in eighteen U.S. states/territories, 2005. *American Journal of Preventive Medicine, 34*(2), 112–118.

Campbell, J. C. (2002). Health consequences of intimate partner violence. *The Lancet, 359*, (9314), 1331–1336.

Campbell, J. C., Abrahams, N., & Martin, L. (2008). Perpetration of violence against intimate partners: Health care implications from global data. *Canadian Medical Association Journal, 179*(6), 511–512.

Campbell, J. C., Webster, D., Koziol-McLain, J., Block, C. R., Campbell, D., Curry, M. A., . . . Wilt, S. A. (2003). Assessing risk factors for intimate partner homicide. *NIJ Journal, 250*, 14–19.

Centers for Disease Control and Prevention. (2008). Adverse health conditions: Health risk behaviors associated with intimate partner violence. *Morbidity Mortality Weekly Report (MMWR), 57*, 113–117.

Centers for Disease Control and Prevention. (2014a). CDC grand rounds: A public health approach to prevention of intimate partner violence. *Morbidity Mortality Weekly Report (MMWR), 63*, 38–41.

Centers for Disease Control and Prevention. (2014b). *Injury prevention & control: Adverse childhood experiences (ACE) study.* Retrieved from www.cdc.gov/violenceprevention/acestudy/

Chamberlain, L., & Levenson, R. (2012). Addressing intimate partner violence, reproductive and sexual coercion: A guide for obstetric, gynecological, and reproductive health care settings (2nd ed.). San Francisco, CA: American Colleges of Obstetricians and Gynecologists and *Futures Without Violence.*

Chibber, K. S., & Krishnan, S. (2011). Confronting intimate partner violence, a global health care priority. *Mount Sinai Journal of Medicine, 78*, 449–457.

Coker, A., Smith, P., Bethea, L., King, M., & McKeown, R. (2000). Physical health consequences of physical and psychological intimate partner violence. *Archives in Family Medicine, 9*, 451–457.

Coker, A. L., Davis, K. E., Arias, I., Desai, S., Sanderson, M., . . . Smith, P. H. (2002). Physical and mental health effects of intimate partner violence for men and women. *American Journal of Preventive Medicine, 23*, 260–268.

Coker, A. L., Sanderson, M., & Dong, B. (2004). Partner violence during pregnancy and risk of adverse pregnancy outcomes. *Pediatric Perinatal Epidemiology, 18*(4), 260–269.

Dahlberg, L. L., & Krug, E. G. (2002). Violence—a global public health problem. In E. Krug, L. Dahlberg, J. Mercy, A. Zwi, & R. Lozano (Eds.), *World report on violence and health.* Geneva, Switzerland: World Health Organization.

Devries, K., Mak, Y., Garcia-Moreno, C., Petzold, M., Child, C., Falder, S., . . . Watts, C. (2013). The global prevalence of intimate partner violence against women. *Science, 340,* 1527–1529.

Dillon, G., Hussain, R., Loxton, D., & Rahman, S. (2013). Mental and physical health and intimate partner violence against women: A review of the literature. *International Journal of Family Medicine, 13,* 1–15. doi:10.1155/2013/313909

Felitti, V., Anda, R., Nordenberg, D., Williamson, D., Spitz, A., Edwards V., . . . Marks, J. S. (1998). Relationship of childhood abuse and household dysfunction to many leading causes of death in adults: The Adverse Childhood Experiences (ACE) study. *American Journal of Preventive Medicine, 14,* 245–258.

Garcia-Moreno, C., Guedes, A., & Knerr, W. (2012). *Understanding and addressing violence against women intimate partner violence.* Geneva, Switzerland: World Health Organization.

Garcia-Moreno, C., Jansen, H., Ellsberg, M., Heise, L., & Watts, C. (2005). *WHO multi-country study on women's health and domestic violence against women: Initial results on prevalence, health outcomes, and women's responses.* Geneva, Switzerland: World Health Organization.

Guruge, S. (2012). Intimate partner violence: A global health perspective. *Canadian Journal of Nursing Research, 44*(4), 37–54.

Hatcher, A. M., Romito, P., Odero, M., Bukusi, E. A., Onono, M., & Turan, J. M. (2013). Social context and drivers of intimate partner violence in rural Kenya: Implications for the health of pregnant women. *Culture, Health and Sexuality, 15*(4), 404–419.

Heise, L., Ellsberg, M., & Gottemoeller, M. (1999). *Ending violence against women.* Population Reports (Series L, No. 11). Baltimore, MD: Johns Hopkins University School of Public Health, Population Information Program.

Heise, L., & Garcia-Moreno, C. (2002). Violence by intimate partners. In E. Krug, L. Dahlberg, J. Mercy, A. Zwi, & R. Lozano (Eds.), *World report on violence and health.* Geneva, Switzerland: World Health Organization.

Institute of Medicine (IOM). (2011). *Clinical preventive services for women: Closing the gaps.* Washington, DC: The National Academies Press.

Jewkes, R. (2002). Intimate partner violence: Causes and prevention. *The Lancet, 359*(9315), 1423–1429.

Joint United Nations Program on HIV/AIDS. (2013). *AIDS by the numbers.* Geneva, Switzerland: Author.

Joint United Nations Program on HIV/AIDS (UNAIDS). (2014a). Global AIDS response progress reporting 2014: Construction and core indicators for monitoring the 2011 UN political declaration on HIV/AIDS. Geneva, Switzerland: Author.

Joint United Nations Program on HIV/AIDS. (2014b). Unite with women. Unite against violence and HIV. Geneva, Switzerland: Author.

Karanja, L. (2003). Just die quietly: Domestic violence and women's vulnerability to HIV in Uganda. *Human Rights Watch, 15,* 1–76.

LoGuidice, J. A. (2014). Prenatal screening for intimate partner violence: A qualitative meta-synthesis. *Applied Nursing Research, 28*(1), 2–9. doi:10.1016/j.apnr.2014.04.004

Miller, E., Decker, M., McCauley, H., Tancredi, D., Levenson, R., Waldman, J., . . . Silverman, J. G. (2010). Pregnancy coercion, intimate partner violence and unintended pregnancy. *Contraception, 81,* 316–322.

National Center for Injury Prevention and Control. (2003). *Costs of intimate partner violence against women in the United States*. Atlanta, GA: Centers for Disease Control and Prevention.

Nelson, H., Bougatsos, C., & Blazina, I. (2012). Screening women for intimate partner violence: A systematic review to update the 2004 U.S. Preventive Services Task Force Recommendation. *Annals of Internal Medicine, 156*(11), 796–808.

Odero, M., Hatcher, A. M., Bryant, C., Onono, M., Romito, P., Bukusi, E. A., & Turan, J. M. (2014). Responses to and resources for intimate partner violence: Qualitative findings from women, men, and service providers in rural Kenya. *Journal of Interpersonal Violence, 29*(5), 783–805.

SafeNetwork. (1999). *Herstory of domestic violence: A timeline of the battered women's movement*. Retrieved from www.vawnet.org/domestic-violence/summary.php?doc_id=828 &find_type=web_desc_GC

Sarkar, N. N. (2008). The impact of intimate partner violence on women's reproductive health and pregnancy outcomes. *Journal of Obstetrics and Gynecology, 28*(3), 266–271.

Seghetti, L. M., & Bjelopera, J. P. (2010). *The violence against women act: Overview, legislation, and federal funding* (R42299). Washington, DC: Congressional Research Service.

Stockl, H., Devries, K., Rotstein, A., Abrahams, N., Campbell, J., Watts, C., & Moreno, C. (2013). The global prevalence of intimate partner homicide: A systematic review. *Lancet, 382*, 859–865.

Stockman, J. K., Lucea, M. B., & Campbell, J. C. (2013). Forced sexual initiation, sexual intimate partner violence, and HIV risk in women: A global review of the literature. *AIDS and Behavior, 17*(3), 832–847.

United Nations General Assembly. (1993, December). *Declaration on the elimination of discrimination against women* (UN Doc A/RES/48/104). New York, NY: Author.

U.S. Preventive Services Task Force. (2013). *Screening for intimate partner violence and abuse of elderly and vulnerable adults*. Retrieved from www.uspreventiveservicetalskforce.org/ uspstf12/ipvelder/ipvelderfinalrs.htm

U.S. 47—113th Congress. (2013). *Violence Against Women Reauthorization Act of 2013*, 42 (2013–2015). Retrieved from http://www.govtrack.us/congress/bills/113/s47

Watts, C., Heise, L., Ellsberg, M., & Garcia-Moreno, C. (1999). *Putting women's safety first: Ethical and safety recommendations for research on domestic violence against women*. Geneva, Switzerland: World Health Organization.

Watts, C., & Zimmerman, C. (2002). Violence against women: Global scope and magnitude. *Lancet, 359*, 1232–1237.

World Health Organization (WHO). (2009). *Violence prevention, the evidence: Changing cultural and social norms that support violence*. Geneva, Switzerland: Author.

World Health Organization. (2013). *Global and regional estimates of violence against women: Prevalence and health effects of intimate partner violence and non-partner sexual violence*. Geneva, Switzerland: Author, Reference number: 978 92 4 156462 5.

CHAPTER 14

Sex Trafficking as a New Pandemic

Mary de Chesnay

*T*he author hopes that this chapter both enrages and inspires the reader: That you will become angry that human and sex trafficking exist today as the fastest-growing and most lucrative of crimes, and inspired to learn more about the lives these people endure in order to help them transcend their unbearable present and have a happier and healthier future. The resilience of the human spirit is proven time after time when we listen to the stories of survivors. Although it might seem impossible, the victims of sex trafficking can become survivors and move beyond it with help. Nurses are likely to be among the few outsiders they will approach. Yet we may not recognize them as being exploited. It is a global problem and nurses worldwide must be proactive in assessment, intervention, and assisting the victims into survivorhood.

CONTEXT

Definitions

Some terms need to be defined in order to understand the complexity of trafficking. This chapter begins with an overview of key terms related to sex trafficking.

Human Trafficking

Article 3, paragraph (a) of the United Nations Protocol (2000) to Prevent, Suppress and Punish Trafficking in Persons defines Trafficking in Persons as the recruitment, transportation, transfer, harbouring, or receipt of persons, by means of the threat or use of force or other forms of coercion, of abduction, of fraud, of deception, of the abuse of power or of a position of vulnerability or of the giving or receiving of payments or benefits to achieve the consent of a person having control over another person, for the purpose of exploitation. Exploitation shall include, at a minimum, the exploitation of the prostitution of others or other forms of sexual exploitation, forced labour or services, slavery or practices similar to slavery, servitude or the removal of organs. (www.unodc .org/unodc/en/human-trafficking/what-is-human-trafficking. html#What_is_Human_Trafficking)

Precise statistics on the extent of the problem are hard to obtain. Bales estimated that 27 million people around the world live in slavery today (Bales, 2004; U.S. State Department, 2012). It is estimated that at any given time, there are about 2.5 million people worldwide who are victims of human trafficking, with 40% to 50% of those being children (International Labor Office, 2005).

In this definition, there are two forms of human trafficking: *forced labor* and *sex trafficking*. *Debt bondage* is a phenomenon common to both in which the traffickers create an increasing debt based on "expenses" for transporting the victims.

Forced Labor

Victims of forced labor might be migrant workers, other agricultural workers such as children who work in the African cocoa plantations, children who work the brick kilns in India, child soldiers (common in India and Africa), and sweat-shop workers. The Restavek children of Haiti can be found in domestic servitude (Nicholas et al., 2012).

Sex Trafficking

Women and children comprise most of the sex trade around the world but adult men are also forced into the sex trade, sometimes directly and sometimes through forced labor, where they encounter torture and rape (Bales, 2005; Jones, 2010).

Commercial Sex Exploitation of Children (CSEC) or Domestic Minor Sex Trafficking (DMST)

These terms refer to sex trafficking of minors. The age of 18 is most commonly the age of majority in the United States and most countries (www.worldlawdirect .com/forum/law-wiki/27181-age-majority.html).

Pathways

In a landmark study for the Department of Justice, Bales and Lize (2005) reviewed cases from Florida, Chicago, and Washington, DC, and identified five stages of the process of human trafficking:

1. Vulnerability
2. Recruitment

3. Transportation
4. Exploitation
5. Exposure, discovery, liberation

The people most *vulnerable* to trafficking tend to be young and fairly healthy, and are likely to be poor and powerless but not necessarily from the poorest class of their societies. They may be educated and are rarely kidnapped. Traffickers are more likely to prey upon their dreams and aspirations because they know that cooperation by their victims eases the process. Traffickers favor victims from marginalized groups or women or children because these people are often looking for a better life for their families.

Selling the dream, or *recruitment*, is easier when traffickers are charismatic. They are expert at reading people and convincing victims that they can deliver on promises of golden opportunities in the destination country or city. They may use a woman or man, even a family member, who has been paid to recruit and who can be trusted to be loyal to the traffickers and lie to the victims about the opportunities. Once the victims arrive at the destination, the trafficker uses bait-and-switch techniques to keep the person. The rules change and threats and violence enforce the new rules.

Transportation might be simple, involving existing legal entities and legal visas or false documents. There might be a transporter who accompanies the victim and provides a safe house during transit. The next level of transportation is a segmented business operation in which the traffickers themselves transport and provide "stash houses." The third level, and most difficult to identify and prosecute, is complex integrated operations in which criminal networks with many resources control the transportation.

Exploitation is final when control is established. How control is established varies from debt bondage to confiscation of documents, threats of arrest or deportation, degradation, and violence. In many cases, traffickers wait until arrival at the destination to establish control because they need the victim's cooperation to pass borders. In the case of children, though, they have control as soon as they take custody of the child since children are more likely to do as they are told by an adult. Traffickers maintain a constant vigilance and may lock their victims in when not working and transport them to their place of work. Keeping victims isolated and disoriented is an effective control tactic.

The last stage is a progression of *exposure*, *discovery*, and *liberation*. Unfortunately, the rates of murder by traffickers and accidental death from injury and suicide are high for this population. Women and children in the sex trade are at risk for contracting HIV/AIDS. Relatively few victims are rescued by law enforcement and some manage to escape. The fortunate ones manage to be found by "Good Samaritans" who may be of their own ethnicity or who are at least able to recognize the signs of trafficking. If victims can connect with the right authorities they may be eligible for change-of-visa status, may be able to help authorities to arrest and prosecute their traffickers, and may be eligible to receive services to reverse the effects of their enslavement.

Stages of Entrapment

While it is true that some children are kidnapped and others are sold by their parents, it is more common for children to be tricked by traffickers who present themselves as a friend, boyfriend, or protective employer. Barnardo's, a children's advocacy charity in the United Kingdom, identified four stages of entrapment into prostitution. These are presented in O'Connor and Healy (2006) and Hawthorne (2011) as the following:

- Stage 1 is *ensnaring*, in which the trafficker gains the child's trust by pretending to be her caring protector/boyfriend. He may buy her presents, give her shelter and food, and clothe her. He may be accepted by her parents as a "nice young man" if she is living at home.
- Stage 2 is *creating dependence*, in which he isolates her from family and friends, changes her name, and generally becomes more possessive. She interprets this possessiveness as his passionate love for her and, as proof that she loves him, she willingly distances herself from her family and friends and engages in prostitution to please him.
- Stage 3 is characterized by *taking control*, in which he exerts increasing control over her daily activities such as what she eats and wears and he may alternate violence with kindness in order to remain unpredictable. He usually becomes increasingly violent at this stage, but she still loves him and maintains hope that he will change. Because she is isolated from support systems and feels shame for her activities, she does not try to escape.
- Stage 4 is *total dominance*, in which he convinces her by force if necessary to have sex with whomever he directs. He may lock her in a room to ensure she does not try to escape and threaten to kill her or her family if she attempts to leave him.

Other authors (McClanahan, McClelland, Abram, & Teplin, 1999) have described pathways to child prostitution as running away and childhood sexual abuse. A study of 1,142 female jail detainees found that running away in early adolescence had a dramatic effect on entry into prostitution, but little effect later in life. However, being sexually abused as a child nearly doubled the odds of entry throughout their lives. The role of drug abuse is inconclusive as some victims begin drug use after they enter "the life" and some are users beforehand.

Sex Tourism

Closely related to sex trafficking is sex tourism (de Chesnay, 2012). Sex tourism describes travel for sex, usually with partners who would be perceived as exotic (different race than the traveler) or with children who might be more accessible in destination countries in which the child sex trade is allowed to flourish. Thailand is so well known for sex tourism with both women and children that *Fielding's Guide* devoted a section of its Thailand book to sex tourism (Dulles, 1996). Child sex tourism flourishes in impoverished areas of the world where parents can delude themselves that the traffickers to whom they sell their children will give them a better life. On the other hand, children who have no families and live on the street survive any way they can. Once the child is in the life, the benefits to the family of the sex trade and the options for leaving the life create a paradox for the child. The more he or she stays in the life, the more the child learns to tolerate the bad parts and becomes numb to any attempts to be rescued.

Scholars have studied cultural aspects of Thailand as a destination for the child sex trade. In an ethnographic study in which she interviewed children in Thailand, Montgomery (2008) concluded that the stereotype of the tourist visiting Thailand on organized sex tours was misleading and that some children did not define themselves as prostitutes, nor did they despise their "johns." Instead, they developed relationships with these men who helped support their families during times of severe economic stress (Montgomery, 2008). While definitely not making the case that sex with children is acceptable, Montgomery cautioned that the phenomenon of sex tourism is much more complex than tawdry advertisements would lead one to believe. Pedophiles succeed in seducing children and can be quite convincing that they love the children.

Solutions such as revoking passports of Americans who travel to Thailand for sex, as suggested by some authors (Hall, 2011), might be effective at stopping the tourists from exploiting children in the destination countries but paradoxically might not be perceived as help by those we define as victims. If the police are corrupt, they will not cooperate with American authorities to detain or deport them because the sex tourists are a source of revenue for the police. Pedophiles flourish in places that allow sex with children. Who will step forward to protect these children if their own police look the other way? Unless governments find ways to reverse the poverty, violence, devaluation of women, and ignorance that underlie the sex trade, women and children, particularly in developing countries, will continue to have few alternatives.

The Caribbean is a destination for sex tourists of both genders. In the Dominican Republic, male sex workers specialize in male sex tourists from North America and Europe (Gigliotti, 2006; Padilla, 2008). Female sex tourists, or "sugar mummies," as well as male tourists to Cuba and the Dominican Republic might define themselves as romance tourists and see themselves in long-term relationships with locals, sometimes leading to marriage and migration for the local to the tourist's home country (Aston, 2008; Cabezas, 2004).

The complexity of relationships in sex tourism masks the exploitation of children who are trafficked for the purpose of commerce. In an Organization of American States (OAS)-funded study of nine countries in Latin America and the Caribbean, researchers found that little has been done to implement the UN Protocol of 2000 that called for initiatives by member countries to halt human trafficking, prosecute traffickers, and provide services to victims (Langberg, 2005).

On a more positive note, though, the tourism industries in a number of countries have signed the Code of Conduct for the Protection of Children From Sexual Exploitation in Travel and Tourism, an industry-driven initiative funded by the Swiss government and private concerns and sponsored under the auspices of an international organization, End Child Prostitution and Trafficking (ECPAT). Notable signers of the code are Delta Airlines, Hilton Hotels, and Wyndham Hotels (ECPAT, 2012). The criteria in the code call for ethical commitment to end child trafficking with training for staff and screening of suppliers. One way to support efforts to abolish modern slavery is to patronize businesses that do not facilitate traffickers.

BEST PRACTICES AND EVIDENCE-BASED RESEARCH

There are no best practices for treating sex trafficking victims in the sense that research is sparse and clinical research is almost nonexistent. The highest order of evidence is traditionally thought to be that derived from randomized clinical trials. However, evidence can also be based on nonrandomized trials, descriptive studies that build testable theory, case reports by clinicians, and qualitative studies that describe in rich detail the experience of members of the population of interest. In the case of sex-trafficked victims, who are difficult to identify and who do not have control of their own bodies or schedules, valid and reliable research data are difficult to acquire.

Several attempts by nurse scholars have been made to identify the key issues and barriers in working with this population. In this sense, Sabella (2011) and Crane (Crane & Moreno, 2011) are two nurses who have pioneered the process of identifying best practices of working with survivors of trafficking. Sabella is a Pennsylvania-based psychiatric/mental health nurse who teaches nurses and works with the population. She taught one of the first courses on human trafficking to assist health care providers to recognize and interact appropriately with victims. Crane (Crane & Moreno, 2011) is a forensic nurse who is instrumental in political advocacy for victims in Texas, one of the early states to pass legislation in the spirit of decriminalizing prostituted children. Both of these leaders in the field have published their work in the nursing literature so that other nurses may benefit from their experiences and they remain active and committed to this most vulnerable population.

Trout (2010) also has published on the need for nurses to identify these victims. McClain and Garrity (2011) addressed the need for nurses who work with adolescents to educate themselves about this growing problem. The American Nurses Association (ANA) and several states have passed resolutions opposing human trafficking (Alabama State Nurses' Association, 2009; Kansas State Nurses' Association, 2008; Trossman, 2008). The American Academy of Nursing appointed a task force (chaired by Dr. Melanie Percy) under the Expert Panel on Global Health to prepare a white paper on human trafficking for presentation in 2012. In 2010, the National Student Nurses Association (NSNA) passed a resolution to increase awareness of human trafficking (NSNA, 2010). These efforts are a good start but need to be expanded.

Even though there is a great need for evidence-based research on human trafficking, there are best practices for treating a variety of health conditions that affect victims. For example, much work on posttraumatic stress disorder (PTSD) has been done to help soldiers readjust to civilian life (Bastien, 2010; Meis, Barry, Kehle, Erbes, & Polusney, 2010; Mulvaney, McLean, & De Leeuw, 2010). Although the issues for CSEC victims are different, some of the same treatments might be helpful. For example, pharmacologic management in concert with trauma-focused cognitive behavioral therapy can lead to better outcomes by alleviating at least one of the three symptom clusters of PTSD: reexperiencing, avoidance, and hyper arousal (Ipser, Seedat, & Stein, 2006). PTSD in child sexual abuse survivors, whether commercially exploited or not, is comorbid with a host of other conditions, necessitating multiple methods of treatment.

Research on torture generated interventions to help victims of state-sponsored atrocities (Genefke, 2002; Glittenberg, 2003; Grodin & Annas, 2007; Levine, 2001; Moreno & Grodin, 2002; Moreno & Iacopino, 2008; Olsen, Montgomery, Bojholm, & Foldspong, 2006; Racine-Welch & Welch, 2000). Many of the signs of torture are similar to those in women or children who have been prostituted. They regularly endure beatings, fractures, sleep and food deprivation, sexually transmitted infections (STIs), and verbal messages that they are worthless. Like torture victims, they live with chronic pain from the many types of injuries suffered during torture and they suffer the effects of malnutrition from being deprived of food and water for long periods. Certainly there are best practices for the health conditions of pregnancy, STIs, physical trauma, and so on.

Primary prevention is one of the most important concepts when discussing best practices in health care. In the United States, great attention is given to teaching people how to stay healthy and prevent illness and injury. However, for the population of trafficked victims who are still in the life, prevention is not only irrelevant but impossible, and trying to teach about prevention could have the paradoxical effect of reinforcing the victim's view that we really have no idea what she is going through. For example, the best prevention practice for vesico-vaginal fistula is not to bear children until beyond adolescence. Wearing condoms goes a long way toward preventing AIDS and STIs and, of course, early pregnancies. How is a prostituted child supposed to follow that advice when she does not get to decide with whom and when she will engage in sex?

Prevention means being able to avoid activities that place one at risk for specific health problems or generalized poor health. However, vulnerability due to poor family resources creates risks for girls who connect with traffickers who promise them or their families a better life. "Romeo pimps" in the United States (men who pretend to be in love with their victims) sometimes deliberately impregnate the girls in order to control them (anonymous, personal communication, 2011). Once the baby comes, they can then alternately hold out the hope that they will be a "real family" or the threat that they will sell the baby if the girl does not stay in line.

Alternatively, some traffickers, particularly in Eastern Europe, take children for organ harvesting (Kambayashi, 2004; Lita, 2007). Yea (2010) reports on two ways children are trafficked in addition to sex trafficking. Some children are taken for begging assignments and these children may be deliberately disabled to create sympathy, or they might be disabled already and then forced to beg for the traffickers. Deaf children are particularly attractive to the traffickers because they are less able to communicate with people who might help them. A second way children are used is to train them as camel jockeys. Male children who are preferably around age 5 are taken from India, Pakistan, and Bangladesh to the Arab Emirates to be camel jockeys for the racing industry. Their parents are told the boys will earn much money to send home, but in reality the children are sent to desert camps where they undergo brutal training and punishment with electric shocks and food deprivation. They are contained within complexes where they sleep in cardboard boxes, making them prone to scorpion bites. They wake at 4 a.m. to exercise the camels and then must care for the camels before the afternoon-to-nightfall exercise periods.

Given the limited outcomes research on sex trafficking, this chapter is an attempt to present the best practices to date with the hope that those working with victims will have some basis on which to set priorities and provide the best care possible under limited conditions. Human trafficking is receiving wide attention from the media, legislators, and prosecutors. Health care professionals need to partner with others in their communities to address the medical and psychological needs of victims holistically. It is hoped that nurses who practice in settings in which victims are likely to appear will recognize their need for help, define them as victims and not criminals, and, in working with them, improve on the ideas presented here.

CULTURAL ASPECTS OF SEX TRAFFICKING

The Culture of the Street

Culture is a set of life-ways, rituals, values, language, and behaviors that are held in common by a people who may or may not live in proximity to one another. Traditionally, culture is discussed in connection with one's geographic home, but culture can also describe the shared values and life-ways of people who share other common characteristics. Nurses are a good example of a group of people who live in many areas of the world but who share a common culture. Whatever our education and wherever in the world we practice, we share that our lives are dedicated to helping our people improve their health. We use both the science and art of intervention to help our patients attain a higher level of health. We have rituals such as pinning ceremonies and protocols such as best practices to guide our work.

Language defines where we live (New Yorkers, Californians); our nationality (Cambodians, Canadians, Australians); what kind of work we do (nurses, police officers, dog groomers, teachers, social workers, carpenters, postal workers); or how we see ourselves in relation to others (child advocates, leaders, advisors, Republicans, retirees). Language is shared by a cultural group, not only in terms of the primary languages of English, French, Japanese, or Swahili, but also in terms of dialects and jargon.

Language expresses power and can be used to exclude or include individuals from a group. For example, jargon is sometimes used to prevent nongroup members from fully understanding in-group members. The language of the street provides a way for people who live "on the street" to exclude members of the "establishment" and to make themselves feel more powerful in relation to powerful people around them.

Similarly, street language of whore, "ho," "hooker," or prostitute—even euphemisms such as "sex workers," "call girls," and "ladies of the night"—are negative labels used to stereotype those who sell their bodies for sex. There is even controversy over the term "selling" since that implies choice on the part of the girl. Linda Smith, a former congresswoman and the founder of Shared Hope International, tells the story of her husband mentioning to her that what really happens is that the pimp rents the child to others for money (Smith, webcast 12/1/2011). Renting is a more descriptive term since it connotes the involvement of the person usually in control of the process. Shared Hope International (2011) sponsors a billboard campaign to fight trafficking in which one billboard shows a picture of a man's torso with his hands (showing a wedding ring) in the process of removing his jacket and with his belt partially undone. The caption is: "This man wants to rent your daughter."

Another example of how language is used is particularly relevant for those who would help commercially sexually exploited people. For the purposes of this chapter, we will sometimes refer to these women and children as victims (almost all are women and children of both sexes) but with the caution that they not only do not always see themselves as victims and, in fact, might become angry at the thought of anyone else calling them victims. Anger at being labeled a victim could be a defense mechanism to exaggerate what little control they have in their lives. The reality is that no matter how demoralized they are, they are all survivors. The term "survivor" is preferred but it is critical to use the term "victim" as well to convey that these children do not choose a life of exploitation, rape, and torture. They may choose to go with a Romeo pimp because they are conned or coerced, but their choice quickly becomes "comply or die." Those who would label them as criminals need to understand the lengths to which these women and children must go in order to survive.

When Rachel Lloyd (2011) founded the Girls' Education and Mentoring Services (GEMS) to assist prostitutes to make the transition out of "the life," she constructed a language model from victim to survivor to leader to capture a sense of hope for these women. Whether they are called victims, survivors, or leaders, and whether we as nurses call them patients or clients, it is critical to understand that they are human beings forced into a life in which their choice is usually to comply or die.

Life-ways and rituals are also part of life on the street and define rules and how they are to be followed for survival. The rules about appropriate behavior for girls in the life are designed by pimps to control every aspect of the girl's life in order to minimize the chance that she will leave. The trafficker or pimp makes rules about where she sleeps, how much she eats, how she obtains basics such as tampons, and how much toilet paper she can use. Rules are enforced brutally with beatings with fists or a pimp stick. A pimp stick can be a cane or coat hanger doubled over itself to form a thin rod. Other common forms of torture are cigarette burns, dragging by the hair until clumps come out, submersing the face in a toilet, and gang rape.

Pimps are businessmen and their goal is to make money for themselves by sexually exploiting women and children. They may work in apparent isolation and competition with each other, but they have informal networks with other pimps. For example, they will trade or sell girls to each other. A girl who looks at or talks to another pimp is likely to be beaten by her pimp, but the pimp may initiate deals to obtain a younger model or a girl may negotiate to be traded. It would be reasonable to assume that pimps would want to protect their investment and protect the girls rather than torture them, but control trumps caring and keeping the girls malnourished, sleep-deprived, and in pain maintains dominance.

Pimps celebrate their accomplishments at exploiting women and children by dressing in their finery and holding an annual convention called the Players' Ball, which is an opportunity to buy and sell women and children (World Famous Players' Ball, 2005). They give an award to the pimp who has made the most money during the year. This author deliberated long and hard about including mention of the Players' Ball here, which might be viewed by some as helping to glorify pimps, but decided to do so in the hope that residents of the cities to which they apply to hold their convention will follow the lead of Mayor Shirley Franklin of Atlanta, who refused to support the convention in Atlanta in 2003. It was moved to a private club outside the city (Interfaith Children's Movement, 2009).

Culturally Competent Care

Cultural competence is a trendy term that has been widely used in nursing, education, and social work to convey the importance of understanding cultural differences when working with diverse groups of people. It can be confusing, though, because some practitioners assume cultural competence means to become proficient in another's cultural behavior. However, trying to be something one is not is more likely to be viewed as insincere and disrespectful, particularly with sex trafficked victims who are likely to have little reason to trust anyone.

In this chapter, cultural competence is defined as the ability to use information about another's culture to provide care that the person can accept comfortably while remaining authentic to one's own culture. For example, in providing care to a Navajo man whose culture teaches that it is rude to look people directly in the eyes, an White nurse who might have been taught that it is rude not to look directly at others when conversing would not interpret his behavior as rude but rather as respectful according to the norms of his culture. Similarly, when treating a young prostituted girl in the emergency department, it would be helpful to understand the culture of sex trafficking and not be frustrated by the patient's fearful or angry resistance to being rescued.

HOW SURVIVORS PRESENT

The following cases were drawn from real people but the identifying information has been changed to protect their privacy. The people represented here are examples of the variety of ways girls enter the life and show the systematic pattern of abuse that destroys their sense of self. The presenting behavior when seeking medical help shows some of the issues that we might expect to encounter with this population.

CASE STUDY: ANGEL

Angel is a 14-year-old African American girl who has been in "the life" for 3 years. At the age of 11, she met a 22-year-old White man named Johnny who was the first person to make her feel special. He listened to her talk about the abuse she endured at home and comforted her by telling her she was pretty and buying her small presents. Johnny told Angel he would help her escape her violent home situation. Her mother worked nights in a bar, often came home drunk, and had a variety of boyfriends, all of whom regularly raped Angel while her mother was at work. Her first sexual encounter was with her stepfather when she was 5 years old, but when she told her mother she was accused of lying, so she never told anyone else about the later abuse until she met Johnny. He said all the right things, comforted her in a tender way, and she immediately fell in love with him. He took her away to another city where they lived together in what was to be a short period of happiness in Angel's life. For 2 weeks, Angel and Johnny lived together in his apartment and gradually Angel realized she was not the only girl in his life. However, she loved him and when he asked her to go on "dates" with his friends she complied in the belief that they were building a future together. When some of his friends got too rough, well, that was nothing new to her and she would do anything to please Johnny. It was almost a month before he seemed to undergo a personality change and started beating her if she did not bring home her quota. He called it his 25/25 rule: $25 a trick at a rate of 25 men a night.

She presented in the emergency department with a fractured rib, multiple hematomas and abrasions, clumps of hair missing, and two broken teeth. She was accompanied by an older woman who said she was Angel's aunt and who insisted on speaking for her. The nurse did not separate the two when conducting the assessment interview and exam, but when she asked the appropriate questions about whether Angel felt safe in her home and whether she had been beaten, Angel lied and insisted she had been hit by a car. The emergency department team decided there was nothing they could do for her if she did not tell the truth, so they treated her for the fractured rib and sent her home with no report to protective services even though they believed she was younger than the 18 years she claimed.

CASE STUDY: STARR

Starr is a 15-year-old White girl whose father sold her at the age of 12 to a pimp to pay off his gambling debt. She was violently beaten on a regular basis by this man, who eventually sold her to another pimp. At the time of admission to the emergency department, she had been trafficked around the country from the East Coast to the West Coast and looked emaciated and depressed, and had bloody urine, rectal bleeding, and one eye was closed. When asked about the reason for coming to the emergency department, she said she had been gang raped. The intake person laughed about this and asked how a whore could possibly have been raped. Starr tried to explain that when a customer takes her by force, that is the same as what happens to women who are not whores. The intake person answered the phone and when she looked up Starr had gone.

CASE STUDY: BOTUM

Botum, whose name means "princess," is a 14-year-old Cambodian refugee who was married at the age of 6 in Cambodia at the insistence of her parents, who struggled to support their family of 10 children and older parents. Her husband sold her to a brothel at the age of 9 when he tired of her and arranged for the brothel owner to send small amounts of money from her earnings back to her parents. Botum experienced many sexually transmitted diseases and has had two pregnancies that were terminated via coat hanger by a woman employed by the brothel. However, she has only had to endure beatings by occasional violent customers and not the brothel owner because Botum quickly understood that if she cooperated she was helping her family, a strong Cambodian cultural value. She came to the United States as part of a container shipment of illegals from Singapore to work in American massage parlors owned by a Chinese gang. The gang tells the girls they will send money home to their families but first they have to repay their expenses to come to America.

Botum was arrested in a raid on a massage parlor and brought to the hospital for medical treatment, but she refuses help escaping "the life" because she would have no way to help her family. In a paradoxical situation, she insists she is ruined and can never go home because she would be shunned for shaming her family by working as a prostitute. Yet, if she stops working as a prostitute she will have no way to earn money to send home. In her culture, the value of helping family trumps individual freedom.

Analysis

These three young women exemplify several difficult issues in trying to help women leave the life. Angel was first sexually abused within her family and had a dysfunctional mother who did not protect her. She came to the life with a desperate hope in the stranger Johnny, whom she decided she loved and whom she believed was her protector. As bad as life with Johnny was, it was better than going home. In the emergency department, the staff failed to separate Angel from her "aunt" (often pimps send a trusted accomplice, called a "bottom girl," with the injured girl), and seemed to expect Angel to trust them immediately although they had given her no reason to do so. The staff not only failed to provide safety, but they failed to follow up. They chose to ignore their own instincts about her age and did not report the situation to protective services as they are mandated to do in cases of child abuse.

What should have happened for Angel is simple: Provide safety for her immediately by separating her from the accompanying person and report the situation to protective services regardless of how old she claimed to be. It would then be the responsibility of protective services to investigate since they employ social workers trained to sort out the truth.

Starr and Botum entered the life as many do—at the hands of their parents. In Starr's case, she endured long-term torture and was trafficked around the United States in such a way that she was disoriented as to where she was at any given point in time. When she sought help in the emergency department, she was treated with cruelty instead of the caring attitude toward all patients that we in health care like to hold as a cherished delusion.

Botum's cultural value of family was much stronger than her need for personal safety and freedom. Without concentrated services, there would be little hope of convincing her she could be trained to earn money she could send home by other means. In her situation it is critical to show her that she would have options. Under the Trafficking Victims Protection Act (TVPA), she would be eligible for a T-visa, one given to victims of trafficking who find themselves in the United States without immigration documents (United States Citizenship and Immigration Services, 2012).

USEFUL INTERVENTION MODELS

Useful intervention models exist that offer theoretical support for applying best practices to victims of human trafficking. Prochaska and DiClemente's (1983) Stages of Change Model is one valuable approach for developing nursing interventions with victims of sex trafficking.

Stages of Change Model

The Stages of Change Model (Prochaska & DiClemente, 1983) was developed for substance abuse cessation but has relevance to the psychotherapeutic process and can be useful in helping the therapist identify the receptivity for change of the client. The original stages are precontemplation, contemplation, action, maintenance, and relapse. Knowing that relapse is normal and to be expected assuages the guilt of the client for not improving because it takes the pressure off the therapist to move the client forward too quickly.

While considering the stage the patient is currently in when she seeks help is critical, it is equally important to conduct a thorough assessment in order to address malnutrition, sleep deprivation, physical injuries, and comorbid diseases. Trauma-focused cognitive behavior therapy and dialectical cognitive behavior therapy are two treatment methods that are evidence-based with survivors of child sexual abuse and PTSD. Eye movement desensitization and reprocessing (EMDR) is a technique that has efficacy in PTSD and can produce results in a short time.

Family therapy is appropriate if the person can be returned to a family or if the person wishes to work on underlying family issues. Reintegrating into the family of origin would not be advisable when the parents have served as the traffickers. Substance abuse treatment will be necessary for a large percentage of victims of trafficking. Traffickers often use drugs to control the victim, making her less likely to run and more likely to do whatever the pimp requires in order to obtain more drugs. Group therapy, particularly the peer support model described by Lloyd (2011), provides a chance for survivors to benefit from the therapeutic relationship with other survivors. Finally, medications can take the edge off symptoms, but should not be used long term or as a substitute for comprehensive services.

ASSUMPTIONS AND EXPECTATIONS

Expect the Unexpected

We might expect trafficking victims to welcome our help with open arms, but the reverse is often true for a variety of reasons. These women and children have been conditioned, often from an early age and certainly by their pimps, to mistrust everyone. As nurses, we are usually thanked profusely for our help not only by our patients, but also by their families and friends. Trafficked victims do not have family and friends they can count on. The person they are closest to is their exploiter, who will certainly not cooperate with us for interfering in his business. Victims bond with their abusers and will defend their abusers to outsiders because they have been conditioned to be totally dependent on them and to mistrust anyone else. The devil one knows is less frightening than the devil one does not know. Victims sometimes exhibit Stockholm Syndrome and will go to great lengths to protect their pimps (Jameson, 2010).

Relapse Is Normal

The Stages of Change Model is useful in understanding this process. With a high rate of physical and psychological abuse by pimps and customers, these women and children become numbed. They usually live with chronic pain from the beatings and rapes. One of their coping mechanisms is denial. They do not have a way to earn money any other way and they cannot save money since the pimp controls the money they earn. If they could scrape together enough for a bus ticket, where would they go? Their original homes are not likely to be seen as a refuge. Even when excellent services are provided, they often have such a poor self-image that they mistrust their ability to do anything else. So they return again and again to the exploiter. The known is less fearful than the unknown.

Respect Their Right to Self-Determination

Sex-trafficked children and women most likely receive continuous messages from their pimps that they are worthless. They are literally slaves. They do not control their own money and are often disoriented by being moved from city to city and forced to work nights, with the result that they are sleep deprived and malnourished. The health care system is designed for compliance—or as it is now fashionable to say, adherence. We are the experts, we care deeply about our patients, and we know how to help people if they will only do as we say and not fight us or argue with us. This approach is a guaranteed way to fail with victims of sex trafficking. What little self-control they have over their bodies they are not likely to relinquish to us if they do not see immediate positive results. And how many medical interventions are that dramatically successful? It is critical to approach these patients in a radically different way than the usual. We need to look for opportunities to demonstrate that we respect their right to self-determination. We need to explain medical procedures thoroughly and ask for their permission to proceed at every step rather than assume they will trust us to do what is necessary to help them. This takes time and patience.

Assume That the First Visit Is the Last

Many health conditions and treatments require follow-up. A broken arm requires a cast, monitoring circulation, and removal of the cast. STIs require a course of medication. Antibiotics usually need to be administered for 10 days. Pregnancy requires prenatal care for months, safe delivery, and follow-up. None of these conditions can be met if the traffickers feel threatened and if the girls cannot be rescued during the first visit. As seen in the case examples, the girls will often resist being rescued. The traffickers will move girls around from city to city to avoid detection. They know they cannot be prosecuted if the victims cannot be found to testify. We must do what we can during the brief time we see these victims. One example is using a single dose of Gardesil rather than the customary three doses to treat HPV (Anne Nichols, personal communication, 2012). Another strategy is to leave the door open by making the patient feel so comfortable that she will return if she can.

CONCLUSION

This chapter is an introduction to the problem of sex trafficking. The culture of the street serves as a framework for how nurses might interact with victims and survivors. Models of care and approaches to intervention are critical to consider in addressing the global urgency and the need for nursing leadership in addressing the problem of sex trafficking.

ACKNOWLEDGMENT

This chapter is a reprint from Mary de Chesnay's text, *Sex Trafficking: A Clinical Guide for Nurses* (2012), published by Springer Publishing.

REFERENCES

Alabama State Nurses' Association. (2009). Human trafficking: 21st century slavery. *The Alabama Nurse, 36*(1), 1, 7.

Aston, E. (2008). A fair trade? Staging female sex tourism and trade. *Contemporary Theatre Review, 18*(2), 180–192.

Bales, K. (2004). *Disposable people: New slavery in the global economy.* Berkeley, CA: University of California Press.

Bales, K. (2005). *Understanding global slavery.* Berkeley, CA: University of California Press.

Bales, K., & Lize, S. (2005). *Trafficking in persons in the United States: A report to the National Institute of Justice.* Retrieved from http://www.ncjrs.gov/pdffiles1/nij/grants/211980.pdf

Bastien, D. L. (2010). Pharmacologic treatment of combat-induced PTSD. *British Journal of Nursing, 19*(5), 318–321.

Cabezas, A. (2004). Between love and money: Sex, tourism, and citizenship in Cuba and the Dominican Republic. *Signs: Journal of Women in Culture and Society, 29*(4), 987–1015.

Crane, P., & Moreno, M. (2011). Human trafficking: What is the role of the health care provider? *Journal of Applied Research on Children: Informing Policy for Children at Risk, 2*(1), 1–27.

de Chesnay, M. (2012). Sex trafficking and sex tourism. In M. de Chesnay & B. Anderson (Eds.), *Caring for the vulnerable: Perspectives in nursing theory, practice and research* (pp. 385–392). Sudbury, MA: Jones and Bartlett.

Dulles, W. (1996). *Fielding's guide to Thailand: Including Cambodia, Laos, and Myanmar.* Redondo Beach, CA: Fielding Worldwide.

ECPAT. (2012). *Code of conduct for the protection of children from sexual exploitation in travel and tourism.* Retrieved from http://www.ecpat.net/ei/Publications/CST/Code_of_Conduct_ENG.pdf

Genefke, I. (2002). Chronic persistent pain in victims of torture. *Journal of Musculoskeletal Pain, 10*(1/2), 229–259.

Gigliotti, S. (2006). "Acapulco in the Atlantic": Revisiting Sosúa, a Jewish refugee colony in the Caribbean. *Immigrants & Minorities, 24*(1), 22–50.

Glittenberg, J. (2003). The tragedy of torture. *Issues in Mental Health Nursing, 24,* 627–638.

Grodin, M., & Annas, G. (2007). Physicians and torture: Lessons from the Nazi doctors. *International Review of the Red Cross, 89*(867), 635–654.

Hall, J. (2011). Sex offenders and child sex tourism: The case for passport revocation. *Virginia Journal for Social Policy and the Law, 18*(2), 153–202.

Hawthorne, E. (2011). Women in Northern Ireland involved in prostitution. *Irish Probation Journal, 8,* 142–164.

Interfaith Children's Movement. (2009). *Child exploitation and trafficking in Georgia.* Atlanta, GA: Interfaith Children's Movement.

International Labor Office. (2005). *A global alliance against forced labor global report under the follow-up to the ILO Declaration on Fundamental Principles and Rights at Work 2005.* Retrieved from http://www.ilo.org/wcmsp5/groups/public/@ed_norm/@declaration/documents/publication/wcms_081882.pdf

Ipser, J., Seedat, S., & Stein, D. (2006). Pharmacotherapy for post-traumatic stress disorder: A systematic review and meta-analysis. *South African Medical Journal, 96*(10), 1088–1096.

Jameson, C. (2010). The short step from love to hypnosis: A reconsideration of the Stockholm Syndrome. *Journal for Cultural Research, 14*(4), 337–355.

Jones, S. (2010). The invisible man: The conscious neglect of men in the war on human trafficking. *Utah Law Review, 2010*(4), 1143–1188.

Kambayashi, T. (2004). Human trafficking plagues vulnerable Moldovans. Interview with Agnes Chan. *Washington Times*, June 18, 2004, pp. A17.

Kansas State Nurses' Association. (2008). Human trafficking. *The Kansas Nurse, 83*(8), 22–23.

Langberg, L. (2005). A review of recent OAS research on human trafficking in the Latin American and Caribbean region. *International Migration, 43*(1), 129–139.

Levine, J. (2001). Working with victims of persecution: Lessons from Holocaust survivors. *Social Work, 46*(4), 350–360.

Lita, A. (2007). *Organ trafficking in Eastern Europe.* Retrieved from http://www .americanhumanist.org/hnn/archives/index.php?id=319&article=6

Lloyd, R. (2011). *Girls like us.* New York, NY: Harper Collins.

McClain, N., & Garrity, S. (2011). Sex trafficking and the exploitation of adolescents. *Journal of Obstetric, Gynecologic & Neonatal Nursing, 40*, 243–252.

McClanahan, S., McClelland, G., Abram, K., & Teplin, L. (1999). Pathways into prostitution among female jail detainees and their implications for mental health services. *Psychiatric Services.* Retrieved from http://ajp.[psychiatryonline.org/article.aspx?articleid=83780&RelatedWidgetarticles=true

Meis, L., Barry, R., Kehle, S., Erbes, C., & Polusney, M. (2010). Relationship adjustment, PTSD symptoms, and treatment utilization among coupled National Guard soldiers deployed to Iraq. *Journal of Family Psychology, 24*(5), 560–567.

Montgomery, H. (2008). Buying innocence: Child sex tourists in Thailand. *Third World Quarterly, 29*(5), 903–917.

Moreno, A., & Grodin, M. A. (2002). Torture and its neurological sequelae. *Spinal Cord, 40*, 213–223.

Moreno, A., & Iacopino, V. (2008). Forensic investigations of torture and ill-treatment in Mexico. *Journal of Legal Medicine, 29*, 443–478.

Mulvaney, S., McLean, B., & De Leeuw, J. (2010). The use of stellate ganglion block in the treatment of panic/anxiety symptoms with combat-related post-traumatic stress disorder; preliminary results of long-term follow-up: A case series. *Pain Practice, 10*(4), 359–365.

National Student Nurses Association (NSNA). (2010). *In support of increasing awareness of human trafficking.* Retrieved from http://www.nsna.org/Portals/0/Skins/NSNA/ pdf/Final%20Resolutions%202010_revised%205-05-10.pdf

Nicholas, P., George, E., Raymond, N., Lewis-O'Connor, A., Victoria, S., Lucien, S. . . . Valcourt, R. (2012). Orphans and at-risk children in Haiti. *Advances in Nursing Science, 35*(2), 182–189.

O'Connor, M., & Healy, G. (2006). *The links between prostitution and sex trafficking: A briefing handbook.* Retrieved from http://www.catwinternational.org

Olsen, D., Montgomery, E., Bojholm, S., & Foldspong, A. (2006). Prevalent musculoskeletal pain as a correlate of previous exposure to torture. *Scandinavian Journal of Public Health, 34*, 496–503.

Padilla, M. (2008). The embodiment of tourism among bisexually behaving Dominican male sex workers. *Archives of Sexual Behavior, 37*, 783–793.

Prochaska, J., & DiClemente, C. (1983). Stages and processes of self-change of smoking: Toward an integrative model of change. *Journal of Consulting and Clinical Psychology, 51*(3), 390–395.

Racine-Welch, T., & Welch, M. (2000). Listening for the sounds of silence: A nursing consideration of caring for the politically tortured. *Nursing Inquiry, 7*, 136–141.

Sabella, D. (2011). The role of the nurse in combating human trafficking. *American Journal of Nursing, 111*(2), 28–39.

Shared Hope International. (2011). *This man wants to rent your daughter.* Vancouver, WA: Author.

Smith, L. (webcast, 2011, December). *Report of the state report cards.* Vancouver, WA: Shared Hope International.

Trossman, S. (2008). The costly business of human trafficking. *American Nurse Today, 3*(12). Retrieved from http://www.americannursetoday.com/article.aspx?id=4134& fid=4104

Trout, K. (2010). The role of nurses in identifying and helping victims. *Pennsylvania Nurse, 65*(4), 18–20.

United Nations Office on Drugs and Crime. (2000). *Human trafficking.* Retrieved from http://www.unodc.org/unodc/en/human-trafficking/what-is-human-trafficking .html#What_is_Human_Trafficking)

United States Citizenship and Immigration Services. (2012). *Victims of human trafficking: T nonimmigrant status.* Retrieved from http://www.uscis.gov/portal/site/uscis/ menuitem.eb1d4c2a3e5b9ac89243c6a7543f6d1a/?vgnextoid=02ed3e4d77d73210VgnV CM100000082ca60aRCRD&vgnextchannel=02ed3e4d77d73210VgnVCM100000082ca 60aRCRD

United States State Department. (2012). *Trafficking in persons report—2012.* Retrieved from http://www.state.gov/j/tip/rls/tiprpt/2012

World Famous Players' Ball. (2005). *A briefing document based on online research and general knowledge.* Retrieved from http://www.crisisconnectioninc.org/pdf/Players_ Ball.pdf

Yea, S. (2010). Human trafficking: A geographical perspective. *Geodate, 23*(3), 2–6.

CHAPTER 15

Complex Issues in Conflict Areas

Antonia Makosky

Nursing students often ask how they can help developing countries around the globe. Perusal of the literature reveals accounts from many nurses who offered their unique skills in conflict zones in Afghanistan, Congo, Darfur, Kosovo, Iraq, Liberia, Sierra Leone, Somaliland, Sudan, and South Sudan. Jennifer Cunningham, an Australian nurse who cared for war wounded from South Sudan, wrote, "What attracted me to this type of work was the opportunity to use my nursing skills in a very different setting and to make a contribution to international health care" (Cunningham, 2000, p. 19). The purpose of this chapter is to review some of the most common problems confronted by nurses working in conflict zones.

FRAMEWORK—NURSING METAPARADIGM AND ENVIRONMENTAL METAPARADIGM

First articulated in the late 1970s by nurse theorist Jacqueline Fawcett, the nursing metaparadigm is an overarching framework that contains the four core concepts of nursing theory: person, environment, health, and nursing (Masters, 2012). Although Florence Nightingale, the founder of modern nursing, addressed all of these concepts in her pioneering work in the 1800s, the environment was foremost: Nightingale believed that in order to help patients to regain health, they must first be placed in a healthy environment (Masters, 2012). The country case exemplars in this chapter are loosely organized using the framework of the nursing metaparadigm: Person is represented as population (with health indicators); environmental factors are described; health challenges are presented; and nursing needs and roles are enumerated.

Significance of Health Indicators for Overview and Health Policy

Eight health indicators are listed in the case examples: population, adult literacy rate, life expectancy at birth, infant mortality, mortality of children younger than 5 years of age, maternal mortality, HIV/AIDS, and health care expenditures. These health indicators provide a structure for evaluating the performance of a health system and may be used to diagnose key health and environmental problems; thus, they are useful for priority setting and budgetary planning by governments and aid groups. Population is a basic demographic health indicator that gives an idea of the size of the country as a whole. Adult literacy rate is a socioeconomic indicator for national educational level and may be used to plan governmental spending on education. Life expectancy, infant mortality, child mortality, maternal mortality, and HIV/AIDS are defined as "state" indicators that help drive responses such as funding for immunization and family planning initiatives (von Schirnding, 2002).

Early Exemplar: Florence Nightingale in the Crimean War

Florence Nightingale was asked to bring nurses to serve in the Crimean War because British soldiers were dying more from disease than from war wounds (Woodham-Smith, 1951). Upon arrival at the British hospital barracks at Scutari, Ms. Nightingale found the soldiers sleeping uncovered on the floor in their battle-soiled uniforms. Nightingale improved the health of the soldiers by instituting nutrition and hygiene reform, in addition to dressing wounds and administering medication. She kept scrupulous records and was one of the first hospital administrators to use statistics for analysis of morbidity and mortality (McDonald, 1998).

Diarrhea and gangrene caused many deaths at the hospital, largely because hygiene was completely inadequate (Woodham-Smith, 1951). Nightingale estimated that for 1,000 men there were 20 chamber pots; most human waste was collected in large wooden tubs on each ward, causing an inescapable stench. After a hurricane in November 1854, military administrators finally conceded Nightingale the authority to arrange cleaning of the floors, compel the emptying of the tubs of human waste, and arrange the provision of clean clothing, cutlery, operations tables, soap, towels, and screens, among other supplies (Woodham-Smith, 1951).

Despite the improved food and cleaner conditions in the hospital, mortality increased, then worsened further still in December 1854 with an epidemic of cholera. In March 1855, a sanitary inspection commission found pools of sewage under the hospital, and the hospital's water supply running through a decaying horse carcass. After 26 dead animals, including two dead horses, were removed and buried, the sewers flushed, and numerous other measures taken, the health of the soldiers began to improve (Woodham-Smith, 1951).

Modern nurses in conflict zones face elements similar to those faced by Florence Nightingale in the 1860s: crowded and unsanitary conditions, political conflict, limited resources, malnutrition, and epidemics. Today's nurse needs to bring the same acumen to her or his work in the global conflict arena as did Florence Nightingale in her day. The nursing scholar Dorothy Kleffel (2006) conceives a more global view of the nursing paradigm, regarding the environment itself as the nursing client. The environment is by far the largest factor influencing health in conflict areas.

PREPARING FOR TRAVEL AND WORK IN CONFLICT AREAS

Personal challenges to the nurse volunteer include communication difficulties due to language differences and misunderstandings due to cultural differences. Feelings of isolation and loneliness are common. Spartan living conditions such as extreme heat or cold and lack of electricity or running water can be physically challenging. The stress of managing a multitude of very sick patients or the boredom of waiting for a looming disaster can take an emotional toll. Although there will certainly be difficult experiences, thorough preparation will help the nurse volunteer cope as these arise.

Skills and Schooling

Preparing for work in a conflict area requires planning and forethought. Most nonprofit or nongovernmental organizations (NGOs) require some prior cross-cultural experience in a nonconflict area to start and prior work with underserved populations. Many small nonprofit or religious organizations in developed countries offer brief 1- or 2-week volunteer medical missions to various countries. Such missions offer an opportunity for nurses new to global health to gain experience and to be mentored by more experienced nurses as well as other visiting and host country staff. Teaching and/or managerial skills are desirable. Foreign language skills are also helpful. The mission may or may not be in a country where the volunteer speaks the language, but the cross-cultural skill of speaking another language is valuable. At the time of this writing, French was in especially high demand for work with Doctors Without Borders (known more commonly as Médecins sans Frontières, or MSF) in Francophone Africa, a region with several ongoing conflicts; Portuguese is also useful in several African countries (MSF, 2014). In addition, Arabic, Chinese, Russian, and Spanish are all World Health Organization (WHO) languages and can be helpful in working with multiple donor agencies (WHO, 2014a).

One can also take courses to prepare for global health work, tropical medicine, and humanitarian aid. Tulane University, University of Virginia, University of Minnesota, and University of Pennsylvania all offer courses in global health. The University of Minnesota offers seven online global health modules and a live global health course in collaboration with the Centers for Disease Control and Prevention (CDC). The London School of Hygiene and Tropical Medicine and the Liverpool School of Tropical Medicine offer 5-month diploma programs in tropical medicine. For a listing of approved diploma courses in clinical tropical medicine and travelers' health, see www.astmh.org/Approved_Diploma_Courses/5711.htm.

Harvard University offers several courses in humanitarian studies as well as shorter 3-day, 4-day, and 2-week workshops in humanitarian response to emergencies (Humanitarian Academy at Harvard, 2014). Several schools in the United Kingdom offer master's programs as well as shorter courses in humanitarian studies, including the London School of Economics and Political Science, the University of Oxford, the University of York, and the Liverpool School of Tropical Medicine (Liverpool School of Tropical Medicine, 2014; London School of Economics and Political Science, 2014; University of Oxford, 2014; University of York, 2014).

In her 2009 account in the *Journal of Emergency Nursing*, "My Journey to Sudan," Canadian nurse author Sue Witt explains the steps she took to prepare herself for work with MSF. Ms. Witt volunteered as a nurse in Ecuador, Ghana, Kenya, and the Northwest Territories of Canada. Further, she obtained a diploma in Tropical Nursing from the London School of Hygiene and Tropical Medicine. Finally, she underwent a week-long MSF training in Amsterdam (Witt, 2009). In order to prepare for work with MSF as a nurse supervisor in Niger and mobile team nurse leader in the Democratic Republic of the Congo (DRC), the author of this chapter, in addition to 3 years of Peace Corps experience in the Congo, also volunteered in Honduras, and worked with homeless and underserved populations in Boston, Massachusetts.

Most countries have many local nurses who need updates in education and skills training. Therefore, international humanitarian organizations such as MSF, International Committee of the Red Cross (ICRC), International Rescue Committee (IRC), and others will expect the global nurse volunteer to act in a supervisory role, as teacher, team leader, or nurse manager. A composite list of preferred skills and experience for nurses from the MSF and ICRC websites includes:

- 2 to 5 years of relevant professional experience
- Availability for 9 to 12 months
- Relevant travel or work
- Experience supervising, managing, and training others
- Language skills
- Organization skills, self-discipline, flexibility, adaptability
- Ability to live and work with a multidisciplinary and multicultural team
- Good communication skills, ability to listen, diplomacy
- Humanitarian commitment
- Able to cope with stress
- Prepared to work under pressure in a potentially dangerous environment (ICRC, 2014; MSF, 2014)

Medical Examination, Immunizations, Medications

Closer to the date of departure, personal medical preparation will be required. Usually this includes a complete physical examination, immunizations (specific to the mission location), any prophylactic medications (e.g., antimalarials), and any personal medications needed by the nurse volunteer. In some cases, the NGO will arrange for the examination and immunizations; in other cases, the individual will be responsible. Planning ahead is important for immunizations such as hepatitis

A and B, which are given in series. For more specific information regarding immunizations, see the CDC website: wwwnc.cdc.gov/travel.

Important Documents and Informing Oneself

Important travel documents include passport, immunization record, and nursing diploma. Sometimes a copy of one's birth certificate is required. Copies of all documents (in addition to any originals) should also be brought on the mission. American nurse volunteers should also consider malpractice insurance and ask whether this is provided by the volunteer organization.

Preparatory study for the mission should include any documents available from the NGO, for example, status reports, country profiles, security protocols, and any human resources materials. More specifically, many NGOs have their own medical protocols for treatment of common conditions. The nurse should thoroughly familiarize herself or himself with these protocols. It is important also to request a job description in order to understand one's role and the expected duties and skill set. If possible, it is extremely helpful to either talk or correspond with someone who has recently returned from or is still stationed at the service site. The job offered may not be the best fit for the nurse volunteer's experience and qualifications; in some cases, it may be wise to wait for a job that is a better fit.

More generally, it is helpful to understand the history and politics of conflict in the area. Often the NGO will have its own website with background, blogs, and so forth, but other helpful sources of information include the websites of UNICEF, Human Rights Watch, NationMaster, the U.S. Department of State, the BBC, the United Nations High Commissioner for Refugees (UNHCR), and WHO. If one is travelling to an area with a long history of armed conflict, it may be painful to read about atrocities and rape used as a weapon of war. However, it will be more helpful to understand the health problems of the affected population with this knowledge in advance of arrival.

Tjoflat and Karlsen (2012) suggest that the expatriate nurse should "have knowledge about the culture, context and hospital, as well as the health educational system in the country" (p. 491). They also suggest that the nurse volunteer should know how education is conducted in the country, how work is organized, and should have knowledge of cultural differences and values (Tjoflat & Karlsen, 2012). Often conflicts exist in the host state or country and may not be evident at first. Some examples of these from the author's experience include conflict between the educated nurses and the less educated patients, often from rural areas and often not literate; conflicts between clans; conflicts between farmers and pastoralists (Makosky, 2010; Tesch, 2006), and conflicts between local and visiting staff. As the nurse volunteer builds relationships with both the expatriate and the national staff, she or he will be able to gain more information about existing conflicts that may be obvious from the start or may be simmering under the surface.

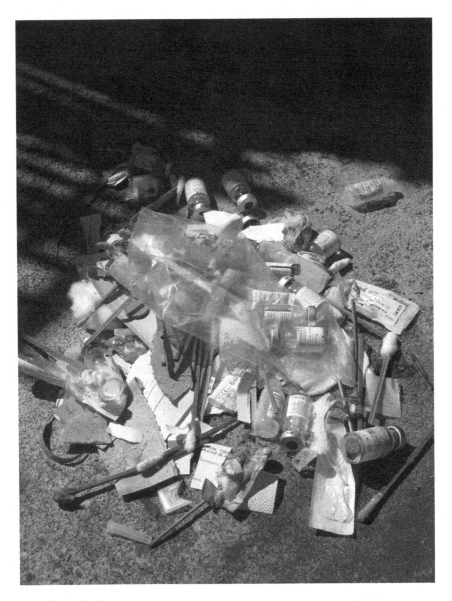

Mixed medical waste.

Major health indicators such as life expectancy; maternal, infant, and child mortality rates; and prevalence of infectious and endemic diseases such as tuberculosis, malaria, and HIV/AIDS also provide insight into the health challenges of the area. Other health problems in conflict areas include gender-based violence; respiratory infections; and infectious and vector-borne diseases such as measles, meningitis, and typhoid fever (Gately, 2005). Treatment protocols will likely be available from the aid organization, and the nurse volunteer should become familiar with these. It is also useful to bring one's own references in both paper and electronic form. There may not be Internet access on arrival; however, it is very useful to bring reference material on a flash drive or hard disk, and to bring spare flash drives in case of infection by computer virus.

Packing: What to Bring

First-time volunteers tend to overpack, but quickly learn that less is more. Often the aid organization will use extra baggage capacity to send supplies to the site. Team members already onsite will appreciate current newspapers, magazines, and edible treats, if available. It is important to bring appropriate clothing for the weather, including warm clothing for winter transit. Some spending money is useful; usually the NGO provides a safe for storage of valuables. Clothing and small equipment for exercise, such as resistance bands for muscle strengthening or a yoga mat, are helpful for stress relief and maintaining fitness. Sunscreen and insect repellent are often needed and usually easier to buy at home before departure. Camping mosquito nets will be necessary in malaria-endemic areas. Toiletries can be heavy to carry and may be available at the local UN commissary or stores in the national or regional capital cities. Both the nurse volunteer and host country colleagues will appreciate looking at pictures of family and friends from home.

Preparing for a Long Absence

Preparing for a long absence from home requires comprehensive planning. It is important to make arrangements for handling of mail and official documents. Questions to consider include should one give up one's home or apartment? Who will pay any bills or loans that are due? Who will receive and open mail? Who will answer summons for jury duty? Will it be necessary to file for extension for income tax? Often it is most expedient to ask a close friend or family member to serve as power of attorney for decisions and document signatures needed in one's absence. Finally, in the unlikely case of accident or death, it is wise to make a simple will and leave instructions for distribution of one's belongings. It is important to leave this information with the emergency contact person who is identified to the health organization.

ENVIRONMENTAL EFFECTS OF CONFLICT

Effect of War on Human Migration

Violent conflict leads to large numbers of displaced persons who have fled their homes for safer settings. In 2013 the United Nations High Commission for Refugees (UNHCR) completed a report titled *Displacement: The New 21st Century Challenge* describing the enormity of the numbers of displaced persons around the world and defining terminology. Persons who flee to another country are "refugees"; those who flee within their own country are "internally displaced persons (IDPs)." In a third category are stateless persons, for whom no government accepts responsibility, and in the fourth category are persons seeking asylum. All are vulnerable to health risks and are dependent on aid (UNHCR, 2013).

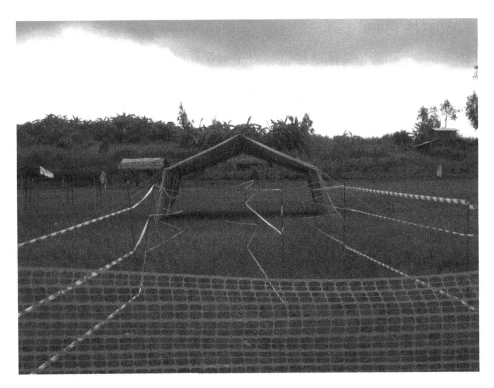

Preparations for community-wide measle vaccination.

At the end of 2012, the UNHCR found that there were 45.2 million forcibly displaced persons worldwide. Of those 45.2 million, approximately 35 million were refugees or IDPs, and 10 million persons were stateless. The UNHCR notes that more than half of refugees reside in low-income countries—defined as gross domestic product (GDP) less than $5,000 per capita—that are ill equipped to bear this human and financial burden. The UNHCR helps defray the cost of these refugees and IDPs. The top five countries of origin of displaced persons are Afghanistan, Somalia, Iraq, the Syrian Arab Republic, and Sudan, respectively. The top three host countries by percentage of GDP are Pakistan, Ethiopia, and Kenya, respectively (UNHCR, 2013). An estimated 48% of refugees are women and girls while 46% are children under 18 (UNHCR, 2013). Children in particular are vulnerable to human trafficking, child labor, prostitution, sexual bartering, and forced military duty (Martone, 2003a).

Health Effects of Displacement

When large populations of persons are displaced and move into crowded living conditions, health hazards quickly increase. Necessary elements of health infra-structure such as clean water sources, sewage water treatment or sanitary facilities, hospitals, clinics, and health care staff are all negatively affected. Ensuing diseases include malnutrition, dehydration, and diarrhea; unsanitary conditions lead to epidemics of communicable diseases such as cholera, measles, and typhoid, and increases in preventable and treatable diseases such as meningitis and tuberculosis (Gately, 2004; Parish, 2002).

CASE STUDY: SIERRA LEONE, WEST AFRICA

Background

Population 6 million; 10-year civil war from 1991 to 2002. War tactics included rape, mutilation, mass murder, and child soldiers.

Health Indicators

Adult literacy rate	43%
Life expectancy at birth	46 years
Infant mortality:	117/1,000 live births
Mortality in children younger than 5	182/1,000 live births
Maternal mortality	1,100/100,000 live births
Prevalence of HIV/AIDS	1,304/100,000 live births
Health care expenditures	18.8% of GDP

Environment

Lack of access to clean water and sanitation
Food insecurity
Damage to health care and educational infrastructure
Significant damage to roads, buildings, and so forth

Health Challenges

Ebola virus disease
Malnutrition
Physical disabilities from violence-related injuries: amputations, disfigurement
HIV/AIDs
Malaria, dysentery, cholera, measles
Mental health issues related to sexual assault, violence exposure

Role of Nurse Volunteer

Health education and raising awareness; for example, safe drinking water, hygiene, protections from sexual violence; effects of trauma on mental health
Planning, providing, and monitoring care; for example, vaccination programs, nutrition programs, services for amputees

Sources: CDC (2014); Kargbo (2002); Martone (2003a); Wallis (2001); WHO (2014b).

Effects of War and Violence on Infrastructure

In war, the damage and destruction of electrical power infrastructure and transportation infrastructure, such as roads and public transport, severely impact life, health, and livelihoods. Destruction of clean water supplies, wastewater treatment, health care infrastructure, and food supplies, including subsistence crops and animals, can lead to malnutrition, dehydration, illness, injury, and death. Health care facilities and schools may be bombed on purpose or by accident. They may be set on fire or looted of medications and supplies (Gately, 2004; Martone, 2003b; Parish, 2002; Salvage, 2004).

CASE STUDY: IRAQ, MIDDLE EAST

Background

Population 32.8 million; three wars in 20 years; first the Iran–Iraq War from 1980 to 1988; then the Gulf War from 1990 to 1991; then U.S. air strike in 2003 with ongoing internal fighting since that time. Nature of the war: bombings, ground warfare, land mines, improvised explosive devices, drones, and special forces.

Health Indicators

Adult literacy rate	78%
Life expectancy at birth	70
Infant mortality	28/1,000 live births
Mortality in children younger than 5	34/1,000 live births
Maternal mortality	67/100,000 live births
HIV/AIDS	—
Health care expenditures	3.6% of GDP

Environment

Damage to health infrastructure; hospitals and medication storage warehouses bombed and/or looted. Prior to these wars the Iraqi health care system was well organized; hospitals were well staffed and equipped. Primary care facilities now greatly reduced. Damage to electrical infrastructure and to water treatment plants; consequently, greatly reduced access to clean water and sanitation since the wars. Disruption of employment and education and high fuel costs due to sanctions.

Health Challenges

Squalid camp living conditions for internally displaced persons
Malnutrition
Cholera, dysentery, typhoid
Malaria, Kala Azar (Leishmaniasis)
Measles, respiratory infections
Lack of supplies: antibiotics, blood for transfusions, pain medications, vaccines, medications used for chronic diseases, such as insulin

Role of Nurse Volunteer

Collection of health data regarding population demographics, birth and death rates, immunization rates
Evaluation of disease frequency
Evaluation of structural damage and access to food, water, shelter, health care providers
Review of nursing curricula, assistance with nurse training

Sources: Gately (2004); IRIN News (2013); Martone (2004); Salvage (2004); Sofer (2003); WHO (2014b).

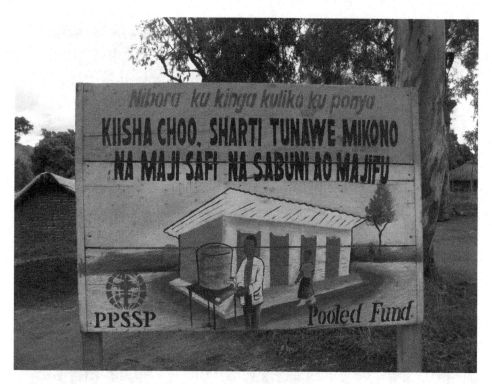

A public health message emphasizing the importance of hand washing.

ONCE IN THE FIELD

Cross-Cultural Encounters

In the author's experience, an approach of cultural humility is beneficial in all settings. Building relationships with all staff, local staff in particular, is crucial to accomplishing goals and enjoying the experience of working with others. National staff will greatly appreciate any efforts to learn the local language, try regional foods, wear national dress, and visit staff and family members in their homes, if appropriate. In this author's experience, national staff were eager to share their knowledge and experience with visiting nurse volunteers. Whatever the task assigned, it is beneficial to ask the local staff about their practice; they are the experts! When this author was asked to plan a measles vaccination campaign in the DRC, local staff were instrumental in recruiting additional nurses and nurses' aides, and in mounting a publicity campaign. If the visiting nurse inquires among the visiting and local staff, it will be easy to learn of acknowledged experts who can serve as mentors. In countries such as the DRC or Niger, there has been a long history of conflict or disasters with many aid agencies involved. There are often many underemployed trained staff who are available for temporary work such as vaccination campaigns, or to fill a new position (Makosky, 2010).

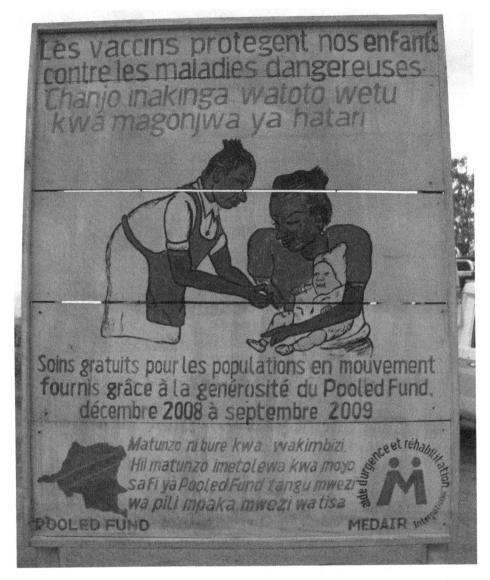

A public health message emphasizing the importance of vaccinations for children.

Despite good intentions, misunderstandings can occur. Tjoflat and Karlsen (2012) describe the challenges of sharing knowledge with a nurse colleague in a Sudanese hospital. A long civil war had destroyed the health infrastructure of the country. The Sudanese nurses had been trained with a curriculum dated from 1956, but had not had the opportunity for continuing education in the 14 years that the ICRC had been providing support to the hospital. In their example, the newly arrived expatriate nurse was assigned to work along with a Sudanese nurse. She explained to the Sudanese nurse that vital signs would need to be taken every 15 minutes. When vital signs had not been checked an hour later, the expatriate nurse became upset (Tjoflat & Karlsen, 2012).

In their analysis, Tjoflat and Karlsen (2012) characterize this encounter as "one way communication," in which the expatriate nurse did not give the

Sudanese nurse a chance to describe their local practice, which was to check the patient's vital signs every hour. The authors also note that the two nurses were communicating in English, a second language for both. In this author's experience, communicating in a second language is fraught with opportunities for misunderstanding, even with good skills and the best of intentions. In this case, it may have been helpful to use an interpreter to clarify. Tjoflat and Karlsen (2012) note that asking about local practice methods would have opened up an opportunity for dialogue and reduce the potential for misunderstandings.

In another example of cross-cultural encounters, Witt (2009) describes an experience in Sudan where she took the mattress out of the night staffing room and gave it to a brain-damaged patient with pressure sores. Her nursing staff became angry. As they were discussing the matter, a dying child was brought in and she left the meeting carrying the child, attempting to resuscitate. She was followed by one of the nursing staff still trying to tell her why she should not have taken the mattress. It was explained to her later that death was more common than mattresses (Witt, 2009).

This author had similar misunderstandings in both Niger and the DRC. In one case in Niger, the author was pressured to give written warnings to nurses who had left work early. The national staff was unionized and scolded the author in a public meeting for not first notifying the nurses' immediate supervisor. In another case in the DRC, an expatriate nurse publicly berated the local health center nurse for not urgently referring a patient with stroke symptoms. Later the local nurse told the expatriate nurse supervisor that this kind of treatment was not respectful. Notably, when the local nurses discussed this case, they took a holistic view and ascribed great importance to the patient's lack of family support as much as her risk factors for disease.

De Jong et al. (2010) published a qualitative research article on mass casualty care by 107 U.S. military nurses who served in the Middle East after September 11, 2001. The authors identified 12 principles for managing mass casualty events in the combat environment, but many of these principles also apply to humanitarian work in conflict zones. Two of these principles address learning as much as possible from outgoing team members. De Jong et al. (2010) recommend that incoming teams "[b]e humble and assume that what they (outgoing team members) learned from their experience will benefit your work" (p. 57) and not to make changes in protocol until it is clear that the present system does not work for the team.

Safety and Risk

Nursing in an area where the population needs urgent help can be very rewarding, but the nurse volunteer should go in clear eyed about the risk involved. The editors of the news section of the *Journal of Advanced Nursing* (Nurses in war zones, 1999) noted that seven nurses were killed throughout the 1990s in Afghanistan, Liberia, and Chechnya. The short article includes comments from Dr. Pierre Perrin, chief medical officer for the ICRC, who notes that respect for health care workers had recently declined. He theorized that White volunteers might stand out more as targets because they are thought to be rich. Perrin stated that, in the future, the

ICRC would be relying more on local staff who were less likely to be targeted. He also noted that nurses would not be expected to provide testimony regarding war crimes, which is one factor that might put them in greater danger of retaliation. In the recent ICRC booklet *Health Care in Danger*, violence against health care workers and facilities is documented in more detail (ICRC, 2011).

As a visiting nurse in a conflict area, one must maintain the practice of neutrality in the work environment. In a personal example, this author was visiting a health center in a border area with known rebel activity in the Eastern DRC. An armed soldier came onto the health center grounds. The operations staff politely asked the soldier to leave his weapon outside the grounds while he made his visit. Fortunately, he complied without further action or violence.

The Geneva Convention of 1949 and the Additional Protocols of 1977 state that health care workers are neutral and must be treated as such (ICRC, 2011). Nurses and other health care workers who enter a conflict area to retrieve the wounded should be allowed to pass without threats to their safety. In order to maintain this practice of neutrality, health care organizations must maintain strict rules of conduct in which ambulances and hospitals are not used for the transport or storage of weapons (ICRC, 2011). Unfortunately, these tenets have been violated multiple times in recent years. In Kosovo, hospitals have been used as weapons storage areas (Raisler & Heymann, 2001); in Afghanistan, ambulances have been used to transport explosives, and in Libya, there have been reports that ambulances have been used to transport arms and armed personnel (ICRC, 2011).

In Abbottabad, Pakistan, the Central Intelligence Agency (CIA) used a fake vaccination campaign to gain information about the family of Osama bin Laden in their compound (Shah, 2011). These kinds of actions have led to the mistrust or willful targeting of health care workers, such as the shooting of polio vaccination workers in Peshawar, Pakistan, in March 2014 (Larson, 2012; *Scientific American*, 2013; Sherazi & Watkins, 2014). Fortunately, the CIA has just announced that it will no longer use fake vaccination campaigns as an intelligence-gathering tactic, but it will take time to repair the damage done to the reputation and safety of community health care workers in the region (Keating, 2014).

CASE STUDY: AFGHANISTAN, CENTRAL ASIA

Background

Population 29.8 million; Soviet invasion 1979 and withdrawal in 1989; civil war followed. Kabul seized by Taliban in 1996; introduction of Sharia law. 2001, U.S. invasion; 2014, U.S. troop withdrawal at press time. War tactics: bombings, ground warfare, land mines, improvised explosive devices, drones, special forces.

Health indicators

Adult literacy rate	28%
Life expectancy at birth	60

Infant mortality	71/1,000 live births
Mortality in children younger than 5	99/1,000 live births
Maternal mortality	400/100,000 live births
HIV and AIDS	—
Health care expenditures	8.4% of GDP

Environment

Displacement: 2.6 million refugees in other countries including Pakistan, and 667,000 IDPs
Environmental Infrastructure: crumbling prior to 1979 war; limited road system; donkeys used in remote areas and mountains; lack of clean water, no electricity.
Financial Infrastructure: no banking; currency worth very little.
Health Care Infrastructure: unregulated medications, drugs sold in the market, quality unknown. No staff, facilities; migration of many qualified health personnel to safer countries.
Very few qualified doctors and nurses. Not enough midwives. Nursing held in low regard. Doctors reluctant to perform what is considered to be nurses' work.

Health challenges

Malnutrition
Mental illness, opium addiction
Diarrhea
Rabies

Role of Nurse Volunteer

Rebuilding of health services including restoration of facilities such as health posts, outreach teams
Inclusion of nurses in planning seminar for reconstruction
Support for curricula in nursing schools reopened after 5-year gap in nurse training
5-year gap in nurse training
WHO priorities: child and reproductive health, communicable disease control, mental health, injuries.

Sources: CIA (2014); IDMC (2014); Martone (2002); Murray (2001); Pickersgill (2002); UNHCR (2014); WHO(2014b).

Personal Security

MSF posts a clear security policy statement on its website, stating that MSF takes security very seriously and expects all employees to adhere to their security protocols (MSF, 2014). This author experienced those rigorous protocols in the Eastern Congo in 2010. At that time there was relative calm, but a security briefing was held every morning for all staff. All movement of staff was tracked by radio during the work week. Limited leisure activities such as local walks, morning runs, and trips to the local market were tracked during the weekend. Names of all departing staff were listed to radio operators when leaving for the day and when leaving health centers or vaccination sites to return after delivering services. These transmissions were then copied to local and regional headquarters. Transportation was not allowed after dark. If there was unrest in a particular area, operations were cancelled. The author was also evacuated to the capital in a prior mission to Niger. It is wise to practice packing a bag of essentials in order to be ready to leave quickly should an evacuation be necessary.

COMMON HEALTH PROBLEMS

Vulnerability of Women and Children

Women and children are most greatly affected by war and armed conflict. Armed conflict leads to increased rates of gender-based violence and sexually transmitted diseases such as HIV infection (UNICEF, 1996). In times of conflict, children are vulnerable to malnutrition, which then lowers resistance to common public health problems such as malaria, measles, and respiratory infections such as pneumonia (Martone, 2003a; Salvage, 2004). Poorer health indicators, such as high maternal, child, and infant mortality, reflect these conditions.

An example from this author's experience illustrates the vulnerability of women and children. While this author was working in the Eastern DRC, a woman came to the local health center with her three children. She had been hiding in the jungle with her rebel husband. Her uncle and aunt died while in the jungle. When she arrived at the health center her second child was severely ill with Kwashiorkor. Her eyes were almost swollen shut from edema. Fortunately for this family, after several weeks of treatment her daughter recovered (Makosky, 2010).

Violent conflict also exacerbates conditions that lead to disease. The pool of unvaccinated people increases, leading to epidemics of preventable diseases such as measles, meningitis, and polio (Gately, 2004). The lack of equipment and manpower for waste removal leads to the accumulation of many kinds of waste, including garbage, human and animal feces, dead animals, and medical waste, causing epidemics of diseases such as typhoid and cholera. There is increased mortality from chronic communicable diseases such as tuberculosis and HIV that, under better conditions, can be controlled. Persons with chronic diseases such as asthma, cancer, depression, diabetes, heart disease, hypertension, and tuberculosis are more vulnerable to breaks in drug supply that occur as a result of the violence (Gately, 2004; Salvage, 2004; Sofer, 2003).

Mental Health

Mental health is adversely affected by violent conflict, and has only recently begun to be addressed by humanitarian relief agencies. At a London conference on mental health in 2007, best practices were shared (Lester, 2008). Aid organizations are beginning to integrate mental health into the services they deliver to target populations by raising awareness of mental health as a clinical need among the local populations. To this end, they have begun training local health workers to identify and treat mental health problems, to facilitate support groups, and to provide counseling, and sometimes these groups have provided education related to medication (Lester, 2008). A mental health component is particularly important for victims and survivors of gender-based violence and atrocities such as mass rape and amputation. It will be important for the nurse volunteer to learn what mental health services, if any, are offered in the services area. MSF offers mental health training to local health workers and support to survivors of gender-based violence (MSF, 2014).

In 2012, *The Guardian* newspaper profiled a Liberian nurse, Dakemue Kollie, who works as a mental health coordinator in the region of Bong County (Ford, 2012). The story highlights not only the importance of providing mental health services, but also illustrates how local providers' lives may have been shaped by violence and violent conflict. In 1994, when he was just 15 years old, Mr. Kollie's father, a hospital cook, was killed in a massacre; his sister and mother have also since died. Nurse Kollie rides his motorcycle to remote villages to provide counseling and treatment for patients with mental health problems. His work is funded by the international aid group Medecins du Monde, or Doctors of the World (Ford, 2012).

War or violent conflict also causes increases in gender-based violence and subsequent mental health problems. In Kosovo, 68% of the women interviewed by the Center for Protection for Women and Children reported a history of domestic violence or sexual assault; long-term depression is also reported, with feelings of shame, guilt, and vindictiveness (Raisler & Heymann, 2001). In a 2008 cross-sectional, population-based study of 1,666 Liberian adults, Johnson et al. (2008) found that both male and female combatants were more likely to report symptoms of posttraumatic stress disorder (PTSD), major depression, and suicidal ideation, and those who had experienced sexual violence had higher rates of those symptoms than those who had not.

Children in conflict areas also need mental health intervention. The University of Missouri, Columbia, has pioneered treatment strategies for children with PTSD and depression. They offer training to mental health workers and teachers in rural areas; they have also sent volunteer teams to Afghan refugee camps in Pakistan, Chechnya, and other areas (Lamberg, 2008). A Dutch mental health aid organization called HealthNet TPO offered classroom interventions to address trauma in Burundi, Sri Lanka, Sudan, and Indonesia; children who participated showed improvement in mood and behavior. HealthNet TPO shows ongoing mental health projects serving Afghanistan, Burundi, Cambodia, the DRC, Nepal, and South Sudan, among others on their website (HealthNet TPO, 2014).

In another example, a screening study of 2,400 children and adolescents in a refugee camp in Darfur showed a 20% prevalence of psychiatric symptoms (Lamberg, 2008). The challenge in Darfur is to identify resources to help the children since funding is so scarce. The WHO/Sudan 2009 Ministry of Health assessment of mental health resources states that only 6% of mental health resources are allocated to children; most treatment centers are located in cities and not rural areas where more children could benefit. Moreover, most treatment centers are inpatient (WHO, 2009). No resources are specifically identified for internally displaced persons despite the fact that, in 2012, in Sudan and South Sudan combined, there were approximately 295,500 IDPs (UNHCR, 2013). WHO has recognized mental health, neurological, and substance abuse disorders as a priority for care and has identified Sudan, as well as Afghanistan, Burundi, Indonesia, the DRC, Nepal, and Cambodia, as regions that meet criteria for intensified support. According to WHO, 14% of the global burden of disease is caused by mental health, neurological, and substance abuse disorders (WHO, 2008).

LEADERSHIP ROLE OF EXPATRIATE NURSES

Understanding the State of Nursing in the Host Country

By inquiring about the history and current state of nursing in the host country, the nurse volunteer may demonstrate interest and gain insight into local practice and the reputation of nursing. In the author's experience in the United States and in the Congo, the complex hierarchical culture of nursing is challenging to understand in one's own language, but even more so in a second language (Makosky, 2010). Host country nurses will appreciate being asked what motivated them to pursue nursing and about their prior work experience, just as with colleagues at home. Long jeep rides or other downtimes provide a good opportunity to ask these kinds of questions. It is also helpful and enlightening to look at the national nursing curriculum, if it exists. This information may be difficult to acquire and will likely require networking and wait time, but will provide valuable insight. Both the DRC and Niger have relatively long histories of nursing education, and nurses earn a high wage compared to other jobs.

Role of the Returning Nurse Educator

Prolonged armed conflict can have devastating effects on the discipline of nursing and on nursing education (Ismail, 2011; Murray, 2001; Raisler & Heymann, 2001). Many nurses are either killed or injured during conflict or flee to safety. In her inspiring account of rebuilding nursing in Somaliland, Fouzia Mohamed Ismail writes that when she returned to her country, "Nursing and midwifery . . . were almost non-existent. They had died" (Ismail, 2011, p. 7). Public confidence in health care workers was low, and the war precluded continuing education. When Ismail formed the first Somaliland Nursing and Midwifery Association (SLNMA), she started with only seven members (2011). She recounts how the registers from the old school of nursing in Mogadishu were rescued by a Somali nurse, and were used to conduct a survey to find other nurses. The SLNMA has now grown to almost 600 members (Ismail, 2011).

Role of the Visiting Nurse Midwife Educator

Tensions between different ethnic groups can also have serious adverse effects on the nursing profession. Michele Heymann, a nurse midwife and family nurse practitioner, describes the health system in Kosovo after the conflict ended between the Serbians and the ethnic Albanians, which she experienced during her work to launch a mother and child health promotion project (Raisler & Heymann, 2001). Her story is another example of how prolonged conflict negatively impacts the availability of competent and skilled nurses.

For more than 10 years, the Serbian government had excluded ethnic Albanians from government-funded health services, so they had a separate system with little or no government support. In Kosovo, as in Somaliland, there was low public confidence in Albanian health workers, in this case because they were deprived of their documents by Serbian forces and had lost access to education during the war. Thus, efforts to rebuild the health system in Kosovo had to begin with standardized training of nurses, midwives, and health care workers. As they gained knowledge and skills, the Kosovar midwives also gained self-esteem, and their public reputation improved (Fisher & Van Rooyen, 2004; Raisler & Heymann, 2001).

TAKING CARE OF OURSELVES

Challenges

During peak disaster conditions, many nurses work long hours under difficult circumstances. Witnessing the death of a young child or the suffering of innocent people can be very upsetting for any health care worker. Seeing these types of cases repeatedly can cause emotional distress that may take on many forms. It is important for the global nurse volunteer to seek help when needed. Colleagues will likely have experienced these same feelings, so debriefing can be helpful. Local or regional barriers to health care, such as corruption or mismanagement, also cause frustration. One may observe symptoms of burnout such as anger, depression, or inappropriate behavior in a colleague who has not found an effective way to deal with bearing witness to such suffering. Most aid organizations have provisions for mental health problems, but the individual may not recognize the issue or feel comfortable asking for help. It is ideal to identify resources before going into the field and, again, before heading home.

Reentry

This author and countless others who have returned from working in resource-poor environments have experienced a feeling of disconnection upon return to their home country. Canadian nurse Sue Witt describes it well, "I did not belong here; I did not belong there. I was not prepared for the length of time it took to adjust to living back in Canada again" (Witt, 2009, p. 567). For this author and many colleagues who have had similar experiences, the luxury of living in a developed country is initially difficult to accept. Coming from a place where many people are suffering can make it difficult to step back into one's old job. Author Lynne Wallis interviewed Kay Anderson, a nurse from the United Kingdom, on her return from Sierra Leone. Ms. Anderson related, "You do get impatient with people who've got minor health problems after you've been in a war zone. I couldn't help thinking, 'God, you don't know what's happening in the world'" (Wallis, 2001, p. 20). Usually these feelings gradually fade, and one is able to adjust. However, many aid organizations provide coverage for mental health services on return. The nurse volunteer should not hesitate to make use of any employee assistance program services that may be available.

CONCLUSION

Nursing work in a conflict zone is a challenging but rewarding experience rife with personal discomforts and emotional highs and lows. Nurses are perfectly positioned to teach healthy behaviors to populations at risk, for example, the importance of clean water, hygiene, nutrition, and immunizations (Martone, 2003a). This author found inspiration in host country health staff members who were smart and eager to learn. Many resources, including training programs, online information, and input from experienced staff, are available for nurses who wish to contribute to global health nursing in conflict areas. Nurses who are interested in relief work will benefit greatly from preparation and research. Because of their expanded worldview, nurses with global health experience are better positioned to care for immigrants and refugees in their new home country. Experienced nurses and nursing students alike are curious to hear about the role of nursing in conflict areas. Take notes and pictures while you are there. Then come back and tell your story.

REFERENCES

Centers for Disease Control and Prevention. (2014). *2014 Ebola virus disease in West Africa—Case counts*. Retrieved from: http://www.cdc.gov/vhf/ebola/outbreaks/2014-west-africa/case-counts.html

Central Intelligence Agency. (2014). *The world factbook*. Retrieved from https://www.cia.gov/library/publications/the-world-factbook/docs/profileguide.html

Cunningham, J. (2000). Nursing near a war zone. *Australian Nursing Journal, 7*(7), 19.

De Jong, M. J., Benner, R., Benner, P., Richard, M. L., Kenny, D. J., Kelley, P. K., . . . Debisette, A. T. (2010). Mass casualty care in an expeditionary environment: Developing local knowledge and expertise in context. *Journal of Trauma Nursing, 17*(1), 45–58.

Fisher, M. L., & VanRooyen, M. J. (2004). Care amid the rubble in Kosovo: An interdisciplinary effort to develop services in a war-ravaged country. *AJN: American Journal of Nursing, 104*(7), 72AA–72FF.

Ford, T. (2012, October 10). Liberia slowly coming to terms with civil war's impact on mental health. *The Guardian*. Retrieved from http://www.theguardian.com/global-development/2012/oct/10/liberia-civil-war-mental-health

Gately, R. (2004). Humanitarian aid to Iraqi civilians during the war: A U.S. nurse's role. *Journal of Emergency Nursing, 30*(3), 230–236.

Gately, R. (2005). Sudan: A humanitarian response to a silent genocide: An American nurse's perspective. *Journal of Emergency Nursing, 31*(3), 325–332.

Hayward, M. (2004). Facing danger. *Nursing Standard, 19*(3), 20–21.

HealthNet TPO. (2014). Retrieved from http://www.healthnettpo.org/en

How the CIA's fake vaccination campaign endangers us all? [Editorial]. (2013). *Scientific American, 308*(5). Retrieved from http://www.scientificamerican.com/article/how-cia-fake-vaccination-campaign-endangers-us-all

Humanitarian Academy at Harvard. (2014). Retrieved from http://www.humanitarianacademy.harvard.edu/about-us/our-programs

Internal Displacement Monitoring Center (IDMC). (2014). Latest IDP numbers by country. Retrieved from http://www.internal-displacement.org/global-figures

International Committee of the Red Cross. (2011). *Health care in danger: Making the case.* Geneva, Switzerland: Author.

International Committee of the Red Cross. (2014). Retrieved from http://www.icrc.org/eng/resources/documents/job/always-in-demand/fd-nurse.htm

IRIN News. (2013, May 2). Iraq 10 years on: War leaves lasting impact on healthcare. *IRIN News.* Retrieved from http://www.irinnews.org/report/97964/war-leaves-lasting-impact-on-healthcare

Ismail, F. M. (2011). *Patience and care: Rebuilding nursing and midwifery in Somaliland.* London, UK: Africa Research Institute.

Johnson, K., Asher, J., Rosborough, S., Raja, A., Panjabi, R., Beadling, C., & Lawry, L. (2008). Association of combatant status and sexual violence with health and mental health outcomes in postconflict Liberia. *Journal of the American Medical Association, 300*(6), 676–690.

Kargbo, K. L. (2002). Limbs of hope: Restoring amputees in Sierra Leone. *Journal of Christian Nursing, 19*(1), 22–24.

Keating, J. (2014, May 19). No more fake vaccination campaigns, says CIA. *Slate.* Retrieved from http://www.slate.com/blogs/the_world_/2014/05/19/cia_promises_no_more_fake_vaccination_campaigns_after_bin_laden_raid_linked.html

Kleffel, D. (2006). The evolution of the environmental metaparadigm in nursing. In L. Andrist, P. Nicholas, & K. Wolf (Eds.), *A history of nursing ideas* (pp. 97–108). Sudbury, MA: Jones & Bartlett.

Lamberg, L. (2008). Psychiatrists strive to help children heal mental wounds from war and disasters. *Journal of the American Medical Association, 300*(6), 642–643.

Larson, H. (2012, May 27). The CIA's fake vaccination drive has damaged the battle against polio. *The Guardian.* Retrieved from http://www.theguardian.com/commentisfree/2012/may/27/cia-fake-vaccination-polio

Lester, N. (2008). An emotionally charged journey. *Mental Health Practice, 12*(2), 18–19.

Liverpool School of Tropical Medicine. (2014). Retrieved from http://www.lstmliverpool.ac.uk/learning—teaching/lstm-courses/professional-diplomas/dha

London School of Economics and Political Science. (2014). Retrieved from http://www.lse.ac.uk/study/graduate/taughtProgrammes2014/MScInternationalDevelopmentAndHumanitarianEmergencies.aspx

Makosky, A. (2010). *Congo global health experience: Summer 2010.* Global health paper. Unpublished manuscript, School of Nursing, MGH Institute of Health Professions, Charlestown, Massachusetts.

Martone, G. (2002). Mission to Afghanistan. *AJN The American Journal of Nursing, 102*(9), 40–43.

Martone, G. (2003a). The crisis in West Africa: A region suffers from war, poverty, and disease. *AJN The American Journal of Nursing, 103*(9), 32–40.

Martone, G. (2003b). Water and health in Iraq: A nurse reports on this crucial link as a country is rebuilt. *AJN The American Journal of Nursing, 103*(11), 46–47.

Martone, G. (2004). Crisis in Darfur, Sudan: In 18 months, more than 1 million people have been uprooted by war. A nurse-photographer documents life in one camp. *AJN The American Journal of Nursing, 104*(7), 54–57.

Martone, G., & Kennedy, M. S. (2012). Scenes from Somalia. *AJN The American Journal of Nursing, 112*(12), 38–39.

Masters, K. (2012). *Nursing theories: A framework for professional practice.* Sudbury, MA: Jones & Bartlett.

McDonald, L. (1998). Florence Nightingale: Passionate statistician. *Journal of Holistic Nursing, 16*(2), 267–277.

Médecins sans Frontières. (2014). Retrieved from http://www.msf.org

Murray, K. (2001). When the bombing stops. *Nursing Standard, 16*(12), 13.

Nurses in war zones are facing growing danger. (1999). *Journal of Advanced Nursing, 30*(4), 779–780.

Parish, C. (2002). The price of war. *Nursing Standard, 17*(14–15), 18–20.

Pickersgill, F. E. (2002). The war against disease. *Nursing Standard, 16*(45), 18–19.

Raisler, J., & Heymann, M. (2001). Reproductive health promotion in Kosovo. *Journal of Midwifery & Women's Health, 46*(2), 74–81.

Salvage, J. (2004). Mass destruction. *Nursing Standard, 19*(12), 12–13.

Shah, S. (2011, July 11). CIA organized fake vaccination drive to get Osama bin Laden's family DNA. *The Guardian.* Retrieved from http://www.theguardian.com/world/2011/jul/11/cia-fake-vaccinations-osama-bin-ladens-dna

Sherazi, Z. S., & Watkins, T. (2014, March 1). Attack targets polio workers in Pakistan, kills 11. Cable News Network. Retrieved from http://www.cnn.com/2014/03/01/world/asia/pakistan-attack/

Sofer, D. (2003). Iraq's health care system: What now? *AJN: American Journal of Nursing, 103*(6), 24–25.

Tesch, P. (2006). In the war zone. *Nursing Standard, 20*(24), 26–27.

Tjoflat, I., & Karlsen, B. (2012). Challenges in sharing knowledge: Reflections from the perspective of an expatriate nurse working in a South Sudanese hospital. *International Nursing Review, 59*(4), 489–493.

United Nations Children's Fund (UNICEF). (1996). *Sexual violence as a weapon of war. The state of the world's children 1996.* Retrieved from http://www.unicef.org/sowc96pk/sexviol.htm

United Nations High Commission for Refugees (UNHCR). (2013). *Displacement: The new 21st century challenge.* UNHCR global trends 2012. Geneva, Switzerland: Author.

United Nations High Commission for Refugees. (2014). *War's human cost: UNHCR global trends 2013.* Retrieved from http://www.unhcr.org/cgi-bin/texis/vtx/home/opendocPDFViewer.html?docid=5399a14f9&query=UNHCR%20Global%20Trends

University of Oxford Refugee Studies Center. (2014). Retrieved from http://www.rsc.ox.ac.uk/study/short-courses/health-and-humanitarian-responses

University of York Overseas Development Institute. (2014). Retrieved from http://www.odi.org.uk/programmes/humanitarian-policy-group/advancedcourse

Von Schirnding, Y. (2002). *Health in sustainable development planning: The role of indicators.* Geneva, Switzerland: WHO.

Wallis, L. (2000). Working in a war zone. *Nursing Standard, 15*(24), 19–20.

Witt, S. (2009). My journey to Sudan. *Journal of Emergency Nursing, 35*(6), 564–568.

Woodham-Smith, C. (1951). *Lonely crusader: The life of Florence Nightingale.* New York, NY: McGraw-Hill.

World Health Organization. (2008). *mhGAP: Mental health gap action programme: Scaling up care for mental, neurological and substance use disorders.* France: Author.

World Health Organization. (2009). WHO-AIMS Report on mental health system in Sudan. Khartoum, Sudan: Author.

World Health Organization. (2014a). *Employment: Required qualifications.* Retrieved from http://www.who.int/employment/who_we_need/requirements/en

World Health Organization. (2014b). *World health statistics 2014.* Retrieved from http://www.who.int/gho/publications/world_health_statistics/EN_WHS2014_Part3.pdf?ua=1

CHAPTER 16

Mental Health of Asylum Seekers

Jayden Nadeau, Patrice K. Nicholas, and Susan Stevens

*T*he United States is a nation that takes tremendous pride in its freedom and the vast diversity of cultures and customs. The thought of living even a piece of the "American dream" is enough to attract people from all over the world. The United States can offer a physically and economically safer environment for people who have never felt safe or even know what safety means. Individuals are willing to risk everything, including their lives and the lives of their children, in order to have a chance to escape situations involving drug-related violence, torture, sexual assault, poverty, and nonstop warfare, among numerous other atrocities.

In trying to start a new life, undocumented immigrants and other nonnatives encounter countless problems and indecencies when entering the United States. Some were brought to the United States as infants and are sent back to their "native" country after a routine traffic stop. Many natives of the United States have focused on the political situation surrounding immigration and are unaware of the problems the United States creates for newcomers, regardless of the outcome of their citizenship. Immigrants face discrimination, humiliation, and other emotional and physical traumas. A large proportion of people seeking help from the United States have already survived horrendous experiences and become retraumatized by the treatment received in the place they believed was their last hope. A person's legal status should not impact his or her right to receive appropriate, decent, and respectful treatment.

In order to help improve the mental health of asylum seekers and detainees in the United States, their treatment and environments need serious change. Our systems to assist them are overwhelmed by the numbers alone of people worldwide who are forced to flee and escape the horror of world violence in its various destructive and damaging forms. Additional problems begin from the day they arrive and may have lifelong effects. Addressing the mental health of these populations is crucial for their rehabilitation and integration into a new environment, wherever it may be. Providing asylum seekers and detainees with appropriate mental health care can help those who are eventually repatriated to have some stability and coping mechanisms in place before being sent back to potentially unstable conditions. The environments, mainly detention centers, are the most influential part of the asylum and detainment processes. Improving the environment for these individuals can have an incredible impact on their long-term mental health.

BACKGROUND

Terminology

In order to understand the issues of asylum seekers and detainees, there are a few terms that need to be defined. Definitions of displaced persons are usually developed by international organizations; however, individual nations can decide upon their own terminology to define those within their boundaries. Internally displaced persons (IDPs) is a term used for individuals or groups of individuals who have fled or been forced to leave their home because of, or to evade, "the effects of armed conflict, situations of generalized violence, violations of human rights, or natural/human-made disasters, and who have not crossed an international border" (United Nations High Commissioner for Refugees [UNHCR], 2011b, p. 37). The admission of refugees to the United States and their resettlement here are authorized by the Immigration and Nationality Act (INA) (1952) as amended by the Refugee Act of 1980. The protocol defines a refugee as a nonnative person who is

> displaced abroad who is unable or unwilling to return to, and is
> unable or unwilling to avail himself or herself of the protection of, that
> country because of persecution or a well-founded fear of persecution
> on account of race, religion, nationality, membership in a particular
> social group, or political opinion. (Wasem, 2005, p. CRS-3)

People seeking refugee status must live outside of the United States and their country of origin. An asylum seeker is defined as a person who has entered or attempts to enter a country other than his or her native, who meets the requirements of a refugee (U.S. Department of Homeland Security [USDHS], 2013a). Asylum seekers have sought international protection, but have not yet been granted refugee status and are awaiting a final determination (UNHCR, 2011a). It is important to note that the country in which the person is seeking asylum is usually the country that determines the approval or denial of refugee status (UNHCR, 2011b). This jurisdiction means that the asylee is subject to the laws and procedures of that country and his or her native country may not be able to intervene.

Although there are many concerns and even stigmas regarding the terminology that refers to immigrants, the terms set forth by the USDHS and the UNHCR are used here to maintain consistency and uniformity. For the purpose of this chapter, the use of the term "immigrant" refers to undocumented immigrants and other undocumented nonnatives. *Detainee* is a much broader term encompassing individuals who are "held in custody in police holding cells or in a prison, or as a suspect" (Wadee, 2006, p. 68). Detainees can include captives of war, native citizens awaiting trial, and undocumented noncitizens who have and have not committed crimes, among others. Essentially, anyone taken into custody by law enforcement from any jurisdiction can be considered a detainee. In order to keep within the focus of this chapter, the use of the term "detainee" will exclude captives of war and those held outside of U.S. territory. Detainee refers only to detained immigrants and asylum seekers.

The importance of including the mental health of detainees is also crucial to an understanding of the challenges of asylum seekers. While their backgrounds and reasons for entering or attempting to enter the United States can be vastly different, how they are processed once inside the states impacts their mental health in similar ways. The majority of asylum seekers and undocumented immigrants picked up by or presenting to authorities (e.g., border patrol) are required to await their trial in a detention center, regardless of the presence of a criminal history. There is some overlap between immigrants' and asylum seekers' plans as immigrants can also apply for asylum. People not seeking asylum may encounter different legal processing and procedures but are also subject to similar situations and stressors while in detention.

Growing Concerns Related to Asylum Seekers

Throughout the world violence and crime have been rising, forcing many people to become vulnerable to displacement and relocation. The refugee crises reached record levels in 2012. UNHCR reports and analyzes statistical trends and changes for the populations for whom UNHCR has been entrusted. These populations include refugees, asylum seekers, returnees, stateless persons, and certain groups of IDPs. These groups are collectively referred to as persons of concern. An average of 3,000 persons per day became refugees in 2012. By the end of 2012, more than 45.2 million people were forcibly displaced due to persecution, conflict, generalized violence, and human rights violations. This number included 10.5 million refugees, 937,000 asylum seekers, and the 28.8 million who were forced to flee within their own countries (UNHCR, 2013a).

Approximately 55% of the refugees were forced out of five countries affected by conflict: Afghanistan, Somalia, Iraq, Syria, and Sudan. An estimated 7.6 million people were newly displaced due to conflict or persecution, including 1.1 million new refugees, representing the highest number since 1999. More than 920,000 people submitted applications for asylum or refugee status in 2012. UNHCR (2013b) registered 13% of these claims. With an estimated 82,000 asylum claims, South Africa had the highest number of new application asylum claims, followed by the United States with 70,400, then Germany with 64,500, and France with 55,100. An estimated 479,300 asylum applications were received in 44 industrialized countries in 2012, an increase of 8% over 2011 (UNHCR, 2013b).

Children younger than the age of 18 represented an average of 49% of the total population of concern to UNHCR, of whom 13% were younger than the age of 5.

Less than half of this population were adults or between the ages of 18 and 59, and 4% were 60 and older. Refugee women and girls accounted for 49% of this population, a proportion that has remained relatively constant over the past decade. Children younger than 18 admitted into the United States in 2012 represented 32.4% of the total admitted (UNHCR, 2013b).

Also of great concern are the internally displaced. About two thirds of the world's forcibly uprooted people are displaced within their own country. UNHCR has been playing an increasingly important role in recent years in assisting these IDPs. There were 28.8 million IDPs dispersed around the world in 2012. This number has steadily increased from a total of around 17 million in 1997 and includes more than 6.5 million newly displaced, almost twice as many as the 3.5 million recorded in the previous year (UNHCR, 2013b). By the end of 2012, the UN Refugee Agency included around 15.5 million of these IDPs in its care, a number greater than the total number of refugees of concern to UNHCR. The conflicts in Syria and the Democratic Republic of the Congo (DRC) were considered responsible for approximately half of the new displacements, with 2.4 million and 1 million, respectively, while an estimated 500,000 people escaped their homes in both Sudan and India (UNHCR, 2013b).

Regionally the largest increase in the number of internally displaced people in 2012 occurred in the Middle East and North Africa, where 2.5 million people were displaced because of violence. With almost 6 million IDPs in this region at the end of 2012, this figure represents an increase of 40% from 2011. Sadly, this number continued to rise in 2013. Asia reported the second highest increase in new displacements after the Middle East and North Africa, with 1.4 million people forced to escape their homes during 2012. The region with the largest total number of IDPs was sub-Saharan Africa with 10.4 million, an increase of 7.5% compared with just the previous year. The Americas identified the second largest number of IDPs in 2012 with a total of 5.8 million, representing an increase of 3% compared with the previous year. Colombia continues to claim the highest number of IDPs in the world, with a total of between 4.9 and 5.5 million. The country's internal armed conflict forced an estimated 230,000 people to flee their homes during 2012 (UNHCR, 2013b).

In 2012, 58,179 refugees were admitted to the United States, a 3.2% increase from 56,384 in 2011. A slight majority of refugees were male (51%), and 38% were married. Of the refugees admitted to the United States in 2012, 32% were younger than 18 years of age (UNHCR, 2013b). In the past few years, the number of unaccompanied children arriving in the United States has risen dramatically, particularly from Central America. The majority of these children arrive from Guatemala, Honduras, and El Salvador. By spring of 2012, U.S. immigration officials had taken into custody nearly double the number of children as in the previous years (UNHCR, 2013b). In 2012 the Office of Resettlement (ORR), the agency charged with the care and custody of unaccompanied children, had a record number in its care with 18,876 children arrivals in the United States alone (USDHS, 2013b; UNHCR, 2013b). The thousands of children who pass through this system come up against a maze of perplexing and confusing obstacles, as do the service providers whose responsibility it is to assist them (Huemer et al., 2009; Johnsson, Zolkowska, & McNeil, 2014; Lustig et al., 2004; Robjant, Hassan, & Katona, 2009).

The demand has been overwhelmingly higher than the numbers of spaces available for refugees. Complicating the problem further, the number of refugee returns has been declining since 2004, with 2010 reporting the lowest returns in more than 20 years (UNHCR, 2011). These data suggest there has been limited improvement in the violence and instability throughout the world, increasing the numbers of people needing homes and decreasing the numbers able to return (USDHS, 2013a).

In 2012, the United States reported there were 643,474 immigrants eligible for deportation, of which 448,697 were from Mexico, 55,307 from Guatemala, 37,197 from El Salvador, and 48,984 from Honduras (USDHS, 2013b). The number of immigrants from Mexico and Central America make up over 94% of the immigrants present in the United States. More Mexicans have also been requesting asylum, but the amount accepted has been declining. In 2011, 6,133 people from Mexico requested asylum in the United States, and 104 were accepted (USDHS, 2012; UNHCR, 2012). In 2010, 4,510 people from Mexico requested asylum and 49 were accepted (USDHS, 2011; UNHCR, 2011). While these numbers are lower than many other countries, it does not mean they are without troubles. The number of people requesting asylum in the United States from Mexico rose to 9,206 in 2012 (UNHCR, 2013). Mexico and Central America have seen dramatic increases in drug-related crime and violence. The Mexican government reported that more than 28,000 people have died due to drug trafficking and related violence since 2006 (Beittel, 2011). It is difficult to obtain accurate statistics since many crimes are unreported due to fear of retaliation or are covered up by drug cartels. Other organizations reported death totals of 2,280 in 2007, 5,153 in 2008, 6,587 in 2009, and over 11,000 in 2010 (Beittel, 2011). The majority of drug-related violence has increased in Mexico's northern border states, with 60% of deaths occurring in Tijuana, Culiacan, and Ciudad Juarez alone, but it is also spreading south to new areas across the country (Beittel, 2011).

Credible Fear

The United States affirms it will not deport nonnationals to their home country if their lives or freedom are at risk, yet the United States has repeatedly rejected valid applications (Wasem, 2011). In order to be considered for asylum, candidates must demonstrate to an officer a "credible fear" of persecution based on "race, religion, nationality, membership in a particular social group, or political opinion" (Immigration and Nationality Act, 1952; Wasem, 2005, 2011). A definition of credible fear is available for officers to reference when determining if someone meets the requirements. However, it is not guaranteed the officer has an appropriate understanding of a person's background or the ability to omit his or her personal opinions from his or her decisions. The terms "credible" and "fear" are both subjective and may be interpreted differently by various audiences. The subjectivity of the term "fear" makes it difficult to distinguish between what is credible and what is not. Fear can be extremely hard to assess, especially if the person conducting the assessment has never feared for his or her life. Interpretation can vary extensively between authority figures and in relation to current events (i.e., September 11, 2001), resulting in variations in how cases are evaluated.

Officers must also determine if the candidate meets criteria for a "well-found fear" of persecution (Wasem, 2005, 2011). The term "well-found fear" contains a more elaborate definition, but it, too, includes a subjective component. It requires a "reasonable possibility" of facing persecution that necessitates an extensive knowledge base of the problems facing other nations (Wasem, 2011). The terms *race, religion, nationality, membership in a social group*, and *political opinion* have been built upon social constructs and are not universally definable (Jan, 2011). For example, a social group in one country may not exist in another, making it difficult to define across borders. Even race and religion are difficult to discern as they, too, are variable and may be seen differently between the persecutor and victim. There is an endless mix of factors, including culture, language, mental status, foreign laws, political stability, and safety, among many others, to evaluate when determining if someone's fear is essentially worth believing. It is difficult to assess if a person's claim is credible if the officer has not witnessed, been educated about, or kept up to date with the extensiveness of problems throughout the world.

Meeting the requirements of an asylum seeker does not guarantee a claim will be granted since acceptance is up to the discretion of an officer or judge (Wilkinson, 2010). Officers are the first people given the ability to determine a nonnative's case based on the culturally biased, complicated, and subjective terminology. If an officer decides the candidate is ineligible, he or she is then referred to a judge who reexamines the case. Approval for asylum can vary considerably between officers, judges, and courts, and by the applicants' country of origin (even within the same court) (Rottman, Fariss, & Poe, 2009; Wasem, 2011). Rottman et al. (2009) found evidence suggesting officers were more likely to grant asylum based on physical abuses and deny claims from English-speaking countries. It also found judges were more likely to grant asylum to people from countries considered to be important to U.S. security and deny claims from countries speaking Arabic and Spanish. After 2001, both officers' and judges' decisions revealed an increase in the number of denied claims for people from Arabic-speaking countries.

Emotions can be expressed in many ways, and persons in authority may easily misperceive the credibility of another based on his or her culture's behaviors and expressions. Being in an unfamiliar land with a different language and culture can make it terrifying to disclose traumatic events to strangers. Many people have grown up in places where they are unable to trust the government, which in turn affects their interactions with authorities foreign to them. Some applicants might have been abused by uniformed officers or militia and experience a tremendous amount of fear and anxiety when presenting to officers as a result of the memories triggered by their uniform.

In order to avoid claims of generalized fear, international refugee laws prohibit larger numbers of people from claiming a well-founded fear of persecution and often require applicants to show how they have been targeted individually (Jan, 2011). This prohibition is confounding considering the definition of refugee includes people who are fearful of persecution based on their involvement in social groups or political opinion (beliefs shared by many). Judges also assess new applicants' risks based on previous reports from others in the same or nearby regions when deciding eligibility for refugee status. Preventing a group of people from applying is counterproductive to U.S. laws and makes it harder for individual asylees and refugees to adapt to a new culture. Denying groups isolates people from their culture and prevents them from being able to help support each other emotionally, financially, and socially in a foreign land.

The legal process can be very intimidating and stressful for anyone, let alone asylum seekers who may have to learn about Western and international laws in addition to having possible cultural, language, and educational differences (Robjant et al., 2009). Asylum seekers frequently have to relive past traumas when explaining their case, triggering posttraumatic stress disorder (PTSD) symptoms and risking severe detriment to their mental health (Human Rights Watch, 2010a). In presenting their case, asylum seekers have to portray their history in a way to convince authorities their fear is credible enough for U.S. standards. Power dynamics also have the potential to play an important role in court proceedings. Some asylees may face a judge of the same race, culture, and so forth as their persecutor, and in presenting their case they are symbolically asking their abuser for help. Asylum seekers and other detainees can wait extended periods of time for their trial, often in prison-like cells with little else to occupy their minds. Knowing they will have to convince an officer or judge of the extensiveness of their fear may force extremely traumatic events to be replayed repeatedly to ensure they do not forget any details. If their first motion is denied, the nonnative may have to again endure the asylum process and court proceedings with other judges and authorities to proclaim their fear. These experiences may feel like reenactments of previous traumas and trigger significant emotional distress.

Predetention Trauma

The reasons for leaving one's country most often include some sort of violence or economic hardships. A study by Piwowarczyk (2007) found 84% of asylum seekers had experienced significant trauma or torture in their country of origin prior to entering the United States. Piwowarczyk also reported 50% had experienced rape or sexual assault and 37% had first-degree family members who were tortured or killed. Another study found 64% of asylum seekers had been physically assaulted, 52% tortured, 52% imprisoned, and 36% witnessed death of someone close to them (Bernardes et al., 2010). Often governments or government-funded organizations have been involved in mass murders, rapes, and other atrocities. Governments have tortured their citizens not only to punish those they feel have done wrong, but also to instill fear in the community for those who question or disagree with their beliefs (Piwowarczyk, 2007).

Although asylum seekers and immigrants have their differences, many immigrants share histories of trauma and abuse. Some of the common traumas experienced by immigrants include sexual assault, physical violence, domestic violence, sexually transmitted infections, human trafficking, detention, combat, deportation/repatriation, drug-related crimes and violence, and political violence, as well as being a witness to violence. Many of the traumas in Mexico have been related to the growing numbers of drug- and gang-related activities (Levers & Hyatt-Burkart, 2011).

Many asylum seekers have not had any psychiatric support prior to their entry into a new country (Piwowarczyk, 2007). There can be numerous reasons as to why they have not tried to seek help in their country prior to fleeing. Access to mental health services and the views surrounding it vary considerably throughout the world. Asylees may not have had any services available in their country, or they may have been too far away or risky to obtain given their resources and the potential for violence. Some may not know about nearby services as militia and rebel groups sometimes isolate families in small areas where leaving could endanger their lives (Woodward & Galvin, 2009). Some may hold the belief that seeking mental health care makes them weak or mentally unsound. Some communities have built strong communications with each other and rely on friends and family for support; however, this affiliation does not mean they are getting the support they need. Cultures with strong community communication may be less willing to discuss their trauma history in fear of information spreading to others or that they will be shamed (Piwowarczyk, 2007). Experiences prior to or leading to someone's migration can have profound effects on his or her mental health. Additionally, placing trauma survivors in detention facilities on arrival in a new country can aggravate trauma histories, placing them at further risk for mental distress (Robjant et al., 2009).

Traumas are not only experienced prior to leaving their homeland, but asylum seekers and immigrants encounter problems during migration. In departing their country they may be leaving behind their home, friends, family, customs, culture, and community. There is, at least, a great deal of uncertainty, and, more likely, fear for these individuals to have to move to a new place with different languages and laws without knowing the outcome. Many travel with little money or resources with no idea of problems they could face during travel, just hoping they will be safer than they were in their home country. Some people encounter enormous struggles when trying to enter the United States. It is not uncommon for women to face sexual violence and for others to run into human trafficking operations (Davies, Borland, Blake, & West, 2011). Immigrants can face physical dangers associated with crossing the border (physical injuries, dehydration, etc.), crowded and unhygienic situations, as well as dangers associated with human trafficking (Beckerman & Corbett, 2008). The majority of immigrants from Mexico are now entering the United States illegally, and many are turning to illegal activities such as drug trafficking and gangs to help them enter (Spring, 2009). These methods of migration place them in numerous traumatic situations and often tie them to gang activity for the rest of their life.

Once inside the United States they are likely to face a whole new set of stressors. Beckerman and Corbett (2008) discuss how acculturative stress has a particularly strong negative impact on immigrants' mental health and that some experience "a profound or incapacitating sense of loss, disassociation, flashbacks or nightmares about separation from the homeland or family of origin" (p. 66). Bernardes et al. (2010) conducted a study on postmigratory stressors among asylum seekers and found 76% had acculturation difficulties, 83% were denied employment,

86% worried about relatives in the country of origin, 69% had difficulties with communication, 52% experienced discrimination, and 52% experienced difficulty accessing health care and welfare services. This study highlights that the complex and multiple difficulties with accommodations, communication, finances, discrimination, and denial of employment significantly affect their mental health. People arriving in the United States have to change their entire life to be able to acculturate into society. Even by changing their lives so drastically, there is no guarantee they will not face discrimination and oppression from others in the community.

SPECIAL POPULATIONS

Women

Women may have a more extensive abuse history and encounter unique problems related to their sex while in detention centers. It is common for women crossing the border to be raped by coyotes, people who are hired to help others cross the border (Human Rights Watch, 2009). It is difficult to escape rapes by coyotes as women have likely given them a significant amount of money to get across the border and may have little to sustain them if they decide to return home. Leaving could also put their life at risk since coyotes can have gang and drug cartel ties and crossing the border alone is extremely dangerous.

Women from any number of countries may present with a violent past, often including rape or sexual assault. The Medical Foundation for the Care of Victims of Torture (MF) (2009) conducted a study on 100 women from various countries who were seeking help in the United Kingdom after experiencing some form of torture. It found 80 women had been raped and six were sexually assaulted. Over two thirds of the rape survivors had been raped by multiple perpetrators, and more than one third were unable to recall the number of times they had been raped. There were also many women who had been raped in front of their children, family, and in public. The majority of women did not seek help from authorities because the perpetrators were part of the police force. Sixteen women reported violent incidents, of which 12 received no further action and four endured abuse and/or detention as a result of reporting. None of the perpetrators were prosecuted.

The risk for domestic violence on women is increased when women are not the primary applicant seeking asylum and when they are on a spousal visa getting support from their spouse (Chantler, 2012). Women may be scared to approach authorities about their abuse because of the fear surrounding domestic abuse and their asylum claim (Chantler, 2012). Abusers often create an extensive amount of fear in their victims to the point where they fear they will be killed if they try to seek help. If a woman is dependent on someone else for her status to get into or remain in the United States, she might be less inclined to seek help. The abuser holds a great deal of power when residence also comes into play. Women may be fearful that they will become homeless or lose their asylum status and be deported. Seeking help from authorities might place them in further danger if the attacker finds out she has told.

Reporting abuse can be difficult both in their country of origin and in the United States. Some women who report sexual crimes, especially if they are seen by others as not having defended themselves, may be ostracized from their spouse, family, children, friends, and community (MF, 2009). Women are sometimes blamed for taking part in rapes and betraying their husband, which can sometimes lead to their death (MF, 2009). Women may be less likely to report the crimes when seeking asylum, preventing them from receiving helpful resources to help them recover.

Immigration and Customs Enforcement (ICE) requires initial medical screening to include asking detainees about past sexual abuse, but only advises other abuses be considered when a detainee needs a mental health referral. There is no current screening for domestic abuse and initial screening procedures are not necessarily conducted by medical providers. Even more concerning is that many women reported not being asked about previous abuse at all (Human Rights Watch, 2009). Abuse can also be difficult to prove, especially if a significant amount of time has gone by since the abuse, which many women may not understand. These issues prevent women from accessing care at a very critical time. Some women may be further subjected to abuse by their domestic partner if she or he is also in the detention center. Detention has the potential to offer women a chance to receive help that they may never have been offered.

Women are also at risk from others in detention centers since any ICE facility that can physically and visually separate female and male detainees is allowed to house females and 68% are housed in state or county jails (Human Rights Watch, 2009). ICE has repeatedly failed to educate detainees about rules and regulations surrounding sexual harassment and abuse. The Human Rights First (2011) has determined that body searches should only be performed by authorities of the same sex to maintain detainees' rights to privacy, yet pat searches have no restrictions. Many times female detainee(s) are transported to other facilities by a single male officer. Women have been forced to undress and have been sexually assaulted, abused, harassed, and raped by other detainees and officers. These problems in detention centers make it very difficult for women, who may already be fearful of authorities, to report abuse that occurred in their past or within the facility (Human Rights Watch, 2010b).

Children

Child asylum seekers are at a great risk of developing mental illnesses in detention due to a range of past high-risk experiences. Unaccompanied children come to the United States from around the world, though primarily from Central and South America. In 2014, there was a dramatic increase in the numbers of unaccompanied children coming to the United States, which President Obama viewed as an urgent humanitarian situation. CNN News (2014) notes that:

> U.S. law prohibits the Department of Homeland Security from
> immediately deporting the children if they are not from Canada or

Mexico. Instead, the children are turned over to Department of Health and Human Services supervision "within 72 hours of DHS taking them into custody," an official said.

While the majority of unaccompanied children are boys between the ages of 15 and 17, unaccompanied children are of both genders and some are infants. Unaccompanied refugee minors are in a highly vulnerable situation with greater psychiatric morbidity than the general population or even accompanied refugee minors. Younger refugee children are more vulnerable to emotional distress than older children. Procedures for dealing with asylum seekers may contribute to high levels of stress and emotional symptoms in children who have been previously traumatized (Huemer et al., 2009). Children of all ages also accompany their parents (USDHS, 2013a, 2013b). Both of these groups are extremely vulnerable, and their needs often go unmet. Children in detention centers may have been through various predetention traumas such as murders, trafficking, female genital mutilation, annihilation of homes, physical and sexual abuse, prostitution, and slavery, among many others (Hodes, 2010; Newman & Steel, 2008; Prasad & Prasad, 2009). Many have also been victimized while in refugee situations while they are away from their families (Newman & Steel, 2008). It is not uncommon for children who have experienced traumas to develop depression, hopelessness, oppositional defiant disorder, behavioral problems, and PTSD at a young age (Hodes, 2010; Newman & Steel, 2008; Prasad & Prasad, 2009). Many are also at heightened risk for suicide and self-harm (Hodes, 2010; Newman & Steel, 2008). In detention they are at increased risk for further traumas due to the conditions of the facilities and their separation from the rest of the world.

Children are often housed in detention centers without their parents (Alayarian, 2009). Removing children from their parents takes away what may be their only comfort in a strange and sometimes hostile place. They have to overcome fears and venture into a new world where they know little about the culture and language (Alayarian, 2009). Children may have received little to no education in their home country and not understand many of the changes they are going through, making it hard to adapt to a new culture (Hodes, 2010). Detention prevents children from developing normal social relationships, which may contribute significantly to attachment disorders (Newman & Steel, 2008). Children housed with their parents sometimes experience role reversal and end up having to care for their parents due to their depression (Newman & Steel, 2008). Role reversal and other stressors in detention can cause distress in families, having an enormous impact on children's' mental health and development (Newman & Steel, 2008).

Children caught in the immigration process also have experienced maltreatment from U.S. immigration authorities (Center for Public Policy Priorities [CPPP], 2008). When being deported, they are often placed in dangerous situations and left in unsafe conditions at their drop-off locations (CPPP, 2008). The returning countries' consulates are frequently unaware of a child's return, which sometimes takes place in the middle of the night and to places outside of regional agreements

(CPPP, 2008). Many children have reported that they were never asked if they were afraid about returning to their home country (CPPP, 2008).

Child Soldiers

A certain population, child soldiers, faces unique problems as a result of their history. One of the exclusions for asylum eligibility in the United States under the INA is engaging in the persecution of another person (Lonegan, 2011). In the United States, persecution is considered to be having "ordered, incited, assisted, or otherwise participated in the persecution of any person on account of race, religion, nationality, membership in a particular social group, or political opinion" (U.S. Department of Justice, 2009). Prosecution can vary considerably depending on the nation that is responsible for discerning their participation in crimes (Grover, 2008). In the United States, children may have to extensively prove their reasons for committing crimes as well as being persecuted themselves.

Roughly 250,000 male and female children younger than 18 years old have been compulsorily persuaded or forced to engage in combat or live in servitude (Lonegan, 2011). International laws, rights, and statutes are often broad and leave a considerable amount of room for subjectivity by determining authorities (Grover, 2008). While some nations have developed protocols for determining the age at which one is considered a child and eligible for asylum, others can range anywhere from younger than 10 years to 18 years old (Grover, 2008). Former child soldiers' lives can be put at great risk when returning to their native country, where they may again face militia groups as well as the families of those they have hurt and/or killed (Woodward & Galvin, 2009). Moving back to the place in which they were recruited can also severely affect their psychological well-being. They may have to live in the same area where they lost their family and were recruited, inviting memories of trauma on a daily basis.

Children who are recruited as soldiers by rebels, militias, and other armed groups have been subject to repeated drugging and extreme physical, mental, and sexual abuse (Grover, 2008). Children are sought out by armed groups for their participation because as children they are malleable and easily succumb to fear (Grover, 2008). One study found a common recruitment method among a group of rebel soldiers was to kill all of the family members of the second oldest son, then give him a choice between murder or joining the soldiers (Woodward & Galvin, 2009). Other groups have forced families into isolated regions without access to food and water, leaving them with no choice but to join or starve to death (Woodward & Galvin, 2009). Former child soldiers in refugee camps are often approached by soldiers offering them money to re-join (Woodward & Galvin, 2009). The thought of joining can be very tempting because it offers them a place to be accepted. Even though it may be psychologically damaging, they are compelled by the thought of being part of a group. Others may feel obliged to join to be able to get revenge on the people who had traumatized them and/or their families (Lonegan, 2011). Some children have joined rebel groups because they felt there was no other place for them in society due to their limited education and resources

(Lonegan, 2011). Former child soldiers have a very difficult time reintegrating into society and being accepted after having committed various atrocities, such as murder and rape (Woodward & Galvin, 2009).

A former child soldier's psychological stressors create extreme difficulty when trying to reintegrate into society (Woodward & Galvin, 2009). Different forms of trauma can have various degrees of long-term psychological impact (Betancourt, Brennan, Rubin-Smith, Fitzmaurice, & Gilman, 2010). Often times, child soldiers have been isolated from everyone they know (Lonegan, 2011). Not being able to trust anyone from such a young age can create tremendous difficulties in maintaining relationships with others. Child soldiers have been deprived of their rights as children, have little or no social support, and have been denied access to services crucial for their growth and development. In addition, they have to live with being perpetrators of violence that may have been committed against their own communities (Drury & Williams, 2012).

Many children have also been beaten until the point where they feel no emotion and are forced to believe everyone else is an enemy (Lonegan, 2011). Armed groups use these tactics as an attempt to create a strong soldier that will follow orders without questioning. It can take a lifetime of intensive therapy to help people experiencing an emotional numbness due to such violent traumatic experiences, to begin to work through their feelings. Experiencing symptoms of PTSD, they may experience nightmares and flashbacks and become hypervigilant, resentful, angry, and possibly psychotic (American Psychiatric Association, 2013). Drug abuse and addiction are common in former child soldiers since many were given drugs by rebel soldiers for initiation and coercion in an attempt to decrease fear and "make them braver" (Woodward & Galvin, 2009, p. 1009).

Gang Exclusion

Child soldiers are not the only children who run into problems with the language of the law; others with ties to gang activity encounter challenges. Families of gang members, people targeted for recruitment, and others indirectly associated with gang activity are often denied asylum under the provision that they are not a socially visible group (Wilkinson, 2010). Wilkinson and others have argued the importance of recognizing the persecutor's view of the targeted asylee's social group, not society. While the general public may see gang activities as nothing more than violence and drug activity, bystanders are often targeted based on their appearance, race, and possibility for ransom (Beittel, 2011). Youth along Mexico's border are especially sought after by gang members for recruitment in gang and drug activity (Beittel, 2011). Car bombings, kidnappings, assassinations, torture, human smuggling, and drug trafficking, among many other crimes, are becoming increasingly more common along the U.S. and Mexico border (Beittel, 2011). Children and other innocent people are becoming caught up in the activity of their neighborhoods, yet they are denied asylum for either not being a socially recognizable group or because of their knowledge of gang activity. Under humanitarian goals, these youth should be protected for their right to deny participation and live their life free from violent criminal activities (Wilkinson, 2010).

Lesbian, Gay, Bisexual, and Transgender

Literature investigating and addressing the needs of lesbian, gay, bisexual, and transgender (LGBT) detainees and asylum seekers is scarce. Most of the literature under review includes a paragraph, at most, about the needs and problems this population encounters. Historically, people who are LGBT have been denied asylum for various reasons, but recent changes in laws have helped more people to be granted asylum (Heller, 2009). Credibility on the basis of sexuality or gender can be difficult to prove since opinions about what is considered a social group can range from one person to the next (Heller, 2009). People who are LGBT have been denied asylum for not exhibiting what an officer or judge feels is LGBT behavior (Heller, 2009). However, many individuals come from places where gays or lesbians are not tolerated and such behaviors could lead to rape, torture, and murder from law enforcement and the general public (Grungras, Levitan, & Slotek, 2009; Heller, 2009). Asylum seekers may then have learned how to disguise their behaviors and feelings in order to remain safe (Heller, 2009). Proving oneself to be LGBT is a ridiculous task because there are no behaviors that are universally determinable.

Transgender detainees are routinely harassed by other detainees and officers (Human Rights Watch, 2010b). Safety often means being locked up in solitary confinement because no other suitable housing has been made available (Human Rights Watch, 2010b). Segregating LGBT individuals into solitary confinement only adds to feelings of rejection and wrongdoing since they are being locked up for the same reasons they are seeking help. LGBT individuals seeking asylum often have experienced significant traumas and have few resources available to help them (Heller, 2009).

MENTAL HEALTH AND RESETTLEMENT

While laws and court processes have an impact on asylum seekers' and detainees' mental health, the opposite is also true. Some people with mental illness may not know where they are, why they are in detention, what deportation is, or even their place of birth (Human Rights Watch, 2010a). It is difficult to accurately assess credible fear if a person is also experiencing symptoms of psychosis. Not only is it hard for a judge to decipher between a detainee's psychotic symptoms and reality, it is also extremely difficult for the detainee. Detainees may have trouble maintaining consistency of their claims due to their mental illness (Human Rights Watch, 2010a).

Some detainees have made mistakes by telling officers and judges their concerns in ways that are actually against their interest and then are unable to mitigate their responses (Human Rights Watch, 2010a). For example, Mamawa, a Liberian refugee who presented to an immigration officer after being beaten by her roommate, asked to be deported (Human Rights Watch, 2010a). ICE proceeded to take her into custody and sent her to a psychiatric hospital for 6 weeks, after which she was placed in a detention center for over 4 months. The stress of detention has caused other mentally ill detainees to voluntarily be deported because they were unable to think beyond the immediate situation to the problems they would face after deportation (Human Rights Watch, 2010a).

Mental illness is likely underreported in detainee populations. Courts may not recognize detainees as mentally ill and are unable to gauge their level of competency, while detainees may not understand they have a mental illness (Human Rights Watch, 2010a). Other reasons, such as stigma or fear of repercussions, prevent detainees from coming forward about mental health problems (Human Rights Watch, 2010a). Some are afraid to disclose, in fear that they will be deported, that their kids will be taken away, or that they will be placed in segregation (Human Rights Watch, 2010a). Even with a diagnosed mental illness, detainees' records from jails, prisons, and medical facilities usually contain little to no information regarding their mental health (USDHS, 2011b). ICE attorneys feel they are ethically required to report any potential or diagnosed mental illness that could hamper their mental competency; however, there is no process in which to file a report (USDHS, 2011b). These problems make it hard for attorneys to create a case or to know about their client's mental illness prior to court. Attorneys then have to rely on their short visits with detainees in detention centers (when possible), conversations with staff, limited records, and their actions in court to formulate their own opinion as to whether their client has a mental illness (USDHS, 2011b).

While attorneys may be able to help in a client's diagnosis, only 16% of detained noncitizens had a lawyer in 2006–2007 (Human Rights Watch, 2010a). Although criminals in the United States have the right to an attorney, noncitizens have the privilege of counsel and a "reasonable opportunity" to present their case (Human Rights Watch, 2010a; Ochoa, Pleasants, Penn, & Stone, 2010). What is considered to be reasonable is up for debate. Lawyers often report problems communicating with clients (through mail and in-person visits), they are not notified when clients are transferred, and transfers often occur to distances well outside of their limits (Schriro, 2009). U.S. immigration has also stated it stands behind its position to deport mentally incompetent individuals unrepresented by counsel (Ochoa et al., 2010). Since there are no standard guidelines relating to competency, mental illness has interfered with deportations of U.S. citizens when courts misinterpret or do not understand the defendant (Packer & Immigration Policy Center, 2010).

According to the USDHS (2011b), in the event that a client is unable to, or refuses to, attend his or her trial, a custodian can take the client's place. There is little guidance surrounding the use of a custodian, and when a family or friend is unavailable, correctional staff members are often used. If correctional staff recommends the detainee be deported, the attorney is then left to defend the case with whatever documentation is present (Packer & Immigration Policy Center, 2010). Courts are frequently overwhelmed with cases and cannot spend adequate time consulting with detainees. Detainees with mental illness may not understand their legal rights or be able to understand the implications of their statements.

Identification of Medical and Mental Health Problems

Medical staff, credentialing, and services vary considerably from one location to another, and there is no collaboration between sites (Schriro, 2009). Medical screening is conducted once detainees have been assigned to a facility; however, those with specific needs (including physical and mental illness) might not be sent to an appropriate facility for their needs (Schriro, 2009). Medical classification (if listed) is marked as "healthy" or "unhealthy" and mental health classification does not exist (Schriro, 2009, p. 25). Detainees' records do not accompany them when transferring; instead, a medical summary is supposed to suffice, yet rarely does that happen (Schriro, 2009). There is no policy with regard to the maintenance of medical records, and a new record is required every time a detainee enters a different facility (Schriro, 2009).

Mental Health and Detention Centers

Detention has now become almost as fearful as deportation because it denies individuals' freedom and access to employment and schooling, and limits their ability to maintain ties with friends and family (Kalhan, 2010). The overwhelming majority of individuals are placed in facilities originally built as prisons and jails with various designs and supervision capabilities (Schriro, 2009). Approximately 50% of detainees (including asylum seekers) are housed in facilities with county prisoners and inmates (Schriro, 2009). When processing, individuals are classified into one of three categories based on their previous history: noncriminal, nonviolent criminal, or violent criminal (Schriro, 2009). Although immigrants are classified based on their history, little is done to separate noncriminals and violent criminals in housing placements (Schriro, 2009). This configuration creates a prison-like environment for detainees to feel like they are criminals even though they are not.

The jail/prison-like structure houses a number of individuals in cells together for the majority of the day and many do not have windows (Schriro, 2009). Other problems include overcrowding, little/no programming, improper ventilation, poor quality of food, unsanitary residences, malfunctioning showers and toilets, as well as verbal and physical abuse from staff and other detainees/inmates (Human Rights First, 2011; Kalhan, 2010; Schriro, 2009). In many detention facilities there is a lack of variation in religious services provided, religious diets and objects are not made available, and religious attire and various hair lengths are not always permitted (Schriro, 2009). Forcing detainees to succumb to these policies takes away any last culture and comfort they may have brought with them.

Asylum seekers have also reported negative experiences with staff and the asylum process. Officers frequently question detainees in a confrontational manner about their history, including traumas (Cleveland, Rousseau, & Kronick, 2012). Detainees have described difficulties accessing interpreters; when they are unavailable, other detainees are used (Schriro, 2009). They have reported difficulty obtaining primary care services, confusion surrounding the asylum process, extended wait times for appointments, frequent riots or abuse between inmates, and discrimination (Bernardes et al., 2010; Robjant et al., 2009). These and other problems have led inmates to feel an overwhelming sense of injustice and hopelessness (Robjant et al., 2009). Being locked up without having committed a crime has caused detainees to feel angry, frustrated, and out of control, and because they have to depend on others, they could not plan to move on without knowing their asylum status (Bernardes et al., 2010).

While most immigrants are housed in one of the over 300 detention centers, some are sent to one of the three Alternatives to Detention (ATD) programs operated by ICE (Schriro, 2009). Designation to one of the programs is based primarily upon an individual's location rather than his or her perceived threat or lack thereof. ATD is available to people within a 50- to 85-mile radius of an ICE field office and/or when funding is sufficient (Schriro, 2009). The ATD programs are split into three different levels based on the type of security. The most restrictive program, the Intensive Supervision Appearance Program, requires reporting over the telephone, radio frequency tracking devices, curfews that are routinely monitored, spontaneous home visits, and employment verification (Schriro, 2009). The next level down, the Enhanced Supervision Reporting, requires the same as the above except it eliminates curfews and employment verification (Schriro, 2009). The least restrictive program, Electronic Monitoring, uses telephone communications and radio frequency tracking devices (Schriro, 2009).

The ICE Health Service Corps (IHSC) is responsible for overseeing the medical and mental health care of detainees in centers staffed by IHSC as well as monitoring the finances of emergency and specialty services (USDHS, 2011b). IHSC staff is present in only 18 of roughly 250 detention centers across the United States, resulting in discrepancies in oversight between those staffed by IHSC and facilities without IHSC-specific staff (USDHS, 2011b). Those lacking IHSC staff do not collaborate with ICE to maintain mental health statistics, keep records up to date regarding the mental health status and treatment of detainees, or maintain an awareness of types of care they can provide (USDHS, 2011b). Significant illness reports are supposed to summarize critical cases of mental illness, but the accuracy of these reports is limited by field personnel's ability to identify relevant cases (USDHS, 2011b). ICE protocol states that a treatment plan will be made for detainees needing mental health care, but treatment is not well defined and is limited by the available services (Human Rights Watch, 2009). Nonemergent treatments are often not covered, and therapy must be approved by a medical director (Human Rights Watch, 2009). These issues prevent IHSC from providing detainees with the most appropriate, efficient, and cost-effective care, especially since noncritical care is not reported. It hinders their ability to know about any critical changes made in the diagnosis and/or treatment of a detainee. The lack of record keeping inhibits IHSC from obtaining accurate data regarding the prevalence and severity of mental illness, disabling them from knowing how to distribute resources. It also does not allow them to monitor the effectiveness of the care provided at facilities without IHSC staff.

The extent of understaffing in mental health providers is also concerning. Staffing was at 50% or less of its capacity in 11 out of the 18 IHSC staffed detention centers (USDHS, 2011b). The lack of proper staffing can create huge problems for detainees that need access to psychiatric care since IHSC has to approve all services from outside providers. IHSC field staff not only needs to submit treatment authorization requests before obtaining services, but all nonemergent requests also need to be reviewed and approved by headquarters (USDHS, 2011b). Lack of staffing has also affected other staff members in the facility. Improperly treated detainees with mental illness can become anxious and aggressive, increasing the potential for safety concerns among all detainees and staff (USDHS, 2011b). As a result, other staff members may be called on to perform duties that are outside of their scope of practice (i.e., medical providers prescribing psychotropic medications they are unfamiliar with), increasing the potential for mistakes as well as fatigue and burnout (USDHS, 2011b).

The report by the USDHS (2011b) revealed staffing at facilities is not adequate to meet the needs of the demand. While 11 detention centers were allotted one psychiatrist, psychologist, and social worker, seven were not. Three facilities were allotted only one social worker despite having up to 76 mentally ill detainees. This inadequacy is concerning considering the extensive time and involvement required in working with detained populations (USDHS, 2011b). Care between providers and detention centers can also vary considerably, and some have treated detainees as if their symptoms were behavior related (Packer & Immigration Policy Center, 2010). Lack of continuity in care can confuse providers and staff members and fails to inform them of potential risks. Receiving inconsistent care can have huge implications for mentally ill detainees if they are being treated for multiple illnesses or the wrong illnesses. It can also prevent detainees from receiving appropriate care if they are not given an adequate length of time for a trial of treatments or medications.

Many ICE detention facilities lack proper housing for detainees with mental health concerns (USDHS, 2011b). Short-stay units are one type of area used to segregate severely mentally ill detainees needing individualized care from the rest of the population. A report released by the USDHS and the Office of Inspector General (2011b) found four out of eight facilities inspected did not have any short-stay units, yet they were treating between 46 and 226 detainees with various mental illnesses. Most of the units that were provided housed anywhere from two to 10 beds. Three facilities had single-cell rooms, but they were most often used to house detainees with tuberculosis. One facility was limited to one of its three rooms, because the other two were used for a medical laboratory and storage. Four facilities did not have single-cell rooms or places to use to monitor patients on suicide watch. Despite receiving recommendations to discontinue using segregation/special management units that are designed to be used as a disciplinary measure or protective custody, many facilities used them for mentally ill detainees. Even facilities with short-stay units continued to use segregation cells for this purpose (USDHS, 2011b).

The report also found a number of detention centers are located in areas where it is difficult to obtain mental health services outside the facility. Detention centers are required to provide treatment for mental illness either in the facility itself or from the community if the facility cannot provide the necessary treatment, such as hospitalization. Four of the eight facilities visited by the USDHS were located 40 to 60 miles from the nearest hospital, where an emergency room was their only option. Even more concerning is that these facilities had no short-stay units and used segregation for psychiatric detainees. Upon discussion with officials at detention centers, the USDHS found community hospitals routinely declined to see detainees, would immediately send detainees back to the facility, and "voiced concerns about detainees appearing in the waiting area in shackles and prison uniforms scaring or intimidating other patients" (USDHS, 2011b, p. 17).

Detainees are usually held for 30 days, but it is not uncommon for cases to be extended anywhere from months to years, especially for those who are seeking asylum (Kalhan, 2010; Schriro, 2009). Interestingly, it is not an individual's criminal history that extends their case, but it is most often due to proceedings for relief statuses such as asylum. Others have been left in detention for extended periods of time after a decision for deportation due to lack of travel documents, poor relations between the United States, and the other country, and/or failure of their native country to accept them for any number of reasons (Human Rights Watch, 2010a). In such cases, a detainee's efforts to cooperate with removal proceedings (pursuing travel documents) can help them to be released after 180 days (Human Rights Watch, 2010a). However, people with mental illness may be unable to understand the documentation needed, especially if they cannot afford an attorney, and end up in a detention center for years.

The longer a detainee spends in a detention center, the more likely he or she is to have a poorer mental health outcome (Robjant et al., 2009). After release they commonly experience nightmares and intrusive thoughts of past traumatic experiences including time served in detention (Cleveland et al., 2012). Even 3 years after being released, asylum seekers who had spent longer times in detention showed poorer mental health outcomes compared with those with lesser periods of detention (Robjant et al., 2009). The process of waiting for asylum status also has significant effects on individuals who are not detained. One study found a higher incidence of depression and anxiety when waiting more than 2 years (43.7% and 30.5%, respectively) as opposed to 6 months (25.2% and 14%, respectively; Ryan, Kelly, & Kelly, 2009).

Mental Illnesses

Asylum seekers and refugees have been found to have more extensive mental health histories than the general population (Heeren et al., 2014; Robjant et al., 2009; Vostanis, 2014). The majority of studies assessing the mental health of detained populations have found depression, PTSD, and anxiety to be the most prevalent mental illnesses. Piwowarczyk (2007) studied diagnoses of asylum seekers at intake using the *Diagnostic and Statistical Manual of Mental Disorders-IV (DSM-IV) (2000)* criteria. The study revealed 96% had been diagnosed with depression and 82% with PTSD. Bernardes et al. (2010) similarly reported 76% of asylum seekers had been diagnosed with PTSD.

There is no doubt that traumas experienced before arriving at a detention center contribute to the prevalence of mental illness. However, Robjant et al. (2009) analyzed 49 studies examining the mental health of current and past detained asylum seekers in Australia, the United Kingdom, and the United States. All of the studies they assessed found marked levels of emotional distress, PTSD, depression, and anxiety in the detained populations compared to the released. Toar, O'Brien, & Fahey (2009) found the most common stressors in a group of asylum seekers was length of time involved in asylum procedure, language barriers, and not knowing their residency status. The study also examined the impact of stressors before and after migrating and concluded that postmigration stressors had the greatest impact in increasing the risk for PTSD, anxiety, and depression. A study by Cleveland et al. (2012) revealed after 18 days in a detention center roughly three quarters of the asylum seekers met clinical criteria for depression, two thirds for anxiety, and a third for PTSD. Detained immigrants tend to experience higher anxiety, depression, and substance abuse disorders as a result of acculturative stress (Levers & Hyatt-Burkart, 2011). Higher levels of psychosis have also been reported in detained populations; however, psychosis tends to be less prevalent than depression, anxiety, and PTSD (Robjant et al., 2009).

These studies show the need for change and how the mental health of detainees needs to be addressed. The legal and detainment processes make for an extremely stressful and frustrating environment that can have a significant effect on a person's mental health. In detention, detainees face humiliation and lose control over their lives and the hope for a better life. In detainees overall, suicidal ideation has been widely reported (Robjant et al., 2009). Bernardes et al. (2010) found three out of 29 participants had tried to commit suicide because they did not feel they had a purpose. Detainees' lives are being impacted tremendously by the way they are treated in the United States, and it is affecting their mental health not only while in detention but for the rest of their lives.

Fear of Repatriation

The most pronounced fear contributing to a great deal of mental distress in detainees is the possibility of repatriation. Bernardes et al. (2010) found participants had the most stress surrounding the fear of being sent back to their native country, to the point where they had physical symptoms strong enough to impact daily living. The United States has been becoming increasingly discriminatory and oppressive over the years, as evidenced by the passing of Arizona Senate Bill 1070 (Levers & Hyatt-Burkart, 2011). Deportation is much more common and authorities have been pressured to uphold immigration policies to the fullest extent (Levers & Hyatt-Burkart, 2011). These policies have instilled fear in individuals, preventing them from seeking help from social, mental, and medical health care services (Levers & Hyatt-Burkart, 2011). As immigration laws force authorities to tighten border security and detain more individuals, the fear of repatriation grows. "In the absence of reform we're left with essentially enforcement on steroids, but that's all we're left with. That is our immigration policy" (Young, 2011). Throughout the United States, immigrants that have not committed crimes (beyond entering the United States.) are being sent to detention and deported more often than criminals for laws designed to target criminal offenders (Hagan, Rodriguez, & Castro, 2011; Young, 2011).

The federal government does not routinely oversee how local law enforcement carries out its policies, leaving the potential for racial profiling (Hagan et al., 2011; Young, 2011). Police in some states, such as North Carolina, frequently set up roadblocks in places they suspect immigrants frequent (Hagan et al., 2011). They check driver's licenses, and since immigrants cannot get a driver's license without a Social Security number, they are found to be criminals and sent to jail. When ICE is informed, the immigrant is soon deported. Instances such as these have ruined the trust law enforcement once had with immigrant communities (Hagan et al., 2011; Young, 2011). Police can no longer gain information from immigrants about crimes because they are afraid to talk in fear of being deported. The threat of deportation has impacted communities by scaring immigrant populations to remain indoors. They have become less likely to be seen in schools, churches, and other public settings (Hagan et al., 2011; Young 2011).

The fear of repatriation is growing, especially for the United States' most prevalent immigrant population—Mexicans. Deported Mexicans are most often released to bus stops at the northern border of Mexico, where some people are hundreds to thousands of miles away from where they had been prior to detention (Goldberg et al., 2011; Packer & Immigration Policy Center, 2010). Repatriation has caused families to separate and has resulted in psychological and emotional stress on children (Hagan et al., 2011; Young, 2011). A quick Google search of a border city such as Ciudad Juarez, Nogales, or Nuevo Laredo, and one can understand why so many people are afraid to return to Mexico.

Few studies have accurately assessed how detainees are deported to Mexico; however, the media has been showing an increased interest. One CNN correspondent, Thelma Gutierrez, investigated how detainees are taken back to Nogales, Mexico, which lies on Arizona's border. She found many deportations occurred at night, after 11 p.m., and included men, women, and children. Deportees in the video reported being scared for their lives due to the amount of gang- and drug-related crime and violence in the area. Gutierrez made a point of walking through Nogales at 10 p.m. to demonstrate the vacancy along the streets because residents are afraid to leave their homes after dark. Many of the individuals did not have any identification, money, phones, or connections to anyone in Mexico. Gutierrez encountered a 19-year-old man who had migrated to San Diego at 2 years old. The man had not been to Mexico and had no resources or direction of where to go. She also met a few people who had recently been kidnapped by drug cartels. Even the camera operator was afraid to film too far from the border. Upon contacting the

Mexican Embassy they were told the only exceptions to night deportations were
". . . pregnant women, unaccompanied minors, sick or elderly people." Gutierrez
reports that over the course of 2 nights they never saw any picked up and taken to
shelters as they had been told is what happens (CNN, 2012).

There are many fears along the Mexican side of the border. Tijuana and Ciudad
Juarez have the highest reported drug use in Mexico and dramatic increases in
HIV (Brouwer et al., 2009; Goldberg et al., 2011; Strathdee & Magis-Rodriguez,
2008). Studies have shown that Mexicans who have been deported from the United
States are more likely to engage in injection drug use, use drugs more frequently,
and engage in risky sexual practices (Brouwer et al., 2009; Strathdee & Magis-
Rodriguez, 2008). HIV risk has been shown to be elevated by social isolation, search
for intimacy, deportation, and migration, and Mexico has been damaged by its
effects (Goldberg et al., 2011). Goldberg et al. (2011) believe the amount of deportations from the United States has contributed significantly to mental and physical
health consequences of Mexicans. Many migrants have reported an increase in
drug use after deportation to cope with economic, emotional, and social stressors
(e.g., trauma, family separation, loneliness) as a result of being deported (Ojeda
et al., 2011).

When they return to Mexico, health care is also a problem. While in the United
States, many immigrants' health declines as they acculturate, and differences in
food, lifestyle, and occupation can cause changes to their health (Davies et al.,
2011; Gonzalez-Block & de la Sierra-de la Vega, 2011). Deported individuals
often do not get appropriate medical and mental health services in detention
centers and then get sent to their home country where there is no assistance as to
where to go (Davies et al., 2011). Some may have been affected with infections or
diseases, such as Lyme disease, that are unfamiliar in Mexico and as a result have
difficulty finding treatment (Davies et al., 2011). Health care services are limited in Mexico and many immigrants do not have money to pay for the services
(Davies et al., 2011).

CONCLUSION

An incredible story of human suffering is revealed by the record numbers of
people forced to flee their homes and countries and confirms a disturbing world
problem: Millions of people all over the world live in extreme fear for their lives
and continue to be forcibly displaced from their homes by world violence and
economic conditions. The often traumatic reasons for leaving their home country,
as well as the potentially long and perilous journey and process of resettlement,
increase the risk for refugees to suffer from a variety of mental health problems.
The sheer numbers of individuals alone, the complex and varied contexts, their
diverse languages, scattered refugee locations, and the relative lack of evidence-
based interventions for their mental health problems have made it difficult to even
address the problem with any consistency or standard.

Among the mental health diagnoses associated with refugee populations
are PTSD, major depression, generalized anxiety, panic disorders, adjustment

disorders, and somatization. The incidence and severity varies accordingly with specific groups within this population and their experiences. The number of traumas, the long and delayed asylum application process, detention, and the loss of culture and support systems exacerbate and further complicate their mental health problems.

Refugees represent all ages of life's spectrum, and each stage poses different vulnerabilities. Children and adolescents are especially vulnerable and may become separated and unaccompanied and, therefore, at the mercy of others for care and protection—care and protection that may not come quickly or easily, or at all. Instead of care and protection, these orphans may be further traumatized and violated at the hands of those into whose care they entrust themselves.

We are faced with many challenges in the detection and effective treatment of mental health problems in refugees. Language and cultural barriers and biases, on both sides of the refugee/provider dyad, can hinder identification of problems and the development of a safe and therapeutic relationship. Further, there is little evidence of the efficacy of interventions and treatments. Although the need is great, much work is necessary to develop culturally competent means of screening and then implementing evidence-based interventions for the debilitating diagnoses and the suffering that affects these marginalized populations.

REFERENCES

Alayarian, A. (2009). Children, torture and psychological consequences. *Torture, 19*(2), 145–156. Retrieved from http://www.ncbi.nlm.nih.gov/pubmed/19920332

American Psychiatric Association. (2000). *Diagnostic and statistical manual of mental disorders* (4th ed., text revision). Washington, DC: Author.

American Psychiatric Association. (2013). *Diagnostic and statistical manual of mental disorders* (5th ed.). Washington, DC: Author.

Beckerman, N. L., & Corbett, L. (2008). Immigration and families: Treating acculturative stress from a systematic framework. *Family Therapy, 35*(2), 63–81. Retrieved from http://www.apa.org/pubs/ databases/psycinfo/index.aspx

Beittel, J. S. (2011). Mexico's drug trafficking organizations: Source and scope of the rising violence. *Congressional Research Service.* Retrieved from http://fpc.state.gov/documents/organization/155587.pdf

Bernardes, D., Wright, J., Edwards, C., Tomkins, H., Dlfoz, D., & Livingstone, A. G. (2010). Asylum seekers' perspectives on their mental health and view on health and social services: Contributions for service provision using a mixed-methods approach. *International Journal of Migration, Health and Social Care, 6*(4), 3–20. doi:10.5042/ijmhsc.2011.0150

Betancourt, T. S., Brennan, R. T., Rubin-Smith, J., Fitzmaurice, G. M., & Gilman, S. E. (2010). Sierra Leone's former child soldiers: A longitudinal study of risk, protective factors, and mental health. *Journal of the American Academy of Child & Adolescent Psychiatry, 49*(6), 606–615. doi:10.1016/j.jaac.2010.03.008

Brouwer, K. C., Lozada, R., Cornelius, W. A., Firestone Cruz, M., Magis-Rodriguez, C., Zuniga de Nuncio, M. L., & Strathdee, S. A. (2009). Deportation along the US-Mexico border: Its relation to drug use patterns and accessing care. *Journal of Immigrant and Minority Health, 11*(1), 1–10. doi:10.1007/s10903-008-9119-5

Center for Public Policy Priorities. (2008). *A child alone and without papers: A report on return and repatriation of unaccompanied undocumented children by the United States.* Retrieved from http://forabettertexas.org/images/A_Child_Alone_and_Without_Papers.pdf

Chantler, K. (2012). Gender, asylum seekers and mental distress: Challenges for mental health social work. *British Journal of Social Work, 42*(2), 318–334. doi:10.1093/bjsw/bcr062

Cleveland, J., Rousseau, C., & Kronick, R. (2012). Bill C-4: *The impact of detention and temporary status on asylum seekers' mental health.* Retrieved from http://oppenheimer.mcgill.ca/IMG/pdf/Impact_of_Bill_C4_on_asylum_seeker_mental_health_full-2.pdf

CNN. (Producer). (2012). *Detainees fear deportation to Mexico* [Online news broadcast]. Atlanta, GA: Turner Broadcasting System. Retrieved from http://www.cnn.com/video/#/video/us/2012/03/30/deportations-after-dark.cnn

CNN. (Producer). (2014). *Obama vows urgent action as children make perilous illegal journey into US.* Atlanta, GA: Turner Broadcasting System. Retrieved from http://www.cnn.com/2014/06/09/us/undocumented-children-immigrants

Davies, A. A., Borland, R. M., Blake, C., & West, H. E. (2011). The dynamics of health and return migration. *PLoS Medicine, 8*(6), 1–4. doi:10.1371/journal.pmed.1001046

Drury, J., & Williams, R. (2012). Children and young people who are refugees, internally displaced persons or survivors or perpetrators of war, mass violence and terrorism. *Current Opinion in Psychiatry, 25*(4), 284. doi:10.1097/YCO.0b013e328353eea6

Goldberg, S. M., Strathdee, S. A., Gallardo, M., Rhodes, T., Wagner, K. D., & Patterson, T. L. (2011). "Over here, it's just drugs, women and all the madness": The HIV risk environment of clients of female sex workers in Tijuana, Mexico. *Social Science & Medicine, 72*, 1185–1192. doi:10.1016/j.socscimed.2011.02.014

Gonzalez-Block, M. A., & de la Sierra-de la Vega, L. A. (2011). Hospital utilization by Mexican migrants returning to Mexico due to health needs. *BioMedCentral Public Health, 11*(241), 1–8. doi:10.1186/1471-2458-11-241

Grover, S. (2008). "Child soldiers" as "Non-combatants": The inapplicability of the refugee convention exclusion clause. *The International Journal of Human Rights, 12*(1), 53–65. doi:10.1080/1364290701725210

Grungras, N., Levitan, R., & Slotek, A. (2009). Unsafe haven: Security challenges facing LGBT asylum seekers and refugees in Turkey. *PRAXIS: The Fletcher Journal of Human Security, 24*, 41–61. Retrieved from http://fletcher.tufts.edu/Praxis/Archives/~/media/Fletcher/Microsites/praxis/xxiv/PRAXISXXIV_4Grungas.pdf

Hagan, J. M., Rodriguez, N., & Castro. B. (2011). Social effects of mass deportations by the United States government, 2000–10. *Ethnic and Racial Studies, 34*(8), 1374–1391. doi:10.1080/01419870.2011.575233

Heeren, M., Wittmann, L., Ehlert, U., Schnyder, U., Maier, T., & Muller, J. (2014). Psychopathology and resident status—comparing asylum seekers, refugees, illegal migrants, labor migrants, and residents. *Comparative Psychiatry, 55*(4), 818–825. doi:10.1016.j

Heller, P. (2009). Challenges facing LGBT asylum-seekers: The role of social work in correcting oppressive immigration processes. *Journal of Gay & Lesbian Social Services, 21*, 294–308. doi:10.1080/10538720902772246

Hodes, M. (2010). The mental health of detained asylum seeking children. *European Child & Adolescent Psychiatry, 19*, 621–623. doi:10.1007/s00787-010-0093-9

Huemer, J., Karnik, N. S., Voelkl-Kernstock, S., Granditsch, E., Dervic, K., Friedrich, M. H., & Steiner, H. (2009). Mental health issues in unaccompanied refugee minors. *Child and Adolescent Psychiatry and Mental Health, 3*(1), 13. doi:10.1186/1753-2000-3-13

Human Rights First. (2011). *Jails and jumpsuits: Transforming the US immigration detention system—a two year review.* Retrieved from http://www.humanrightsfirst.org/wp-content/uploads/pdf/HRF-Jails-and-Jumpsuits-report.pdf

Human Rights Watch. (2009). *Detained and dismissed: Women's struggles to obtain health care in United States immigration detention.* Retrieved from http://www.hrw.org/sites/default/files/reports/wrd0309webwcover_1.pdf

Human Rights Watch, American Civil Liberties Union. (2010a). *Deportation by default: Mental disability, unfair hearings, and indefinite detention in the US immigration system.* Retrieved from http://www.aclu.org/files/assets/usdeportation0710_0.pdf

Human Rights Watch. (2010b). *Detained and at risk: Sexual abuse and harassment in the United States immigration detention.* Retrieved from http://www.hrw.org/sites/default/files/reports/us0810webwcover.pdf

Immigration and Nationality Act, 208 U.S.C. §1158 (1952).

Jan, M. N. (2011). The criteria for determination of refugee status in international law: A critical appraisal. *Journal of Applied Sciences Research, 7*(13), 2292–2304. Retrieved from http://irep.iium.edu.my/16225

Johnsson, E., Zolkowska, K., & McNeil, T. (2014). Prediction of adaptation difficulties by country of origin, cumulate psychosocial stressors, and attitude to integrating: A Swedish study of first-generation immigrants from Somalia, Vietnam, and China. *International Journal of Social Psychiatry,* 1–9. doi:10.1177/002076401437639

Kalhan, A. (2010). Rethinking immigration detention. *Columbia Law Review Sidebar, 110,* 42–58. Retrieved from http://www.columbialawreview.org/sidebar/volume/110/42_Anil_Kalhan.pdf

Levers, L. L., & Hyatt-Burkart, D. (2011). Immigration reform and the potential for psychosocial trauma: The missing link of lived human experience. *Analyses of Social Issues and Public Policy, 00,* 1–10. doi:10.1111/j.1530-2415.2011.01254.x

Lonegan, B. (2011). Sinners or saints: Child soldiers and the persecutor bar to asylum after Neguise v. Holder. *Boston College Third World Law Journal, 31*(1), 71–99. Retrieved from http://lawdigitalcommons.bc.edu/cgi/viewcontent.cgi?article=1003&context=twlj

Lustig, S. L., Kia-Keating, M., Knight, W. G., Geltman, P., Ellis, H., Kinzie, J. D., ... Saxe, G. N. (2004). Review of child and adolescent refugee mental health. *Journal of the American Academy of Child and Adolescent Psychiatry, 43*(1), 24–36.

Medical Foundation for the Care of Victims of Torture. (2009). *Justice denied: The experiences of 100 torture surviving women of seeking justice and rehabilitation.* Retrieved from http://www.freedomfromtorture.org/sites/default/files/documents/Justice_Denied.pdf

Newman, L. K., & Steel, Z. (2008). The child asylum seeker: Psychological and developmental impact of immigration detention. *Child and Adolescent Psychiatrics of North America, 17*(3), 665–683.

Ochoa, K. C., Pleasants, G. L., Penn, J. V., & Stone, D. C. (2010). Disparities in justice and care: Persons with severe mental illnesses in the U.S. immigration detention system. *The Journal of the American Academy of Psychiatry and the Law, 38*(3), 392–399. Retrieved from http://jaapl.org/content/38/3/392.full.pdf+html

Ojeda, V. D., Robertson, A. M., Hiller, S. P., Lozada, R., Cornelius, W., Palinkas, L. A., & Strathdee, S. A. (2011). A qualitative view of drug use behaviors of Mexican male injection drug users deported from the United States. *Journal of Urban Health: Bulletin of the New York Academy of Medicine, 88*(1), 104–117. doi:10.1007/s11524-010-9508-7

Packer, T. (2010). *Non-citizens with mental disabilities: The need for better care in detention and in court.* Washington, DC: American Immigration Council. Retrieved from http://76.227.221.63/articles/ 2011,0224-packer.pdf

Piwowarczyk, L. (2007). Asylum seekers seeking mental health services in the United States: Clinical and legal implications. *The Journal of Nervous and Mental Disease, 195*(9), 715–722. doi:10.1097/NMD.0b013e318142ca0b

Prasad, A. N., & Prasad, P. L. (2009). Children in conflict zones. *Medical Journal Armed Forces India, 65*(2), 166–169. doi:10.1016/S0377-1237(09)80134-2

Refugee Act of 1980, Pub. L. 96–212. 94 Stat. 102 (1980).

Robjant, K., Hassan, R., & Katona, C. (2009). Mental health implications of detaining asylum seekers: Systematic review. *British Journal of Psychiatry, 194*, 306–312. doi:10.1192/bjp.bp.108053223

Rottman, A. J., Fariss, C. J., & Poe, S. C. (2009). The path to asylum in the US and the determinants for who gets in and why. *International Migration Review, 43*(1), 3–34. Retrieved from http://papers.ssrn.com/sol3/papers.cfm?abstract_id=1625617

Ryan, D. A., Kelly, F. E., & Kelly, B. D. (2009). Mental health among persons awaiting an asylum outcome in Western countries. *International Journal of Mental Health, 38*(3), 88–111. doi:10.2753/IMH0020-7411380306

Schriro, D., U.S. Department of Homeland Security, Immigration and Customs Enforcement. (2009). *Immigration detention overview and recommendations.* Retrieved from http://www.ice.gov/doclib/about/offices/odpp/pdf/ice-detention-rpt.pdf

Spring, U. O. (2009). Social vulnerability and geopolitical conflicts due to socio-environmental migration in Mexico. *IOP Conference Series: Earth and Environmental Science, 6*(56), 1–2. doi:10.1088/1755-1307/6/56/562005

Strathdee, S. A., & Magis-Rodriguez, C. (2008). Mexico's evolving HIV epidemic. *Journal of the American Medical Association, 300*(5), 571–573. doi:10.1001/jama.300.5.571

Toar, M., O'Brien, K. K., & Fahey, T. (2009). Comparison of self-reported health & healthcare utilization between asylum seekers and refugees: An observational study. *BioMed Central Public Health, 9*(214). doi:10.1186/1471-2458-9-214

United Nations High Commissioner for Refugees, The UN Refugee Agency. (2011a). *Asylum levels and trends in industrialized countries 2010.* Retrieved from http://www.unhcr.org/cgi-bin/texis/vtx/home/opendocPDFViewer.html?docid=4d8c5b109&query=asylum_levels_and_trends

United Nations High Commissioner for Refugees, The UN Refugee Agency. (2011b). *Global trends 2010.* Retrieved from http://www.unhcr.org/4dfa11499.html

United Nations High Commissioner for Refugees, The UN Refugee Agency. (2012a). *Asylum levels and trends in industrialized countries 2011.* Retrieved from http://www.unhcr.org/4e9beaa19.html

United Nations High Commissioner for Refugees, The UN Refugee Agency. (2012b). *UNHCR Global trends 2011.* Retrieved from http://www.unhcr.org/4fd6f87f9.html

United Nations High Commissioner for Refugees, The UN Refugee Agency. (2013a). *UNHCR Global trends 2012.* Retrieved from http://unhcr.org/globaltrendsjune2013/UNHCR%20GLOBAL%20TRENDS%202012_V08_web.pdf

United Nations High Commissioner for Refugees, the UN Refugee Agency. (2013b). *UNHCR Statistical yearbook 2012* (12th ed.). Retrieved from http://www.unhcr.org/52a7213b9.html

U.S. Department of Homeland Security, Office of Inspector General. (2008). *ICE policies related to detained deaths and the oversight of immigration detention facilities* (Report No. OIG-08-52). Retrieved from http://www.oig.dhs.gov/assets/Mgmt/OIG_08-52_Jun08.pdf

U.S. Department of Homeland Security, Office of Immigration Statistics. (2011). *2010 Yearbook of immigration statistics.* Retrieved from http://www.dhs.gov/xlibrary/assets/statistics/yearbook/2010/ois_yb_2010.pdf

U.S. Department of Homeland Security, Office of Immigration Statistics. (2012). *2011 yearbook of immigration statistics.* Retrieved from http://www.dhs.gov/xlibrary/assets/statistics/yearbook/2010/ois_yb_2010.pdf

U.S. Department of Homeland Security, Office of Immigration Statistics. (2013a). *Annual flow report 2012.* Retrieved from http://www.dhs.gov/sites/default/files/publications/ois_rfa_fr_2012.pdf

U.S. Department of Homeland Security, Office of Immigration Statistics. (2013b). *2012 yearbook of immigration statistics.* Retrieved from http://www.dhs.gov/sites/default/files/publications/ois_yb_2012.pdf

U.S. Department of Homeland Security, Office of Inspector General. (2011b). *Management of mental health cases in immigration detention* (Report No. OIG-11-62). Retrieved from http://www.oig.dhs.gov/assets%5CMgmt%5COIG_11-62_Mar11.pdf

U.S. Department of Justice, Office of Justice Programs, Bureau of Justice Statistics. (2008). *Census of state and federal correctional facilities, 2005* (BJS Publication No. NCJ 222182). Retrieved from http://bjs.ojp.usdoj.gov/content/pub/pdf/csfcf05.pdf

U.S. Department of Justice, Executive Office for Immigration Review, Office of Legislative and Public Affairs. (2009). *Asylum and withholding of removal relief convention against torture protections: Relief and protections based on fear of persecution or torture* (fact sheet). Retrieved from http://www.justice.gov/eoir/press/09/AsylumWithholdingCATProtections.pdf

Vostanis, P. (2014). Meeting the mental health needs of refugees and asylum seekers. *British Journal of Psychiatry, 204*(3), 176–177. doi:10.1192/bjp.bp113.134742

Wadee, S. A. (2006). Examination of detainees. *Continuing Medical Education, 24*(2), 68–71. Retrieved from http://www.cmej.org.za/index.php/cmej/article/download/302/187

Wasem, R. E., Congressional Research Service. (2005). *US immigration policy on asylum seekers* (Order code RL32621). CRS Report for Congress, Congressional Research Service, The Library of Congress. Retrieved from www.fas.org/sgp/crs/misc/rl32621.pdf

Wasem, R. E., Congressional Research Service. (2011). *Asylum and "credible fear" issues in US immigration policy* (CRS Report No. 7-5700). Retrieved from http://fpc.state.gov/documents/organization/168099.pdf

Wilkinson, E. (2010). Examining the Board of Immigration Appeals' social visibility requirement for victims of gang violence seeking asylum. *Maine Law Review, 62*(1), 387–419. Retrieved from http://mainelaw.maine.edu/academics/maine-law-review/pdf/Vol62_1/Vol62_me_l_rev_387.pdf

Woodward, L., & Galvin, P. (2009). Halfway to nowhere: Liberian former child soldiers in a Ghanaian refugee camp. *Annals of the Association of American Geographers, 99*(5), 1003–1011. doi:10.1080/00045600903245698

Young, R. (Writer & Director). (2011). Lost in detention [Television series episode]. In D. Fanning (executive producer), *Frontline.* Boston, MA: Public Broadcasting System. Retrieved from http://video.pbs.org/video/2155873891

CHAPTER 17

Childhood Malnutrition in India

Diane E. Hazel, Elissa C. Ladd, and Ansuya Bengre

Childhood malnutrition has repeatedly been identified as one of the largest, if not the largest, contributors to deaths of those younger than age 5 worldwide; nearly half of these deaths occur in the poorest countries of the world, including India. The Indian government, with support from international organizations such as the World Health Organization (WHO), has made impressive strides in reducing the burden of childhood malnutrition and disease. This chapter provides a comprehensive assessment of the current state of malnutrition in children younger than age 5 in India, and will examine WHO and National Family Health Survey (NFHS) trends; contributing factors such as maternal health, environment, and feeding practices; current government initiatives, including immunization, deworming, and nutritional programs; and future directions. Many components of child malnutrition in India fit within the conceptual framework of undernutrition established by the United Nations Children's Fund (UNICEF) in1990.

In addition to a review of the extant literature, our assessment of childhood malnutrition was informed by field-based observations conducted within a 20-km radius of Manipal, India. Observations included visits to local health care centers and hospitals, government-run day care facilities, interviews with mothers and children residing in a small rural village, and interviews with local faculty and experts in childhood malnutrition at Manipal University College of Nursing. Finally, a series of case studies was generated and is presented here to illustrate the current state of child nutrition in a rural village of southern India, providing support for the theory that children in India are in a better state of health than in previous years, and are continuing to improve.

TRENDS, RISK FACTORS, CONSEQUENCES, INTERVENTIONS, AND FUTURE DIRECTIONS

Childhood malnutrition is responsible for more than one third of the total worldwide deaths in children younger than age 5 (Imdad, Sadiq, & Bhutta, 2011). More than half of malnourished children reside in the poorest countries of the world, with the majority located in India, Pakistan, and Bangladesh (Goulet et al., 2006). In India alone, it is estimated that 1 in 11 children die every year before the age of 5 due to malnutrition (Antony & Laxmaiah, 2008). The NFHS, a large national survey conducted in three iterations in 1991, 1999, and 2006, utilized standardized growth curves to estimate percentages of malnutrition. The NFHS conducted a study in 2006 that showed that 47% of children younger than age 5 were underweight, 46% were stunted, indicating a state of chronic maltnutrition, and 17% were wasted, indicating acute malnutrition (Mamidi, Shidhaye, Radhakrishna, Babu, & Reddy, 2011). We explore recent trends in childhood malnutrition based on the hypothesis that the overall health of children, as defined by nutritional status, has greatly improved in recent years.

Significant efforts have been made by private and government researchers to understand the risk factors for developing malnutrition. In 1990, UNICEF established a conceptual framework for understanding these risk factors for undernutrition (see Figure 17.1).

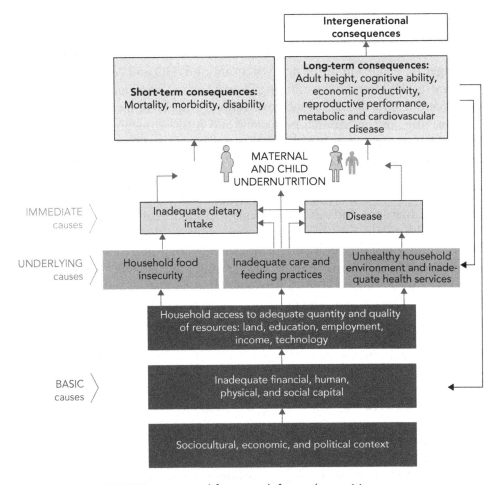

FIGURE 17.1 UNICEF conceptual framework for undernutrition.

These are discussed in the context of India as a developing nation, using UNICEF's framework to highlight the level at which each component predicts overall child health (UNICEF, 2013). Identification of the root causes of malnutrition is essential to the development of targeted, effective interventions.

Background

The term *malnutrition* encompasses both overnutrition and undernutrition. Undernutrition is measured by three parameters: *underweight, wasting,* and *stunting.* Each term is assessed through the use of (WHO) growth standards. Underweight is measured by plotting weight against age. Wasting is measured by plotting weight against height, and stunting is measured by plotting height against age (WHO, 2006). Underweight, wasting, and stunting each represent different levels and causes of malnutrition. Until recently, underweight was regarded as the best indicator of child nutrition. However, in recent years the international community has placed greater emphasis on tracking of stunting as an indicator of chronic nutritional status (UNICEF, 2013).

The consequences of acute and chronic malnutrition have been well documented. It has been widely recognized that childhood stunting is indicative of chronic malnourishment, whereas underweight is indicative of acute malnourishment. Wasting indicates severe acute malnourishment (SAM) (Sachdev, 2012). Stunting and underweight during childhood have been shown to correlate with reduced adult height, impaired cognitive development, reduced IQ, fewer years of completed education, and reduced adult income potential (Ade, Gupta, Maliye, Deshmukh, & Garg, 2010; Ahmed, Michaelsen, Frem, & Tumvine, 2012; Imdad et al., 2011). Several authors have suggested that these negative consequences become irreversible when they persist beyond 24 months of age (Ahmed et al., 2012; Sachdev, 2012). Additionally, children suffering from poor nutrition are more likely to contract respiratory, gastrointestinal, and infectious diseases during childhood (Sarkar et al., 2013).

UNICEF CONCEPTUAL FRAMEWORK

UNICEF established the Conceptual Framework for the Determinants of Child Undernutrition in 1990. The framework is revisited periodically, and small additions have been made, but the basic concepts have remained the same. The framework is based on the notion that undernutrition is predicted at three distinct levels of risk; basic, underlying, and immediate causes. Basic causes of undernutrition include sociocultural, economic, and political factors. The existence of poor governmental organization, widespread poverty, and/or political unrest lead to economic and social disadvantages for lower class populations, making it difficult to fulfill essential needs such as housing, education, land, technology, employment, and income. The presence of inequity at the basic level leads to the next level of risk factors, described as underlying causes, which include household food insecurity, inadequate care and feeding practices, unhealthy living environment, and inadequate access to health care. Underlying risk factors then lead to immediate causes of undernutrition, including inadequate dietary intake of macro- and micronutrients, and the presence of disease. These risk factors directly lead to both short- and long-term health consequences for children (UNICEF, 2013). Our focus is on identification of risk factors at the "underlying" and "immediate" levels of the framework and discussion of interventions at these levels.

WHO AND NFHS TRENDS

The United Nations Development Programme (UNDP) established the Millennium Development Goals (MDGs) in 1990, which were reexamined and expanded upon in the year 2000. Currently there are eight MDGs, each aimed at improving global public health and quality of life. MDG 4 aims to reduce childhood under-5 mortality by 66% between 1990 and 2015. More specifically, the goal aims to reduce under-5 deaths from 93 per 1,000 to 31 per 1,000 by 2015 (UNDP, 2013). As previously stated, malnutrition contributes substantially to global under-5 mortality. As such, it is important to establish and utilize standardized measures for assessing malnutrition and progress.

WHO, in collaboration with the U.S. National Center for Health Statistics (NCHS), established standards for childhood growth and development and routinely recommended them for international use beginning in the 1970s (WHO, 2014a). These growth standards were based on observations of growth and development under optimal conditions in one country. In 1994, the WHO and United Nations (UN) undertook a decade-long investigation into the patterns of growth and development globally. In 2006, new growth standards were released that reflected optimal growth and development for all children, of any age, in any country (Fenn & Penny, 2008; WHO, 2014b).

The government of India utilized the new growth standards in the most recent version of the NFHS in 2006, which collected data on 41,306 children younger than the age of 5. Mamidi et al. (2011) compared data from this survey to that of the first NFHS in 1991 through the use of z scores. They found significant improvements in weight-for-age (WAZ) and height-for-age (HAZ) z scores at every time point, including birth, 6, 12, 24, and 36 months of age. For example, the average HAZ at 36 months of age improved from -2.63 in 1991 to -1.94 in 2006 ($p < 0.001$). WAZ at 36 months improved from -2.08 in 1991 to -1.72 in 2006 ($p < 0.001$). Despite these improvements, the 2006 data still reveal an average z score just above the threshold for malnutrition. The data also reveal that up to 44% and 23% of the total losses in weight and height, respectively, have already occurred at the time of birth. By age 6 months, 71% of WAZ loss and 41% of HAZ loss have occurred. These findings suggest that a larger focus must be placed on interventions during the prenatal and early infancy time periods.

RISK FACTORS FOR MALNUTRITION

Maternal Factors

Data from multiple studies suggest that a large percentage of childhood malnutrition is predicted by care received in utero (Mamidi et al., 2011; Ozaltin, Hill, & Subramanian, 2010). The 2012 report from the Federation of the Societies of Pediatric Gastroenterology, Hepatology, and Nutrition (FISPGHAN) supported these data. They concluded that childhood undernutrition is frequently predicted by maternal undernutrition as measured by maternal stunting and insufficient weight gain during pregnancy (Ahmed et al., 2012). As a result, the FISPGHAN group has prioritized maternal care and education as a central means of preventing childhood undernutrition.

The report states that efforts to promote maternal care must include micronutrient supplementation, antenatal visits with a health care provider including community-based providers, family planning services, and promotion of gender equality. Maternal supplementation and access to health care would fall mainly into the middle tier of underlying causes of child undernutrition; several interventions have been implemented in India at this level. Gender equality as defined by education and access to services has been identified by other authors as an important area for childhood health promotion (Antony & Laxmaiah, 2008; Goulet et al., 2006). Gender issues as predictors for undernutrition fall into the basic tier of the UNICEF framework. An advanced discussion of gender issues is beyond the scope of this chapter but it is important to note that it has been identified by the UNDP as MDG 3 (UNDP, 2013).

Nutrient supplementation is one of the most important methods for promoting healthy fetal development. Zinc, calcium, iron, and folic acid, in particular, are essential for fetal development. Zinc is essential for protein synthesis and cell growth and differentiation. Calcium reduces gestational diabetes and hypertension and promotes healthy bone growth. Iron is essential for maintenance of healthy red blood cells. Folic acid aids in the prevention of neural tube defects (Imdad et al., 2011). As such, the government of India has allocated significant financial support toward providing these essential micronutrients for the full duration of the pregnancy to all women receiving care through public health facilities at no cost to the mother or family. Pregnant women that are identified as underweight or with insufficient weight gain may also be provided with protein supplementation, not to exceed 25% of total caloric intake in addition to micronutrient supplementation (Imdad et al., 2011).

Finally, the Indian government has stressed the importance of regular antenatal care and facility-based deliveries. In 2006, the NFHS 3 reported that up to 20% of pregnant women did not receive any prenatal care, and 25% completed less than or equal to two prenatal visits. Since that time, the government has increased its funding and support for more frequent prenatal appointments. They recommend and provide monthly antenatal check-ups for the first 28 weeks of pregnancy; biweekly check-ups are provided through week 32, and weekly check-ups thereafter until delivery (A. Shetty, personal communication, January 21, 2014).

Many of these health checks are provided by physicians or by trained community health workers including auxiliary nurse midwives (ANMs) and accredited social health workers (ASHWs). At the time of delivery, all pregnant women are encouraged to deliver in medical facilities rather than having home births. To promote hospital births, the government introduced the Janani Suraksha Yojana (JSY) program in 2007, which provides cash incentives for families to deliver in government hospitals. The success rates of the JSY program have been mixed but Dr. Shetty reports that southern India again leads northern India in reducing home birth rates since the inception of the program (Sachdev, 2012).

Environmental Factors

The child's environment is an important risk factor for malnutrition. For the purposes of this analysis, the term "environment" includes sanitation and hygiene; toileting facilities; built environment; and water, air, and soil quality. Similar to maternal factors, this class of risk would be defined as an underlying cause of malnutrition in the UNICEF framework.

India is the second most populous country in the world, with more than 1.2 billion people. As the population has expanded, there has been a rapid shift from rural to urban living, resulting in large populations living in slum conditions where sanitation and hygiene problems yield high rates of infectious disease (Sarkar et al., 2013). Several studies have found associations between poor maternal and child health and several environmental risk factors, including crowding, poor access to clean water, toileting facilities, electricity, stable housing (i.e., rental vs. permanent residency), and housing constructed of weak or hazardous materials (Osrin et al., 2011; Sarkar et al., 2013). These poor health conditions have been found in both rural and urban communities of India. Dr. Troy A. Jacobs (2010) of the Maternal and Child Health Division of the U.S. Agency for International Development (USAID) speaks to the spread of health problems associated with all living environments. He warns that while developed nations such as the United States have paid increasingly more attention to the role of "built environment" in predicting health and development, poorer countries such as India have yet to prioritize this burgeoning field in their public health interventions.

Within poor living environments, both infectious and chronic diseases are prevalent. Respiratory and diarrheal diseases are the most common illnesses found among children living in low-income areas where municipal water is routinely contaminated by human and urban waste. Persistent diarrhea can cause rapid fluid and weight loss, and reduces the body's ability to absorb essential nutrients, thus contributing to high rates of malnutrition (Goulet et al., 2006; Imdad et al., 2011). The FISPGHAN working group has thus recommended that governments in developing countries, such as India, place high importance on maintenance of clean municipal water (Ahmed et al., 2012). Additionally, Indian health workers are working to educate mothers on prevention and management of diarrhea, including hand hygiene, exclusive breastfeeding through age 6 months, boiling water through age 12 months, use of proper toileting facilities, cleaning cooking utensils, and thoroughly cooking foods to kill bacteria (Subba Rao et al., 2007). Agencies such as USAID have undertaken efforts to ensure adherence to the recommended guidelines for diarrhea management, including the use of zinc and oral rehydration tablets (USAID, 2010). Along with USAID, other agencies such as UNICEF and WHO, are also working with private industries to increase access to both affordable medical care and medications.

Another environmental hazard commonly faced by children of low- and some middle-income families is indoor air pollution. As stated earlier, respiratory infections comprise one of the largest categories of childhood disease. In many developing countries, including India, direct links have been found between acute respiratory infections and poor indoor air quality from cooking fuels. In many of the homes visited in the rural village of Malpe, the primary source of cooking fuel was firewood; cleaner biofuels such as kerosene or butane may be unaffordable or impractical for low-income families (Emmelin & Wall, 2007). Furthermore, many of these homes perform all cooking in enclosed kitchen areas. Daily exposure with poor ventilation significantly increases the risk of inhaling toxic chemicals and gases such as carbon monoxide and hydrocarbons (Emmelin & Wall, 2007).

Finally, another environmental risk factor for childhood malnutrition in India is gastrointestinal infestations of soil-borne worms and helminths. Some of the most common worm infestations include hookworm, schistosomiasis, and, in children, *Trichuris trichiura*. It is estimated that nearly 50% of all people living in developing nations are infected with at least one type of soil-transmitted parasite (Humphries, Nguyen, Boakye, Wilson, & Cappello, 2012). Chronic parasitic infestations cause anemia, malabsorption of nutrients, and colitis, and can lead to cognitive delays. All of these outcomes lead to reduced growth and development, especially during early childhood (Humphries et al., 2012). It could be argued that intestinal infections from contaminated water or soil represent both environmental and direct disease risk factors, thereby bridging the second and third levels of the UNICEF framework. Regardless of the level of risk, soil-borne infections are an important area for intervention.

Feeding Practices

UNICEF clearly identifies feeding practices as an underlying cause for malnutrition. Feeding practices in infancy and childhood include both breast and complementary feeding. Cultural and family beliefs, education about safe practices, access to clean water and quality food, and illness history all impact a mother's ability to make healthy choices for her child. Breastfeeding in particular has garnered much attention from national and international public health communities.

The FISPGHAN Working Group has identified exclusive breastfeeding through 6 months of age as an effective and direct method of reducing childhood malnutrition (Ahmed et al., 2012). The health benefits of exclusive breastfeeding have been extensively studied and include increased childhood survival, growth, and development; and reduced risk for both chronic and infectious diseases, including gastrointestinal and respiratory tract infections (Goulet et al., 2006; Imdad et al., 2011; Sachdev, 2012).

Unfortunately, it is believed that many mothers do not follow these recommendations due to cultural and family pressures from older generations. Conversations with Manipal College of Nursing faculty and several women in Malpe village revealed that many mothers introduce complementary foods earlier than 6 months under the belief that their breast milk is not adequate (A. Shetty, personal communication, January 21, 2014; Ansuya, personal communication, January 14, 2014; Lahkshmi, personal communication, January 13, 2014). Other reasons for inappropriate complementary food introduction include maternal employment, commercial advertising, lack of education and support from hospitals and providers, and emotional stress (Imdad et al., 2011).

Complementary foods must be introduced at the right time and with the right balance of nutrients, carbohydrates, fats, and proteins for proper digestion. As previously stated, most experts recommend initiation of simple complementary foods at 6 months of age. Similar to practices in the United States, the Integrated Child Development Services (ICDS) recommends initial feeding with soft cereal called porridge, which may be made with wheat, rice, ragi, or millet mixed with water or milk. Sugar and clarified butter (known as ghee) may be added to increase caloric value. Chapatis, flour-based breads that closely resemble tortillas, may also be introduced as early as 6 months. After successful introduction of grains, ICDS recommends soft fruits such as banana, papaya, mango, or any other fruit that can be mashed for a soft consistency. As infants grow and demonstrate tolerance to an increasing variety of foods, mothers may introduce other traditional Indian foods such as idli, curd, lassi, eggs, fish, and soft vegetables (Mother and Child Health and Education Trust, 2014).

The ICDS and WHO have increased their efforts to educate mothers about exclusively breastfeeding through age 6 months followed by safe and progressive introduction of complementary foods. These efforts have yielded improvements in maternal knowledge and overall child growth. However, there are still many rural areas of India where outreach efforts have much room for improvement (Vazir et al., 2013).

INITIATIVES FOR IMPROVEMENT

ICDS and Anganwadi Centers

The Indian government established the ICDS sector in the 1970s. It is one of the largest national initiatives for maternal and child health in the world

(Kapil & Pradhan, 1999). It currently offers nutritional, educational, and health care support to children ages 6 months through 6 years and their mothers, as well as lactating and pregnant women. One of the most important and innovative steps taken by the ICDS was the conceptualization and implementation of Anganwadi centers (AWCs).

AWCs are government-run day care facilities that can be found in every state of India. Ideally, there is one fully funded AWC for every 1,000 population (Avula, Frongillo, Arabi, Sharma, & Schultink, 2011), yielding an estimated 1.2 million AWCs nationally. These centers offer a package of services for children ages 3 to 5 years. This package addresses risk factors at all three levels of UNICEF-identified risk, making it a remarkably comprehensive government initiative.

Services include informal education such as numbers, colors, shapes, sanitation and hygiene, immunization tracking, basic annual health check-ups, sick referrals, supplementary nutrition, and health education for mothers and pregnant and lactating women (Avula et al., 2011). Free day care is available for full or half days and includes one snack, one hot meal, and warm milk for all participating children. Additionally, pregnant and lactating women, and children identified as malnourished according to the WHO growth standards, are provided with take-home supplementation of milk powder, egg powder, or grains based on specific needs. Each AWC is staffed with one government-trained teacher, as well as one cook to aid in meal preparation (Avula et al., 2011).

In addition to providing standardized services, free of charge, to children and families across India, AWCs have been a rich source of information regarding trends in maternal and child health, nutrition, knowledge, and community perceptions and utilization. A 2011 study examined height, weight, and correlates for undernutrition among Anganwadi children and their siblings in Andhra Pradesh. Results revealed that the prevalence of underweight, stunting, and wasting increases with age; risk for adverse outcomes are higher among children from low-income households and also seemed to be higher among boys (Meshram et al., 2011).

Savitha and Kondapuram (2012) found similar results when they examined children in AWCs in Mysore City. Varma et al. (2007) and Kapil and Jain (2011) have also utilized data from AWCs to assess the prevalence of iron, vitamin A, and zinc deficiencies. Agrawal et al. (2012) utilized AWCs to show that increased knowledge of Anganwadi workers and ability to connect with the surrounding community resulted in increased knowledge of early breastfeeding, postnatal temperature control, and cord care among mothers. Studies such as these provide insight into successful programs and areas for improvement.

Several authors have also utilized data from AWCs to demonstrate opportunities for improvement. Ade et al. (2010) conducted a matched case control trial to examine the impact of improved education for Anganwadi workers through monthly government-run training sessions. The study also included additional funds for toys and learning materials that were developmentally appropriate. Results demonstrated a statistically significant increase in development and IQ among students enrolled in the intervention group compared with standard Anganwadi offerings. A similar study by Avula et al. (2011) looked at the impact of improved nutrition in AWCs rather than improved educational support. Nutritional supplementation included fortification with micronutrient powders, inclusion of more locally grown foods, and more frequent monitoring of height and weight changes among children ages 6 to 30 months. They found that HAZ and WAZ scores and total calorie intake were higher at each assessment point for children in the intervention group.

Davey, Davey, and Datta (2008) examined another aspect of Anganwadi care: utilization and satisfaction. In their Delhi-based study, they found that 52.5% of mothers who were surveyed were dissatisfied with Anganwadi services for one or more reasons. The most commonly cited reasons were lack of accessibility, inadequate classroom space, poor quality food, and subpar education. Finally, a 2007 study enrolled families from AWCs to examine maternal knowledge of food contamination. They found that most mothers felt that home-cooked meals were safer than meals prepared outside the home. They also found that mothers were generally aware of common food contaminants but did not take appropriate measures to prevent gastrointestinal infection. The authors concluded that Anganwadi workers could provide education on safe food practices as part of their services (Subba Rao et al., 2007). These studies provide a few examples of how AWCs can offer excellent opportunities for data collection and analysis. More importantly, they demonstrate important areas for improvement in maternal and child nutrition and education.

Immunizations

Malnutrition is often preceded or compounded by infectious diseases, particularly those of the gastrointestinal or respiratory systems. Illness affects malnutrition by suppressing appetite and thus reducing caloric intake, increasing fluid loss and poor nutrient absorption from diarrhea, and increasing energy expenditure from fever (Anekwe & Kumar, 2012). Immunization against common childhood diseases plays an important role in reducing infection and preventing new onset or worsening of malnutrition.

India's Universal Immunization Program (UIP) operates with the mission of reducing incidence of vaccine-preventable diseases. According to the UNICEF framework, disease prevention reduces child undernutrition at the highest and most individual level of risk. The UIP began as the Expanded Program on Immunization (EPI) in 1978. This program offered immunization against tuberculosis (BCG), polio, diphtheria, tetanus, pertussis, and typhoid (DTaP). The EPI was replaced by the UIP in 1985 and the government set a specific goal of 85% immunization rates among all infants by the year 1990; complete immunization was defined as having received one BCG, one measles, three polio, and three DTaP vaccine injections by age 12 months. To support these goals, UIP provided the vaccines, along with staffing and proper vaccine storage and transportation materials (Anekwe & Kumar, 2012). Results from one study published in 2012 suggest that immunization rates have improved under the new UIP but have not reached the targeted goal. These authors estimated a total vaccination rate of 20% in the mid-1980s, increasing to approximately 60% at the time of publication (Bairwa et al., 2012).

Currently, India provides a series of vaccinations free of charge to all children seeking care at government-run hospitals. Children receiving care from private hospitals are more likely to receive vaccinations according to the Indian Academy of Pediatrics schedule at a charge. The two schedules are outlined in Table 17.1 (Shah, 2014; Vashishtha et al., 2013).

A study done by Anekwe and Kumar (2012) investigated the benefits of India's vaccination programs on improved nutritional status. This is one of a very few studies to attempt to link vaccination with reduced malnutrition in an Asian country. The study found that consistent and complete vaccination leads to an overall increase in average WAZ z scores of 0.29 and an overall increase in average HAZ z scores of 0.50 among children younger than age 4 years in the first NFHS.

TABLE 17.1 Immunization Schedules

	UNIVERSAL IMMUNIZATION PROGRAM (GOVERNMENT-RUN FACILITIES)	INDIAN ACADEMY OF PEDIATRICS (PRIVATE FACILITIES)
Birth–15 days	BCG + OPV (zero dose)	BCG + OPV (zero dose) + Hep B1
6–8 weeks	OPV1 + DTP1 + HepB1 + Hib1	IPV1 + DTP1 + HepB2 + Hib1 + Rotavirus1 + PCV1
10–12 weeks	OPV2 + DTP2 + HepB2 + Hib2	IPV2 + DTP2 + Hib2 + Rotavirus2 + PCV2
14–16 weeks	OPV3 + DTP3 + HepB3 + Hib3	IPV3 + DTP3 + Hib3 + Rotavirus3 + PCV3
6 months		HepB3 + OPV1
9 months	Measles	Measles + OPV2
12 months		HepA1
15–18 months	OPV + DTP + MMR	MMR1 + Varicella1 + PCV + DTP + IPV + Hib
2 years		Typhoid1
5–6 years	DTP	DTP + OPV + MMR2 + Varicella2 + Typhoid2
10 years	TT	TDap/Td + HPV (girls only)
16 years	TT	

BCG, Bacillus Calmette-Guerin; OPV, oral polio vaccine; IPV, inactivated polio vaccine; DTP, diphtheria, tetanus, pertussis; HepB, hepatitis B; HepA, hepatitis A; Hib, haemophilus influenza B; PCV, pneumococcal conjugate vaccine; MMR, measles, mumps, rubella; TT, tetanus toxoid; HPV, human papilloma virus

They also found that families from higher socioeconomic groups experienced greater gains in anthropometric measures with vaccination than children from lower socioeconomic groups (Anekwe & Kumar, 2012). A repeat of this study, utilizing data from the more recent NFHS surveys, might provide more evidence for the benefits of immunization in reducing malnutrition.

Deworming

It is estimated that nearly 60% of the world's population live in countries with endemic soil-transmitted nematode (STN) and helminth infections (Humphries et al., 2012). Research suggests that between 33% and 50% of children living in these endemic countries are infected with intestinal parasites at any given time (Awasthi et al., 2008; Humphries et al., 2012). WHO has suggested that such infections may be linked to decreased nutritional status, poor height and weight gain, reduced hemoglobin concentrations, impaired development and cognition, and reduced school attendance (Humphries et al., 2012; Taylor-Robinson, Maayan, Soares-Weiser, Donegan, & Garner, 2012). While claims about the association of STN infections and cognitive and developmental delays have been questioned (Taylor-Robinson et al., 2012), the impact of infection on projected growth has garnered more support. Several studies have been conducted among children enrolled in AWCs in northern India to examine the effectiveness of routine deworming prophylaxis with albendazole at 6-month intervals for children ages 1 through 5 years. These studies have shown statistically significant increases in weight ranging from 0.58 to 1.0 kg weight differences between treated and untreated children (Awasthi et al., 2008; Taylor-Robinson et al., 2012).

Routine prophylaxis against intestinal helminth infections is offered by the ICDS in India under their routine health care programs. As previously stated, intestinal diseases borne from contaminated soil could be classified as both underlying and immediate risk factors for malnourishment; therefore, addressing this component of undernutrition may generate improvements at multiple levels of the UNICEF framework. Typical prophylaxis includes albendazole or other available antihelmintic medication at 6-month intervals starting between 9 and 12 months and continuing at least through age 5 years (Awasthi et al., 2013). Unfortunately, a 2011 report from the Institute for Financial Management and Research (IFMR) on the current financial utilization by ICDS estimated that less than 4% of the funds allocated for deworming protocols are used (IFMR, 2011). This represents a large gap in services that could be provided to children across India to prevent infection and increase growth potential.

Family Planning

The Indian government has placed high importance on family planning. Doing so improves maternal health, reduces financial and resource burdens experienced by families with higher numbers of children, and aids in population control. At a personal interview, Dr. Avinesh Shetty, Chief Medical Officer at the TMA Pai Rotary Hospital in Karkala, explained the various aspects of family planning currently supported by the Indian government and, more importantly, the Indian culture. Most health professionals have recommended birth spacing of at least 36 months between pregnancies; benefits of birth spacing include better maternal recovery between pregnancies and reduced competition for resources among young siblings (Imdad et al., 2011). Education regarding the importance of birth spacing is provided at postnatal health visits. The primary means of contraception utilized by Indian women between pregnancies is the Copper T intrauterine device.

Another important component of family planning includes number of children. The Indian government has advocated for a maximum of two children per couple. They are supporting this recommendation by offering permanent sterilization following the birth of a second child via tubectomy or vasectomy, at no cost to the patient. An estimated 98% of all sterilization occurs in women and many families are taking advantage of this government-funded procedure to promote health and reduce population growth (A. Shetty, personal communication, January 21, 2014). He also notes that south Indian states are experiencing more success with these government programs due to overall higher education and quality of life, as compared with northern states (A. Shetty, personal communication, January 21, 2014).

Supplementation

Lack of proper dietary nutrient intake is clearly identified as a distinct immediate cause of child undernutrition in the UNICEF framework. There has been an abundance of research published in the past decade on the pros and cons of micro- and macronutrient supplementation for pregnant women and children in developing countries, including India. Supplementation in pregnancy has already been discussed previously, but it is important to understand the current benefits in providing supplementation to young children.

The author of a large study comparing healthy and malnourished children to understand the recommendations for nutrient intake for children suffering from moderate malnourishment asserted that previous recommendations were no longer valid as of 2006 when the WHO changed their definitions of malnourishment (Golden, 2009). Furthermore, the need for revised recommendations was based on the notion that previous recommendations were written for children living in clean environments, with reliable access to nutritious foods, and healthy growth and development. The author writes,

> In order to derive the requirements of each nutrient for moderately
> malnourished children, the lower and upper boundaries were
> assumed to lie between the requirement for a normal, healthy child

> living in a clean environment and the requirement for treatment of a severely malnourished child living in a contaminated environment. (Golden, 2009, p. S267)

Finally, a summary of findings from this study outlines the benefits of currently available supplementation programs in various countries. They indicate that programs that focus solely on macronutrients (fats, proteins, carbohydrates) generally lead to increased weight gain, but do not guarantee an improvement in overall health; micronutrient supplementation is required to ensure growth of "functional tissues" to maintain physiologic stability, cognitive development, and upward growth potential (Golden, 2009).

Identifying essential micronutrients for supplementation continues to generate much discussion. In recent literature, the most commonly cited micronutrients in preventing malnutrition are zinc, iron, folic acid, calcium, iodine, and vitamin A (Ashong et al., 2012; Imdad et al., 2011; Sachdev, 2012). Zinc is perhaps most beneficial in shortening episodes of diarrhea and promoting protein synthesis and absorption, thereby reducing stunting (Ashong et al., 2012; Golden, 2009; Imdad et al., 2011). Iron is essential for production of hemoglobin, which carries oxygen in red blood cells. While anemia may be common among women and children of low- and middle-income countries (Ashong et al., 2012), Golden (2009) points out that iron-deficiency anemia is more common among normally developing children; he cautions against oversupplementation with iron, stating that malnourished children typically have higher iron stores than healthy children and require only mild iron doses.

Further, folic acid is important in prevention of neural tube defects in utero but also plays an important role in many other physiological processes including blood production, heart health, fertility, and neurotransmitter regulation. The WHO recognizes that folic acid deficiency is common among developing nations and recommends supplementation and fortification (Golden, 2009). Calcium is essential for healthy bone development; while supplementation has not been shown to increase growth, it has been recommended in severely malnourished children to prevent bone demineralization and subsequent injury (Golden, 2009). Iodine deficiency has been linked with brain damage in infancy and is routinely corrected through provision of iodized salts in the diet (Ahmed et al., 2012). Like folic acid, vitamin A (retinol) has been linked to many physiological processes, including vision, function of mucosal surfaces, immune function, and gene expression. The controversy of vitamin A supplementation is grounded in identifying proper dosage; too little leads to dysfunction, while too much has been shown to increase mortality and respiratory infections in children with SAM in some studies (Golden, 2009).

There are several approaches to providing the essential nutrients in developing countries. Characteristics that contribute to the relative success of supplementation programs include energy density, nutrient density, cost, acceptability on behalf of the child (i.e., taste, texture, etc.), preparation time, and risk of contamination (de Pee & Bloem, 2009). Some currently available options include fortification of commercial foods, particularly infant foods and formulas, micronutrient powders, lipid-based micronutrient supplements (i.e., spreads, creams), and ready-to-use therapeutic foods (RUTF) such as pastes, biscuits, and bars (Ahmed et al., 2012; Golden, 2009). RUTF has been found to be the most effective in the management of SAM, due to its high nutrient density and ability to be consumed without water, thereby removing potential for bacterial infection from contaminated water and improving shelf life.

Unfortunately, RUTF is costly and has not been found to be a feasible option in extremely resource-poor areas (Ahmed et al., 2012). India has developed their own formulation for RUTF including chick peas, rice flour, and oil (type not specified), and lower concentrations of dried skim milk. Long-term outcomes of this product are yet to be published (de Pee & Bloem, 2009). Fortification of foods such as grains, juices, and dairy products has been more commonly used by many developing and developed nations. AWCs in India utilize fortified rice, cereals, and milk to provide essential nutrients to enrolled children; however, as seen in Case Study 3, this is not always sufficient to prevent malnutrition.

CASE STUDY 1: AJIT AND JOWAR

Demographics

Ajit, male, age 2 years, 10 months, and Jowar, male, age 6 years, 6 months, are brothers living with their mother and father in a fishing village bordering the Arabian Sea, in the Indian state of Karnataka. The mother is a housewife. The father works in the fishing industry nearby.

Environment

They live in a three-room house made of cinder blocks that includes a kitchen and two living spaces. The kitchen uses wood burning as its primary fuel source and all cooking is done indoors. The mother, father, and two boys sleep together on a set of padded blankets on the floor each night. Jowar attends school during the day. Ajit stays home with his mother

Maternal History

Both boys were born at 8.5 months in a hospital via spontaneous vaginal delivery. She had monthly prenatal visits for both pregnancies. The pregnancy with Ajit included first-trimester bleeding leading to bed rest for several months. Otherwise, both pregnancies and deliveries were unremarkable. The mother was 24 and 27 years of age at the birth of Jowar and Ajit, respectively.

(continued)

CASE STUDY 1: AJIT AND JOWAR (*continued*)

She took government-provided iron, calcium, and folic acid supplements for the duration of her pregnancy. She did not require protein supplements.

Child Illness History

The mother reports use of Ayurvedic syrups for fever (both) and respiratory infections (Ajit). She denies frequent gastrointestinal illnesses.

Feeding Practices

The mother exclusively breastfed both boys until age 2 months. At this time she felt that her breast milk was inadequate because the boys would cry so she began complementary foods with biscuits. Ajit continues with breastfeeding in addition to complementary foods at 34 months. Jowar was breastfed until age 3.5 years when Ajit was conceived. Both boys eat whatever the mother cooks and are generally good eaters. The main source of protein is milk and fish due to father's occupation. Watermelon makes Ajit sick.

Family Planning

The deliveries were spaced approximately 4 years apart. The mother had laparoscopic tubal ligation after the birth of Ajit.

Immunizations

Both boys are up-to-date on vaccines according to the government-recommended immunization schedule.

Deworming

Both boys initiated deworming tablets at age 24 months, with routine deworming every 6 months until 5 years of age. These are provided by the government.

Growth Monitoring

See Table 17.2 for current field anthropometrics. See Table 17.3 for weight history. Height and middle upper arm circumference (MUAC) was not routinely recorded in the history.

Analysis of Case

Ajit and Jowar come from a low-income family in a rural area. They are an excellent example of the effects of government interventions on childhood growth and nutrition. Maternal care included monthly prenatal visits as well as government-recommended iron, calcium, and folic acid supplementation. Family planning was also managed well, including a minimum of 3 years between

CASE STUDY 1: AJIT AND JOWAR (continued)

births and permanent sterilization after the second child. Breastfeeding is extensive in both boys; however, complementary feeding began earlier than is recommended by health professionals. This mother would have benefited from stronger counseling in this area. Each boy began life below optimal weight requirements but they have managed to catch up to recommended growth curves within the first few months of life. Both boys have fluctuated in height and weight velocity but are both considered normal and do not meet the criteria for malnourishment.

TABLE 17.2 Current Anthropometric Measurements as of 01/13/14 for Ajit and Jowar

	AJIT AGE: 2 YEARS, 10 MONTHS			JOWAR AGE: 6 YEARS, 6 MONTHS		
	VALUE	z SCORE (APPROX)	%ILE (APPROX)	VALUE	z SCORE (APPROX)	%ILE (APPROX)
Weight (kg)	12.5	−0.9	16	25	+1.0	85
Height (cm)	93.5	−0.5	37	124	+1.0	85
Middle upper arm circumference (MUAC) (cm)	16	+0.25	65	21	NA	NA

TABLE 17.3 Growth Monitoring for Case Study 1

	AJIT (DOB: 03/20/2011)			JOWAR (DOB: 02/08/2007)		
	WEIGHT (kg)	z SCORE (APPROX)	%ILE (APPROX)	WEIGHT (kg)	z SCORE (APPROX)	%ILE (APPROX)
Birth	2.8	−1.0	10	Missing	NA	NA
6 weeks	4.6	−0.5	30	4.3	−1.0	15
10 weeks	5.9	+0.1	49	5.3	−0.9	22
14 weeks	7.1	+0.9	70	6.3	−0.2	30
9 months	10.1	+1.1	86	10.8	+1.8	98
12 months	Missing	NA	NA	Missing	NA	NA
15 months	10.8	+0.6	65	12.0	+1.4	92
19 months	11.0	−0.1	49	12.6	+1.1	86
2 years	Missing	NA	NA	15.0	+1.5	96
5 years	NA	NA	NA	19.0	+0.3	63
TODAY	12.5	−0.9	20	25.0	NA	NA

CASE STUDY 2: LEKISHA

Demographics

Lekisha, female, age 3 years, lives with her mother and father, also in a fishing village bordering the Arabian Sea on the southwest Indian coast. The mother is a housewife. The father is an electrician. She has no siblings. They are of the Hindu religion.

Environment

The family lives in a five-room house that includes a kitchen, two bedrooms, and two living spaces. All cooking is done indoors but the primary cooking fuel is unknown. Lekisha stays home with her mother during the day.

Maternal History

The mother married at age 24 and delivered Lekisha at age 27. This has been her only pregnancy. She received monthly prenatal visits and a full government supply of iron, calcium, and folic acid. She received the recommended two tetanus toxoid (TT) shots during pregnancy. The mother was identified as being of short stature at 140 cm. She delivered Lekisha via planned caesarian section at 9 months.

Child Illness History

Lekisha has a ventricular septal defect (VSD). The resulting murmur can be described as nearly holosystolic at a grade V out of VI. The mother reports that her pediatric cardiologist is hopeful that the VSD will close spontaneously. If it does not, she will be evaluated for surgery at age 5 years. She takes digoxin, spironolactone, enalapril, and furosemide. The mother reports that she gets fevers when the season changes, with occasional diarrhea. She is otherwise very active and has reached all developmental milestones for her age.

Feeding Practices

The mother reports that Lekisha was exclusively breastfed until age 24 months. She introduced complementary foods, starting with chapatis, rice, and roti. She is a good eater.

Family Planning

Unknown.

Immunizations

She is up to date on all government-recommended immunizations.

Deworming

She receives routine deworming tablets every 6 months.

Growth Monitoring

Lekisha was born at 2.75 kg (WAZ ≈ −1.0, WA% ≈ 13th). Growth monitoring records were not available at the time of the interview. The last known weight at 3 years, 3 months was 9.5 kg, which places her below the first percentile for weight. The height of the child is unknown. The mother is of short stature; as such, it is possible that the child is also of short stature and her weight-for-height may be closer to the normal range.

Analysis of Case

There is less information available on physical parameters for growth and development for this case; however, Lekisha comes from a family with higher education and income potential. She lives in a larger home and has no siblings competing for resources. Due to her cardiac condition she is likely to receive more medical care than the children presented in Case Study 1, however, her ability to thrive is reduced. Her mother is well educated in caring for her child and she seems content with having only one child. Lekisha's medical condition may factor into the mother's decision to delay or avoid a second pregnancy. Unlike Case Study 1, Lekisha's mother maintained exclusive breastfeeding for longer than recommended. This likely played a large role in slowing her weight gain. However, it is reassuring to know that she is currently taking all foods well and has had no other significant illnesses. It would be helpful to have more information on Lekisha's growth, particularly her height measurements. The literature supports the notion that mothers of short stature are likely to produce children of short stature. It is difficult to accurately assess the normalcy of Lekisha's weight gain without comparing it to her height gain. She is otherwise developmentally healthy.

CASE STUDY 3: PRAVEEN

Praveen is a student at a local Anganwadi day care center. Approximately 2 hours were spent observing him and his classmates. With the exception of drop-off, his parents were not present. Information for this case study came from observation and his teacher, with translation assistance by nursing faculty from a local university. Little is known about his living environment, maternal history, illness history, family planning, or deworming regimen; as such, these sections are not included in this case study.

Demographics

Praveen is a 5-year-old male. He lives in a rural district in the state of Karnataka and attends a local AWC for day care. He attends 5 days per week. On the day of

(continued)

CASE STUDY 3: PRAVEEN (*continued*)

data collection, he was dropped off by his father. He lives with his mother, father, and sister, who is 14 years old.

Feeding Practices

While he attends the AWC, Praveen receives one snack, one meal, and warm milk prepared by the Anganwadi worker. Because he meets the criteria for severe malnourishment, he receives supplemental nutrition through the AWC. This includes egg and milk protein powders and rice. The center provides only enough for Praveen, not his mother, father, or older sister.

Immunizations

He is up to date on all government-recommended immunizations.

Growth Monitoring

At birth, Praveen weighed 2.5 kg (WAZ = -2.0, WA% = 3rd). At birth, he qualified as malnourished based on his weight. At the time of observation, at age 5 years, 1 month, Praveen weighs 11.8 kg with a height of 97 cm. His WAZ is less than -3.0, placing him below the WAZ threshold for severe malnourishment. His HAZ score is approximately -2.8, just barely above the HAZ threshold for severe malnourishment. Furthermore, monitoring of his height and weight according to the WHO standard curves reveals that Praveen has not gained weight since his fourth birthday. A comparison of his growth curve with the WHO growth standards is available in Figure 17.2. Because of Praveen's continued failure to thrive, he has been reported to the Women and Social Welfare Office, according to standard procedure.

Analysis of Case

Praveen represents a case of severe childhood malnourishment, despite advances in government programming. His Anganwadi teacher explained that he eats well in the classroom and always goes home with supplemental nutrition. However, it is difficult to know what his feeding practices are at home, or how these nutritional supplements are used by the family. It would also be helpful to know his bowel patterns and any deworming regimens, his sleeping habits, and his interaction with his mother and sister. When he was dropped off at the start of the day, he exhibited a strong bond with his father as evidenced by hugging and trust that his father would return to pick him up later. His Anganwadi teacher explained that Praveen is socially and cognitively delayed when compared with his classmates of the same age. Upon observation in the classroom, Praveen did not interact with his peers and preferred to observe classroom activities rather than participate in them. He did not sing along with prayer and required frequent direction for exercises. The AWCs play a key role in managing child nutrition; however, with only one Anganwadi worker present in a classroom of 25 children and no way of

CASE STUDY 3: PRAVEEN (*continued*)

knowing if and how nutritional supplements are being taken, it is unlikely that the Anganwadi alone can reverse Praveen's nutritional status. He requires direct observation and individualized intervention from health care providers if there is any hope of reaching a healthy weight. His social, developmental, and cognitive delays will also require specific intervention.

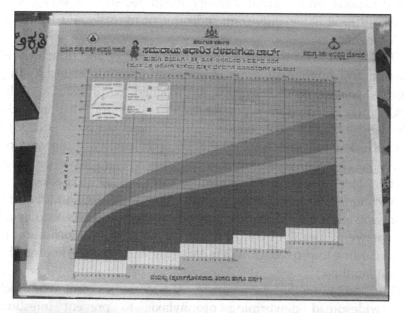

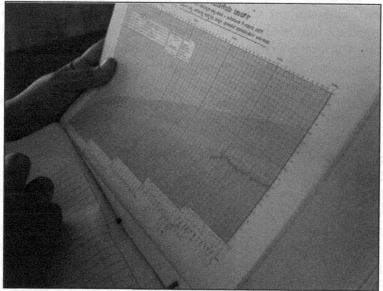

FIGURE 17.2 WHO weight-for-age standard growth curve. Praveen's weight-for-age growth.

CONCLUSION

When WHO altered the definitions of childhood malnutrition in 2006, the result was an increase in the number of children meeting the definition of being malnourished, thus increasing the number of children and families in need of public health support. India has consistently ranked among the poorest countries in the world and has struggled to conquer problems of poverty such as infectious disease, access to clean water and safe housing, educational and socioeconomic gaps between genders, economic equality, and poor child and maternal health. Several national and international organizations, such as WHO, have identified proper nutrition as an important indicator of overall child health, growth, and development.

The Indian government has heeded their advice and utilized available funds to design and implement some impressive programs to tackle the problem of childhood malnutrition. They have approached the problem at each level of the UNICEF conceptual framework for childhood undernutrition, including basic, underlying, and immediate contributors. Some of the more successful initiatives have included the efforts of the ICDS, particularly those services provided by AWCs. These government-run day care centers have provided access to preschool-level education, immunization tracking, health check-ups and referrals, and nutritional support and supplementation to children and their families. This nationwide effort has reached millions of children and has been demonstrated to improve overall health of children. Yet, there are still opportunities for improvement including improved growth monitoring and expanded outreach to rural and migrant families.

Other programs that have seen great success in recent years include India's UIPs, widespread deworming prophylaxis to prevent intestinal helminth infections, and support for family planning. Benefits and efforts to promote macro- and micronutrient supplementation have received a lot of attention in the literature. Current government funding for maternal supplementation appears to be improving the health of both mother and child. Information on child supplementation, including zinc, iron, folic acid, vitamin A, iodine, and calcium, have revealed positive effects on overall childhood growth and development, but more research is needed to determine effective doses for public administration and government funding.

As a developing nation, India continues to face many obstacles in achieving health equity. Despite these struggles, information collected and reviewed in this chapter suggests an overall uptick in India's overall state of health, including that of young children. Their multitiered, comprehensive approach to the problem incorporates important components outlined in the UNICEF framework, suggesting that this framework indeed offers appropriate guidance to populations struggling with childhood malnutrition. To maintain this upward motion, international and national government figures will need to continue to place emphasis and funding on several public health efforts, including community-based programs to supplement acute facility-based care for both healthy and malnourished children; promotion of exclusive breastfeeding through age 6 months followed by appropriate introduction of complementary foods; improved sanitation, including proper toileting facilities, clean water, and reduction of indoor air contaminants from cooking fuels; promotion of general and health education for women, including mothers, and pregnant and lactating women; and ongoing support for direct interventions to prevent malnutrition including nutritional supplementation and proper growth monitoring. If India can continue to promote these activities, they may continue to improve the health of children now and in the future.

ACKNOWLEDGMENT

The authors acknowledge Mrs. Ansuya, Ms. Sudha, and the students and faculty at Manipal University College of Nursing, Manipal, India, for their contributions to data collection.

REFERENCES

Ade, A., Gupta, S. S., Maliye, C., Deshmukh, P. R., & Garg, B. S. (2010). Effect of improvement of pre-school education through Anganwadi center on intelligence and development quotient of children. *Indian Journal of Pediatrics, 77*(5), 541–546. doi:10.1007/s12098-010-0056-7

Agrawal, P. K., Agrawal, S., Ahmed, S., Darmstadt, G. L., Williams, E. K., Rosen, H. E., . . . Baqui, A. H. (2012). Effect of knowledge of community health workers on essential newborn health care: A study from rural India. *Health Policy & Planning, 27*(2), 115–126. doi:10.1093/heapol/czr018

Ahmed, T., Michaelsen, K. F., Frem, J. C., & Tumvine, J. (2012). Malnutrition: Report of the FISPGHAN working group. *Journal of Pediatric Gastroenterology & Nutrition, 55*(5), 626–631. doi:10.1097/MPG.0b013e318272b600

Anekwe, T. D., & Kumar, S. (2012). The effect of a vaccination program on child anthropometry: Evidence from India's universal immunization program. *Journal of Public Health, 34*(4), 489–497. doi:10.1093/pubmed/fds032

Antony, G. M., & Laxmaiah, A. (2008). Human development, poverty, health & nutrition situation in India. *Indian Journal of Medical Research, 128*(2), 198–205.

Ashong, J., Muthayya, S., DeRegil, M. L., Laillou, A., Guyondet, C., MoenchPfanner, R., . . . PenaRosas, P. J. (2012). Fortification of rice with vitamins and minerals for addressing micronutrient malnutrition. *Cochrane Database of Systematic Reviews, 6.*

Avula, R., Frongillo, E. A., Arabi, M., Sharma, S., & Schultink, W. (2011). Enhancements to nutrition program in Indian integrated child development services increased growth and energy intake of children. *Journal of Nutrition, 141*(4), 680–684. doi:10.3945/jn.109.116954

Awasthi, S., Peto, R., Pande, V. K., Fletcher, R. H., Read, S., & Bundy, D. A. (2008). Effects of deworming on malnourished preschool children in India: An open-labelled, cluster-randomized trial. *PLoS Neglected Tropical Diseases, 2*(4), e233. doi:10.1371/journal.pntd.0000223

Awasthi, S., Peto, R., Read, S., Richards, S. M., Pande, V., & Bundy, D. (2013). Population deworming every 6 months with albendazole in 1 million pre-school children in north India: DEVTA, a cluster-randomized trial. *Lancet, 381*(9876), 1478–1486. doi:10.1016/S0140-6736(12)62126-6

Bairwa, M., Pilania, M., Raiput, M., Khanna, P., Kumar, N., Nagar, M., & Chawla, S. (2012). Pentavalent vaccine: A major breakthrough in India's universal immunization program. *Human Vaccines & Immunotherapeutics, 8*(9), 1314–1316. doi:10.4161/hv.20651

Davey, A., Davey, S., & Datta, U. (2008). Perception regarding quality of services in urban ICDS blocks in Delhi. *Indian Journal of Public Health, 52*(3), 156–158.

de Pee, S., & Bloem, M. W. (2009). Current and potential role of specially formulated foods and food supplements for preventing malnutrition among 6- to 23-month-old children and for treating moderate malnutrition among 6- to 59-month-old children. *Food & Nutrition Bulletin, 30*(Suppl 3), S434–S463.

Emmelin, A. B., & Wall, S. (2007). Indoor air pollution: A poverty-related cause of mortality among the children of the world. *Chest, 132*(5), 1615–1623. doi:10.1378/chest.07-1398

Fenn, B., & Penny, M. E. (2008). Using the new World Health Organization growth standards: Differences from 3 countries. *Journal of Pediatric Gastroenterology & Nutrition, 46*(3), 316–321. doi:10.1097/MPG.0b013e31815d6968

Golden, M. H. (2009). Proposed recommended nutrient densitites for moderately malnourished children. *Food and Nutrition Bulletin, 30*(3), S267–S342.

Goulet, O., Lebenthal, E., Branski, D., Martin, A., Antoine, J., & Jones, P. J. (2006). Nutritional solutions to major health problems of preschool children: How to optimise growth and development. *Journal of Pediatric Gastroenterology & Nutrition, 43*(Suppl 3), S1–S3. doi:10.1097/01.mpg.0000255843.54164.af

Humphries, D., Nguyen, S., Boakye, D., Wilson, M., & Cappello, M. (2012). The promise and pitfalls of mass drug administration to control intestinal helminth infections. *Current Opinion in Infectious Disease, 25*(5), 584–589. doi:10.1097/QCO.0b013e328357e4cf

Imdad, A., Sadiq, K., & Bhutta, Z. A. (2011). Evidence-based prevention of childhood malnutrition. *Current Opinion in Clinical Nutrition & Metabolic Care, 14*(3), 276–285. doi:10.1097/MCO.0b013e328345364a

Institute for Financial Management and Research (IFMR). (2011). *Integrated child development services (ICDS) scheme brief.* Retrieved from http://cdf.ifmr.ac.in/wp-content/uploads/2011/03/ICDS-Scheme-Brief.pdf

Jacobs, T. A. (2010). Rethinking hard-to-reach communities in the realm of global pediatrics: The urban poor and community health workers. *Archives of Pediatrics & Adolescent Medicine, 164*(3), 294–296.

Kapil, U., & Jain, K. (2011). Magnitude of zinc deficiency among under five children in India. *Indian Journal of Pediatrics, 78*(9), 1069–1072. doi:10.1007/s12098-011-0379-z

Kapil, U., & Pradhan, R. (1999). Integrated child development services scheme (ICDS) and its impact on nutritional status of children in India and recent initiatives. *Indian Journal of Public Health, 43*(1), 21–25.

Mamidi, R. S., Shidhaye, P., Radhakrishna, K. V., Babu, J. J., & Reddy, P. S. (2011). Pattern of growth faltering and recovery in under 5 children in India using WHO growth standards—A study on first and third national family health survey. *Indian Pediatrics, 48*(11), 855–860.

Meshram, I. I., Laxmaiah, A., Gal Reddy, C., Ravindranath, M., Venkaiah, K., & Brahmam, G. N. (2011). Prevalence of under-nutrition and its correlates among under 3-year-old children in rural areas of Andhra Pradesh, India. *Annals of Human Biology, 38*(1), 93–101. doi:10.3109/03014460.2010.498387

Mother and Child Health and Education Trust. (2014). *Complementary feeding guidelines—India.* Retrieved from http://motherchildnutrition.org/india/complementary-feeding-guidelines.html

Osrin, D., Das, S., Bapat, U., Alcock, G. A., Joshi, W., & More, N. S. (2011). A rapid assessment scorecard to identify informal settlements at higher maternal and child health risk in Mumbai. *Journal of Urban Health, 88*(5), 919–932. doi:10.1007/s11524-011-9556-7

Ozaltin, E., Hill, K., & Subramanian, S. V. (2010). Association of maternal stature with offspring mortality, underweight, and stunting in low- to middle-income countries. *Journal of the American Medical Association, 303*(15), 1507–1516.

Sachdev, H. P. (2012). Overcoming challenges to accelerating linear growth in Indian children. *Indian Pediatrics, 49*(4), 271–275.

Sarkar, R., Sivarathinaswamy, P., Thangaraj, B., Sindhu, K. N., Ajjampur, S. S., Muliyil, J., . . . Kang, G. (2013). Burden of childhood diseases and malnutrition in a semi-urban slum in southern India. *BMC Public Health, 13*, 87. doi:10.1186/1471-2458-13-87

Savitha, M. R., & Kondapuram, N. (2012). Comparison of 2006 WHO and Indian Academy of Pediatrics recommended growth charts of under five Indian children. *Indian Pediatrics, 49*(9), 737–739.

Shah, I. (2014). *Immunization schedule.* Retrieved from http://www.pediatriconcall.com/forpatients/vaccination/article.aspx?artid=390#

Subba Rao, G. M., Sudershan, R. V., Rao, P., Vishnu Vardhana Rao, M., & Polasa, K. (2007). Food safety knowledge, attitudes and practices of mothers: Findings from focus group studies in south India. *Appetite, 49*(2), 441–449.

Taylor-Robinson, D. C., Maayan, N., Soares-Weiser, K., Donegan, S., & Garner, P. (2012). Deworming drugs for soil-transmitted intestinal worms in children: Effects on nutritional indicators, haemoglobin and school performance. doi:10.1002/14651858. CD000371.pub5

United Nations Children's Fund (UNICEF). (2013). *Improving child nutrition: The achievable imperative for global progress.* New York, NY: Author.

United Nations Development Programme. (2013). *Millennium development goals.* Retrieved from http://www.undp.org/content/undp/en/home/mdgoverview.html

United States Agency for International Development. (2010). *Treating childhood diarrhea in India with ORT and zinc: Engaging the pharmaceutical industry and private providers. Lessons learned from the POUZN/AED project.* Washington, DC: AED Center for Private Sector Health Initiatives.

Varma, J. L., Das, S., Sankar, R., Mannar, M. G., Levinson, F. J., & Hamer, D. H. (2007). Community-level micronutrient fortification of a food supplement in India: A controlled trial in preschool children aged 36-66 mo. *American Journal of Clinical Nutrition, 85*(4), 1127–1133.

Vashishtha, V. M., Kalra, A., Bose, A., Choudhury, P., Yewale, V., Bansal, C. P., & Gupta, S. G. (2013). Indian Academy of Pediatrics (IAP) recommended immunization schedule for children aged 0 through 18 years—India, 2013 and updates on immunization. *Indian Pediatrics, 50*, 1095–1108.

Vazir, S., Engle, P., Balakrishna, N., Griffiths, P. L., Johnson, S. L., Creed-Kanashiro, H., . . . Bentley, M. E. (2013). Cluster-randomized trial on complementary and responsive feeding education to caregivers found improved dietary intake, growth and development among rural Indian toddlers. *Maternal & Child Nutrition, 9*(1), 99–117. doi:10.1111/j.1740-8709.2012.00413.x

World Health Organization (WHO). (2006). *The WHO child growth standards.* Retrieved from http://www.who.int/childgrowth/standards/en

World Health Organization. (2014a). *How different are the new standards from the old growth charts?* Retrieved from http://www.who.int/childgrowth/faqs/how_different/en/index.html

World Health Organization. (2014b). *Why are the new growth standards needed?* Retrieved from http://www.who.int/childgrowth/faqs/why/en/index.html

CHAPTER 18

End-of-Life Care in a Global Health Context

Inge B. Corless, Rana Limbo, Regina Szylit Bousso, and Kim Rochon

*E*nd-of-life (EOL) care received renewed attention by health care professionals with the development of the hospice movement in the latter part of the 20th century. Hospice care programs were initiated to improve EOL care for persons suffering largely from chronic noncommunicable diseases (NCDs), and in particular, cancer (Mor & Masterson-Allen, 1987). Knowledge of symptoms typically experienced by those suffering from end-stage cancer helped hospice professionals develop a toolkit of approaches for ameliorating this distress. The recognition that care encompasses more than attention to the soma but also concern with the psychological, social, and spiritual realms of individuals incorporated a nursing perspective into what characterizes hospice and now palliative care. The terms *hospice* and *palliative care* were initially used interchangeably to refer to care at the EOL. Currently hospice care still has this meaning, referring to care given by a hospice program at the last 6 months of life. Palliative care now refers to holistic care given when a patient is diagnosed with a potentially life-limiting disease.

BACKGROUND

It may be no accident that a physician with training as a nurse and a social worker, Dame Cicely Saunders, initiated the first modern hospice program, St. Christopher's Hospice in London, England, in 1967 (Saunders, 1999). The development of hospice programs led by nurses, doctors, social workers, and others with a holistic approach to care of the patient was initiated in the United States as a home care program in New Haven, Connecticut, in 1974 by Florence Wald, RN, former dean of the Yale School of Nursing (Corless, 1983). The first dedicated unit in an acute care hospital was established at the Royal Victoria Hospital in Montreal, Canada, in 1975 by Dr. Balfour Mount and his associates, Dr. Ina Cummings Ajemian and Dr. John Scott. There were other early hospice programs, notably at St. Luke's Hospital in New York, New York; Hillhaven Hospice in Tucson, Arizona; and the Hospice of Marin in Marin County, California, among other places in the United States (Corless, 1983). Many of the leaders of these programs were from nursing, with notable exceptions from medicine including, among others, William Lamers, Frank Ferris and Charles von Gunten and, from social work, in particular, Zelda Foster.

The hospice movement spread across the United States and elsewhere and produced the call for an association of hospice programs. In 1978, the National Hospice Organization, now known as the National Hospice and Palliative Care Association, was incorporated (Beresford & Connor, 1999). Efforts to further the recognition of hospice programs and to obtain reimbursement for hospice care resulted in legislation introduced to Congress by Congressman Leon Panetta of California, Representative Bill Gradison of Ohio, and Senator Bob Dole of Kansas (Beresford & Connor, 1999). Attached to the Tax Equity and Fiscal Responsibility Act, the Hospice Medicare benefit was approved by Congress in 1982. This legislation, originally scheduled to sunset in 4 years, was made permanent in 1986.

The emphasis of those defining the Hospice Medicare benefit was that the cost of hospice not be an add-on to the prevailing expenditures of Medicare. Consequently, those "electing" hospice could not simultaneously be receiving, that is, be reimbursed for, care aimed at cure. Exceptions to this rule, for example, were care for a fracture as a result of an accident or palliative chemotherapy. It should be noted here that if a patient elects hospice care over curative care, it does not mean that the patient may not have a change of mind and/or heart and want to engage in further curative care. That clearly is a possibility and the hospice benefit can be rescinded for that person.

The concern with fiscal frugality (with regard to the design of the Hospice Medicare benefit) or responsibility, depending on one's perspective, isolated the approaches used by hospice professionals in the last 6 months of life. This financial decision may be responsible in large part for the delay in incorporating palliative approaches into the care of all patients with life-threatening conditions. There are other barriers to the further development of palliative care apart from fiscal concerns and these have to do with the popular vision of hospice care as being for those who are dying, as well as the interchangeable use of the terms *hospice* and *palliative care* in the first decades of the hospice movement.

Underutilization of hospice care may be due to prognostic uncertainty and discomfort with EOL discussions on the part of the health care provider as well as the patient and family (McAteer & Wellbury, 2013). There is also the concern that hope will be lost if hospice referral is made. It is well worth asking whether it is the patient's loss of hope, the physician's loss of hope, or both? The question to be asked about the patient is "hope for what?" Is it hope for a lengthier life; hope for a return to a life before diagnosis; or hope for freedom from discomfort? For the physician, is it hope for a cure for the patient; hope for a remission; hope for the patient to have a life without discomfort; or hope not to have to deal with a dying patient? The latter hope may be the result of fondness for a given patient or an attempt to avoid having to confront the sequelae of terminal illness. For various reasons, both patient and physician may want to "put off" the discussion of EOL choices about care. "Failure" may be a specter for the patient who vowed to win the battle for continued life and for the physician who feels a sense of failure in not being able to conquer the cancer. Death also may not be in the physician's lexicon, just as failure is not for the competitive athlete. These barriers make it difficult for both patient and provider.

If the role of the physician is first to do no harm, how is this to be enacted so that the physician is free to accept that given the state of the science, a specified intervention will not halt the progression of the disease? And, further, given that the side effects of the therapy may have a negative impact on the quality of the life remaining, continuation of the protocol or any other protocol is not in the best interests of the patient. Under such circumstances, a decision not to continue with care aimed at cure is not a failure on the part of the physician but an acknowledgment of an unfortunate reality. In fact, such a decision is in keeping with the principle to first do no harm.

When the decision is reached to have an EOL discussion with a patient, the provider also needs to assess the decision-making capacity of the patient. Zaros, Curtis, Silveira, and Elmore (2013) have expounded on the four criteria that should be met to assess decision-making capacity as outlined by Applebaum and Grisso (1988, 1989). Namely, "Does the patient (1) communicate a clear consistent choice; (2) understand the relevant information surrounding that decision; (3) appreciate the consequences of that decision; (4) communicate reasoning for that decision?" (p. 334). If the physician has the EOL discussion with the patient when the cancer is refractory to care but the patient is not moribund, there is a greater likelihood that these criteria will be met.

The concern that enrollment in hospice or palliative care results in a shortened life has been refuted by research. In a study of patients with nonsmall cell lung cancer, those receiving palliative care had better survival rates than the controls who received standard care (Temel et al., 2010). Results such as these are helpful in countering the supposition that acceptance of hospice and/or palliative care is "giving up" and that fruitful life is no longer a possibility. Quite the contrary, attention to the physical, psychological, social, and spiritual aspects of care is foundational to fruitful life whether one has the diagnosis of a terminal illness or not. For the naysayers, a disease for which cure is not possible will likely result in a life where one has a sounder appreciation for the limitations in length of life, whether that be days, weeks, months, or years. Palliative care does not change the prognosis. It does provide the support to enable the individual to make the most of whatever time remains. And for palliative care initiated at the diagnosis of a life-threatening illness when it is not clear whether a cure is possible, the support enables the patient to confront the multiple challenges in treatment for such a disease. Indeed, receiving such care is what patients in hospice care always commented about; namely, why couldn't I have received this care earlier in the disease process? Palliative care makes that possible. Indeed, the World Health Organization (WHO) now includes communicable diseases as appropriate for palliative care (eHospice, 2014).

PALLIATIVE CARE

The recognition of palliative care globally has taken a major step forward in 2014. Although acknowledged for decades by hospice and palliative care professionals as an essential component of care for persons with life-threatening diseases, it is only recently that WHO has developed a new resolution on palliative care (Worldwide Palliative Care Alliance [WPCA], 2014). This report and the accompanying resolution, *Strengthening of Palliative Care as a Component of Integrated Treatment Within the Continuum of Care*, was considered by the World Health Assembly at its meeting in May 2014. The significance of this report and resolution were noted by Connor, who stated:

> WHO has affirmed that palliative care is needed for people suffering
> from many communicable and non-communicable diseases and
> calls on member states [to] develop policies, multilevel education,
> essential medicines, access, and adequate funding for palliative care.
> (eHospice, 2014, para 4)

An interesting component of the WHO approach is the inclusion of both communicable and NCDs. More will be said about this shortly.

WHO (2002) defined palliative care for adults as having a focus on quality of life for:

> . . . patients and their families facing the problems associated with life
> threatening illness, through prevention and the relief of suffering by
> means of early identification and impeccable assessment and treatment
> of pain and other problems, physical, psychosocial and spiritual.
> (para 4)

The WPCA (2014) cites WHO Global Estimates in stating that there were approximately 54.6 million deaths in 2011 worldwide, of which 66% were due to NCDs, 25% due to "communicable maternal, perinatal and nutritional conditions"(p. 11) and 9% due to injuries for which palliative care could have been helpful. The vast majority (69%) of such deaths occur in people 60 years and older, with 25% occurring in those 15 to 59 years of age and 6% in children 0 to 14 years old (WPCA, 2014, p. 12). In persons 15 to 59 years of age, the need for palliative care is greatest in those diagnosed with HIV/AIDS (> 97%), whereas the greatest need for palliative care in those 60 years and older is for those suffering from Alzheimer's disease and other dementias, as well as Parkinson's disease (> 97%; WPCA, 2014, p. 14). Adults who could have benefitted from palliative care died largely from cardiovascular disease (38.5%), cancer (34%), chronic respiratory diseases (10.3%), HIV/AIDS (5.7%), and diabetes (4.6%; WPCA, 2014, p. 13).

With a focus on EOL care, diseases requiring palliative care were grouped as cancer, HIV/AIDS, and progressive nonmalignant diseases (WPCA, 2014). The need for palliative care was greatest for those with progressive nonmalignant diseases, with the exception of Africa where the need was greatest for those living with HIV/AIDS. It was also noted that the need for palliative care is greatest in upper middle-income countries (41%) followed by lower middle income countries (29%), high-income countries (22%), and last by low-income countries (8%) (WPCA, 2014, p. 16). And in what seems a paradox, the highest rate of those in need of palliative care per 100,000 adults was in the high-income countries (WPCA, 2014, p. 17). The answer is likely related to the age structure of the populations, with higher income countries having a proportionately older population.

Palliative Care in Brazil

When faced with the challenge of having to incorporate palliative and hospice care into its health care system, Brazil enacted an incipient, unarticulated EOL policy (Bousso, Misko, Mendes-Castillo, & Rossato, 2012). This EOL and palliative care policy was developed in the context of Brazil's universal health care system, or the Sistema Único de Saude (Unified Health System, SUS).

The SUS is one of the largest public health systems globally and provides comprehensive care from primary care to complex critical care. SUS provides access to health care through a full, universal, free-access health system. This system was created in 1988 through the Brazilian Federal Constitution and offers care to more than 190 million Brazilian citizens (Ministério da Saúde, 2014).

But despite SUS advocating full access for all Brazilians, this does not occur in practice. There is a private health system that is used primarily by the more privileged classes because of access difficulties, especially access to high-complexity services, such as treatment in intensive care units (ICUs), for example.

There are countless differences with regard to the care received in public and private hospitals. For example, in public hospitals, there is no clear definition of who is responsible for admitting the patient to the hospital, whereas in teaching hospitals linked to universities, the patient is accompanied by students and residents. In private hospitals, the family's doctor deals with the hospitalization of the patient and is responsible for all of the care during the patient's time in the hospital.

There are important aspects of the Brazilian health system that are worth emphasizing. Hospital care is very selective and access for admission depends on the availability of the necessary resources for patient treatment; importantly, health care services are better in developed urban centers. Thus, the socioeconomic differences and the clinical needs of the patients both play a role in the choice of a public or private hospital, and determine the quality and quantity of patient care and assistance for patients and their families in EOL situations (Baliza, 2013).

Within the context of the SUS, as previously noted the first palliative care services appeared in Brazil in the 1990s, and despite the increase in the number of available units, the services are still insufficient to meet the country's needs. Most of the current palliative care groups began in about 2000, with significant progress in the growth of services in the past 4 years. However, the practice still lacks regulations, definitions, and policies for practice. There are no statistics on the number of patients undergoing this type of care in Brazil. However, as is the case in other parts of the world, it is known that, given the advance in therapies for the various chronic illnesses, the number of palliative care services in both inpatient and home care settings is growing (Bousso et al., 2012).

Regarding the needs and barriers to good quality palliative care, Brazil is classified as Level 1 by WPCA (2014). There are no hospice programs in Brazil and palliative care is not recognized as an area of expertise, which prevents the adequate training of professionals. Currently, there is a palliative care "Consultant Group Team" in some hospitals that consists of an interprofessional team trained to be at the disposal of physicians of different specialties. The goal of the palliative care consultation is to elaborate a plan of care for the patient and family that will result in a smooth transition to palliative care.

At present, the greatest challenge in Brazil is health care professionals' willingness to accept the palliative care team. Medical professionals are concerned about interference in their decisions and personal conduct, an issue not isolated to Brazil. This is compounded by the decision-making process in EOL situations, which is difficult and involves ethical questions related to moral, cultural, and social values. Within the context of ICUs, this scenario is even more challenging; health professionals must incorporate EOL care and palliative care when assisting patients and members of their families.

The challenges of differences in care based on location of the hospital or clinic, economic differences of the patient/family, as well as the values of patients, families, and health care providers make the provision of palliative care a continuing challenge. The good news is that there are health care professionals who see the need and importance of doing so.

Palliative Care in South Africa

In South Africa, the second country in Africa to introduce palliative care, the hospice movement has taken hold, with approximately 138 hospices and other programs offering hospice care according to the Hospice Palliative Care Association of South Africa (HPCA, 2012). In addition, there are 23 satellite hospice programs so that key hospice programs can provide hospice and palliative care from offices located closer to the recipients of care (HPCA, 2012). A number of the leaders of well-developed, well-known hospice programs, including St. Luke's Hospice in Cape Town, were inspired by Dame Cicely Saunders, who visited South Africa in 1982 and encouraged South African hospice leaders in their efforts (Merriman, 2006).

The HPCA was formed in 1987 as a national association in South Africa, the purpose of which was to share best practices (Gwyther, 2012). The African Palliative Care Association (APCA) was formed in Tanzania in 2004 with the purpose of providing information to increase knowledge and awareness; integrating palliative care at all levels of the health care system; and building an evidence base about palliative care throughout Africa (APCA, 2004). Although there has been a renewed emphasis by international organizations regarding palliative care for

NCDs, the needs in Africa include not only NCDs but also infectious diseases such as HIV, TB, and malaria. These health issues require a more encompassing perspective.

South Coast Hospice/Palliative Care nurses engage in palliative care by providing the injections required by patients with multidrug-resistant tuberculosis (MDR-TB). These daily visits allow patients to remain at home after their initial in-patient treatment with hope for full recovery. Such care is in response to a Department of Health request to HPCA to "support treatment and provide care to TB patients" and in particular MDR-TB patients (Gwyther, 2012, p. 2). This is also in keeping with WPCA (2014), which emphasizes that "palliative care should in no way become a substitute for appropriate curative care" (p. 8). In this example, they are one and the same.

Children and Palliative Care

For children in need of palliative care worldwide, the greatest percentage of children die from congenital anomalies (25.06%), followed by neonatal conditions (14.64%), protein energy malnutrition (14.12%), meningitis (12.62%), and HIV/AIDS (10.23%; WPCA, 2014, p. 20). The majority of children in need of palliative care are in the African region (49%), the Southeast Asia region (24%), and the Eastern Mediterranean region (12%), with the least requiring such care in the Western Pacific region (7%), the American region (5%), and the European region (3%; WPCA, 2014, pp. 19–20).

Stillbirths

Less mentioned in discussions of palliative and EOL care is the subject of stillbirths. And while care for the deceased depends on gestation and other factors, the family can benefit from bereavement care. Approximately 2.6 million stillbirths occurred worldwide in 2009, with 98% in low- and middle-income countries (Cousens et al., 2011). In the United States, where stillbirth in most states is defined as no signs of life at birth occurring at or after 20 weeks of completed gestation, figures indicate that there were 25,894 stillbirths in 2005 (Macdorman, Kimeyer, & Wilson, 2012). If the U.S. definition were applied worldwide, one would expect a substantially higher number than 2.6 million. Stillbirth remains a relatively disenfranchised death, not included in Millennium Development Goals or the Global Burden of Disease estimates (as cited in Kelley, 2011). Lawn et al. (2011) write, "Stillbirths are invisible in many societies and on the worldwide policy agenda, but are very real to families who experience a death" (p. 1448).

The WHO policy brief (2009), using data from the Cousens et al. (2011) study, noted needs in four specific areas to reduce the number of stillbirths: (a) strengthening access to good-quality reproductive health care; (b) continued research on causes and determinants; (c) improved quality and quantity of data sources; and

(d) appropriate training of those completing death certificates in the use of the International Classification of Diseases (ICD) coding.

In 2011, *The Lancet* launched a series on stillbirth in London, New York, Hobart, Geneva, New Delhi, Florence, and Cape Town, demonstrating the global interest in and concern about babies who die before or at birth. *The Lancet* (2011) series featured numerous international researchers, clinicians, and known experts writing about the broad continuum of stillbirth and its effects, including statistics, causes, and determinants to psycho-emotional care of the bereaved families (e.g., bereavement photography).

Whether in high-income or low-income countries, disparities (however they are measured) are critical components of stillbirth causation (Flenady et al., 2011). In the United States, the rate of stillbirth in non-Hispanic Black women is more than double that of non-Hispanic White women (Macdorman et al., 2012). Similarly, even in the Scandinavian countries, which include relatively homogeneous populations, those who are poorer with more deprivation have higher rates of stillbirth (Flenady et al., 2011). Frøen et al. (2011) made a strong case for why stillbirth matters from a psycho-emotional perspective. Families are left with intense grief, sometimes without support from their own families and close friends and a cadre of professionals.

A study conducted in Brazil by Bousso and Coelho Rodrigues (2011) examined the mother's experience of having a stillbirth. They found that for the mother, the news of her baby's death during the period of pregnancy was traumatic, since instead of an expectation of life, mothers found desperation and sadness. In addition, mothers in their study experienced many emotions, including shock, numbness, denial, deep sadness, guilt, anger, and depression. The grieving process was experienced in a lonely way, since the participants' sadness was not shared with families and friends. Bousso and Coelho Rodrigues (2011) found that the mothers preferred to be alone due to feeling shame for failing to produce a healthy child. For the authors of the study, this process can be represented by four epiphanies: the destruction of a dream; having a meaningless childbirth; leaving empty-handed, and having a lack of recognition of her grief and stigmatization. A mother who has had a stillbirth needs time to grieve. These mothers form a bond with their child long before birth, so they may feel intense loss when their unborn baby dies (Bousso & Coelho Rodrigues, 2011).

Although perinatal bereavement has the potential for transformative growth through intense suffering and connection (Black & Sandelowski, 2010), the negative sequelae of stillbirth on the mother and those close to her can be long-lasting if she is discouraged from doing what she needs and wants to do, such as providing care to her baby (Cacciatore, Rådestad, & Frøen, 2008; Limbo & Lathrop, 2014). Although women and families around the world grieve the death of a stillborn child, most published work on all types of perinatal loss (miscarriage, stillbirth, newborn death, and perinatal palliative care [PPC]) are authored by Euro-Americans (Callister, 2014).

WHAT NURSES AND OTHER HEALTH CARE PROVIDERS CAN DO

In 2011, a group of leaders in perinatal bereavement care wrote a position paper titled *Caring for Families Experiencing Stillbirth: A Unified Position Statement on Contact With the Baby* (Warland, Davis, & the International Stillbirth Alliance Parent Advisory Committee, 2011). The statement provides a standard of care that reflects the parents' natural desire to see and hold their baby after birth. The statement, written by 20 clinical experts, scholars, and parent advocates representing 16 organizations from nine countries, provides a worldwide standard that recognizes the baby born still as a person, valued and loved, and acknowledges the pain and grief of parents who experience such a death. The statement also offers to those caring for bereaved parents and families, including the baby who died and other children, a framework for expressing empathy, developing trust, and guiding difficult decisions. Because of its international applicability and uniqueness, the statement is printed in its entirety in Appendix 18.1.

Perinatal Palliative Care

PPC is a worldwide phenomenon. Amy Kuebelbeck (2003), author of *Waiting With Gabriel: A Story of Cherishing a Baby's Brief Life*, and co-author (Kuebelbeck & Davis, 2011) of *A Gift of Time: Continuing Your Pregnancy When Your Baby's Life Is Expected to Be Brief*, established the website perinatalhospice.org, which lists PPC programs in 44 states and 18 countries. Tammy Ruiz (2011), bereavement coordinator and PPC provider at Mary Washington Hospital in Fredericksburg, Virginia, created a film showing how she supported a family during the delivery of a baby with a life-threatening condition. The film has been translated into six languages and viewed more than 40,000 times.

Wool (2013) and Belaguer Martín-Ancel, Ortigoza-Escobar, Escribano, and Argemi (2012) summarized the state of the science/art in PPC. In the past decade, PPC research has increased exponentially, with physicians, nurses, genetic counselors, social workers, chaplains, and others publishing findings that guide clinicians in their care of bereaved families. Belaguer et al. (2012), who are from Spain, also noted that most studies they reviewed were conducted in the United States. The research delineates care in five primary areas: (1) prenatal diagnosis, (2) advance care planning, (3) labor and delivery care, (4) genetic counseling, and (5) ongoing care for babies who survive the perinatal period (Kobler & Limbo, 2011; Limbo, Toce, & Peck, 2008/2009). Both Wool (2013) and Belaguer et al. (2012) highlight the importance of care that is family-centered, begins at the time of diagnosis, provides options for method of delivery (e.g., cesarean delivery by choice), and focuses on the relationship between parents and providers that is based on empathic communication. Based on the number of published articles, Belaguer (2012) noted that interest in neonatal and palliative care is strongest in the United States and Europe. However, they also remind the reader that PPC in other areas of the world may have different sociological and clinical contexts. But despite these possibly different contexts, the significance to parents and families worldwide is important to recognize, particularly since child and infant mortality continue to be a global issue.

Finally, Belaguer et al. (2012) emphasize that PPC needs to be integrated, moving seamlessly among curative and palliative measures. Milstein (2014) and Kobler and Limbo (2011) proposed that both "bereavement" and "hope" be encased in such an integrative model. This integrative model presents an approach that can be utilized not only for PPC but for palliative care in general. Being aware of the prior losses faced by persons with life-threatening diseases and their families, and how they coped with these challenges, can provide valuable insights as to how best to support patients and families currently. While cultures influence how illness and death are approached, persons confronting EOL care deserve to have their wishes respected by their caregivers, whether lay or professional. And for nurses, wherever they may practice, this is part of their credo.

REFERENCES

African Palliative Care Association (APCA). (2004). Retrieved from www .africanpalliativecare.org/about/about-apca/

Applebaum, P. S., & Grisso, T. (1988). Assessing patients' capacities to consent to treatment. *New England Journal of Medicine, 319*(25), 1635–1638.

Applebaum, P. S., & Grisso, T. (1989). Assessing patients' capacities to consent to treatment. Erratum. *The New England Journal of Medicine, 320* (11), 748.

Baliza, M. G. (2013). *The nurse's experience in decision-making processes in end-of-life situations lived in intensive care units* (Dissertation). University of Sao Paolo Nursing School, Sao Paolo, Brazil.

Belaguer, A., Martín-Ancel, A., Ortigoza-Escobar, D., Escribano, J., & Argemi, J. (2012). The model of palliative care in the perinatal setting: A review of the literature. *BMC Pediatrics, 12*(25), 1–7.

Beresford, L., & Connor, S. R. (1999). History of the National Hospice Organization. In I. B. Corless & Z. Foster (Eds.), *The hospice heritage: Celebrating our future* (pp. 15–31). Philadelphia, PA: Haworth Press.

Black, B., & Sandelowski, M. (2010). Personal growth after severe fetal diagnosis. *Western Journal of Nursing Research, 32*(8), 1011–1030.

Bousso, R. S., & Coelho Rodrigues, M. M. (2011). *The mother's experience of having a stillborn child*. EUA 33rd Annual Conference; Miami, Florida, June 21–22, 2011.

Bousso, R. S., Misko, M. D., Mendes-Castillo, A. M., & Rossato, L. M. (2012). Family Management Style Framework and its use with families who have a child undergoing palliative care at home. *Journal of Family Nursing, 18*(1), 91–122.

Cacciatore, J., Rådestad, I., & Frøen, J. F. (2008). Effects of contact with stillborn babies on maternal anxiety and depression. *Birth, 35*(4), 313–320.

Callister, L. C. (2014). Global perspectives on perinatal loss. *American Journal of Maternal Child Nursing, 39*(3), 207. doi:10.1097/NMC.0000000000000033

Corless, I. B. (1983). The hospice movement in North America. In C. A. Corr & D. M. Corr (Eds.), *Hospice care principles and practice* (pp. 335–351). New York, NY: Springer Publishing.

Cousens, S., Blencowe, H., Stanton, C., Chou, D., Ahmed, S., Steinhardt, L., . . . Lawn, J. E. (2011). National, regional, and worldwide estimates of stillbirth rates in 2009 with trends since 1995: A systematic analysis. *The Lancet, 377*(9774), 1319–1330. doi:10.1016/S0140-6736(10)62310-0

eHospice. (2014). *World Health Organization (WHO) Executive Board adopts resolution on palliative care.* Retrieved from http://www.ehospice.com/ArticleView/tabid/10686/ArticleId/8580/language/en-GB/View

Flenady, V., Middleton, P., Smith, G. C., Duke, W., Erwich, J. J., Khong, T. Y., . . . *Lancet's* Stillbirths Series steering committee. (2011). Stillbirths: The way forward in high-income countries. *The Lancet, 377,* 1703–1717.

Frøen, J. F., Cacciatore, J., McClure, E. M., Kuti, O., Jokhio, A. H., Islam, M., . . . *Lancet's* Stillbirths Series steering committee. (2011). Stillbirths: Why they matter. *The Lancet, 377*(9774), 1353–1366.

Gwyther, L. (2012). Introduction. In S. Ameron et al. (Eds.), *HPCA's best practice series* (pp. 2–3). Retrieved from www.hospicepalliativecare.SA.CO.ZA/pdf/HPCA_Best_Practices_Series_final_print.pdf

Hospice Palliative Care Association of South Africa (HPCA). (2012). *Hospice palliative care association of South Africa.* Retrieved from http://www.hospicepalliativecaresa.co.za

Kelley, M. (2011). Counting stillbirths: Women's health and reproductive rights. *The Lancet, 377,* 1636–1637.

Kobler, K., & Limbo, R. (2011). Making a case: Creating a perinatal palliative care service using a perinatal bereavement program model. *The Journal of Perinatal & Neonatal Nursing, 25,* 32–41.

Kuebelbeck, A. (2003). *Waiting with Gabriel: A story of cherishing a baby's brief life.* Chicago, IL: Loyola Press.

Kuebelbeck, A., & Davis, D. L. (2011). *A gift of time: Continuing your pregnancy when your baby's life is expected to be brief.* Baltimore, MD: Johns Hopkins Press.

Lancet. (2011). Stillbirths. Retrieved from http://www.thelancet.com/series/stillbirth

Lawn, J. E., Blencowe, H., Pattinson, R., Cousens, S., Kumar, R., Ibiebele, I., . . . Stanton, C. (2011). Stillbirths: When? Where? Why? How to make the data count. *The Lancet, 377,* 1448–1463.

Limbo, R., & Lathrop, A. (2014). Caregiving in mothers' narratives of perinatal hospice. *Illness, Crisis, & Loss, 22*(1), 43–65.

Limbo, R., Toce, S., & Peck, T. (2008/2009). *Resolve through sharing position paper on perinatal palliative care.* Retrieved from bereavementservices.org/position papers

Macdorman, M. F., Kimeyer, S., & Wilson, E. C. (2012). Fetal and perinatal mortality. U.S., 2006. *National Vital Statistics Reports, 60*(8). Retrieved from http://www.cdc.gov/nchs/data/nvsr/nvsr60/nvsr60_08.pdf

McAteer, R., & Wellbery, C. (2013). Palliative care: Benefits, barriers, and best practices. *American Family Physician, 88*(12), 811–813A.

Merriman, A. (2006). The development of palliative care in Africa. In E. Bruera, I. Higginson, & C. F. von Gunten (Eds.), *Textbook of palliative medicine* (pp. 42–48). Boca Raton, FL: CRC Press, Taylor & Francis Group.

Milstein, J. M. (2014). Our moral imperative: Finding a path to wholeness. *Clinical Pediatrics,* 1–3. doi:10.1177/0009922814527506

Ministério da Saúde. (2014), Retrieved from http://portal.saude.gov.br/portal/saude/cidadao/area.cfm?id_area=1395

Mor, V., & Masterson-Allen, A. (1987). *Hospice care systems–structure, process, costs, and outcome.* New York, NY: Springer Publishing.

Ruiz, T. (2011). Perinatal hospice video (English, Spanish, Italian) [Video file]. Retrieved from http://www.youtube.com/watch?v=tY7mq1g9pGk

Saunders, C. (1999). Origins: International perspectives, then and now. In I. B. Corless & Z. Foster (Eds.), *The hospice heritage: Celebrating our future* (pp. 1–7). Philadelphia, PA: Haworth Press.

Temel, J. S., Greer, J. A., Muzikansky, A., Gallagher, E. R., Admane, S., Jackson, V. A., . . . Lynch, T. (2010). Early palliative care for patients with metastatic non-small cell lung cancer. *New England Journal of Medicine, 363*(8), 733–742.

Warland, J., Davis, D. L., & the International Stillbirth Alliance (ISA) Parent Advisory Committee. (2011). *Caring for families experiencing stillbirth: A unified position statement on contact with the baby.* ISA Baltimore. Retrieved from http://www.gundersenhealth.org/resolve-through-sharing/publications-and-research/position-papers

Wool, C. (2013). State of the science on perinatal palliative care. *Journal of Obstetric, Gynecologic, & Neonatal Nursing, 42,* 372–382. doi:10.1111/1552-6909.12034

World Health Organization (WHO). (2002). *WHO definition of palliative care.* Retrieved from http://www.who.int/cancer/palliative/definition/en

World Health Organization. (2009). National, regional, and worldwide estimates of stillbirth rates in 2009 with trends since 1995. *World Health Organization Policy Brief.* Retrieved from http://www.who.int/reproductivehealth/topics/maternal_perinatal/stillbirth/en

Worldwide Palliative Care Alliance (WPCA). (2014) *World Health Organization adopts ground breaking palliative care resolution.* Retrieved from http://www.thewpca.org/latest-news/who-adopts-palliative-care-resolution

Zaros, M. C., Curtis, J. R., Silveira, M. J., & Elmore, J. G. (2013). Opportunity lost: End of life discussions in cancer patients who die in the hospital. *Journal of Hospital Medicine, 8*(6), 334–340.

APPENDIX 18.1

CARING FOR FAMILIES EXPERIENCING STILLBIRTH: A UNIFIED POSITION STATEMENT ON CONTACT WITH THE BABY

Preamble

Stillbirth is recognized as one of the most traumatic experiences a parent can go through and may be associated with long-lasting psychosocial effects. Additionally, parents may have had limited or no previous experience with death. They are typically fearful and confused about what to expect and normal response, and there is much evidence that doing so can be a valuable and cherished experience. Parents benefit from support and individualized guidance as they make their own decisions about how much time to spend with their baby, and as they determine when and how to use this time.

Position Statement

Prior to the 1970s, standard hospital practice in the aftermath of stillbirth was to discourage or disallow bereaved parents from seeing their deceased baby. However, in the late 1970s, providers of maternity care began to pay attention to bereaved parents' requests to see their expected baby, and a body of research emerged, which resulted in a shift of practice standards.[1-3] For the next 30 years in most western countries, bereaved families were encouraged to see and hold their baby.

Since 2002, this practice has been questioned following publication of one study which concluded that for some parents, seeing their baby's body results in long-term negative psychological outcomes.[4] This small study has affected bereavement care in some countries, such that some providers of maternity care no longer encourage or guide bereaved parents to have contact with their stillborn baby. This reversal of practice standards is troubling because there is virtually no evidence that discouraging parents from seeing their baby is helpful to their long-term emotional health.

In fact the many studies and guidelines published both before and since 2002[5-24] demonstrate that parents can benefit from spending time with their baby, as they acquire affirming experiences and cherished memories. Conversely, when parents do not see and hold their baby, many express deep regret. Furthermore, in many cultures there are widely accepted customs and rituals involving holding and caring for the body of a deceased loved one of any age. These traditions assist the bereaved in recognizing the reality of the death, saying goodbye, and grieving the loss.[25-30]

Parents normally see and hold their baby after a live birth. It is therefore counterintuitive to suggest that parents would not benefit from nor wish to see their baby after stillbirth. Whether and how to spend time with their deceased baby is a very personal decision, and it is important to ensure that all parents are given enough support and information to enable them to make informed choices.

Recommendations

As international leaders in the perinatal bereavement caregiving community, we make the following recommendations to policy makers and practitioners who work with families experiencing stillbirth. These recommendations are based on: (a) empirical studies, (b) anecdotal wisdom, (c) direct practice experiences of interdisciplinary clinicians, and (d) the advocacy work of grassroots organizations led by bereaved parents.

1. Provide a standard of care that reflects the parents' natural desire to see and hold their baby after birth. This means not asking closed-ended questions such as, "Do you want to . . . ?" Parents will usually reply "no" to such questions but they don't mean "no" forever, just "no" for now.

2. **After bad news is broken**: Begin by aiming to foster a sensitive relationship with the parents. Gauge their needs by having open-ended conversations about their experience, their baby, and their care. Understand that parents will be shocked and will not be able to take in or say too much at this time. Keep information about their options simple and offer it in both written and verbal forms. During this time, if parents express reluctance to see or hold their baby, sensitively explore their fears and concerns, including the likely appearance of their baby. Assure them that you will be with them as they meet their baby.

3. **During labor and birth**: If parents have not raised any concerns about contact with their baby, then proceed just as naturally and respectfully as you would with any parents who wish to see and hold their expected newborn.

4. **Following the birth:** Provide gentle, individualized guidance when parents are meeting their baby. Most parents feel emotionally overwhelmed and this can affect their ability to make prudent decisions, consider the long-term consequences of their actions, or advocate for themselves. If necessary, normalize contact with their infant by sharing how other parents find that saying hello to their babies affirms the baby's importance and offers cherished memories. Modeling, such as cuddling and speaking softly to their baby, can be a powerful, affirming demonstration that may offer parents a path to spending time with their infant.

5. If parents decline to see or spend time with their baby, respect and fully support their wishes. Continue to engage in sensitive conversations with the parents about their baby and experience. Explain that they can change their minds at any time up to burial or cremation. Collecting mementos for these families may still be appropriate, with their consent. The family may choose to take the mementos with them, or the facility can keep them for possible collection at a later date.

When acting on these recommendations, be mindful of the shock, trauma, and grief inherent in experiencing the death of a baby. Consider the parents' need to take their time with emotional processing, decision making, and desired contact with their baby. Each parent's personal values, cultural traditions, and religious beliefs may also influence the amount of time spent with a deceased baby or occasionally preclude contact. Provide care in a manner that is intentional, unhurried, calm, respectful, and culturally sensitive.

Ideally these recommendations would be conducted by well-trained, experienced personnel, with mentoring in place for inexperienced personnel. We also recommend that those providing direct care participate in ongoing professional development and study resources offering ways to support families, build relationships, and discuss options in open-ended conversations. Finally, we recommend the establishment of well-planned, evidence-based bereavement care policies, protocols, and guidelines in all clinics and hospitals where stillbirth might occur, and administrative support for ongoing implementation.

REFERENCES

1. Giles PF. Reactions of women to perinatal death. *Aust N Z J Obstet Gynaecol.* 1970;10(4):207–210.
2. Kennell JH, Slyter H, Klaus MH. The mourning response of parents to the death of a newborn infant. *N Engl J Med.* 1970;283(7): 344–349.
3. Lewis E. Mourning by the family after a stillbirth or neonatal death. *Arch Dis Child.* 1979;54(4):303–306.
4. Hughes P, Turton P, Hopper E, Evans CD. Assessment of guidelines for good practice in psychosocial care of mothers after stillbirth: a cohort study. *Lancet.* 2002;360(9327):114–118.
5. Lovell A. Some questions of identity: late miscarriage, stillbirth and perinatal loss. *Soc Sci Med.* 1983;17(11):755–761.
6. Rådestad I, Steineck G, Nordin C, Sjögren B. Psychological complications after stillbirth—influence of memories and immediate management: population based study. *BMJ.* 1996;312(7045):1505–1508.
7. Trulsson O, Rådestad I. The silent child—mothers' experiences before, during, and after stillbirth. *Birth.* 2004;31(3):189–195.
8. Cacciatore J, Rådestad I, Frederik Frøen J. (2008). Effects of contact with stillborn babies on maternal anxiety and depression. *Birth.* 2008;35(4):313–320.
9. Barr P, Cacciatore J. Problematic emotions and maternal grief. *Omega (Westport),* 2007;56(4):331–348.
10. Cacciatore J. Stillbirth: patient-centered psychosocial care. *Clin Obstet Gynecol.* 2010;53(3):691–699.
11. Cacciatore J. The unique experiences of women and their families after the death of a baby. *Soc Work Health Care.* 2010;49(2):134–148.
12. Wijngaards-de Meij L, Stroebe M, Stroebe W, et al. The impact of circumstances surrounding the death of a child on parents' grief. *Death Stud.* 2008;32(3):237–252.
13. Cacciatore J. The silent birth: a feminist perspective. *Soc Work.* 2009;54(1):91–95.
14. Rådestad I, Christoffersen L. Helping a woman meet her stillborn baby while it is soft and warm. *British Journal of Midwifery.* 2008;19(9):588–591.

15. Schott J, Henley A, Kohner N. *Pregnancy Loss and the Death of a Baby: Guidelines for Professionals.* 3rd ed. Sands UK/Bosun-Publications; 2007.

16. Flenady V, Wilson T. Support for mothers, fathers and families after perinatal death. *Cochrane Database Syst Rev.* 2008;(1):CD000452. doi:10.1002/14651858.CD000452.pub2

17. Pregnancy Loss and Infant Death Alliance. Practice Guidelines: Offering the Baby to Bereaved Parents. 2008. http://www.plida.org/pdf/PLIDA%20Guidelines%20 Offering%20Baby.pdf. Accessed May 4, 2011.

18. Primeau MR, Lamb JM. When a baby dies: rights of the baby and parents. *J Obstet Gynecol Neonatal Nurs.* 1995;24(3):206–208.

19. Rådestad I, Surkan PJ, Steineck G, Cnattingius S, Onelov E, Dickman PW. Long-term outcomes for mothers who have or have not held their stillborn baby. *Midwifery.* 2009;25(4):422–429.

20. Limbo R, Kobler K. The tie that binds: relationships in perinatal bereavement. *MCN Am J Matern Child Nurs.* 2010;35(6):316-321; quiz 321–323.

21. Gold KJ, Dalton VK, Schwenk TL. Hospital care for parents after perinatal death. *Obstet Gynecol.* 2007;109(5):1156–1166.

22. Brabin PJ. To see or not to see: that is the question. Challenging good-practice bereavement care after a baby is stillborn: the case in Australia. *Grief Matters: Australian Journal of Grief and Bereavement.* 2004;7(2):28–33.

23. Christoffersen L. Parents experience and the use of the Norwegian public health service previous to, during and after stillbirth: a pilot project. 2009 [link to English abstract http://www.lub.no/id/22706C42B07BE677C1257689004ED9EB, Paper in Norwegian] Accessed May 4 2011.

24. Davis DL. Reflections on the *Lancet* Stillbirth Study. *The Forum: Newsletter of the American Association of Death Education and Counseling.* 2004;30(2):4–5.

25. Beder J. Mourning the unfound: how we can help. *Fam Soc.* 2002;83(4):400–404.

26. Boss P. *Ambiguous loss: learning to live with unresolved grief.* Cambridge, Massachusetts: Harvard University Press; 1999.

27. Worden JW. *Grief counseling and grief therapy: a handbook for the mental health practitioner.* New York: Springer Pub; 2008.

28. Cooke MW, Cooke HM, Glucksman EE. Management of sudden bereavement in the accident and emergency department. *BMJ.* 1992;304(6836):1207–1209.

29. Chapple A, Ziebland S. Viewing the body after bereavement due to a traumatic death: qualitative study in the UK. *BMJ.* 2010;340:c2032.

30. Paul R. Viewing the body and grief complications: the role of visual confirmation in grief reconciliation. In: Cox GR, Bendiksen R, Stevenson RG, eds. *Complicated grieving and bereavement: understanding and treating people experiencing loss.* Amityville, New York: Baywood; 2002.

Contributors

Joanne Cacciatore, PhD, MSW
Assistant Professor, Arizona State University
Founder, MISS Foundation International, USA

Jillian Cassidy
Bereaved parent, Parent advocate
Cofounder, Umamanita, Spain

Line Christoffersen, PhD
Bereaved parent, Parent advocate
Associate Professor, Oslo School of Management, Norway

Liz Conway
Bereaved parent, Parent advocate
SANDS Australia

Mairie Cregan, MIITD, MSW
Bereaved parent, Lecturer
University College Cork, Feileacain, Ireland

Vicki Culling, PhD, MSW
Bereaved parent, Co-chair, PAC/ISA & ISA Board
Sands New Zealand

Deborah Davis, PhD
Psychologist, Writer, *Empty Cradle, Broken Heart*
www.NICUparenting.org, USA

Pat Flynn, PhD
Bereaved parent, Parent advocate
CEO, 1st Breath, Treasurer ISA Board, USA

Sue Hale
Bereaved parent, Parent advocate
Group Development Manager, Sands, United Kingdom

Suzanne Helzer, RNC-OB, LCCE
Bereavement Services/RTS Program Coordinator
Banner Desert Medical Center, Mesa, AZ, USA

Sherokee Ilse
Bereaved parent/Advocate; Int'l speaker; Author, *Empty Arms*
Babies Remembered Co-chair PAC/ISA, ISPID Board, USA

Cathi Lammert, RN
Bereaved parent; President, PLIDA; Executive Director,
Share Pregnancy & Infant Loss Support, Inc., USA

Rana Limbo, PhD, RN
Director, Bereavement Services
Gundersen Lutheran Medical Foundation, Inc., USA

Joann O'Leary, PhD, MPH, MS
Parent/Infant Specialist; Field Faculty,
Center for Early Education and Development, University of Minnesota, USA

Suzanne Pullen
Bereaved parent, Parent advocate, Communication educator
PAC/ISA, Doctoral student, Arizona State University, USA

Ingela Rådestad, RN, RM, PhD
Professor, Sophiahemmet University College
President, Swedish National Infant Foundation, Sweden

Claudia Ravaldi, MD, MSc
Psychiatrist, Psychotherapist, ISA Board and PAC member, Founder and President
CiaoLapo Charity for Perinatal Grief Support, Italy

Janne Teigen, RN, RM
Bereaved parent, Parent advocate, Author, Midwife,
Hospital of Telemark, Norway

Alfredo Vannacci, MD, PhD
ISA PAC member, Founder and Vice-President,
CiaoLapo Charity for Perinatal Grief Support, Italy

Jane Warland, RN, RM, PhD
Bereaved parent, Midwife, Author, Faculty (Nursing and Midwifery)
University of South Australia, Australia

Organizations Supporting This Statement

1st Breath (USA)
Babies Remembered (USA)
Bereavement Services (USA)
CiaoLapo Onlus (ITALY)
Feileacain (SANDAI) (IRELAND)
International Society for the study and prevention of Perinatal and Infant Death (ISPID)
Norwegian SIDS and Stillbirth Society
Pregnancy Loss and Infant Death Alliance (International)
Sands (New Zealand)
Sands (UK)
SANDS (Australia)
Share Pregnancy & Infant Loss Support, Inc. (USA)
Star Legacy Foundation (USA)
Swedish National Infant Foundation
The MISS Foundation International (USA)
Umamanita (SPAIN)

Acknowledgments

This position statement was initiated by Sherokee Ilse and the Parent Advisory Committee (PAC) of the International Stillbirth Alliance (ISA). It was developed by a group of bereaved parents, health care professionals, international scholars, and other experts in the area of perinatal loss and bereavement led by Jane Warland and Deborah L. Davis. For editorial expertise, the authors thank Cathy Fischer, Managing Editor/Writer, Department of Medical Research, Gundersen Lutheran Medical Foundation, Inc., USA. © 2011 This Position Paper may be copied in its entirety with no alterations. The recommended citation is Warland, J., Davis, D. L., et al. (2011). Caring for Families Experiencing Stillbirth: A Unified Position Statement on Contact With the Baby. An International Collaboration.

Achieving Global Health

Inge B. Corless

*A*chieving global health is akin to achieving nirvana. Unfortunately, unlike mathematics, solutions to the challenges in global health are not typified by elegance but rather by pragmatics. There is not one problem or one approach.

The chapters in this section exemplify the efforts of dedicated professionals in meeting an array of health care challenges. These illustrations are not exhaustive of the excellent programs that have been implemented in the past or are currently in progress.

In Chapter 19, von Zinkernagel, Palen, and Kaplan focus on approaches to increasing access to primary care, notably enhancing the competencies and, in particular, the scope of practice of the nursing workforce. To achieve the goal of expanded access to care, they discuss such strategies as improving nursing education to focus on primary care nursing, approaches to strengthening the systems supporting the provision of nursing care, and societal level structural changes.

The challenges posed by international nurse migration are addressed by Huston in Chapter 20. The push-and-pull factors fueling migration include an exploration of the needs of both destination and donor nations. The rights of nurses to emigrate and how this may conflict with the societal needs of donor nations is followed by a discussion of approaches to resolving this conundrum—approaches that would promote greater health equity.

Hoffart, Brown, and Farrell, in Chapter 21, detail an initiative aimed at achieving this goal and describes the role of nurse leaders in this effort. The initiative occurred in Lebanon in the newly established School of Nursing and School of Medicine. Reported in this chapter is how the new deans of these schools plus the dean of Pharmacy traversed the territory between an idea and the reality of implementation of interprofessional education.

Continuing education is a necessary component of the intellectual life of any professional. It becomes all the more vital when the education concerns the enhanced care of patients and populations. In Chapter 22, Tyer-Viola addresses this topic and its application to nursing, and gives particular emphasis to countries with fewer resources. The various types of continuing education are delineated together with the argument that the rationale for continuing education is practice change that results in improved patient outcomes. The challenges to achieving this goal are elaborated.

Chapter 23 considers the development of nursing in China and Thailand and the historical, political, and economic factors, together with the cultural embrace of Confucianism, affecting this development. The analysis by Chaiphibalsarisdi, Meedzan, Nicholas, and Meedzan focuses on the history of nursing in each country given the particularities of that country as well as the transition in emphasis from acute care to health promotion and well-being.

As a further contrast, the development of professional nursing education in South Africa is detailed by Klopper and Uys in Chapter 24. Here, too, the influence of the political structure is considered. The nurse leaders and organizations that have played an important role are described, as are the lessons learned—the most significant of these being the importance of leadership and an appreciation for the length of time required for sustainable change.

Chapter 25 discusses another issue: how nursing programs produce graduates who are culturally competent. Meedzan reviews theories of cultural competence and the evidence of the success of various global immersion programs for enhancing cultural humility, and hopefully competence, in the participants of such experiences. Given that health disparities are pronounced in many countries and between countries, the importance of such efforts cannot be overstated.

The role of faith-based organizations in closing the gap in "health achievements" is discussed in Chapter 26 by Lindgren, Rankin, and Schell, with a particular emphasis on Malawi. Recognizing the importance of religion for people worldwide but particularly in Africa, the authors focus on their work in HIV prevention with faith-based organizations, sharing the lessons they have learned in this chapter.

Lessons learned are also a contribution by Hickey, Lou, and Hsu who review the history of the collaboration between the Shanghai Children's Medical Center and the Boston Children's Hospital in Chapter 27. The goal of the collaboration is to increase nursing knowledge and improve the care, and subsequently the lives, of youngsters with cardiovascular disease.

A similar concern is the focus of Chapter 28 where Patton-Bolman, Bigirimana, and Carragher examine their efforts to improve cardiovascular care in Rwanda for both children and adults. The role of partnerships is made explicit in this chapter, as it also has been in some of the preceding chapters. The distinctive role of TeamHeart is described, as are plans for future initiatives. The importance of such efforts fitting with national priorities is stressed.

Problem Solving for Better Health is a model used by the Dreyfus Foundation as the basis for their work in 32 countries (including the United States). In Chapter 29, Hoyt-Hudson, Tsai, Fitzpatrick, and Smith detail these efforts and the central role of nursing in achieving a reduction in the burden of disease. Their plans for the future include evaluation of various aspects of the program in their efforts to improve their collaborative endeavors in enhancing health.

Like earlier chapters, Chapter 30 is replete with lessons learned by the author as a Fulbright scholar in Swaziland. In his efforts to assist with capacity building, advance professionalism, and engage in research, among other activities, Mallinson puts a human face, as have other chapter authors, on living and working in another country with the goal of assisting in the improvement of health care.

In the final chapter in this section and in the book, Kurth, Squires, Shedlin, and Kiarie encapsulate many of the themes of previous chapters. The title of Chapter 31 is Interdisciplinary Collaborations in Global Health Research, and while this is the only chapter explicitly about research, the explication of the challenges and benefits of collaboration and the important role of nursing is germane to all of the chapters in this section and to this book. Given that research is where it starts and ends and is the basis for evidence-based practice, Chapter 31 is an appropriate coda for this book.

The collective hope of the authors and editors of this text is that the approaches reported in these chapters inspire the development of other collaborations in our efforts to improve the health and well-being of the world's people. As the editors of *Global Health Nursing in the 21st Century*, we express our appreciation to the authors of these chapters for their work and the inspiration they provide to all of us.

CHAPTER 19

Expanding Access to Address Priority Health Needs in Low-Resource Settings

Deborah von Zinkernagel, John Palen, and Avril Kaplan

The severe shortage of the current health care workforce, including physicians, nurses, and midwives, has contributed to elevated rates of morbidity and mortality from commonly preventable or managed illnesses in many low- and middle-income countries (LMIC; Buchan & Calman, 2004; International Council of Nurses/Florence Nightingale International Foundation [ICN/FNIF] 2006; Lozano et al., 2012). The burden and pressures on health systems continue to rise as a result of numerous interconnected factors, including growing and ageing populations; the rising prevalence of noncommunicable diseases (NCDs) such as heart disease, cancer, and diabetes, and those related to risk factors such as obesity and alcohol abuse; and environmental and urban health issues linked with climate change, poverty, conflicts, greater mobility, and globalization (Bryar, Kendall, & Mogtlane, 2012; ICN/FNIF, 2006; Lozano et al., 2012). In response to expanding need and rising demand, there has been a global movement to expand primary health care (PHC) in LMIC to deliver services at the community level (Keleher et al., 2007; Laurant et al., 2005). The World Health Organization's (WHO) Declaration of Alma Ata in 1978 and World Health Report 2008, *Primary Health Care Now More Than Ever*, both stress the importance of strengthening universal access to care by deploying health workers at the community level and delivering patient-centered services (WHO, 1978, 2008b).

The majority of health services in LMICs are delivered by nurses and other trained cadres, serving as the primary point of contact within communities (WHO, 2009b). The Chiang Mai Declaration of 2008 focuses specifically on the role of nursing and midwifery staff, and stresses that primary health care and the Millennium Development Goals will not be achieved without scaling up these two cadres (Chiang Mai Declaration, 2008). The declaration calls for new legislation that will expand the scope of practice for nurses and midwives operating in communities, and for the health system to focus on primary health care. Multiple World Health Assembly (WHA) Resolutions[1] call for a renewed focus on primary health care with a strong reliance on nurses as the primary care givers. The resolutions show the importance that WHO member states attach to nursing and midwifery services as a means for achieving better health for all.

This chapter explores and identifies essential policy and programmatic options to increase access to primary health care services through improved training and expanded competencies of the nursing cadre. In doing so, attention needs to be paid to the nature of the nursing education experience and professional environment; the alignment of nursing competencies with local community population health needs; availability of a functional service delivery system including facilities, drugs, equipment, and other vital elements; and the policy and programmatic elements and leadership provided by national governments and other key stakeholders, such as training institutions and regulatory bodies.

THE CASE FOR NURSING

As countries act to expand primary health care for their citizens, they can build from the strong foundation of PHC nursing. Nurses in LMICs are a unique cadre within the health system: They are the main providers of care and frequently serve in multiple roles as clinicians, counselors, educators, case managers, advocates, and consultants, often concurrently (WHO, 2010a). With appropriate training and support, nurses are uniquely positioned to manage complex conditions and their associated risk factors that contribute to the leading causes of death and disability in LMICs (Lozano et al., 2012). Box 19.1 provides information on the burden of disease with particular reference to low-income countries. Furthermore, nurses are positioned to coordinate care from the community up to higher levels of the system (Keleher et al., 2007). Many interventions have been used to expand the reach of nurses serving in the community. For example, there has been an increase in the number of nurse-led clinics and walk-in centers, health advice delivered by nurses over the telephone, and more often, nurses taking on the role of general practitioners to care for minor illness and to manage chronic conditions (Keleher et al., 2007).

Supporting this trend, evidence is growing that shows a positive impact of nurses serving as providers of PHC. In a study by Keleher et al. (2007) on community nursing, the authors found that nurse-led services in a primary care

BOX 19.1 GLOBAL BURDEN OF DISEASE FACTS

- The leading causes of death in low-income countries are pneumonia, heart disease, diarrhea, HIV/AIDS, and stroke
- The leading risk factors of death in low-income countries are childhood malnutrition; high blood pressure; unsafe sex; unsafe water, sanitation, and hygiene; high blood glucose; indoor smoke from solid fuels; tobacco use; physical inactivity; suboptimal breastfeeding; and high cholesterol
- As a result of injuries, violence, conflict, and higher levels of heart disease, men aged 15 to 60 years have higher risks of dying than women of the same age in every region of the world
- Depression is the leading cause of years lost due to disability
- Alcohol dependence and problem use is among the 10 leading causes of disability across all income strata (WHO, 2009a)

setting resulted in higher patient satisfaction and quality of life as compared with physician-led services in the same setting. A WHO report in 2010 found that nurse-led care at the community level increases the cost-effectiveness of services; contributes positively to disease prevention by increasing surveillance, early detection of disease, and health promotion; and reduces newborn, infant, and maternal mortality (WHO, 2010d). Finally, in light of increasing NCDs, which are responsible for 60% of deaths worldwide, a second WHO study found that nurses have provided successful follow-up to address the key risk factors of certain NCDs (WHO, 2012).

To date, some LMICs have used task shifting as an approach for nurses to expand the delivery of PHC services in a community setting (McCarthy, Zuber, Kelley, Verani, & Riley, 2010). Task shifting involves substitu-ting tasks among different professionals, or delegating roles and responsibilities from one employee to another with less training (Fulton et al., 2011). Recent evidence shows that task shifting affords quality, cost-effective care to more patients than a physician-centered model (Callaghan, Ford, & Schneider, 2010). In countries with high prevalence rates of HIV, such as South Africa, Rwanda, and Ethiopia, task shifting was found to be a successful approach to increasing access to HIV services and improving adherence to treatment regimens (Callaghan et al., 2010; Dohrn, Nzama, & Murrman, 2009; Fairall et al., 2012; Johns et al., 2014; Petersen, Lund, & Alan, 2012; Shumbusho et al., 2009; Zuber, McCarthy, Verani, Msidi, & Johnson, 2014). WHO supports task shifting as a central approach to scaling up HIV services in Africa, and released global recommendations and guidelines for task shifting in 2008 (WHO, 2008a). In terms of NCDs, a study by Lekoubou, Awah, Fezeu, and Pascal Kengne (2010) found that task shifting improves access to care for hypertension and diabetes in sub-Saharan Africa (Lekoubou et al., 2010).

While task shifting has produced positive results, the sustainability and adequacy of this approach has been at the center of the debate (Lehmann, Van Damme, Barten, & Sanders, 2009; Zachariah et al., 2009). Oftentimes, to prepare nurses to take on more responsibility, training workshops that may result in higher absenteeism in health facilities are used to scale up select nursing competencies (Zachariah et al., 2009). These new skills are usually not regulated, and payment and management structures do not adjust for the new role of the nurse within the health system (Lehmann et al., 2009; Zachariah et al., 2009). Expanding the supply of nurses for delivery of health care is therefore not just an issue of increasing the absolute number of workers or expanding their tasks to meet health needs; it relies more broadly on the adequacy of training, labor market dynamics, and regulatory and support structures in place for nurses (McPake, Maeda, Araujo, Maghraby, & Cometto, 2013). To achieve a durable and well-grounded impact on population health outcomes, there is both opportunity and need to incorporate a focus on PHC needs and address commonly preventable diseases as a part of preservice nursing training, thereby equipping nurses for expanded scopes of practice. The parameters of an expanded scope of practice would be defined by "the range of roles, functions, responsibilities and activities, which a registered/ licensed professional is educated for, competent in, and is authorized to perform" (Affara, 2009, p. 6), identifying both the accountability for, and limits of, practice.

Once nurses are prepared to carry out expanded scopes of practice in primary care, they also need adequate organizational and regulatory support systems throughout their career to ensure that new skills are maintained and translated into higher quality patient care.

This chapter discusses advancing the goal of expanding access to PHC by focusing and investing in the nursing workforce through three strategies: transforming nursing education to train primary care nurses, strengthening delivery and support systems, and revising a country's policy and regulatory environment. As outlined in Figure 19.1, this chapter also considers specific

Goal: Implement a framework for nursing practice that affords increased access to primary health care services within the community		
Strategy Transform using education to train primary care nurses	Strengthen delivery and support systems	Revise policy and regulatory environment
Objectives • Establish primary care competencies, critical thinking, and learning skills relevant to public health needs • Drive transormative learning • Establish interdependence of learning environment with primary care setting • Establish professional education opportunities that include management and leadership	• Nurses are motivated and supported in their roles • Clear career pathways for professional development are in place • Nurses work in multidisciplinary teams • Adequate resources and infrastructure to fulfill role are in place	• Greater political commitment to nursing for expansion of access to primary care • Legal and regulatory framework to support expanded scopes of practice • Professional associations and councils role advance nursing
Implementation • Develop priorities for education reform • Revise curriculum and establish competency-based learning • Train and retain faculty • Continued professional education to advance primary health care • Identify sources of financing for education	• Use of supportive supervision and clinical mentors • Interdisciplinary care teams • Financial and non-financial incentives that motivate staff • Referral systems to connect community to the health system • Define opportunities for professional development • Adequate infrastructure and materials for delivery of care	• Government leadership and key stakeholder consensus around expanded scope of practice • Implement regulatory framework for expanded scope of practice and career opportunities • Document outcomes and best practices • Include nurses in policy and planning decisions

FIGURE 19.1 Strategy to increase access to primary health care services within the community.

objectives for each strategy and makes recommendations for how countries can begin implementing a more sustainable model for PHC through community-level nursing care.

NURSING COMPETENCIES FOR EFFECTIVE DELIVERY OF PHC SERVICES AT THE COMMUNITY LEVEL

There are a number of key issues for consideration in promoting the engagement of PHC nurses in health care delivery systems in LMIC, including (a) sufficient pre- and in-service training to ensure skills are current and based on acceptable norms of practice; (b) competencies in the prevention, diagnosis, and management of common illnesses—acute and chronic—and across the life span; (c) communication and leadership and management skills; (d) recognition and application of legal and regulatory frameworks to practice settings, and (e) an ability to apply quality assurance practices within the practice setting.

PHC nurses often serve in community settings or rural facilities without sophisticated technologies or resources (Kwansah et al., 2012). It is necessary to have the skills to plan, implement, and evaluate plans of care for their patients, with an understanding of major treatment modalities, pharmacology, medication, and treatment-prescribing protocols as well as those clinical procedures and interventions most commonly needed by their patient population (Affara, 2009). Key to effective practice is the recognition of when a patient needs to be referred to a higher level of care, or when the nurse needs to seek consultation in managing a patient problem (Affara, 2009). Optimizing the benefit of community-level access to care involves treating what can be managed at the periphery of the health delivery system, with a primary care nurse knowledgeable and skilled in appropriate referrals and/or linkages to manage the complex patient jointly with distance support.

Both in their role of providing patient care and frequently supervising trained and volunteer community health workers, important competencies of the PHC nurses are strong communication and interpersonal skills (Affara, 2009). As a primary provider of care, the nurse holds the responsibility for a trusted relationship with patients and their families to promote health and manage illness.

The International Council of Nurses (ICN) has highlighted two additional crosscutting components important in PHC nursing, which may apply at the level of the community facility or at higher levels of practice or management responsibility (Affara, 2009). These are employing an effective leadership and management style, and team building, which contribute to a positive practice environment optimizing the skills of all team members (Affara, 2009). ICN notes the responsibility PHC nurses have to enhance their profession by promoting quality assurance and improvement practices, such as establishing and monitoring practices, tracking health outcomes goals for providers and clients, and engaging in continuing education. In addition, primary care nurses should be comfortable promoting the dissemination of information and the mentoring and supervision of other nurses as an element of quality control and management (Affara, 2009).

STRATEGIES TO EXPAND NURSING SCOPES OF PRACTICE

To expand nursing scopes of practice for primary care in a sustainable manner, the education system for nurses needs to be transformed to incorporate new competencies (Affara, 2009; Bryar et al., 2012; WHO, 2009b, 2010c). Once nurses enter the workforce, the delivery and performance systems should be structured to provide support for the expanded role of nurses throughout their career (Bryar et al., 2012). In addition, the policy and regulatory environment needs to reflect the expanded scopes of practice of nurses (ICN, 2009; WHA, 2011). The next section of this chapter considers specific objectives and approaches to implement each of these strategies.

Strategy 1: Transforming Nursing Education for PHC Nursing

A first step to implement a national model for expanded access based on PHC nursing is examining the core competencies underlying nursing practice. In 2003, the ICN developed a set of international competencies for the generalist nurse (Alexander & Runciman, 2003). A study by Hlahane, Van Rensburg, and Claassens (2006) found that generalist nurses working in PHC facilities perceived their own ability to provide comprehensive primary care as limited due to their initial training. While they had adequate assessment, diagnosis, and management skills, they felt restricted in their ability to provide preventive services, treatment of common skin conditions, management of pregnancy, and infant care. Public health and community nursing have been identified by ICN as two areas where advanced skills and training have major benefits for the patient (Affara, 2009; Bryar et al., 2012).

To provide appropriate and effective care to patients, primary health care nurses also need to be equipped with skills to promote healthy behaviors and to implement health promotion and disease prevention activities, in addition to diagnosis and medical management of illness (Affara, 2009). This is important not only for the increasing burden of NCDs, but for the prevalent infectious diseases that remain a leading cause of death across Africa (Lozano et al., 2012). Knowledge of the determinants of health and specific tools and approaches for disease prevention, including screening and counselling, is central to designing effective interventions (Affara, 2009). Another component of health promotion is designing community awareness and education campaigns. Primary health care nurses play an important role in providing their patients, families, and communities with relevant and up-to-date information about diseases and their associated risk factors and how to minimize these (Affara, 2009).

Competencies for nurses working in the community setting differ substantially from those working in acute care settings (Keleher et al., 2007). To expand the scope of nursing practice to manage complex cases at the community level, preservice education will need to be reviewed and modified appropriately. In 2010, *The Lancet* commissioned a report on education of health professionals for the 21st century (Frenk et al., 2010). The report was developed by a commission of 20 professionals from multiple countries and set forth a vision for improving postsecondary education in medicine, nursing, and public health. The commission found that globally, curricula for clinicians was fragmented, outdated, and static, producing graduates who were unprepared to address population health needs (Frenk et al., 2010). Furthermore, on the whole, the report found that graduates had limited teamwork and leadership skills and a narrow perspective of how their discipline is affected by the broader health system (Frenk et al., 2010). Since the focus of most preservice programs is on hospital-based care as opposed to primary health care, there is limited emphasis placed on the importance of the continuum of care at the community level and interdisciplinary relationships.

Objectives for Strategy 1

Establish Primary Care Competencies, Critical Thinking, and Learning Skills Relevant to Public Health Needs

The commission's vision for the future of health education for a new century is for "all health professionals in all countries [to] be educated to mobilize knowledge and to engage in critical reasoning and ethical conduct so that they are competent to participate in patient and population-centered health systems as members of locally responsive and globally connected teams" (Frenk et al., 2010, p. 2). To meet this vision, both instructional and institutional reforms are required to ensure transformative learning and interdependence in education (Frenk et al., 2010).

Essential clinical competencies for the primary health care nurse include an advanced set of assessment skills to diagnose their patients and demonstrate sound clinical reasoning, judgment, and decision making throughout the diagnostic and treatment process (Affara, 2009). In order to acquire these competencies in settings relevant to future practice, clinical practicum training in community settings, including health centers or district hospitals, is called for. The practicum training should provide the nurse student with direct hands-on experience in diagnosing, treating, managing, and counseling on common conditions such as cardiovascular disease, diabetes, diarrheal and pulmonary diseases, and common community-acquired infections. Relevant to the scope of practice and environment of service, this requires a good understanding of the epidemiology, physiology, and social aspects that are relevant to the health of the populations they are serving (Affara, 2009).

Within the context of primary care, which is inclusive of health promotion and disease prevention, recognizing the extent to which the social, economic, and physical environment, as well as an individual's characteristics and behaviors, determine their health outcomes informs a more holistic response (Commission on Social Determinants of Health, 2008). Nurses need to be aware of these social determinants of health, and how they affect the development of prevention, treatment, and rehabilitation plans for their patients (WHO, 2010c). Interprofessional education can equip nurses with skills to better understand social determinants of health and incorporate this knowledge into nursing care. Interprofessional education occurs when nursing students interact and learn about other professions, and have opportunities to identify how both groups can collaborate to improve the delivery of services and promote good health outcomes (WHO, 2010c). Nursing students may benefit from learning new perspectives from other fields, such as sociology, economics, psychology, anthropology, and education as part of their training.

Drive Transformative Learning

Transformative learning involves students moving away from memorizing facts and toward developing skills to critically analyze information and applying it to real life situations (Frenk et al., 2010). Transformative learning requires a change in instructional approach. It allows nursing students to gain relevant competencies that can then be applied in team settings to address health system constraints and improve health outcomes. To ensure that competencies are absorbed, students need time to reflect critically on new material and discuss their perspectives in team settings. The output of a more transformative model to education is nurses who have better skills to react to complex environments and find solutions to unique problems.

Establish Interdependence of Learning Environment With Primary Care Settings

Interdependence in education is an institutional reform whereby schools move away from their own silo to work within networks, alliances, or consortiums to share educational resoures (Frenk et al., 2010). Schools can become more interdependent by expanding their reach to include networks of hospitals and primary health centers. These relationships may extend in several directions—between education and training systems including schools and facilities, providers, service sites, and community service organizations. The primary purpose of integrating the education and practice systems into coherent, collaborative, and efficient systems is to ensure quality training matched to the delivery of health services at multiple levels of care. Creating an institutional culture that promotes collaboration along with critical thinking when interacting with multiple learning environments also lays the groundwork for multidisciplinary models of care.

Establish Professional Education Opportunities That Include Management and Leadership

Developing clinical nurse leaders with management skills is particularly important to improving the quality and efficiency of services while also increasing access to and controlling the rising cost of health care (Baernholdt & Cottingham, 2010). Clinical education usually does not incorporate management competencies, and nurses often hold responsibility for running clinic facilities, organizing and supervising community health workers without the benefit of training in basic management skills of staff. Equipping primary health care nurses with fundamental management and leadership skills, such as working effectively with teams, supervision and communication skills, and how to monitor and improve patient care outcomes, can positively enhance the impact of the health team (Baernholdt & Cottingham, 2010). Continuing professional development for primary care nurses may draw in additional skills, such as financial management, how to translate new evidence into practice, use of available information technology to improve both care and administrative management, and broader understanding of factors, policies and regulations impacting care at the local level.

Implementation of Strategy 1

Develop Priorities for Education Reform

Transforming nursing education is a long-term process that requires buy-in from stakeholders in the health and education systems at both the government and training institution level (WHO, 2013). An assessment of the health care needs of the country, conducted in partnership with the professional regulatory councils and associations and the leaders at the training institutions, should inform reforms of nursing education, the number of new nurses that need to be trained, and recruitment strategies that favor retention (Bandazi et al., 2013). The national plan for nursing education and curriculum reform should be well aligned with the national strategic plans for health.

Revise Curriculum and Establish Competency-Based Learning

A component to transforming nursing education is revising the curriculum to make it competency based and relevant to addressing prevalent community health issues, including health promotion and disease prevention and managing acute and chronic conditions. Competencies should be aligned with understanding, diagnosing, and managing common community health problems and addressing the social determinants of health with clients, families, and communities (WHO, 2010a). The process should commence with an open forum for these stakeholders to share lessons learned from use of the existing curriculum and determine priorities for developing the revised version. Building consensus on new nursing competencies can be a long process. For example, to scale up community nurses in the Zhejiang Province of China, a working group of 13 technical experts from government public health departments, colleges, and primary health care service centers was created to develop instructive standards for health education (Fu, Bao, & Meng, 2010). A second working group was organized to write textbooks for community nurse training. Once the textbooks were drafted, they were piloted in select training centers, and after 2 years, five new textbooks were developed for widespread use in training for community nurses. While this process was long, it secured buy-in from government and other stakeholders, and ultimately led to successful implementation of the community nursing program. Over a 4-year period, the number of community health nurses increased by 56% in the Zhejiang Province (Fu et al., 2010).

Train and Retain Faculty

A challenge to reforming nursing education is having sufficient nursing faculty to cover courses in basic sciences and clinical care (Bandazi et al., 2013; WHO, 2013). Development of nursing faculty is a lengthy process: Nursing professors require advanced degrees, a strong foundation in nursing theory, and experience in a practicum training of students in the clinical setting. Oftentimes, nurses with advanced degrees are difficult to retain within a country, or to recruit from clinical practice back to teaching positions. The critical shortages of nurse tutors and clinical mentors for clinical practicum sites in many LMIC must be addressed at both the institutional and national level as part of the investment in building a well-trained and competent primary health care nursing workforce. Nursing institutions need to identify and provide adequate incentives (both financial and nonfinancial) for nurses with appropriate credentials to return to teaching. Opportunities for professional advancement and peer mentoring to help faculty participate in research and publishing have been proposed to encourage retention of faculty in some countries.

The quality of professors is a critical yet often overlooked component to transforming nursing education. Nursing faculty need to be adequately trained in teaching and pedagogical education to nurture critical thinking and physical assessment skills in students, and have manageable workloads and class sizes, particularly in clinic-based courses, so that content taught in the classroom can translate into everyday nursing practice. Faculty members also need ongoing access to professional training opportunities to stay current in the classroom regarding new approaches and methods for diagnosis, management, and treatment of patients (WHO, 2013).

Continued Professional Education to Advance PHC

Opportunities for nurses to continue their professional education and gain new skills, both in primary care management and as instructors and educators, not only lays the groundwork for continued quality improvements in care but can also support individual motivation and satisfaction in work (Willis-Shattuck et al., 2008). The importance of available continuing education offerings, accessible and structured in a manner that can count toward professional development or certification, is reviewed in Chapter 22 (Tyer-Viola).

Identify Sources of Financing for Education

One of the greatest challenges to reforming nursing education is securing the necessary financial resources (Soucat, Scheffler, & Ghebreyesus, 2013). Due to the notion that education is a public good, many countries are reluctant to allow private nursing schools to educate nurses. Scaling up the public budget for education and training is also a challenge since it is often managed by the Ministry of Education, rather than the Ministry of Health (Soucat et al., 2013). Therefore, even if the Ministry of Health prioritizes the scale up of preservice education, they may have limited control to allocate more funds toward the initiative. To increase investment in preservice education, countries need to consider all financing sources available (Soucat, Scheffler, & Ghebreyesus, 2013). Donors, nongovernmental organizations (NGOs), faith-based organizations, and private investors may be willing to invest in preservice education and, in many cases, already do. For example, through the Nursing Education Partnership Initiative (NEPI), the U.S. government partnered with host country governments to provide support to strengthen the public training institutions in four countries (Bandazi et al., 2013).

In Uganda and Malawi, 70% of nurses and midwives are trained in faith-based institutions (Tran, Luoma, & Ron, 2013). Ethiopia and the Democratic Republic of the Congo have also experienced a dramatic scale-up of nursing students, with the government allowed private sector schools to open in the 1990s and in 2001, respectively (Soucat et al., 2013). Another consideration to increase the bandwidth of existing resources for preservice education is to assess the value for money of various approaches to improving educational and student outcomes, and then to use this information to inform and prioritize more efficient and effective investments in future programs.

Tuition fees are a barrier to entry for many students, particularly in developing countries where students may have difficulty accessing finance through loans or other sources (Soucat et al., 2013). An assessment completed by the U.S. Agency for International Development (USAID)-funded Strengthening Health Outcomes through the Private Sector (SHOPS) project in 2013 examined how to finance medical and nursing education through the private sector using Malawi, Rwanda, Tanzania, and Zambia as case studies (Tran et al., 2013). The assessment concludes that there is strong student demand for financing, but understanding the dimensions of demand, such as a student's willingness and ability to pay loans and his or her attitude toward borrowing and repaying, is critical to structuring loan programs (Tran, Luoma, & Ron, 2013). On the supply side, private financial institutions are often willing to provide long-term loans for education, but this is heavily influenced by government policies as well as their general support of the private sector's involvement in education (Tran et al., 2013). A national commitment to investment in educating primary health care nurses as a strategic pillar in expanding universal access to care is fundamental in reducing leading factors associated with high morbidity and mortality rates.

Strategy 2: Strengthen Delivery and Support Systems

Once primary care nurses have gained expanded competencies and completed their education, an adequate clinical practice environment and support for their professional role can directly impact their effectiveness in achieving public health goals. In many circumstances, nurses do not have adequate support to fulfill their roles and responsibilities, which compromises the quality of care delivered and also professional morale (Bryar et al., 2012; ICN/FNIF, 2006). In addition, financial remuneration typically falls below a living wage, and incentives to remain in practice in the public sector, or in the country at large, are often minimal (Franco, Bennett, & Kanfer, 2002; Willis-Shattuck et al., 2008). To address these challenges, delivery and support systems need to be bolstered.

Objectives for Strategy 2

Nurses Are Motivated and Supported in Their Roles
Clinical competency is one of several drivers of high performance, but motivation also plays a key role in the quality, efficiency, and equity of population health

services (Willis-Shattuck et al., 2008). Health worker motivation can be defined as "an individual's degree of willingness to exert and maintain effort towards organizational goals" (Franco et al., 2002, p. 1255). They have classified health worker motivation into three categories: individual motivation, which depends on personal goals and expectations; organizational factors, such as management structure, resources, culture, and feedback loops; and community influences, such as expectations that clients have of their health care providers to deliver services (Franco, Bennett, & Kanfer, 2002). These three categories combined have profound impacts on how health workers deliver care. In advancing primary care nursing as a pillar of expanded access to health services, strategies to foster and enhance each aspect of motivation should be taken into account.

Clear Career Pathways for Professional Development Are in Place
As nurses expand their clinical primary care competencies, clear scopes of work and pathways for professional development from basic to more advanced nursing roles should be in place (Bryar et al., 2012). Nurses should understand the roles and responsibilities associated with being a primary health care provider, and have an opportunity to gain feedback on their performance and patient clinical outcomes. They also need to know the roles and responsibilities of their team members so that patient care can be efficiently planned and delivered. As part of a national strategy built around nurses as core to expanding health services, career pathways that allow primary care nurses to advance in their profession and assume greater roles and responsibilities as they develop greater skills and competencies have the potential to positively impact retention, particularly in rural areas (Mbemba, Gagnon, Pare, & Cite, 2013). Nurses should be knowledgeable of steps and opportunities to advance their practice and career, both in terms of taking on more responsibility and complex work, as well as obtaining greater remuneration.

Nurses Work in Multidisciplinary Teams
Primary health care nurses should be positioned as a central part of a multidisciplinary team that puts the patient's care and wellness at the center of its focus (Institute of Medicine [IOM], 2001). Roles that were traditionally led by physicians can be undertaken by nurses with training matched to expanded scopes of practice. It is vital that systems placing primary care nurses as a first point of contact with health care include a system for consultation and referral with more experienced clinicians and physicians, both for quality of patient care and for the morale of nurses facing complex clinical situations. The availability of mobile health, cell phone, and other communication technologies extends the reach of quality health care to rural and remote areas anchored by a knowledgeable primary health care nurse who can link with physicians and other members of the community health team (Baernholdt & Cottingham, 2010; Bryar et al., 2012).

Adequate Resources and Infrastructure to Fulfill Role Are in Place
The physical infrastructure of the health facilities and conditions where nurses work cannot be overlooked. This is particularly problematic in LMICs and often a key barrier to providing access to quality and safe health care services within

communities (ICN/FNIF, 2006). When primary health care nurses do not have access to adequate medical infrastructure—including running water, power source, medications, medical equipment, and supplies—they are at increased risk for occupational hazards, have less satisfaction with their position, and are often unable to provide appropriate and safe care to their patients (ICN/FNIF, 2006). Attention to these components supporting access to effective primary care can positively impact health outcomes nurses can achieve. As noted earlier, countries planning to extend health care access out to the periphery or down to the community level can leverage information technology (IT) and make it available to primary health care nurses to support their practice. In addition to facilitating timely consultation, nurses are able to better record patient outcomes and services provided, and collate and report this information to higher levels of the health system, where it is relevant to policy makers (Baernholdt & Cottingham, 2010).

Implementation of Strategy 2

Use of Supportive Supervision and Clinical Mentors

Supportive supervision and clinical mentorship are vital tools to ensure that primary health care nurses have adequate support, particularly when they take on more responsibilities (Federal HIV/AIDS Prevention and Control Office, Ministry of Health, 2007; Frimpong, Helleringer, Awoonor-Williams, Yeji, & Philips, 2011). Effective supportive supervision involves a more clinically experienced supervisor providing guidance and training to supervisees, evaluating their performance, and ensuring that they have necessary skills to complete their job. Supportive supervision also enables staff to have a feedback loop with their managers, as an effective supervisor will set performance objectives for his or her staff and provide regular and constructive, rather than intermittent and critical, feedback on performance. In LMIC, the shortage of nurses working at the community level may drive different models for supervision and mentoring, in light of difficulty in taking time away from patient care, and further compounded by transportation challenges. Innovative mHealth may be utilized to offer these oversight and mentoring supports, brought to scale through the system for primary health care services at the community level (Appiah, 2013). Supportive supervision is associated with increased productivity of health workers and can help ensure that primary health care nurses adhere to clinical protocols and standards (Frimpong et al., 2011).

Clinical mentors provide primary health care nurses with ongoing support and professional development opportunities (Andrews et al., 2006). While supportive supervision and clinical mentoring overlap in many ways, clinical mentors are typically more directly focused on clinical care, and should be experienced and practicing clinicians. Ideally, clinical mentoring continues beyond preservice education and should be seen as a form of education. Clinical mentors can serve either onsite, providing feedback on patient care, or off-site, or providing consultation by phone or Internet. Some countries are taking steps to standardize clinical mentoring within their health system. For example, in 2007, the government of Ethiopia developed a set of guidelines for clinical mentorship within the context of HIV care (Federal HIV/AIDS Prevention and Control Office, Ministry of Health, 2007). The government developed the guidelines because, in light of the country's severe HIV epidemic, when doctors were unavailable, nurses were providing care that went beyond their scope of practice (Federal HIV/AIDS Prevention and Control Office, Ministry of Health, 2007). After developing a national curriculum to rapidly train over 400 nurses to initiate antiretroviral therapy (ART), the government chose to standardize clinical mentorship to formalize best practices. The mentors are now available onsite and also over the phone to provide guidance to the newly trained nurses (Federal HIV/AIDS Prevention and Control Office, Ministry of Health, 2007).

Interdisciplinary Care Teams

Implementing interdisciplinary care teams will provide clients with timely access to a range of health care providers, from community health workers to nurses and physicians, in a structured and efficient manner. The constitution of these teams will in part be determined by the constellation and roles of health sector workers in each country, under the direction of the Ministry of Health. Often nurses play a pivotal role as a point of contact between clients and these teams at the community level, helping the client navigate through a complex set of health interventions and providers, including facility and community care sites. The importance of working consultation and referral linkages between primary health care nurses and more sophisticated medical expertise and technical resources cannot be underestimated and is essential in providing access to appropriate health services at the right time and in the right place. The nurse may play an organizing role within the team structure. For example, community health care workers are frequently placed under the direction of the nurse at the clinic, and can be extremely valuable in visiting patient homes and bringing back real-time assessments of home environments, as well as barriers and constraints to following prescribed care. It is important to include both traditional health workers within these teams given they are often sought out as an initial source of health care. The role of local traditional healers should also be considered, as prevailing beliefs and practices and community trust in these providers can positively or negatively impact health outcomes. Primary health care nurses will be most effective when recognizing and understanding the complementary roles of other health workers and establishing a structured and well-defined team in order to maximize access to essential health services while being comfortable assuming the primary responsibility of advocating for the health care needs of their patients.

Financial and Nonfinancial Incentives That Motivate Staff

To stabilize and retain a core nursing workforce for expansion of primary health care, attention to health worker motivation with incentives, financial and nonfinancial, is part of good management (Mathauer & Imhoff, 2006; McCoy et al., 2008). Incentives, which may include professional awards and public recognition, should be linked to added responsibilities and performance expectations and any additional managerial responsibilities assigned to the primary health care nurse. Low wages affect motivation, and are one of several factors cited by health care workers to influence their decisions to migrate from the public to private sector or to other countries (Hernandez-Pena et al., 2013). Financial incentives can be designed to adjust for situations where salaries are inequitable or low, or where there are shortages of health workers. Multiple evaluations on the use of financial incentives and increased salaries demonstrate their profound impact. For example, a 60% increase in salaries in Swaziland and a 52% increase in salaries in Malawi resulted in substantial workers moving back to the public sector from the private sector (Kober & Van Damme, 2006; Palmer, 2006).

In addition to financial incentives, organizational conditions and nonfinancial incentives can also influence health worker motivation and retention. In 2007, the Regional Network for Equity in Health in East and Southern Africa (EQUINET) and the East, Central, and Southern African Health Community (ECSA-HC) completed a study of the types of nonfinancial incentives provided to health workers in 16 countries in East and Southern Africa (Dambisya, 2007). The study found that to improve motivation and retention of clinicians, governments were using national budgets or funds from their sector-wide approach to provide additional training opportunities for staff, improve working conditions, and provide health care for clinicians and their families (Dambisya, 2007). Managers in the 16 countries reviewed the impact of these schemes, and found that they resulted in greater satisfaction among workers and higher retention in the public sector (Dambisya, 2007). These may have particular relevance for countries committed to expanding primary health care nursing at the community level.

Referral Systems to Connect Community to the Health System
As primary health care nurses with expanded scopes of practice provide more services within the community, referral systems need to be strengthened to afford linkages with other knowledgeable providers in the community and at higher facility levels. A tenet of universal access to primary care is that patients should obtain the best possible services at a location close to their home (Pan American Health Organization, 2007). Primary health care nurses, particularly those in more remote or isolated rural areas, may often be confronted with patient medical illnesses or trauma that exceed their clinical knowledge, and both a communications capacity and a system of transportation needs to be identified by health authorities. Effective referral capacity both improves the chances for a good health outcome and frees up the primary health care nurse to serve the population presenting for primary care (WHO, n.d.). National guidelines and protocols outlining appropriate criteria for referral to higher levels of care are of use and acknowledge the defined scope of practice of the primary health care nurse.

Define Opportunities for Professional Development
An initial step in creating a national system for professional development opportunities for primary health care nurses is to develop categories of practice with consistent definitions, clear responsibilities, and minimum qualifications (Currie & Carr-Hill, 2012). Developing standard positions enables supervisors to rate performance between staff members, and to transparently promote staff within the

established system (Currie & Carr-Hill, 2012). As nurses take on expanded scopes of practice, job descriptions need to be updated so that they remain accurate and can be used to evaluate performance (Callaghan et al., 2010). Once roles and responsibilities are outlined, transparent career ladders that outline the path for career progression and set goals for advancement also have the benefit of being benchmarks to ensure that promotions are equitable (TACMIL Health Project, 2009). For employers, career ladders ensure that staff meet set criteria and have sufficient experience before they take on more responsibility, thereby also serving as a quality improvement tool (TACMIL Health Project, 2009). The lack of professional development opportunities is consistently mentioned as a reason for frustration and disillusionment among nurses, and therefore merits thoughtful inclusion as part of an overall plan to build a primary health care workforce (Kingma, 2007).

Strategy 3: Revised Policy and Regulatory Environment

The global push for universal health coverage (UHC) was solidified by the 2012 UN resolution urging governments to move toward UHC and provide affordable, equitable, and high-quality services, "especially through primary health care and social protection mechanisms" (United Nations, 2014, p. 3). Also in 2012, multiple countries began to adopt policies and declarations related to achieving UHC.[2] With nurses serving as the main providers of health care, additional policy and regulatory changes are recommended to ensure a robust and durable supply of nurses to support expanded access to primary health care throughout each country (WHO, 2014).

Objectives for Strategy 3

Greater Political Commitment to Nursing for Expansion of Access to Primary Care
Government leadership is crucial to developing and implementing a vision and strategic plan to scale up the nursing workforce as a critical means to expand access to primary care services (Lehmann et al., 2009). While leadership should come from the Ministry of Health, which oversees health sector planning, multiple stakeholders from across the health sector should be engaged for the intervention to be a system-wide approach. These stakeholders may include nurses and other clinicians from public, private, and faith-based health organizations; academic institutions and leadership; ministries of education, public service, finance, and labor; professional associations; regulatory councils; and civil society (WHO, 2010d). Given the complexity of expanding scopes of practice within an existing delivery system and complementary to other health cadres in the health care system, it is imperative to gain sufficient input and consensus from a diverse array of stakeholders associated with the training, management, credentialing, and financing of nurse cadres.

Legal and Regulatory Framework to Support Expanded Scopes of Practice
National legal and regulatory frameworks need to be adjusted in most LMIC to reflect an expanded scope of practice for primary health care nurses (ICN, 2009).

Regulations establish the roles and responsibilities of advanced practice nurses, including the level of independence that they have in diagnosing and treating patients. As put forward by the ICN, regulatory mechanisms for nurses with expanded scopes of practice should define whether a nurse has the authority to diagnose and treat patients, prescribe medications, refer patients to other clinicians at different levels of the health system, and admit patients to hospitals (ICN, 2009).

Professional Associations' and Councils' Role in Advance Nursing
Professional associations and nursing councils have played a vital role in representing the perspectives of nurses within the policy and regulatory dialogue, and setting and maintaining codes of conduct for professional practice (ICN, 2009). Thus, the support and inclusion of the input of nursing professional bodies is essential to ensure proper expertise and awareness of the nursing workforce in planning, implementing, and managing any health service reforms at the PHC level. Areas of engagement include, but are not limited to, developing and reviewing practice standards, regulatory and policy reforms, revisions to training curriculum and practicums; establishing roles and authorities for nurse's supervisors and mentors; and establishing referral and other reporting systems within the health network. Documenting prevalent health care problems at the community level, and linking the trend in outcomes with specific nursing reforms, is essential in determining the effectiveness and efficiency of expanding the role of nurse primary care. Information on health care utilization patterns, quality of services, costs, and health care provider practice patterns are important in informing current and future nursing practices, and to health policy makers and budget officers in charge of health sector spending.

Implementation of Strategy 3

Government Leadership and Key Stakeholders Consensus Around Expanded Scope of Practice
Both the organization of health care services and planning for the health workforce require high-level political engagement and commitment to achieve the goal of universal access to primary health care. Reforming the health system to better support nurses and expand their scope of practice requires high level political commitment that would ideally be championed from within the Ministry of Health, and garner support from nursing associations and civil society (Dussault et al., 2009). In making the case to policy makers and Ministries of Finance, a clear articulation of the benefits of investing in primary health care for the population, and therefore in the nursing workforce to deliver that care, must be prepared and taken forward to political leadership and decision makers.

The partnership between the Government of Malawi and the President's Emergency Plan for AIDS Relief/Nursing Education Partnership Initiative (PEPFAR/NEPI) demonstrates the power of collaboration (Bandazi et al., 2013). The PEPFAR/NEPI program was a targeted intervention to improve the quantity and quality of nurses (Bandazi et al., 2013). The initiative was integrated into the government's nursing and midwifery operational plan and the Ministry of Health's strategy to address HIV/AIDS. PEPFAR/NEPI collaborated with other donors to support a national assessment of nursing and midwifery that informed the way forward for the intervention. Throughout the implementation of the program, PEPFAR/NEPI provided ongoing capacity-building support to the ministry, as well as the Midwives Council of Malawi and nursing institutions (Bandazi et al., 2013).

A unique problem in LMICs are the many donors and development partners working in the health sector. Progress has been made in recent years through the initiation of the sector-wide approach to better coordinate donor activities and resources (Hutton & Tanner, 2004). This effort of coordination is essential to long-term sustainability of interventions to strengthen and expand the scope and practice of primary health care nursing as a means of improving universal access to care. More importantly, donors and development partners need to work within the country's existing priorities and planning framework, instead of pursuing separate and unconnected programs that are not sustainable (Dambisya, 2007). This not only maximizes the efficiency and impact of the donor investment and intervention, but ensures that it is aligned with the government's own planning and investment.

Despite being the largest cadre of health workers in most countries, nurses are rarely involved in higher level policy making (WHO, 2009b). Furthermore, even though nurses deliver the majority of health care, they are often the first cadre to be cut when budgets are under pressure (ICN/FNIF, 2006). In the future, nurses need to be involved in the development of policies that directly impact their practice and profession so that they can advocate for their needs, and the needs of the clients they serve (WHA, 2011; WHO, 2009b, 2010d). National nursing councils, nursing associations, and academic institutions are all potential resources to reach and engage nurses in matters impacting their lives and practice. Leaders from these organizations have a responsibility to engage decision makers in matters impacting the profession, while the government leadership also benefits from both input and buy-in from the largest component of the health workforce when developing national and local policies and strategies.

Regulatory bodies and professional associations play an important role in safeguarding the nursing profession. In addition to establishing standards of practice and a framework for professional recognition of excellence and advancement, they can establish and evaluate policies on workplace safety, standardized leave, social security benefits, and working hours (WHO, 2010b). These nongovernmental groups can also improve the quality of nursing care by accrediting nursing training institutions and health facilities (Bandazi et al., 2013; WHO, 2013). Accreditation is a tool to ensure that training institutions graduate well prepared and professional nurses, and that these nurses practice in facilities meeting quality standards (WHO, 2013).

Implement Regulatory Frameworks for Expanded Scope of Practice and Career Opportunities

Reforming professional practice standards for either expanding the professional scope of practice or promoting career opportunities often requires reforms to existing laws. Although there are examples of nonlegal adjustments, such as in-service training to implement new practice standards based on current skills/competencies, substantial modifications to existing standards of practice or the establishment of new skills, competencies, or levels of autonomy are instituted relative to the legal conditions set forth in the country's professional standards acts. For nurses, expanding the role of the nurse in the areas of clinical diagnosis, treatment, and patient management may require amending the country's Nurse Practice Act in order to authorize the nurse to perform clinical care duties. These laws are then implemented through a regulatory framework to address the issues of preservice training requirements and competency training, certification and licensing standards, and ongoing professional education requirements. There are essentially four regulatory issues that require consideration when reforming the practice standards for health care workers: (1) establishment of new roles and responsibilities; (2) assessing, credentialing, and licensure; (3) level of autonomy and/or supervisory relations with other health professionals; and (4) levels of practice sites—hospital, clinic, and community or home. In regards to advancing career opportunities, a regulatory framework based on current practice laws and practices is needed to identify professional pathways based on ongoing education and certification (or degree) requirements and practice activities.

Regulatory mechanisms should be enforced through licensure processes, and also define an officially recognized title for nurses who have an expanded scope of practice (ICN, 2009). It is common for nurses to informally expand their duties, responding to community needs and trainings they have received, before countries have revised the regulatory structure. For example, in Jordan, the Ministry of Health piloted a new program where midwives were able to insert intrauterine devices (IUDs; Abdelmohsen et al., 2013). From 2004 to 2009, the number of health centers that allowed midwives to insert IUDs increased from 119 to 193. However, in 2010, legal complications arose because midwives were not allowed by law to administer this service, resulting in a decrease in IUD insertion by 20% the following year (Abdelmohsen et al., 2013). Similarly, in Botswana, family nurse practitioners run clinics in underserved areas (Pulcini, Jelic, Gul, & Loke, 2010). While these nurses are able to legally prescribe drugs, their prescribing authority is not consistent among all employers. Without a defined and regulated scope of work, this new and essential cadre of health workers has faced many challenges in being able to diagnose and treat patients (Pulcini et al., 2010).

Document Outcomes and Best Practices

As governments revise standards of practice for primary care nursing and develop regulatory mechanisms to improve nursing quality, multiple stakeholders need to be brought into the process (WHO, 2010d). Nursing functions as part of multidisciplinary health teams that include physician organizations and grassroots community interests, where clarity and a collaborative environment are critical to good patient care and outcomes. As new standards are created to evaluate nurse training institutions, nurses, and health facilities, a wide range of stakeholders, such as policy makers, nurses, physicians, midwives, academic institutions, facility administrators, nursing associations, and patients, need to be included. When evaluating those functions and roles that primary health care nurses need codified in legal documents, policy makers require some understanding of the epidemiologic data and social determinants of health to match nurses' skills and roles with the health needs of the population (WHO, 2010b).

As steps are taken by governments to strengthen their support for primary care nursing, data on health outcomes and best practices should be fed back to policy makers. Progress toward the goal of expanding universal access to care, and documented positive impact on health outcomes, may contribute to sustaining support for investments in nursing. Optimal models for nurse-led primary care may vary across geographic regions. Mechanisms to capture and evaluate lessons learned and best practices open the door for continued improvement and refinement of how best to reach patients and communities with quality health care.

Once regulatory and legal frameworks have been updated to reflect expanded scopes of practice for primary health care nurses, the updates need to be evaluated and communicated to civil society and patients. Patients in particular need to have confidence in their health care providers, and be reassured that nurses have undergone sufficient training and mechanisms are in place to assure a minimum level of quality. Patients should also be involved in continuous quality improvement processes (IOM, 2001). They should have the opportunity to provide feedback on the care they receive from primary care nurses, and information on patient safety should be transparent for patients to review (IOM, 2001).

Include Nurses in Policy and Planning Decisions

There has been increased attention to nurses participating in policy- and program-planning forums where their input is important to improving quality of services and health outcomes (Currie & Carr-Hill, 2012; WHO, 2009b, 2010d). Inclusion of nurses in the role of chief nursing officers or as participants in strategic planning led by the human resources department in the Ministry of Health can anchor and advance the needs of nurses serving at the primary care level in communities. Both the academic nurse training community and practitioners at all levels of the service delivery system need to perceive and act upon the opportunity to ensure representation of nursing perspectives and concerns in formal and informal forums. It is also important for donors to recognize the value of this large cadre of health providers in any planned investment or expansion of services, as nurses can inform and guide effective responses to the health delivery system at the community level (WHO, 2010d).

CONCLUSION

In recent years, global progress has been made to expand access to health care services and medicines, and many of the leading causes of death in resource-limited settings have changed (Lozano et al., 2012). As countries continue along their epidemiological transition, patients will present with more complex chronic conditions that require more coordinated and patient-centric care that is delivered as close to their home as possible (Bryar et al., 2012; Lozano et al., 2012). With persistent shortages of health workers, countries have a clear choice to expand the scopes of practice of nurses so that they can deliver more relevant and effective primary health care services enhancing universal access to care.

To meet the goal of universal access and build on this largest cadre of trained providers, countries need to transform their systems for nursing education and ensure that these respond to the dominant health needs of the population and prepare nurses to work effectively within decentralized health systems. Once out in the community, attention to the basic infrastructure, including equipment and supplies, for primary health care nurses will increase the effectiveness and positively impact the morale of nurses as well as enhance patient outcomes. Clear pathways for professional development serve to reinforce motivation for nurses to perceive value in their work and to remain in the workforce. Finally, primary health care nurses need to be supported in their expanded practice with legal and regulatory frameworks that define their new role and set clear parameters around which procedures they can complete and treatments they can prescribe.

As countries transition into the 21st century, implementing these strategic changes will be a long-term process. To ensure that each strategy is country owned, a clear vision is needed for nurses and within nursing, with scopes of practice adjusted to meet specific national, regional, and community health demands. While the reforms need to be championed from a high level within the health system, they also need support from nurses, other clinicians, regulatory bodies, associations, and civil society. Only then will progress be made to develop a sustainable nurse-led model of care that ensures the delivery of higher quality and more efficient services within the community.

ACKNOWLEDGMENT

The findings and conclusions in this chapter are those of the author(s) and do not necessarily represent the official positions of the United States government or any other affiliate organization(s).

NOTES

1. The WHA Resolutions include WHA 42.27, 45.5, 47.9, 48.8, 49.1, 54.12, and 59.27.
2. Mexico City Political Declaration on UCH, April 2012; Bangkok Statement on UHC, January 2012; Tunis Declaration on Value for Money, Sustainability, and Accountability in the Health Sector, 2012.

REFERENCES

Abdelmohsen, A., Jrassat, M., As-Sayaideh, A., Mowaswas, A., Hamza, S., Wright, S., & Kawaa, K. (2013, November 13). A decade of task sharing in Jordan; lessons for policy and service delivery. *International Conference on Family Planning*. Addis Ababa, Ethiopia.

Affara, F. (2009). *ICN framework of competencies for the specialist nurse*. Geneva, Switzerland: International Council of Nurses (ICN).

Alexander, M., & Runciman, P. (2003). *ICN framework of competencies for the generalist nurse*. Geneva, Switzerland: International Council of Nurses.

Andrews, G., Browdie, D., Andrews, J., Hillan, E., Thomas, G., Wong, J., & Rixon, L. (2006). Professional roles and communications in clinical placements: A qualitative study of nursing students' perceptions and some models for practice. *International Journal of Nursing Studies, 43*(7), 861–874.

Appiah, B. (2013, January 8). Africa's cellular solution to TB. *Canadian Medical Association Journal, 185*(1), E11–2.

Baernholdt, M., & Cottingham, S. (2010). The clinical nurse leader—New nursing role with global implications. *International Nursing Review, 58*(1), 74–78.

Bandazi, S., Nakata, A., Palen, J., von Zinkernagel, D., Dohrn, J., & Yu-Shears, J. (2013). Building nurse and midwifery capacity in Malawi: A partnership between the government of Malawi and the PEPFAR/Nursing Education Partnership Initiative (NEPI). In M. A. DeLuca & A. Soucat (Eds.), *Transforming the global health workforce*. New York, NY: New York University.

Bryar, R., Kendall, S., & Mogtlane, S. M. (2012). *Reforming primary health care: A nursing perspective*. Geneva, Switzerland: International Council of Nurses.

Buchan, J., & Calman, L. (2004). *The global shortage of registered nurses: An overview of issues and actions*. Geneva, Switzerland: ICN.

Callaghan, M., Ford, N., & Schneider, H. (2010). A systematic review of task-shifting for HIV treatment and care in Africa. *Human Resources for Health, 88*. Retrieved from http://www.human resources-health.com/content/8/1/8

Chiang Mai Declaration: Nursing and Midwifery for Primary Health Care. (2008, February). Chiang Mai.

Commission on Social Determinants of Health. (2008). *Closing the gap in a generation: Health equity through action on the social determinants of health*. Geneva, Switzerland: World Health Organzation.

Currie, E., & Carr-Hill, B. (2012). What is a nurse? Is there an international consensus? *International Nursing Review, 6*(1), 67–74.

Dambisya, Y. M. (2007). *A review of non-financial incentives for health worker retention in east and southern Africa*. Harare, Zimbabwe: ESCA.

Dohrn, J., Nzama, B., & Murrman, M. (2009). The impact of HIV scale-up on the role of nurses in South Africa: Time for a new approach. *Journal of Acquired Immune Deficiency Syndromes, 52*(Suppl. 1), S27–S29.

Dussault, G., Fronteria, I., Prytherch, H., Dal Poz, M. R., Ngoma, D., Lunguzi, J., & Wyss, K. (2009). *Scaling up the stock of health workers: A review*. Geneva, Switzerland: ICN.

Fairall, L., O'Bachmann, M., Lombard, C., Timmerman, V., Uebel, K., Zwarenstein, M., . . . Bateman, E. (2012). Task shifting of antiretroviral treatment from doctors to primary-care nurses in South Africa (STRETCH): A pragmatic, parallel, cluster-randomised trial. *Lancet, 380,* 889–898.

Federal HIV/AIDS Prevention and Control Office, Ministry of Health. (2007). *Guidelines for HIV care/ART clinical mentoring in Ethiopia.* Addis Ababa, Ethiopia: Ministry of Health.

Franco, L., Bennett, S., & Kanfer, R. (2002). Health sector reform and public sector health worker motivation: A conceptual framework. *Social Science Medicine, 54*(8), 1255–1266.

Frenk, J., Chen, L., Bhutta, Z. A., Cohen, J., Crisp, N., Evans, T., . . . Zurayk, H. (2010). Health professionals for a new century: Transforming education to strengthen health systems in an interdependent world. *The Lancet, 376,* 1923–1958.

Frimpong, J., Helleringer, S., Awoonor-Williams, J., Yeji, F., & Philips, J. (2011). Does supervision improve health worker productivity? Evidence from the Upper East Region of Ghana. *Tropical Medicine and International Health, 16*(10), 1225–1233.

Fu, W., Bao, J., & Meng, J. (2010). Development of community nursing in Zheijian Province, China: A report of the driving measures. *International Nursing Review, 57*(2), 265–268.

Fulton, B. D., Scheffler, R. M., Sparkes, S. P., Auh, E. Y., Vujicic, M., & Soucat, A. (2011). Health workforce skill mix and task shifting in low income countries: A review of recent evidence. *Human Resources for Health, 9*(1), 1.

Hernandez-Pena, P., Poullier, J., Van Mosseveld, C., Van de Maele, N., Cherilova, V., & Indikandahena, C. (2013). Health worker remuneration in WHO member states. *Bulletin of the World Health Organization, 91,* 808–815.

Hlahane, M., Van Rensburg, H., & Claassens, D. (2006). Professional nurses' perceptions of the skills required to render comprehensive primary health care services. *Curationis, 29*(4), 82–94.

Hutton, G., & Tanner, M. (2004). The sector-wide approach: A blessing for public health? *Bulletin of the World Health Organization, 82*(12). Retrieved from www.who/int/bulletin/volumes/82/12/en/1893.pdf

Institute of Medicine (IOM). (2001). *Crossing the quality chasm: A new health system for the 21st century.* Washington, DC: The National Acadamies Press.

International Council of Nurses (ICN). (2009). *Nurse practitioner/advance practice nurse: Definition and characteristics.* Geneva, Switzerland: Author.

International Council of Nurses/Florence Nightingale International Foundation (ICN/FNIF). (2006). *Global nursing shortage: Primary areas for intervention.* Geneva, Switzerland: Author.

Johns, B., Asfaw, E., Wong, W., Bekele, A., Minior, T., Kebede, A., & Palen, J. (2014, April 1). Assessing the costs and effects of antiretroviral therapy task shifting from phys-icians to other health professionals in Ethiopia. *Journal of Acquired Immune Deficiency Syndromes, 65*(4), e40–e47.

Keleher, H., Parker, R., Abdulwadud, O., Francis, K., Segal, L., & Dalziel, K. (2007). *Review of primary and community care nursing.* Austrailia: Australian Primary Health Care Research Institute.

Kingma, M. (2007, June). Nurses on the move: A global overview. *Health Services Research, 42*(3, Pt. 2), 1281–1298.

Kober, K., & Van Damme, W. (2006). Public sector nurses in Swaziland: Can the downturn be reversed? *Human Resources for Health, 4,* 13.

Kwansah, J., Dzodzomenyo, M., Mutumba, M., Asabir, K., Koomson, E., Gyakobo, M., . . . Rachel, S. C. (2012). Policy talk: Incentives for rural service among nurses in Ghana. *Health Policy and Planning, 27*(8), 669–676.

Laurant, M., Reeves, D., Hermens, R., Braspenning, J., Grol, R., & Sibbald, B. (2005). Substitution of doctors by nurses in primary care. *Cochrane Database Systamatic Reviews*, (2), CD001271.

Lehmann, U., Van Damme, W., Barten, F., & Sanders, D. (2009). Task shifting: The answer to the human resources crisis in Africa? *Human Resources for Health, 7,* 49.

Lekoubou, A., Awah, P., Fezeu, L., & Pascal Kengne, A. (2010). Hypertension, diabetes mellitus and task shifting in their management in sub-Saharan Africa. *International Journal of Environmental Research and Public Health, 7,* 353–363.

Lozano, R., Naghavi, M., Foreman, K., Lim, S., Shibuya, K., Aboyans, V., . . . Aggarwal, R. (2012). Global and regional mortality from 235 causes of death for 20 age groups in 1990 and 2010: A systematic analysis for the Global Burden of Disease Study 2010. *Lancet, 380*(9859), 2095–2128.

Mathauer, I., & Imhoff, I. (2006). Health worker motivation in Africa: The role of non-financial incentives and human resource management tools. *Human Resources for Health, 4,* 24.

Mbemba, G., Gagnon, M-P., Pare, G., & Cite, J. (2013). Interventions for supporting nurse retention in rural and remote areas: An umbrella review. *Human Resources for Health, 11,* 44.

McCarthy, C. F., Zuber, A., Kelley, M. A., Veranl, A. R., & Riley, P. L. (2010). A systematic review of task-shifting for HIV treatment and care in Africa. *Human Resources for Health, 8,* 8.

McCoy, D., Bennett, S., Witter, S., Baker, B., Gow, J., Chand, S., . . . McPake, B. (2008). Salaries and incomes of health workers in sub-Saharan Africa. *Lancet, 23*(71), 675–681.

McPake, B., Maeda, A., Araujo, E. C., Maghraby, A. E., & Cometto, G. (2013). Why do health labour market forces matter? *Bulletin of the World Health Organization, 91,* 841–846.

Palmer, D. (2006). Tackling Malawi's human resources crisis. *Reproductive Health Matters, 14*(27), 27–39.

Pan American Health Organization. (2007). *Renewing primary health care in the Americas.* Washington, DC: Author.

Petersen, I., Lund, C., & Alan, F. J. (2012). A task shifting approach to primary mental health care for adults in South Africa: Human resource requirements and costs for rural settings. *Health Policy and Planning, 27,* 42–51.

Pulcini, J., Jelic, M., Gul, R., & Loke, A. (2010). An international survey on advanced practice nursing education, practice and regulation. *Journal of Nursing Scholarship, 42*(1), 31–39.

Shumbusho, F., Van Friensven, J., Lowrance, D., Turate, I., Weaver, M. A., Price, J., & Binagwaho, A. (2009). Task shifting for scale-up of HIV care: Evaluation of nurse-centered antiretroviarl treatment at rural health centers in Rwanda. *PLoS Medicine, 6*(10), e1000163.

Soucat, A., Scheffler, R., & Ghebreyesus, T. (2013). *The labor market for health workers: A new look at the crisis.* Washington, DC: The World Bank.

TACMIL Health Project. (2009). *Career ladders for midwives in Pakistan.* Bethesda, MD: Abt Associates Inc. and TACMIL Health Project.

Tran, N.-A., Luoma, M., & Ron, I. (2013). *Financing medical education through the private sector: Emerging insights from the SHOPS project (Draft).* Bethesda, MD: Abt Associates Inc, SHOPS Project.

United Nations General Assembly. (2014, May 15). *Global health and foreign policy, Sixty-seventh session (Agenda item 123).* Geneva, Switzerland: Author.

Willis-Shattuck, M., Bidwell, P., Thomas, S., Wyness, L., Blaauw, D., & Ditlopo, P. (2008). Motivation and retention of health workers in developing countries: A systematic review. *BMC Health Services Research, 8,* 247.

World Health Assembly. (2011). *Strengthening nursing and midwivery, WHA 64.7.* Geneva, Switzerland: Author.

World Health Organization (WHO). (1978). *Declaration of Alma-Ata.* Alma-Ata, Kazakhstan: Author.

World Health Organization. (2008a). *Task shifting: Rational redistribution of tasks among health workforce teams: Global recommendations and guidelines.* Geneva, Switzerland: Author.

World Health Organization. (2008b). *The World Health Report 2008—primary health care (now more than ever).* Geneva, Switzerland: Author.

World Health Organization. (2009a). *Global health risks: Mortality and burden of disease attributable to select major risks.* Geneva, Switzerland: Author.

World Health Organization. (2009b). *Global standards for the initial education of professional nurses and midwives.* Geneva, Switzerland: Author.

World Health Organization. (2010a). *A framework for community health nursing education.* Geneva, Switzerland: Author.

World Health Organization. (2010b). *A global survey monitoring progress in nursing and midwifery.* Geneva, Switzerland: Author.

World Health Organization. (2010c). *Framework for action on interprofessional education and collaborative practice.* Geneva, Switzerland: Author.

World Health Organization. (2010d). *Nursing and midwifery services strategic directions, 2011–1015.* Geneva. Switzerland: Author.

World Health Organization. (2012). *Enhancing nursing and midwifery capacity to contribute to the prevention, treatment and management of noncommunicable diseases.* Geneva, Switzerland: Author.

World Health Organization. (2013). *Transforming and scaling up health professionals' education and training.* Geneva. Switzerland: Author.

World Health Organization. (2014). Nursing and midwifery workforce and Universal Health Coverage (UCH). *Global Forum for Government Chief Nursing and Midwifery Officers.* Geneva, Switzerland: Author.

World Health Organization. (n.d.). *Referral systems—A summary of key processes to guide health services managers.* Geneva, Switzerland: Author.

Zachariah, R., Ford, N., Philips, M., Lynch, S., Massaquoi, M., Janssens, V., & Harries, A. (2009). Task shifting in HIV/AIDS: Opportunities, challenges and proposed actions for sub-Saharan Africa. *Royal Society of Tropical Medicine and Hygiene, 103*(6), 549–558.

Zuber, Z., McCarthy, C. F., Verani, A. R., Msidi, E., & Johnson, C. (2014). A survey of nurse-initiated and -managed antiretroviral therapy (NIMART) in practice, education policy and regulation in East, Central, and Southern Africa. *Journal of the Association of Nurses in AIDS Care, 25,* 520–531. doi:http://dx./.org/10.1016/j.jana.2014.02.003

CHAPTER 20

The Challenges of International Nurse Migration: Seeking Global Solutions

Carol L. Huston

M*igration* can be defined simply as the movement of someone or something from one place to another. International law clearly guarantees an individual the right to freedom of movement and residence, as established in the Universal Declaration of Human Rights (United Nations General Assembly, 1948) and the International Covenant on Civil and Political Rights (Office of the United Nations High Commissioner for Human Rights, 1976). Indeed, the individual's right to migrate is central to self-determination.

International nurse migration is the movement of nurses from one country to another in search of employment. While nurse migration has always existed, migration patterns have changed dramatically in the past 10 to 15 years, with more nurses migrating internationally than ever before. Indeed, Kingma (2010) notes that over time, international migrants have represented a steady 3% of the world's population, but their numbers have doubled in the past four decades and this number continues to increase.

Migration numbers have increasingly become feminized as well, with women now representing almost half of international immigrants (Kingma, 2010). "The immigration of highly skilled women is higher when the source country is poorer. This impacts negatively on three key education and health indicators in source countries: infant mortality rate, under-5 mortality, and secondary school enrollment rate by gender" (Finnish Medical Society, 2013, p. 6).

In addition, resource-limited nations have overwhelmingly become donor countries, resulting in a "brain drain" of their already inadequate numbers of highly educated health care professionals. This is especially true for countries like South Africa, Ghana, India, and Pakistan, where nurses are central to the health care systems and indeed are the most visible health care providers in those systems (Delucas, 2014). The consequences of this large-scale and nonstrategic migration are far-reaching, including a breakdown of national health care infrastructures and the inability of many donor countries to meet the health care needs of their own citizens.

Rosamond (2010) argues, however, that these concerns must be weighed against the value of the remittances (money migrating nurses send back home) that go back to families in donor countries who might otherwise not have access to basic necessities such as food, shelter, or health care. The International Center on Nurse Migration (ICNM, 2014, para 2) agrees, noting that "nurses' remittances represent an important source of added income and stability for individuals, families and communities around the world. These funds lessen the burden on health systems by improving access to food, housing, and education—all three significant social determinants of health."

In addition, the ICNM (2008) suggests that the traditional migration perspective is changing from migrants from the sending country being considered a loss while a gain for the receiving country to "a transnational framework, where migrants continually forge and sustain multiple attachments across nation-states and/or communities. As transnational migrants return home, they can facilitate the transfer of the critical financial and human capital . . . reversing 'brain drain' into 'brain gain'" (p. 2).

A recent issue of *Nursing Outlook* focused on globalization of the nursing workforce. Shaffer (2014) noted that "there is a myriad of legal, economic, cultural, social, and educational ramifications associated with the globalization of the nursing workforce" (p. 1). Thompson et al. (2014) discussed the efforts of the Honor Society of Nursing, Sigma Theta Tau International (STTI), and the International Council of Nurses (ICN) and their summit aimed at addressing the complex forces that drive nurse faculty migration. Brewer and Kovner (2014) examined the concepts related to turnover theory and the intersection with migration theory. They suggest that turnover theory, which includes "a variety of predictors of turnover (e.g., autonomy and physician—nurse relationships)" (p. 32), may strengthen the views of the migration framework. Jones and Sherwood (2014) note that "nurse mobility and migration will require nations and health care organizations to continue working to better understand workforce models and the employment, integration, assimilation, and regulation of an international nursing workforce" (p. 62).

This chapter examines the forces that encourage nurses to migrate; the consequences of uncontrolled migration (particularly in developing countries); and the global interventions that are occurring or need to occur to balance the right of individual nurses to seek positive global economic, social, and professional development with the goal to ensure all nations can provide, at a minimum, basic health care for their own citizens.

PUSH–PULL FACTORS OF NURSE MIGRATION

To understand what is driving the global migration of nurses, it is first necessary to examine what are known as the "push" and "pull" factors of nursing migration. Huston (2014) suggests that *push factors* are those factors that push or drive nurses to want to leave their countries to go to another. Low pay, inadequate opportunities for career advancement or continuing education, sociopolitical instability, and unsafe workplaces are examples of push factors. Other factors that may act as push factors in some countries include the risk of HIV and AIDS to health system workers, concerns about personal security in areas of conflict, and economic instability. Research by Zander, Blumel, and Busse (2012) suggests that a poor work environment is one of the most powerful push factors for nurse migration.

Pull factors are those factors that draw the nurse toward a different country. Huston (2014) notes that pull factors typically include higher pay, more-developed career structures, opportunities for further education and professional development, and, in some cases, safety from the threat of violence (more prevalent in less-developed countries). Other pull factors, such as the opportunity to travel or to participate in foreign aid work, also influence some nurses. Common push–pull factors in nurse migration are noted in Table 20.1.

Nurses migrate for many reasons and the push–pull factors to migrate are in constant imbalance. For example, nurses have migrated from Germany to other European Union (EU) countries in search of lower patient loads. A typical German nurse might be expected to care for 10 patients while a nurse in Norway has a patient load of only four patients (Zander & Busse, 2012). In addition, only 35% of nurses in Germany feel recognized for their nursing work (compared with 61% in Switzerland) and burnout rates are among the highest in the EU. As a result, these push factors encourage the migration of nurses from Germany to other countries.

Similarly, a recent study of South Korean nursing students found that 69.8% of respondents intended to migrate abroad, if possible, or absolutely in the future (Lee & Moon, 2013). The two most common reasons for their intended migration were economic (salary; 29.7%) and professional development (28.2%).

TABLE 20.1 Common Push–Pull Factors in Nurse Migration

PUSH FACTORS	PULL FACTORS
Low pay	High pay
Inadequate opportunities for career advancement or continuing education	More developed career structures or opportunities for further education and professional development
Sociopolitical instability	Political stability
Unsafe workplaces	Safety from the threat of violence
Practice restrictions	Family members in destination country
High workloads	Adventure/love of travel
Poor living conditions (housing, food, water)	Humanitarian motives
Remittance income	Recognition and status
Economic instability	Improved quality of life

Working conditions, however, was the most prevalent reason for the decision regarding the destination and the place to work.

In addition, destination countries increase their incentives for migration (pull factors) whenever nursing shortages exist. For example, Kodoth and Jacob (2013) noted that the estimated 6 million nurses and midwives in the World Health Organization (WHO) European Region are inadequate to meet current and projected workforce needs. As a result, incentives encouraging migration within the EU have increased. An increased import of nurses from India is expected to address this demand, even though at the government levels, the EU countries have voiced "ethical" concerns about shortages of health care providers in the source country (Kodoth & Jacob, 2013).

While approximately 50% of skilled workers do return to their countries of origin, usually after about 5 years, a sense of change, particularly change for the better, is critical if return migration is to occur (ICNM, 2008). If the economic and political conditions that encouraged migration in the first place have not changed then there will be little impetus to return.

DESTINATION AND DONOR COUNTRIES

Historically, nurse migration has followed previous colonial ties (i.e., Philippines to the United States; South Africa and Australia to the United Kingdom; India and Pakistan to England; Algeria to France, etc.). Indeed, people from the colonized countries tend to gravitate and immigrate to their "mother" countries, even after their native countries are granted independence (Rodis, 2013).

For the past decade, however, there has been active planning of large-scale international nurse recruitment, often from developing countries. Developed countries, such as the United States, Canada, Australia, and the United Kingdom, are the primary recipients of migrant nurses, although New Zealand also has a high dependence on nurses trained in other countries, a trend recently seen in Ireland as well. Approximately 5% to 10% of the nurses in the United States, United Kingdom, Canada, and Australia have been trained abroad (Global Health Policy, n.d.). That number rises to 21% in New Zealand and reaches an astounding 40% in Switzerland (Global Health Policy, n.d.).

New destinations have recently gained prominence as recipient countries as well, including Hong Kong and South Africa, which are exploring foreign nurse recruitment in response to workforce shortages (National Nursing Research Unit, 2011). In addition, Jamaica has begun recruiting Cuban nurses and Japan has established special arrangements to allow nurses from Southeast Asian countries (the Philippines, Indonesia, and Vietnam) to enter and practice in Japan (National Nursing Research Unit, 2011). The success of this new venture in Japan, however, is in question since the number of Indonesians who have come to Japan to work as care workers or nurses was 101 in 2012, compared with 362 in 2009. Similarly, the number from the Philippines dropped from 283 in 2009 to 101 in 2013 (ICNM, 2013). Cultural and language barriers are significant and applicants must pass a stringent Japanese language exam within 3 to 4 years. No foreign applicants passed the exam in 2009, and only 3 out of 254 passed in 2010 (ICNM, 2013, p. 2).

Destination Countries

The United States

Despite widespread belief, the United States is not the largest importer of nurses, although foreign-trained nurse entrants to the U.S. nurse workforce have increased at a rate faster than that of U.S.-educated new nurses for the past 15 years (Aiken, Buchan, Sochalski, Nichols, & Powell, 2013). Still, the United States is a high-demand destination country due to its excellent wages, good working conditions, and high standard of living. In fact, the number of foreign-trained nurses passing the licensing examination in the United States quadrupled between 2001 and 2007, before decreasing significantly in the past 2 years (Finnish Medical Society, 2013).

Currently, about 4%, or about 900,000, of the employed nurses in the United States are foreign trained (Aiken et al., 2013). Note, however, that if the United States follows the recent trends in the United Kingdom and Ireland and doubles its supply of foreign-trained nurses to 8% over the coming decade, some 100,000 additional nurses could be recruited from predominantly developing countries, such as the Caribbean or other countries with limited numbers of nurses.

In addition, the use of foreign nurses in the United States appears to be uneven geographically. Rodis (2013) notes that 20% of all the RNs in California are Filipinos, a considerably large percentage since Filipinos number only 2.3 million (officially 1.2 million) in a state population of 38 million. Rodis suggests that the main push factor from the Philippines has been the poor economy, where an average RN earns only about 5% of what an RN is paid in the United States. Many Filipino nurses entered the United States on H-1 work visas and gained permanent resident status under the Nursing Relief Act of 1989 (Rodis, 2013). When that law sunset in 1995, nurse immigration declined, and the passage of the Illegal Immigration Reform and Immigrant Responsibility Act of 1998 further discouraged Filipino nurse immigration to the United States.

Canada

Canada is both a recipient and donor country in terms of nurse migration. The United States is the primary destination of Canadian nurses. With a predicted 60,000 nurses needed by 2022, however, in order to fill labor shortages in both urban and rural areas, the demand for nurses throughout Canada is high. Recent immigration changes (Quebec Skilled Worker Program) made it possible for nurses to immigrate to Canada without a job offer and apply for a Canadian Permanent Residency Visa (Canada Immigration Newsletter, 2013). As a result, the permanent migration of foreign nurses to Canada since the year 2000 has increased threefold (Finnish Medical Society, 2013).

Australia/New Zealand

Australia has long imported foreign nurses to supplement its health care workforce and the numbers are only increasing. In fact, the permanent migration of foreign RNs to Australia has increased sixfold since the year 2000 (Finnish Medical Society, 2013). The majority of foreign nurses come from India, the Philippines, Saudi Arabia, United Arab Emirates, the United States, Kuwait, Singapore, Ireland, and Bahrain (Abraham, 2012). Recently, however, United Kingdom–educated nurses began migrating to Australia in significantly larger numbers (National Nursing Research Unit, 2011).

In addition to the obvious pull factors, Australia also offers both temporary and permanent visas to assist overseas nurses who wish to work there. A business long-stay visa allows RNs to stay for up to 4 years, with full work rights for themselves and accompanying family members (*Visa Options for Nurses*, 2014). In addition, a business short-stay visa allows nurses to undertake an approved bridging or preregistration program that runs for less than 3 months. Upon completion of this program, these nurses may be able to apply for a business long-stay visa. It also assists them in acquiring the English-speaking skills they need to relocate to other English-speaking countries.

New Zealand has been both a source and destination country since the beginning of the 21st century (Huston, 2014). Almost 25% of the workforce in New Zealand as of 2010 comes from overseas (Questioning the Ethics of Nurse Migration, 2010), with India providing a rapidly increasing number of migrants (Woodbridge & Bland, 2010). The movement of New Zealand RNs to Australia is expedited by the Trans-Tasman Agreement, whereas the entry of foreign RNs to New Zealand is facilitated by nursing being an identified *priority occupation*.

United Kingdom/Europe

The United Kingdom has historically relied heavily on international recruits to fill its nursing vacancies. However, as a result of recent economic downturns as well as stricter registration and work permit regulations, the number of non-EU nurses entering the United Kingdom workforce has decreased consistently since 2005 (National Nursing Research Unit, 2011). Indeed, the number of foreign nurses in the United Kingdom has decreased from between 10,000 and 16,000, to between 2,000 and 2,500 per year because the new regulations do not allow recruiters to hire nurses from foreign countries who receive United Kingdom financial aid (*Visato*, 2012).

In Sweden, Denmark, and Switzerland, the influx of foreign-trained nurses peaked around 2003 before decreasing significantly until 2006. Since then, increases in migration flows seem to have resumed (Finnish Medical Society, 2013).

Germany is also continuing to actively seek foreign nurses. In 2013, the German Minister for Labor and Social Affairs and the Philippine Labor Secretary signed an agreement to facilitate hiring of Filipino health care professionals in Germany beginning in 2014 (ICNM, 2013). Agencies from both countries will work together to select nurses, who will complete a basic German language course and attend seminars on German culture and professional practice in Manila. Nurses would then be matched to potential employers in Germany.

Donor Countries

Common donor countries include Fiji, Jamaica, India, Mauritius, Cuba, and the Philippines. The English-speaking Caribbean countries, in particular, are experiencing a nursing shortage as a result of the widespread migration of their nursing workforce to Canada, the United States, and the United Kingdom (International Center on Nurse Migration [ICNM], 2010a). In addition, intraregional nurse migration will likely increase with the implementation of the Caribbean Single Market and Economy (CSME), as the free movement of labor will draw nurses to the highest-paying countries. The Caribbean Community (CARICOM) Free Movement of Persons Act has also allowed nurses free movement across the region since 2006 (ICNM, 2010b).

The Philippines

The Philippines is the leading donor country for nurses internationally by design and with the support of the government (Aiken et al., 2013) because for many years, the Philippines government has actively endorsed and facilitated initiatives aimed at educating, recruiting, training, and placing nurses around the world to encourage the generation of remittance income (migrating nurses often send remittances back home to support their families and bolster the economy). Rosamond (2010) notes that newly migrated nurses can earn up to 100 times what their annual income would be back home and that many migrated nurses send home, at a minimum, 26% of their income.

Indeed, the export of labor is the Philippines' most profitable export for that country, with almost 10% of the population working around the globe and generating more than US$15 billion in remittance income annually (Kaelin, 2011). This includes the export of at least 10,000 nurses annually (Kaelin, 2011). In addition, there is a labor market oversupply of nurses in the Philippines, with that country producing 100,000 to 150,000 nurses every year. Less than 5% of Filipino nurses are employed in the Philippines, either by the government or the private sector (Gamolo, 2008). The Philippine Overseas Employment Administration deployed a total of 13,525 licensed nurses around the world in 2006 (James, 2008), and, according to the Trade Union Congress of the Philippines, more than 21,000 new Filipino nurses sought U.S. jobs in 2007 (Gamolo, 2008). The Trade Union continues to encourage the deployment of surplus nurses and other highly skilled workers rather than unskilled workers, whose skills are more easily replaceable.

Huston (2014) notes that national opinion in the Philippines regarding health care worker migration generally focuses on the improved quality of life for individual migrants and their families and on the benefits of remittances to the nation; however, a shortage of highly skilled nurses and the massive retraining of physicians to become nurses elsewhere has created severe problems for the Filipino health system, including the closure of many hospitals.

Masselink and Lee (2013) agree that resultant impacts on the Filipino health care infrastructure appear to be less important philosophically than perceived potential benefits, noting that "Philippine government officials cast nurses as global rather than domestic providers of health care, implicating them in development more as sources of remittance income than for their potential contributions to the country's health care system" (p. 90). Masselink and Lee suggest this orientation is motivated not simply by the desire for remittance revenues, but also as a way to cope with overproduction and lack of domestic opportunities for nurses in the Philippines.

China

China, with the second-largest nursing workforce in the world, is another country actively seeking to export nurses. Yet Fang (2007) suggests there is actually a severe shortage of nurses in China, with only one nurse per 1,000 population, as well as a very high level of unemployment and underemployment of nurses. This creates an artificial surplus of nurses who can and do want to migrate. Fang suggested that even if the Chinese government were to increase the nursing jobs available and improve working conditions, some surplus would still exist. He concluded that China will likely become an important source of nurses for developed nations in the coming years.

India

India is also gaining ground as one of the world's leading nurse exporters, despite having an extremely low nurse-to-population ratio, with the major destinations being the Gulf countries and the Organization for Economic Cooperation and Development (OECD; Kodoth & Jacob, 2013). Poor remuneration and socioeconomic and living conditions, and the lack of civic amenities such as schools for children, electricity, piped water, and telephone connections in remote areas, are push factors for nurses in India (Issac & Syam, 2009). Bhalla and Meher (2010) agree, suggesting that low wages, heavy workloads, bad working conditions, and a sense of sometimes not being treated with respect have resulted in many Indian nurses migrating to the United States, the United Kingdom, and other countries.

Issac and Syam (2009) note that most migrant Indian nurses initially migrate to large cities within India, such as New Delhi and Mumbai, to get work experience, then to countries in the Persian Gulf, and finally to Europe and America. The internal migration to these cities is through networks of friends and relatives; international travel is then typically arranged through a recruiter. Remittances from nurses overseas have emerged as a stable source of foreign exchange inflows for the country, with India being one of the highest remittance receiving countries in the world.

Africa/Malawi

African countries, particularly those in sub-Saharan Africa, have lost a substantial proportion of their skilled work force through migration. In fact, a recent study suggested that more than a third (37%) of the medical and nursing student respondents intended to work or specialize abroad and the majority intended to leave South Africa within 5 years of completing their medical or nursing studies (George & Reardon, 2013). Poor working conditions within the health sector, such as long work hours, high patient loads, inadequate resources, and occupational hazards, influenced these students' decisions to consider migration. Similarly, research by George, Atujuna, and Gow (2013) found that the migration of health workers in South Africa was not occurring as a result of lower salaries. Instead, the consideration to move was determined by other factors, including age, levels of stress experienced, and the extent to which health workers were satisfied at their current place of work.

The movement of health workers both within and outside of South Africa has been recognized as a major problem for the health sector, increasing the strain on the already burdened public health sector, increasing the workload for those who stay, and leading to a shortage of skills and subsequent loss of capacity for health systems to deliver adequate health care (George, Atujuna, & Gow, 2013). The consequences of uncontrolled migration are apparent when one considers that the sub-Saharan African countries have 25% of the world's disease burden, and yet possess only 1.3% of trained human resources for health. Remittances from migrants are recognized, however, as an important source of resilience for households in African countries, especially in light of the fact that the monetary value of remittances to Africa now exceeds that of aid (United Nations University, 2012).

In Malawi, prior to 2005, strong education links and established migrant networks encouraged large numbers of nurses to migrate to the United Kingdom. While stricter regulations stemmed this outflow during the first decade of this century, recent findings suggest that this did not lead to improved retention of nurses in Malawi (National Nursing Research Unit, 2011). Instead, Malawian nurses have found alternative pathways to migration, with some leaving the profession completely and others choosing nonnursing administrative roles with a nongovernmental organization (NGO) in Malawi itself. On an individual level, many Malawian nurses perceive these United Kingdom regulations to be discriminatory since the United Kingdom is importing other EU nurses and since those doors had been open to them before.

CONSEQUENCES OF UNCONTROLLED MIGRATION

Freeman, Baumann, Blythe, Fisher, and Akhtar-Danesh (2012) suggest that the consequences of migration are positive or negative depending on the viewpoint and its effect on the individual and other stakeholders such as the source country, destination country, health care systems, and the nursing profession. Issac and Syam (2009) agree, noting that the economic gains from migration may translate into greater financial resources to be invested in improving the public health services in the country. It can also ensure that migrant health professionals return with improved skills that can be internalized and applied widely, thereby improving the quality of health services (Issac & Syam, 2009).

Yet others argue that migration has an inherently negative implication on the availability of health professionals in developing countries. Indeed, a review of the literature suggests that different countries have experienced different effects as a result of the push–pull of international nurse migration.

Huston (2014) notes that in some cases, aggressive recruitment, by which large numbers of recruits are sought, may considerably deplete a single health facility or contract a significant number of newly graduated nurses from a single educational institute. This has important local and regional implications. For example, Aiken et al. (2013) note that nurse migration from developing countries is occurring at the same time that international resources are finally available to address HIV/AIDS and improve immunization coverage around the world. However, this effort has been undermined by the severe shortage of health personnel in countries like Botswana.

One of the most significant consequences, though, of uncontrolled migration is the inability of donor countries to develop sustainable health care systems and provide appropriate care to their citizens. Indeed, few donor nations are prepared to manage the loss of their nurse workforce to such widespread migration. "When a country has a fragile health system, the loss of its health workforce can bring the whole system close to collapse, with the consequences measured in lives lost" (WHO, 2010, para 10).

It is *brain drain*, however, that is one of the most critical negative consequences of widespread nursing migration from developing countries. Brain drain refers to the loss of skilled personnel and the loss of investment in education that is experienced when those human resources migrate elsewhere. The Federation for American Immigration Reform (FAIR, 2014) defines brain drain as the flow of skilled professionals from less developed countries to more developed countries and suggests that this practice results in developing countries losing the individuals they can least afford to lose because they are the ones "who are skilled and educated, who perform crucial services contributing to the health and economy of the country, and who create new jobs for others."

Recent reports from South Africa, Ghana, China, the Caribbean, and even the Philippines highlight that the significant outflow of nurses has had negative effects, including reductions in the level and quality of services and the loss of specialist skills. Indeed, Brush (2010) suggests that the continued exodus of nurses from the Philippines now threatens the public health of that country itself, since so many of the country's most experienced nurses are migrating, leaving the care of the local populace (particularly those in rural communities) in the hands of lesser experienced, and lesser qualified, personnel.

Similarly, African ministers of health have repeatedly brought resolutions to the World Health Assembly, stating that health care worker migration is crippling their health care systems. Taiwan too has expressed concerns about the brain drain that has occurred as a result of the migration of nurses from there (Brush, 2008).

Kingma (2010) suggests that recruiting nurses from abroad does not address the basic causative factors for national nursing shortages and, instead, simply redistributes the shortage globally. In addition, if the nurses' education was publicly funded in the source country, this represents a significant loss of investment for the population and government left behind. In essence, then, developing countries are supporting the health care infrastructure of more developed countries, often at the expense of their own country (Huston, 2014).

ADDRESSING THE PROBLEM

Given the current extent of nurse migration and the potentially negative impacts on donor countries, nurse leaders from around the world have weighed in on the issue. Aiken et al. (2013) suggest that a twofold approach is required to address the threat of nursing migration, induced shortages in developing countries and their resultant inability to meet global health initiatives. The first approach requires greater diligence by developing countries in creating a largely sustainable domestic nurse workforce. In fact, many OECD countries have made efforts to increase training rates for doctors and nurses. Since the year 2000, the number of nursing graduates has increased by at least 50% in Australia, France, and the United Kingdom, and has doubled in Canada (Finnish Medical Society, 2013).

The second approach, identified by Aiken et al. (2013), requires a greater investment through international aid in building nursing education capacity in the less developed countries that supply developed countries with nurses. A summit convened by STTI and the ICN in 2012 agreed, concluding that a significant impact could be achieved if all countries worked to attain self-sufficiency in producing and retaining their workforces rather than relying on international recruitment (Thompson et al., 2013).

In addition, some global and national professional associations/organizations have provided formal position statements to guide both donor and importer countries. Others have attempted to provide guidance to the individual nurse considering global migration.

The International Council of Nurses

For example, the ICN has issued several position statements arguing for ethics and good employment practices in international recruitment. The *ICN Position Statement: Nurse Retention and Migration*, authored in 1999 and revised in 2007, confirms the right of nurses to migrate, as well as the potential beneficial outcomes of multicultural practice and learning opportunities supported by migration, but acknowledges potential adverse effects on the quality of health care in donor countries (ICN, 2007b).

The ICN (2007b) position statement also condemns the practice of recruiting nurses to countries where authorities have failed to implement sound human resource planning and to seriously address problems that cause nurses to leave the profession and discourage them from returning to nursing. The position statement also denounces unethical recruitment practices that exploit nurses or mislead them into accepting job responsibilities and working conditions that are incompatible with their qualifications, skills, and experience. The ICN and its member national nurses' associations call for a regulated recruitment process, based on ethical principles that guide informed decision making and reinforce sound employment policies on the part of governments, employers, and nurses, thereby supporting fair and cost-effective recruitment and retention practices.

In addition, the ICN adopted a second position paper on ethical nurse recruitment in 2001 that was also revised and reaffirmed in 2007 (ICN, 2007a). This document identifies 13 principles necessary to create a foundation for ethical recruitment, whether international or intra-national contexts are being considered. The ICN suggests that all health-sector stakeholders—patients, governments, employers, and nurses—will benefit if this ethical recruitment framework is systematically applied.

The International Center on Nurse Migration (ICNM)

Another organization, the ICNM, established in 2005, represents a collaborative project launched by the ICN and the Commission on Graduates of Foreign Nursing Schools (CGFNS). The ICNM serves as a global resource for the development, promotion, and dissemination of research, policy, and information on global nurse migration (ICNM, 2010a). The ICNM website includes commissioned papers on nurse migration, fact sheets, and e-newsletters. In addition, there are links for global nurse migration research.

The World Health Organization (WHO)

Another international organization involved in establishing guidelines for nurse migration is WHO. In an effort to balance the right of workers to migrate with a need to assure that global health care needs are met, the WHO Global Code of Practice on the International Recruitment of Health Personnel was finalized in the 63rd World Health Assembly on May 21, 2010 (Finnish Medical Society, 2013). The Code aims to establish and promote voluntary principles and practices for the ethical international recruitment of health personnel. Though voluntary and nonbinding for member states, it aims to provide a framework for global dialogue on issues relating to global health workforce migration. It may guide the formulation of bilateral or multilateral agreements or legal instruments. It may also be used to mitigate the adverse effects of active recruitment by developed countries.

Thus, the code promotes ethical recruitment, protects migrant health workers' rights, and encourages governments in both developed and developing nations to actively address the push and pull factors that promote nurse migration. The Code of Practice was the first of its kind on a global scale for migration.

The Commonwealth of Nations

The Commonwealth of Nations is a voluntary association of 54 sovereign states, most of which are former British colonies or dependencies of these colonies (includes Australia, Canada, and the UK, among others) (Finnish Medical Society, 2013). In 2003, the Commonwealth adopted a Code of Practice in the international recruitment of health care workers. While not a legal document, it does provide a framework for policy making among member nations, as well as other nations.

The United States

Within the past few years, many countries, including the United States, have published national nursing strategies for dealing with staff shortages. Academy Health, funded through a grant from the John D. and Catherine T. MacArthur Foundation in collaboration with the O'Neill Institute for National and Global Health Law at Georgetown University, convened a task force of recruiters, hospitals, and foreign-educated nurses to develop draft standards of practice about global nurse recruitment, as well as recommendations on how to institutionalize these standards. In late 2007, Academy Health released a report on year 1 of its 2-year project—the *Voluntary Code of Ethical Conduct for the Recruitment of Foreign-Educated Nurses to the United States* (Aliason et al., 2008).

This Code is designed to increase transparency and accountability throughout the process of international recruitment and ensure adequate orientation for foreign-educated nurses. It also provides guidance on ways to ensure recruitment is not harmful to source countries. This document was endorsed by the National Council of State Boards of Nursing (NCSBN) in 2008 (NCSBN, 2011).

Europe

The Netherlands, Ireland, and the Scandinavian countries also have good-practice guidelines on international recruitment or are looking at developing guidelines. In addition, Norway issued a policy statement on the ethics of international recruitment, and in 2007 "instituted a new health worker recruitment policy committed to reducing its contribution to the 'pull' of health workers from their home countries by pursuing a policy of self-sufficiency for its own needs, while also helping to reduce 'push' factors through development assistance to support the strengthening of low-income countries' health systems" (Finnish Medical Society, 2013, p. 10).

The United Kingdom in 2005 began limiting nurse recruitment to the EU countries and only granting work permits to nurses from non-EU countries if National Health Services institutions showed that jobs could not be filled by United Kingdom or EU applications. In fact, the United Kingdom Code of Practice is one of the oldest Codes of Practice in existence. It was initially enacted into law in 2001 after a decade of shortage in human health resources and revised in 2004 (Finnish Medical Society, 2013).

The Caribbean

Some countries have initiated or examined various policy responses to reduce outflow, such as requiring nurses to work in their home countries for a certain amount of time after education completion or by charging the nurse a fee to migrate to another country. For example, the Nurses Association of Jamaica has demanded that the Jamaican government raise salaries in an effort to retain nurses in their home country (Brush, 2008).

Another response has been to recognize that outflow cannot be halted if principles of individual freedom are to be upheld, but that the outflow that does occur must be managed and moderated. The "managed migration" initiative being undertaken in the Caribbean, which has provided regional support for addressing the nursing shortage crisis and developed initiatives such as training for export and temporary migration, is one example of a coordinated intervention to minimize the negative effects of outflow while realizing at least some benefit from the process (Salmon, Yan, Hewitt, & Guisinger, 2007).

CONCLUSION

"Today's search for labor is a highly organized global hunt for talent and nurses are increasingly part of the migratory stream. Critical nursing shortages in industrialized countries have generated a demand that is fuelling international recruitment campaigns. At the same time, structural adjustments in the developing countries have resulted in severe workforce imbalances—shortfalls often coexisting with large numbers of unemployed health professionals" (Kingma, 2010, para 2). Kingma concludes that international nurse migration is simply an exaggeration of the larger system problems that make nurses leave their jobs and their profession.

Huston (2014) agrees, suggesting that one must consider whether recruiting foreign nurses to solve acute staffing shortages is simply a poorly thought out quick fix to much greater problems and whether, in doing so, not only are donor nations harmed, that the issues that led to the shortages in the first place are never addressed. She goes on to suggest that one must at least question whether wholesale foreign nurse recruitment would even be necessary if importer nations made a more concerted effort to improve the working conditions, salaries, empowerment, and recognition of the home-born nurses they already employ. Clearly, there must be some sort of a balance between the right of individual nurses to choose to migrate (autonomy), particularly when push factors are overwhelming, and the more utilitarian concern for the donor nations' health as a result of losing scarce nursing resources (Huston, 2014).

Delucas (2014) agrees, suggesting that both destination and source countries are challenged by poorly controlled nurse migration. Destination countries must address the ethical implications of aggressive recruitment and their failure to develop a sustainable, self-sufficient domestic workforce. Source countries struggle to fund and educate adequate numbers of nurses for domestic needs and migrant replacement.

Many nursing organizations and nursing leaders have begun to recognize the negative effects of uncontrolled international migration but efforts to address the problem have been inadequate. In some countries, national governments and regulatory agencies are beginning to address the issue. Yet, in the meantime, what may be hundreds of thousands of nurses are migrating internationally, and the potentially negative effects of this increasing trend on both the migrant nurse and the donor nation are becoming ever more apparent (Huston, 2014).

Delucas (2014) argues passionately that more work must be done to engage nurses at leadership and grassroots levels to establish international treaties regarding foreign nurse migration that work collaboratively for justice and health equity. She suggests that inertia is not an option as nurses must adopt a broader sense of responsibility in addressing global disparities of health and health care and the need to develop a sustainable nursing workforce.

Freeman et al. (2012) conclude that nurse migration will continue to be a growing global phenomenon as a result of the RN shortage in most countries and that the consequences of this movement will affect nursing practice and health care throughout the world. Huston (2014) agrees, arguing that nurse migration and its associated ethical dilemmas are among the most serious issues facing the nursing profession and there is little sign that this significant issue will abate anytime soon.

REFERENCES

Abraham, G. K. (2012). *10 countries with the most nursing migration to Australia.* Ezine articles. Retrieved from http://ezinearticles.com/?10-Countries-With-the-Most-Nursing-Migration-to-Australia&id=6896590

Aiken, L. H., Buchan, J., Sochalski, J., Nichols, B., & Powell, M. (2013, December). Trends in international nurse migration. *Health Affairs, 32*(12). Retrieved from http://content.healthaffairs.org/content/23/3/69.full

Aliason, V., Bednash, G., Bentley, J., Conpas, L., Foster, P., Gabriel, S., . . . Wilson, A. (2008). *Voluntary code of ethical conduct for the recruitment of foreign-educated nurses to the United States.* Academy Health, MacArthur, and O'Neill Institute. Retrieved from http://www.nursingworld.org/MainMenuCategories/ThePracticeofProfessional Nursing/workforce/ForeignNurses/CodeofConductforRecruitmentofForeign EducatedNurses.aspx

Bhalla, J. S., & Meher, M. A. (2010, March 3). Nursing a foreign dream. *Hindustan Times.* Retrieved from http://www.hindustantimes.com/India-news/NewDelhi/Nursing-a-foreign-dream/Article1-514546.aspx

Brewer, C. S., & Kovner, C. T. (2014). Intersection of migration and turnover theories. *Nursing Outlook, 62,* 29–38.

Brush, B. (2010). The potent lever of toil: Nursing development and exportation in the postcolonial Philippines. *American Journal of Public Health, 100*(9), 1572–1581.

Brush, B. L. (2008). Global nurse migration today. *Journal of Nursing Scholarship, 40*(1), 20–25.

Canada Immigration Newsletter. (2013, August). *Nurses in high demand throughout Canada.* Retrieved from http://www.cicnews.com/2013/08/nurses-high-demand-canada-082809.html

Delucas, A. C. (2014). Foreign nurse recruitment: Global risk. *Nursing Ethics, 21*(1), 76–85. Retrieved from http://nej.sagepub.com/content/21/1/76.full.pdf+html

Fang, Z. Z. (2007). Potential of China in global nurse migration. *Health Services Research, 42*(3, Pt. 2), 1419–1428.

Federation for American Immigration Reform. (2014) *Glossary of immigration terms: Brain drain*. Retrieved from http://www.fairus.org/Default.aspx?PageID=12578841&A=SearchResult&SearchID=5902049&ObjectID=12578841&ObjectType=1

Finnish Medical Society. (2013). *Migration: Destination and source countries*. Retrieved from http://www.duodecim.fi/kotisivut/sivut.nayta?p_sivu=143597

Freeman, M., Baumann, A., Blythe, J., Fisher, A., & Akhtar-Danesh, N. (2012). Migration: A concept analysis from a nursing perspective. *Journal of Advanced Nursing, 68*(5), 1176–1186.

Gamolo, N. O. (2008). RP nurses seen as prime export commodity. *The Manila Times*. Retrieved from http://philnurse.com/?p=10

George, G., Atujuna, M., & Gow, J. (2013). Migration of South African health workers: The extent to which financial considerations influence internal flows and external movements. *Bio Med Central Health Services Research, 13*, 297. Retrieved from http://www.ncbi.nlm.nih.gov/pmc/articles/PMC3765273

George, G. & Reardon, C. (2013, May). Preparing for export? Medical and nursing student migration intentions post-qualification in South Africa. *African Journal of Primary Health Care and Family Medicine, 5*, 1. Retrieved from http://www.phcfm.org/index.php/phcfm/article/view/483

Global Health Policy. (n.d.). *Nurse migration*. Retrieved from http://nurs901globalhealthpolicy.blogspot.com/p/nurse-migration.html

Huston, C. (2014). *Importing foreign nurses*. In C. Huston (Ed.), *Professional issues in nursing* (3rd ed.). Philadelphia, PA: Lippincott, Williams, and Wilkins.

International Center on Nurse Migration (ICNM). (2008). *Return migration of nurses. Fact sheet 2008*. Retrieved from http://www.intlnursemigration.org/assets/pdfs/ReturnMigrationfactsheetA4.pdf

International Center on Nurse Migration (ICNM). (2010a). *Homepage*. Retrieved from http://www.icn.ch/projects/international-centre-on-nurse-migration

International Center on Nurse Migration (ICNM). (2010b, August). The nurse labor and education markets in the English-speaking CARICOM: Issues and options for reform. *Ebrief*. Retrieved from http://www.intlnursemigration.org/assets/pdfs/eBrief_CARICOM.pdf

International Center on Nurse Migration. (2013). New agreement for Filipino nurses in Germany. *ICNM enews* (19). Retrieved from http://www.intlnursemigration.org/assets/enews/ICNMeNews2013May.pdf

International Center on Nurse Migration. (2014). *International nurse migration and remittances*. Retrieved from http://www.intlnursemigration.org/assets/pdfs/NurseMigrationRemitfactsheet2014.pdf

International Council of Nurses (ICN). (2007a). *Position statement: Ethical nurse recruitment*. Retrieved from http://www.icn.ch/publications/position-statements

International Council of Nurses (ICN). (2007b). *Position statement: Nurse retention and migration*. Retrieved from http://www.icn.ch/publications/position-statements

Issac, A., & Syam, N. (2009). *Migration of healthcare professionals from India: A case study* (pp. 1–66). New Delhi, India: WHO India Office.

James, E. (2008). *Global brain drain. Advance perspective: Nurses*. Retrieved from http://community.advanceweb.com/blogs/nurses3/archive/2008/04/10/global-brain-drain.aspx

Jones, C. B., & Sherwood, G. D. (2014). The globalization of the nursing workforce: Pulling the pieces together. *Nursing Outlook, 62*, 59–63.

Kaelin, L. (2011). A question of justice: Assessing nurse migration from a philosophical perspective. *Developing World Bioethics, 11*(1), 30–39.

Kingma, M. (2010). *Nurses on the move: Worldwide migration*. Berlin Institute. Retrieved from http://www.berlin-institut.org/online-handbookdemography/nurses-on-the-move-worldwide-migration.html

Kodoth, P., & Jacob, T. K. (2013). *International mobility of nurses from Kerala (India) to the EU: Prospects and challenges with special reference to the Netherlands and Denmark* (CARIM-India Research Report No. 2013/19). Retrieved from http://www.india-eu-migration.eu/media/CARIM-India-No.2013-19.pdf

Lee, E., & Moon, M. (2013, December). Korean nursing students' intention to migrate abroad. *Nurse Education Today, 33*(12), 1517–1522. Retrieved from http://dx.doi.org/10.1016/j.nedt.2013.04.006

Masselink, L. E., & Lee, S. (2013). Government officials' representation of nurses and migration in the Philippines. *Health Policy and Planning, 28*, 90–99. Retrieved from http://heapol.oxfordjournals.org/content/28/1/90.full.pdf+html

National Council of State Boards of Nursing (NCSBN). (2011). *NCSBN partners with group to help prevent unethical recruitment of foreign-educated nurses (9/4/2008).* Retrieved from http://www.nursingcenter.com/lnc/JournalArticle?Article_ID=848819&Journal_ID=260876&Issue_ID=848807

National Nursing Research Unit. (2011, December). What are the implications of changes in nurse migration? *Policy Plus Evidence, Issues, and Opinions in Healthcare,* (30). Retrieved from http://www.kcl.ac.uk/nursing/research/nnru/Policy/Policy-Plus-Issues-by-Theme/Nursescareers%28andstayinginnursing%29/PolicyIssue33.pdf

Office of the United Nations High Commissioner for Human Rights. (1976). *International covenant on civil and political rights.* Retrieved from http://www.ohchr.org/EN/ProfessionalInterest/Pages/CCPR.aspx

Questioning the ethics of nurse migration. (2010). *Kai Tiaki: Nursing New Zealand, 16*(6), 7.

Rodis, R. (2013, May 14). *Telltale signs: "Why are there so many Filipino nurses in the US?"* Retrieved from http://www.asianweek.com/2013/05/14/telltale-signs-why-are-there-so-many-filipino-nurses-in-the-us

Rosamond, R. L. (2010, May 21). Letter to the Editor by Rosamond to International nurse migration: Facilitating the transition. *The Online Journal of Issues in Nursing.* Retrieved from http://www.nursingworld.org/MainMenuCategories/ANAMarketplace/ANAPeriodicals/OJIN/LetterstotheEditor/Response-by-Randy-Lynn-Rosamond-.html

Salmon, M., Yan, J., Hewitt, H., & Guisinger, V. (2007). Managed migration: The Caribbean approach to addressing nursing services capacity. *Health Services Research, 42*(1), 1354–1372.

Shaffer, F. A. (2014). Ensuring a global workforce: A challenge and opportunity. *Nursing Outlook, 62*, 1–4.

Thompson, P. E., Benton, D. C., Adams, E., Morin, K. H., Barry, J., Prevost, S. S., . . . Oywer, E. (2014, July 08). The global summit on nurse faculty migration. *Nursing Outlook.* Retrieved from http://www.nursingoutlook.org/article/S0029-6554(13)00104-8/fulltext

United Nations General Assembly. (1948). *The universal declaration of human rights.* Retrieved from http://www.un.org/en/documents/udhr

United Nations University. (2012, September 19). *Migration, remittances and resilience in Africa.* Retrieved from http://unu.edu/publications/articles/migration-remittances-and-resilience-in-africa.html#info

Visa options for nurses. (2014). Retrieved from http://www.australia-migration.com/page/Options_for_Nurses/39

Visato. (2012). United Kingdom's immigration policies affect foreign nurses' migration. *Immigration News.* Retrieved from http://news.visato.com/england/united-kingdom%E2%80%99s-immigration-policies-affect-foreign-nurses%E2%80%99-migration/20120109

Woodbridge, M., & Bland, M. (2010). Supporting Indian nurses migrating to New Zealand: A literature review. *International Nursing Review, 57*(1), 40–48.

World Health Organization (WHO) Media Center. (2010, July). *Migration of health workers.* Retrieved from http://www.who.int/mediacentre/factsheets/fs301/en

Zander, B., Blumel, M., & Busse, R. (2012). Nurse migration in Europe—Can expectations really be met? Combining qualitative and quantitative data from Germany and eight of its destination and source countries. *International Journal of Nursing Studies, 50,* 210–218. Retrieved from http://www.mig.tu-berlin.de/fileadmin/a38331600/2013. publications/IJNS-Nurse-Migration-Germany_with_pages.pdf

Zander, B., & Busse, R. (2012). *RN4CastResearch.* Retrieved from http://nurse-migration.com

CHAPTER 21

Nursing Leadership in Interprofessional Education

Nancy Hoffart, Elizabeth J. Brown, and Susan E. Farrell

Unless you instill in the next generation a commitment and expectation that collaboration is normal and will be accomplished, it can never be accomplished. We have to believe in interprofessionalism for it to become possible
—Sioban Nelson (Nelson, Tassone, & Hodges, 2014, p. 55).

*I*n this chapter, we examine the case of an interprofessional education (IPE) initiative in order to highlight the significant role that nursing can play in building a new program for interprofessional learning. Though we recognize that many forces and stakeholders are necessary to the success of transforming health professions education and health care delivery locally and globally, we use this case to illustrate nursing's role in supporting and leading these efforts at one institution. Through this case study and discussion, we consider how nursing leadership can influence the development of a new IPE program, subsequently enhancing the profile of nursing and strengthening the current and future leadership capacity of the participating nursing students and faculty.

The need to radically improve health care delivery and substantially strengthen workforce capacity across the world is vast and expanding. Leadership at all levels of nursing is vital in ensuring that nurses play a significant role in implementing and evaluating transformative changes. High-profile reports from within and outside of the nursing profession have underscored the need for nursing leadership and nurse leaders to shape the future for nursing and improvements in delivery of health care services and health professions education (Institute of Medicine [IOM], 2011; Prime Ministers Commission, 2010; World Health Organization [WHO], 2013b).

> As nurses and midwives are at the forefront of health service delivery globally, maximizing their roles not only as practitioners but also as leaders, is essential to effectively address the variety of challenges posed by evolving health and demographic changes in society . . . . (WHO, 2013b, p. 119)

The Lancet Commission (Frenk et al., 2010) offered a new vision for health professions education, one with a global perspective, and one that incorporates a multidisciplinary systems approach to considering the connections between education and the health system. To achieve this vision, the commission proposed transformative learning and interdependence in education and offered several recommendations, including the promotion of "interprofessional and transprofessional education that breaks down professional silos while enhancing collaborative and nonhierarchical relationships in effective teams" (p. 3). Other recent reports from groups such as WHO (2010) and the IOM (2013b), as well as a number of regional associations (Table 21.1), substantiate the worldwide attention to IPE. The primary argument in favor of IPE is its potential to increase the quality and continuity of patient care through the promotion of learning and teamwork competencies.

The Lancet Commission promoted a competency-driven and team-based approach in transforming health professions education to strengthen health systems, highlighting leadership as an integral competency. "Transformative learning is about developing leadership attributes; its purpose is to produce enlightened change agents" (Frenk et al., 2010, p. 1924). The IOM report (2011) suggested that nursing education programs embed leadership development into their curricula and increase the emphasis on IPE. Transformative and interprofessional learning and collaborative practice (CP) not only require nursing leadership, but also serve as vehicles to develop and strengthen leadership competencies in nursing students and faculty.

The question arises: How can the profession of nursing contribute to and shape efforts to promote and achieve IPE and CP? The IOM's 2011 report, *The Future of Nursing: Leading Change, Advancing Health*, advocated for nurses to become full partners with physicians to lead improvements in the U.S. health care system (IOM, 2011). A number of initiatives around the world have brought health professions students together to learn about each other's professions and contributions in an interprofessional approach to learning and work on behalf of systems that succeed

TABLE 21.1 Regional Interprofessional Education Associations

ASSOCIATION	WEBSITE
Australasian Interprofessional Practice and Education Network (AIPPEN)	http://www.aippen.net/australia
Canadian Interprofessional Health Collaborative (CIHC)	http://www.cihc.ca
Centre for the Advancement of Interprofessional Education (CAIPE)	http://caipe.org.uk
European Interprofessional Education Network (EIPEN)	http://www.eipen.eu
Interprofessional Education Collaborative (IPEC, USA)	https://ipecollaborative.org
Japan Interprofessional Working and Education Network (JIPWEN)	http://jipwen.dept.showa.gunma-u.ac.jp/?page_id=3
Nordic Interprofessional Network (NIPNET)	http://www.nipnet.org

in providing patient-centered care (Brandt & Schmitt, 2011; Kowitlawakul, 2014; WHO, 2013a, 2013c). These novel approaches to teaching and learning in health care have moved IPE forward; nurse leaders have a significant role to play in furthering that effort. Clarke and Hassmiller (2013) highlighted the responsibility of nurse leaders in promoting the role of nursing through IPE:

> The opportunity for the profession to demonstrate leadership in interprofessional education and practice will create systems of care that monitor health needs of individuals, families and populations in relation to complex evolving health care systems. (p. 335)

In countries such as Lebanon, where nursing is not widely recognized as a profession, IPE faces the challenge of disabusing stereotypes about nurses as assistive and subsidiary to physicians. Lebanon is not alone in facing the challenge of enhancing nursing's professional identity. The WHO (2013b) *Nursing and Midwifery Progress Report 2008–2012* cites poor professional image as a key global challenge to strengthening nursing and midwifery services. El-Zubeir, Rizk, and Al-Khalil (2006) conducted a study to validate the Readiness for Interprofessional Learning Scale (RIPLS) in the Middle East context, specifically United Arab Emirates, and examined attitudes and readiness for IPE among undergraduate medical and nursing students in schools where the approach to learning was uni-professional. While they found that both groups saw benefits in interprofessional learning in the curricula, particularly around teamwork, collaboration, and communication, nursing students were significantly more positive about the benefits than medical students. Additionally, a qualitative analysis of students' statements about the role of nurses and therapists raised questions about their own role identities and the role identities of others. These findings indicated that stereotypes of nurses and therapy students being subordinate to physicians were still perceived. In summary, in addition to the intended benefit to patients of IPE and interprofessional collaborative care, another benefit is that interprofessionalism can help break down hierarchies and promote better understanding of all disciplines' roles in providing health care (WHO, 2010).

The following case report describes how simultaneous development of a new school of nursing and an IPE program is helping to raise the profile of nursing in a developing country. The case also serves as an exemplar in highlighting nursing leadership across multiple levels—from the role of a dean as a change agent, to faculty facilitation and role modeling, and finally, to student competency development.

ENHANCING THE PROFILE OF NURSING THROUGH PRELICENSURE INTERPROFESSIONAL EDUCATION

Setting

Lebanon is a small country on the eastern shore of the Mediterranean Sea with varied geography and a beautiful natural environment: 225 km (140 mi) of Mediterranean coastline, mountain peaks as high as 3,088 m (10,131 ft), and the fertile Bekaa Valley. Economically it is considered a developing country and receives aid from many high-income countries to support improvements in infrastructure and services in the health, education, environment, and national defense sectors. The estimated census is 4 million Lebanese plus a large refugee population from Palestine and, more recently, from Syria. Education is a high priority in the country; the literacy rate among the Lebanese is over 87%.

Lebanese citizens have access to health care through a wide array of academic medical centers, general and specialty hospitals, and ambulatory settings. Payment for care is through a mix of private and governmental insurance. A large number of nongovernmental organizations (NGOs) address specific health needs and offer preventive services. Citizens can access care ranging from primary prevention to tertiary care, although continuity of care along the continuum is not well developed. The least developed type of service is community-based care. Data on the incidence and prevalence of disease is not readily available, although the Ministry of Health and a few NGOs periodically collect and disseminate statistics about specific health conditions.

The Alice Ramez Chagoury School of Nursing (ARCSON) at the Lebanese American University (LAU) admitted its first students into the bachelor of science in nursing (BSN) program in fall 2010. LAU is chartered in the state of New York and has campuses in Beirut and Byblos, Lebanon. It is accredited by the New England Association of Schools and Colleges. ARCSON is a small school, with six full-time faculty (excluding the dean); all are Lebanese, yet each has studied in the United States. Three faculty completed internships at a university in the United States as part of their master's of science in nursing (MSN) degree, and the other three earned doctoral degrees at American universities. The school is ambitious and proactive. For example, in 2013 ARCSON earned accreditation for the BSN program through the Commission on Collegiate Nursing Education (CCNE).

In most regions where IPE is flourishing, nursing is already a duly recognized health profession. This is not the case in Lebanon or, for that matter, in many Middle Eastern countries (Kronfol, 2012). Nursing's social status in Lebanon suffers because of misconceptions both within the health sector and by the general public. Nurses often are stereotyped as "medical maids" or doctor's assistants rather than knowledge workers and professionals. Many perceive nursing as sad and depressing work, focused on tasks related to patients' personal hygiene. These stereotypes are reinforced by relatively low pay and few advancement opportunities. Nurses who complete any of three types of training—high school–level training, technical school training, and a university-based BSN degree—are eligible to work as RNs (Huijer, Noureddine, & Dumit, 2005). Nursing as a career choice for young women and men interested in the health sciences is too often a distant last after medicine and pharmacy, which are viewed as highly professional fields of study. Complicating such perceptions is that curriculum standards, instructional approaches, and quality of hospital nursing departments vary considerably. For example, in addition to ARCSON, the Rafic Hariri School of Nursing at the American University of Beirut has achieved CCNE accreditation for its BSN and MSN programs, and one hospital, the American University of Beirut Medical Center, has earned Magnet Hospital Recognition. But there are many nursing programs and hospitals that do not meet such rigorous standards.

LAU's IPE Program

ARCSON was established simultaneously with a new school of medicine and a new bachelor of science (BS) in nutrition program. LAU already offered a BS in pharmacy, a PharmD program accredited by the Accreditation Council for Pharmacy Education (ACPE) of the United States, and a bachelor of arts (BA) in social work. When the LAU Board of Trustees approved the new schools of nursing and medicine it set an expectation for interdisciplinary education. In spring 2010 the deans of pharmacy, medicine, and nursing began planning the IPE program. An IPE Work Group was established with faculty from all five health and social care programs; it was led by the dean of nursing. The Work Group developed a mission, educational goals, and student learning outcomes for IPE, and used the *Framework for Action on Interprofessional Education & Collaborative Practice* (WHO, 2010) to guide program development.

The main component of LAU's IPE program is IPE Days, which bring students from the five health and social care majors together several times over the course of their enrollment (see Table 21.2). Students are leveled for participation based on the point at which they begin their clinical training, which helps ensure their readiness for the content, a positive perception of its value, and the ability to link IPE content with clinical practice. IPE Days are extracurricular but students are required to attend. Each 3-hour IPE Day includes a brief presentation (e.g., minilecture, video, or role-play) on the day's topic, followed by breakout sessions of 12 to 15 students per group, each having students from at least three majors. In the faculty-facilitated small-group session, students apply the presentation content to a case study. The IPE program also includes clinical activities where students apply their IPE learning to practice; there are two such activities at present and an aim to develop several more.

TABLE 21.2 Interprofessional Education Day Topics and Sequencing

STEP	TOPIC	WHEN OFFERED
1	Introduction to IPE and Collaborative Practice	Semester before students begin clinical rotations in their major
2	Interprofessional Communication	Semester during which students in each major are in their first clinical rotations
3	Interprofessional Teamwork and Conflict Management	Third semester of clinical rotations
4	Improving Quality of Care Through Collaborative Practice	Final semester before graduation
5	Ethics: An Interprofessional Approach	Final semester before graduation

RAISING THE PROFILE OF NURSING THROUGH IPE

Involvement in the IPE program has given nursing faculty and students an on-campus venue to provide more accurate information about professional nursing practice. This helps dispel misconceptions that even faculty and students from other health programs may have about nursing. Providing accurate information about the nursing profession happens formally through the IPE Days content and learning activities as well as incidentally through faculty and student participation in IPE.

Formal Opportunities

Content presented during IPE Days is the formal way in which others gain a more accurate understanding of professional nursing. The first IPE Day lays the groundwork for the later programs by presenting content on the role and responsibilities of each of LAU's five health and social care majors, through a handout and a role-play of an interprofessional care planning conference. The American Nurses Association definition of nursing and *Scope and Standards of Professional Nursing Practice* (ANA, 2010) are the sources for the content presented about nursing. The other four professions have developed their content for the handout and role-play using their respective American or international standards. The small-group case study requires students to apply the content about each role to a simple client case; students are expected to represent their own role, guided by a faculty facilitator. Nursing students are in their first nursing course (Fundamentals of Nursing and Health Assessment), so they are quite reliant on the content handout when discussing the nurse's contribution.

Each IPE Day follows a similar structure. The IPE Work Group plans content to accurately represent all five professions. Presenters for the programs are selected from the five professions. For example, a nutritionist leads the introductory IPE Day. The IPE Day program on teamwork uses a video that includes nurses, social workers, and dietitians, as well as a health administrator, to present the content and explain key concepts about teamwork. A physician leads the last IPE Day on ethics. As students progress through the IPE Days, they have gained clinical experience so they can portray their profession's role in greater detail during the case-study discussion in the small groups. The nursing students gain stature as professionals when they portray nurses' holistic assessment of patients, their clinical reasoning approaches, and use of evidence in planning and delivering care.

Prior to starting the IPE Days a half-day retreat was held for faculty from all five majors. This program introduced them to IPE using IPE leaders from England and presented the Work Group's plans for the LAU IPE program. Since then, for each IPE Day, participating faculty receive a facilitator's guide in advance so they can prepare for their role as facilitator. The guides were developed by the IPE Work Group, with members from each profession respectively contributing the appropriate practice-specific content. This is another formal means of conveying accurate information about nursing as well as the other four professions. The nurses on the IPE Work Group contribute the content about nursing for each IPE Day topic and case, outlining nursing's perspective, knowledge, and role in each case. Facilitators from the other professions thus have an accurate resource for fostering discussion during the break-out sessions, but moreover gain a better understanding of nursing as well as the other health professions.

Incidental Opportunities

The IPE Work Group now has three RN members: the dean of nursing (chair), one faculty representative, and ARCSON's assessment officer. In addition, there are three faculty from the School of Medicine, three from the School of Pharmacy, two from the nutrition program, and one from the social work program. The interactions of the nursing representatives with the other nine members of the Work Group exemplify the professionalism, knowledge, and clinical expertise of nurses, which has served to raise the profile of nursing incidentally. Nursing faculty who volunteer as IPE Day presenters or small-group facilitators also portray nursing as a knowledge-based profession.

A natural offshoot of the students' IPE classroom and clinical interactions has been their collaboration through the student clubs of each major. They have jointly planned health awareness campaigns for the campus community and with local NGOs. Examples include a breast cancer awareness day on campus and an international diabetes day in a low socioeconomic community. Through these activities students learn more about each others' roles and gain experience in collaborating across the disciplines.

Impact of the IPE Program

Because our IPE program is so new (only two classes of students who have participated in the entire IPE program have graduated), we have not been able to assess its long-term impact yet. Analysis of evaluation data from the IPE Days is under way. This includes analysis of data collected from students in all majors prior to their first IPE Day and after they had completed the series of programs, using the Readiness for Interprofessional Learning Scale (Mattick & Bligh, 2005). Methods to assess whether or not perceptions about nursing specifically have been changed, however, will require much study beyond these analyses. The results of the graduate exit survey for the first two classes of nursing students show that they perceive their ability to work within an interprofessional team as very high. The first class rated this ability as 6.56/7 (1 = very poor, 7 = exceptional) and the second class rated it as 6.57/7.

Anecdotal information about IPE's influence has been positive. For example, having an IPE program has reinforced the need for faculty to thread the concept throughout the nursing curriculum. The concept of collaboration is introduced in the first professional nursing concepts course. In later health and illness courses, students are taught about collaborative disease management for all health and illness concepts. In their own class assignments, many students incorporate interprofessional collaboration. Nursing students have been responsive to opportunities to work with students in the other health majors. For example, senior nursing students willingly presented their projects about health care ethics to a class of third-year pharmacy students.

During IPE Days, students across different majors meet each other, breaking the ice for later interactions. In the clinical setting they can be observed discussing patient cases on the units. Nursing students are reminded of disease pathophysiology from medical students, or consult pharmacy students when not sure of a medication. Medical students have asked nursing students to help them practice skills like blood pressure measurement and injections. There is also anecdotal feedback from medical residents and physicians that the first cohort of nursing graduates are functioning confidently as members of interprofessional teams.

Because the IPE program provides a forum for faculty to become more acquainted with each other, it has fostered their collaboration on other educational, research, and service initiatives. For example, two nursing faculty are collaborating with two nutrition faculty on research projects, and one nursing faculty is collaborating with a pharmacy faculty member to test a web-based approach for teaching evidence-based practice. Two nursing faculty are preparing a manuscript with a pharmacy faculty member about an innovative active-learning approach that all three have used in their respective courses. There also has been sharing about community clinical sites between nursing and pharmacy and between nursing and medicine. All of these activities serve to clarify perceptions and raise understanding about professional nursing.

Summary

As an American expatriate moving to Lebanon to start a new school of nursing, the dean of nursing (NH) understood that nursing was perceived quite differently in Lebanon than in her home country. Soon after arriving she realized that misunderstandings about nursing were not limited to the public, but were embedded also in the health and higher education systems. It was clear that launching a successful nursing school would require changing these misunderstandings. The prelicensure IPE program is one approach, along with others, to achieve that aim. The early experience of the nursing school has shown that through IPE the valuable intellectual contributions of nurses in caring for patients could be portrayed. (This is true for other members of the health care team that also are undervalued in the Lebanese context, e.g., social work.) Some initial indications show that the IPE program has helped nursing students gain the confidence needed to practice as a colleague, not as a subordinate, to other health professionals. Nonetheless, additional experience and further study is needed to understand if and how IPE will contribute in a longstanding way to raising the profile of nursing within the health sector, in the higher education system, and among the public.

REFLECTIONS FROM THE ACTING DEAN OF THE LAU SCHOOL OF MEDICINE
N. LYNN ECKERT, MD, MPH, DrPH

LAU opened a School of Medicine in 2009 and a School of Nursing in 2010. As the only university outside of the United States with a doctoral-level pharmacy program approved by the U.S. accrediting body, Accreditation Council for Pharmacy Education, LAU's first step in health professions education was extraordinarily successful. Since the schools were new and all wished to promote innovative programs, there was a natural synergy in wanting to work together on programs that would make a difference to the education of the next generation of health professionals.

From the first days, students at the Gilbert and Rose-Marie Chagoury School of Medicine were immersed in social medicine in the classroom, in the cases, and in community facilities that would become central to IPE. A new health professions building planned to accommodate the new styles of learning, housing the nursing, medical, and pharmacy schools, reinforced IPE by promoting interaction among faculty and students from the initial three health disciplines.

As students became more involved in clinical rotations in hospitals it became very clear to me that the culture was different from that in the United States. Coming from an academic health center in the United States, we expected teamwork and depended on highly qualified nurses, PharmDs, and other allied health professionals. They were part of the team and there was an expectation that they would actively participate in the care of patients and provide recommendations for improving patient care. In Lebanon, nurses in particular did not have the same training, nor were there similar expectations of their capabilities or of their participation. It quickly became evident that this new generation of health professionals could benefit from experiences designed to learn together. Since LAU was opening bachelor degree programs in nursing and nutrition the timing for collaborating was perfect.

The leaders of the schools, American-educated, were cognizant of the global movement to IPE, and recognized the opportunity of applying this innovation to the LAU schools. Their work was endorsed by the board of trustees, as one member was a strong proponent of IPE and supported the concept to the Board. The dean of the School of Nursing took the lead in organizing this effort. The School of Medicine provided several faculty members who revised some of the curriculum offerings so as to promote IPE, examined ways to integrate IPE learning into ongoing activities, and participated in the overall planning and teaching activities.

Through the social medicine program, medical students began service learning experiences at the Palestinian camps around Beirut, where pharmacy students were already working. The enthusiasm of the medical students for learning alongside pharmacy students in resource-poor settings made it easy to incorporate this experience into the School of Medicine curriculum. As soon as they were able, the nursing students also joined the work in the camps.

I believe IPE worked well because the deans of the schools valued it as a learning strategy and there were a sufficient number of faculty from the health

(continued)

REFLECTIONS FROM THE ACTING DEAN OF THE
LAU SCHOOL OF MEDICINE,
N. LYNN ECKERT, MD, MPH, DrPH (continued)

professions schools who were committed to IPE and wanted to see it adopted at LAU. Although LAU is in the early stages of adopting IPE across the health disciplines I believe that the initial foray has been successful as students have a better understanding of their own roles and responsibilities, as well as those of students from the other health and social care professions. Given the tendency in Lebanon to undervalue the role of nursing I believe the IPE experience has been positive for nursing at two levels: individually, the nursing students are gaining confidence in their roles, and at the institutional level, the School of Nursing is recognized for its advancement of nursing education from a technical school level to the level of bachelor of science in nursing.

CASE ANALYSIS

The LAU case of the development of IPE across the health professions schools is a demonstration that consideration of contextual factors and characteristics, as has been suggested, is necessary for successful implementation of this new educational model. Historically, despite growing calls and enthusiasm for IPE, bringing this concept to operational stages faced a number of challenges. These challenges consist of lack of administrative support; insufficient human, time, and physical space resources; inflexible curricular structures and timetables; inconsistent use and understanding of language; preexisting stereotypes; and education cultures that were resistant to change (Bennett et al., 2011; Gilbert, 2005; WHO, 2013a).

Early leadership from the deans of nursing, medicine, and pharmacy played an instrumental role in promoting interest in IPE at the university and minimizing reluctance to change. Subsequent success was based on the commitment of time and effort by the dean of nursing to convene a group of faculty from the five professions to plan and implement the initial IPE learning opportunities. From its early planning stages and despite a small faculty, ARCSON engaged other LAU health professions schools in the Work Group that wrestled with the challenges of obtaining resources, developing faculty expertise, creating IPE curricula, allocating time given faculty were busy developing new courses in their own programs, and organizing clinical training sites. Other enabling factors that supported IPE and CP at LAU were a shared vision for IPE, common goals and desired student outcomes, faculty from different disciplines cocreating the learning experiences, support for faculty facilitators, creation of new teaching space, and integrated and experiential opportunities to learn, for both students and faculty (Barnsteiner, Disch, Hall, Mayer, & Moore, 2007; Bennett et al., 2011; Nelson et al., 2014; WHO, 2013a).

The LAU planning team was fortunate to have opportunities to collaborate and create this novel training early in the formation and establishment of the health professions schools. Because the schools were all relatively new, profession-specific training silos were not engrained. Their early work was supported by the leadership of the university and its board, with allocation of resources for teaching space and budget reallocation for students' clinical activities. In addition, the LAU programs were not overly constrained by external accreditation requirements that would hamper the development of novel IPE curricula. In fact, the opposite is true. Both CCNE and ACPE accreditation criteria include elements related to IPE.

Administrative support and leadership are instrumental in guiding and sustaining energy for this work. Several faculty champions emerged within the nursing school and across the other schools at LAU through their efforts on the Work Group. Bennett et al. (2011) published a qualitative study of the perceptions of academic faculty about IPE across a multicampus health faculty and noted that "innovation captures the interest and energy of faculty staff" (p. 573) and was a perceived strength of IPE. Innovation can also capture the energy of students.

> There is one more strategy that can be very influential in fostering leadership development in students. . . . Exposure to faculty who embrace change and support others in introducing innovation in the curriculum can be a powerful influence on the socialization of students. (Halstead, 2013, p. 4)

This combination of leadership and a willingness to be innovative in designing new education models was key to the successful implementation of IPE at LAU. Its impact has been felt at both faculty and student levels.

The LAU case describes benefits in terms of how IPE provided a forum for faculty collaboration across education, practice and research; specific examples are in web-based teaching, collaboration in community clinics, and nutrition research. The IPE Work Group members are currently working on a series of manuscripts based on analysis of the evaluation and assessment data collected to date. These positive outcomes are in keeping with the opportunities for professional growth through IPE described by Bennett et al. (2011):

- Potential for scholarship and research in IPE
- Potential for research across disciplines and with external partners
- Peer learning and new partnerships at every level of the enterprise
- Skills and capacity of staff that have emerged through the recent audit of interest and engagement (p. 573)

Faculty members' work in collaborating and creating a novel program such as IPE can enhance their own leadership development. At LAU, an initial faculty retreat with faculty from all five disciplines and external leaders in IPE from England helped launch the IPE Days and advance the IPE Work Group's plan. The IPE Work Group at LAU developed tools and guides to assist faculty in their new teaching and mentoring roles. Such methods of faculty development, specifically designed to assist faculty in acquiring and strengthening their skills in order to meet student-centered outcomes, are important for the promotion of lifelong learning, both for faculty and students.

Globally, faculty development programs and reforms in IPE and collaborative practice focus on stronger partnerships between education, service, and clinically based experiential learning as synergistic methods for developing interprofessional competencies (Barwell, Arnold, & Berry, 2013; Nelson et al., 2014; Thistlethwaite, Forman, Matthews, Rodgers, Steketee, & Yassine, 2014). LAU uses and is developing additional clinical activities and sites to better bridge education-practice gaps and to integrate IPE and collaborative patient care for students, faculty, and current practitioners.

Calls for assessment that will provide evidence as to the efficacy of IPE are increasing, yet assessment of learning outcomes and IPE program evaluation is not yet universal (Ashton et al., 2012; Reeves, Perrier, Goldman, Freeth, & Zwarenstein, 2013; Rodger & Hoffman, 2010). Rodger and Hoffman (2010), in a global environmental scan of IPE and CP, wrote, "only 37% of participants reported that they assessed learning outcomes for IPE" and "over a third did not formally evaluate IPE" (p. 487). The Toronto Model, recognized for its contributions to IPE globally, underscores that it is critical to consider the impact and sustainability of IPE programs, and to have education and service partners at the decision table when the design of an IPE and CP journey begins (Nelson et al., 2014).

Similarly, the team at LAU has developed mechanisms for assessment of student outcomes and is in the early stages of evaluating the impact of the IPE program through multiple approaches. Baseline data have been collected as each new class begins their IPE experiences, and are being coupled with assessment and evaluation data collected at each IPE Day. All facilitators were recently surveyed to solicit their input for IPE Day improvements. Another data point specific to nursing is the school's exit survey, which showed that the nursing students perceived their ability to work within an interprofessional team as very high. Early indications are that the nursing students have gained confidence in collaboration and that the knowledge and skills that nursing (and other professions) bring to the patient and health care team are portrayed though IPE in the clinical settings at LAU.

IPE provides opportunities for students to gain awareness of their own role on the health care team and better understand the roles of others, to practice and improve communication skills, and to foster relationship building and team skills (Hudson, Sanders, & Pepper, 2013; Lumague et al., 2006; Solomon & Salfi, 2011). These skills and behaviors also contribute to enhanced leadership capacity and professionalism in students (Bianco, Dudkiewicz, & Linette, 2014; IOM, 2013a; Scott & Miles, 2013).

The IPE Collaborative Expert Panel (2011) recommended four competency domains for health professionals to engage successfully in CP: values/ethics, roles and responsibilities, interprofessional communication, and teamwork, domains represented in the LAU case. Hudson et al. (2013) conducted an integrative literature review of intervention studies of IPE among prelicensure baccalaureate nursing students and found that the domain of "roles and responsibilities" was most frequently evaluated (p. 77). Their findings "suggest that nursing students' professional development may be enriched through IPE and that students in other professions may develop an appreciation of the unique contributions of nursing" (p. 79).

Interdisciplinary students across seven disciplines involved in IPE at the University of Toronto and Toronto Rehabilitation Institute articulated the perceived benefits of the program as directly experiencing how colleagues applied their expertise, enhancing confidence in approaching other team members, fostering new respect for each other as colleagues through collaborative learning, gaining a more holistic view of the patient, and improving communication by breaking down professional jargon (Lumague et al., 2006). An authentic understanding by physicians of the role of nurses in patient care was seen as contributing to effective communication between nurses and physicians practicing in the United States (Robinson, Gorman, Slimmer, & Yudkowsky, 2010).

In summary, the LAU case demonstrates the contextual factors that favored the development of an IPE program, many of which are significant barriers in well-established traditional training programs. However, the role of nursing leadership in communicating across traditional health professions boundaries cannot be understated. Successful academic nurse leaders embody the competencies of communication and conflict resolution, which are both necessary for equalizing professional power differentials that inhibit interprofessional learning (Bennett et al., 2010; Boykins, 2014; Price, Doucet, & Hall, 2014). Through role modeling a vision of change, challenging resistance, and respectfully communicating and collaborating, nurse leaders can contribute to the continuing efforts to move IPE initiatives into the early learning experiences of all health professions students. The LAU experience is an example of one institution applying global standards in the local context to improve health professions education and local patient care. Through the process, the potential to raise the long-term profile of the profession of nursing in Lebanon is enhanced.

ACKNOWLEDGMENTS

The authors appreciate the helpful comments from Maha Habre, MSN, CEN, and Tala Hasbini-Danawi, BSN, MS, on an earlier version of this manuscript. The authors acknowledge and appreciate the reflections by N. Lynn Eckhert, MD, MPH, DrPH.

REFERENCES

American Nurses Association. (2010). *Public health nursing: Scope and standards of professional nursing practice*. Washington, DC: Author.

Ashton, S., Rheault, W., Arenson, C., Tappert, S., Stoeker, J., Orzoff, J., . . . Mackintosh, S. (2012). Interprofessional education: A review and analysis of programs from three academic health centers. *Academic Medicine, 87*(7), 949–955.

Barnsteiner, J., Disch, J., Hall, L., Mayer, D., & Moore, S. (2007). Promoting interprofessional education. *Nursing Outlook, 55*(3), 144–150.

Barwell, J., Arnold, F., & Berry, H. (2013). How interprofessional learning improves care. *Nursing Times, 109*(21), 14–16.

Bennett, P., Gum, L., Lindeman, I., Lawn, S., McAllister, S., Richards, J., . . . Ward, H. (2011). Faculty perspectives of interprofessional education. *Nursing Education Today, 31*(6), 571–576.

Bianco, C., Dudkiewicz, P., & Linette, D. (2014). Building nurse leader relationships. *Nursing Management, 45*(5), 42–48.

Boykins, A. (2014). Core communication competencies in patient-centered care. *The Official Journal of the Association of Black Nursing Faculty, 25*(2), 40–45.

Brandt, B., & Schmitt, M. (2011). *Interprofessional education and training in the United States – resurgence and refocus,* 1–8. Retrieved from http://rcpsc.medical.org/publicpolicy/imwc/Interprofessional_Education_US_Brandt_Schmitt.PDF

Clarke, P., & Hassmiller, S. (2013). Nursing leadership: Interprofessional education and practice. *Nursing Science Quarterly, 26*(4), 333–336.

El-Zubeir, M., Rizk, D., & Al-Khalil, R. (2006). Are senior medical and nursing students ready for interprofessional learning? Validating the RIPL scale in a Middle Eastern context. *Journal of Interprofessional Care, 20*(6), 619–632.

Frenk, J., Chen, L., Bhutta, Z. A., Cohen, J., Crisp, N., Evans, T., . . . Zurayk H. (2010). Health professionals for a new century: Transforming education to strengthen health systems in an interdependent world. *The Lancet, 376*(9756), 1923–1958.

Gilbert, J. (2005). Interprofessional education for collaborative, patient-centered practice. *Nursing Leadership, 18*(2), 32–38.

Halstead, J. (2013). Seeking disruptive leaders in nursing education! *Nursing Education Perspectives, 31*(1), 4.

Hudson, C., Sanders, M., & Pepper, C. (2013). Interprofessional education and pre licensure baccalaureate nursing students. *Nurse Educator, 39*(2), 76–80.

Huijer, H. A. S., Noureddine, S., & Dumit, N. (2005). Nursing in Lebanon. *Applied Nursing Research, 18,* 63–64.

Institute of Medicine (IOM). (2011). *The future of nursing: Leading change, advancing health.* Washington, DC: The National Academies Press.

Institute of Medicine. (2013a). *Establishing transdisciplinary professionalism for improving health outcomes: Workshop summary.* Washington, DC: The National Academies Press.

Institute of Medicine. (2013b). *Interprofessional education for collaboration: Learning how to improve health from interprofessional models across the continuum of education to practice: Workshop summary.* Washington, DC: The National Academies Press.

Interprofessional Education Collaborative Expert Panel. (2011). *Core competencies for interprofessional collaborative practice: Report of an expert panel.* Washington, DC: Author.

Kowitlawakul, Y., Ignacio, J., Lahiri, M., Khoo, S., Zhou, W., & Soon, D. (2014). Exploring new health professionals' roles through interprofessional education. *Journal of Interprofessional Care, 28*(3), 267–269.

Kronfol, N. M. (2012). Historical development of health professions' education in the Arab world. *Eastern Mediterranean Health Journal, 18*(11), 1157–1165.

Lumague, M., Morgan, A., Mak, D., Hanna, M., Kwong, J., Cameron, D., . . . Sinclair, L. (2006). Interprofessional education: The student perspective. *Journal of Interprofessional Care, 20*(3), 246–253.

Mattick, K., & Bligh, J. (2005). An e-resource to coordinate research activity with the Readiness for Interprofessional Learning Scale (RIPLS). *Journal of Interprofessional Care, 19*(6), 604–613.

Nelson, S., Tassone, B., & Hodges, B. (2014). *Creating the health care team of the future.* Ithaca, NY: Cornell University Press.

Price, S., Doucet, S., & Hall, L. (2014). The historical social positioning of nursing and medicine: Implications for career choice, early socialization and interprofessional collaboration. *Journal of Interprofessional Care, 28*(2), 103–109.

Prime Minister's Commission on the Future of Nursing and Midwifery in England. (2010). *Front line care: The future of nursing and midwifery in England. Report of the Prime Minister's Commission on the Future of Nursing and Midwifery in England.* Retrieved from http://webarchive.nationalarchives.gov.uk/20100331110400/http:/cnm.independent.gov.uk

Reeves, S., Perrier, L., Goldman, J., Freeth, D., & Zwarenstein. M. (2013). Interprofessional education: Effects on professional practice and health care outcomes (update). *Cochrane Database of Systematic Reviews, 3*, 1–47.

Robinson, F., Gorman, G., Slimmer, L., & Yudkowsky, R. (2010). Perceptions of effective and ineffective nurse-physician communication in hospitals. *Nursing Forum, 45*(3), 206–216.

Rodger, S., & Hoffman, S. (2010). Where in the world is interprofessional education? A global scan. *Journal of Interprofessional Care, 24*(5), 479–491.

Scott, E., & Miles, J. (2013). Advancing leadership capacity in nursing. *Nursing Administration Quarterly, 37*(1), 77–82.

Solomon, P., & Salfi, J. (2011). Evaluation of an interprofessional education communication initiative. *Education for Health, 24*(2), 1–10.

Thistlethwaite, J. E., Forman, D., Matthews, L. R., Rodgers, G. D., Steketee, C., & Yassine, T. (2014). Competencies and frameworks in interprofessional education: A comparative analysis. *Academic Medicine: Journal of the Association of American Medical Colleges, 89*(6), 869–875. doi:10.1097/ACM.0000000000000249

World Health Organization (WHO). (2010). *Framework for action on interprofessional education & collaborative practice.* Geneva, Switzerland: Author. Retrieved from http://www.who.int/hrh/nursing_midwifery/en

World Health Organization. (2013a). *Interprofessional collaborative practice in primary health care: Nursing and midwifery perspectives: Six case studies.* Geneva, Switzerland: Author. Retrieved from http://www.who.int/hrh/resources/observer13/en

World Health Organization. (2013b). *Nursing and midwifery progress report 2008–2012.* Geneva, Switzerland: Author. Retrieved from http://www.who.int/hrh/nursing_midwifery/progress_report/en

World Health Organization. (2013c). *Transforming and scaling up health professionals' education and training: WHO Guidelines 2013.* Geneva, Switzerland: Author. Retrieved from http://www.who.int/hrh/resources/transf_scaling_hpet/en

CHAPTER 22

The Importance of Continuing Education in Global Health Nursing

Lynda Tyer-Viola

The quality and quantity of nursing education varies from country to country and may or may not prepare nurses adequately to care for their patients and families. In some settings, nurses learn from other medical providers; in others, they provide care alone on a daily basis. Although nurses everywhere are nimble in solving problems for their patients with available resources, resources alone cannot ensure good nursing practice. Given the variation in education and practice settings and the challenges confronting nurses, continuing education (CE) is essential to ensure expert global health nursing care.

The profession of nursing is dependent on nurses and midwives having the competency and confidence to practice. To sustain a competent workforce and safe and quality care for patients, it is imperative that health systems and government agencies create opportunities for nurses to receive ongoing education. The availability of CE, also known as continuous professional development (CPD), is important for achieving this global health nursing goal. As frontline providers in many settings and as members of interprofessional teams, it is important that nurses recognize their social obligation to seek out new knowledge that supports their practice and their role in health care.

CE provides the necessary link to good practice and creates opportunities for nurses to participate in the development of discipline-specific knowledge. The presence of CE programs in a range of modalities creates the opportunity for poor habits to be deconstructed and replaced with knowledge and proven skills. Recognizing that CE should be a cornerstone of professional practice must be an imperative for global health nursing in the 21st century. This chapter explores the role of education and professional development in nursing and different methods of achieving knowledge assessment and education, and provides examples of how focused attention on nursing and CE have improved care globally and has the potential for even greater improvement.

EDUCATION AND LICENSURE TO PRACTICE

Even as the profession of nursing has become more visible globally, there continues to be a lack of international consensus as to what a nurse is, with the definition and scope of practice varying from country to country (Currie & Carr-Hill, 2013). Nursing education and license to practice varies, contributing to disparities in care (Global Knowledge Exchange Network, 2009; Robinson & Griffiths, 2007). The profession, however, is making great strides. Nurses now receive more education, and are viewed as influential and sought out by neighbors and elders as a source of authority on health matters. Yet in settings where cultural norms are in opposition to the practice of nursing, despite a community need and higher education, nurses continue to struggle with recognition of their education and licensure (Tyer-Viola, Timmreck, & Bhavani, 2013). Ensuring that education continues past basic preparation can help to decrease these variations and improve practice.

Nurses migrate frequently, creating a need for understanding the various levels of nursing education and how licensure is obtained and maintained. In-country nurses have gained status as they are sought out by nongovernment organizations (NGOs) as the local authorities that bridge the gap between (ex-patriot) health care providers and local health care practitioners. Nurses are able to articulate the needs of a community, local health habits, and how the local system works, and can pave the way for NGOs trying to partner with a community. With the demand for and growth of international health care providers in diverse settings, it will become more important for nurses to participate in CPD to ensure they meet the qualifications needed for their local scope of practice.

Primary education for nurses and midwives varies globally, as do local demands for health care, creating differences in the practice of nursing (World Health Organization [WHO], 2009). In many global settings, nursing education ends with basic training in their home country, leaving the nurse at a disadvantage that affects their role in providing care and their ability to influence patient outcomes. Physicians and midlevel providers, on the other hand, often are educated outside their home countries and/or receive education from international educators. How and where they are educated affects how they perceive the role of the nurse. There is often a mismatch between a physician's knowledge of the role of the nurse, nursing practice, education, and competency, and the reality of their local scope of practice (Currie & Carr-Hill, 2013). Physicians and midlevel providers may undervalue nurses' knowledge and skills. If nurses were given the opportunity to improve their clinical decision making and skills, they could excel as interprofessional partners. This gap in basic and CE and needed skills can affect quality outcomes and harm patients, which is why it is imperative to foster the concept of CPD in nurse practice globally.

Although the nursing profession recognizes that there should be a standard set of competencies to be called a nurse, there has been a debate over the educational standard for entry into practice (WHO, 2009). Without this standardization, the label of "nurse" cannot signify a given level of education and knowledge. In countries where the profession is more developed and often has a governing body to foster and encourage advancing education and skills, the practice of nursing has flourished. Formal recognition of nurses is evidenced by the establishment of boards of registration/registrars of nursing and midwifery (McCarthy et al., 2013; WHO, 2002). The role of regulatory bodies is important as it ensures that the scope of practice is clearly defined relative to the qualifications of the professional. As noted earlier, these government entities vary globally and the resultant requirements to be licensed as a nurse and to renew a license to practice are not well defined. McCarthy et al. (2013) examined the role of legislation and regulation of nursing and midwifery in Africa and found a wide variation in the requirements for licensure, preservice accreditation, and CPD. Although all RNs were mandated to register with their country council to practice and require renewal of their registration at a minimum of 1 year, there were no common requirements for education and CPD.

To become an RN in many countries requires only the completion of a nursing curriculum. It may also include passing an examination and/or interview. Once registered, there is wide variation in continued registration requirements. Today, many countries do require relicensure; however, it is not universal. In the United Kingdom, the Nursing and Midwifery Council maintains the largest registry of health care professionals in the world (Nursing and Midwifery Council, 2013). The qualifications for nursing and midwifery are based on countrywide standards for hours of training set forth by the Higher Education Institute. The Nursing and Midwifery Council recognizes other European Union training as well as global education; however, it requires that all applicants meet the specified hours of education. In addition, any midwife not trained in the United Kingdom must take an adaptation course offered in England. This requirement recognizes the unique skills of midwives and their advanced training in many countries, yet ensures that those who practice in the United Kingdom do so from the same basic level of knowledge. To continue to be registered, nurses and midwives must complete continuing professional development requirements.

In the United States, the National Council of State Boards of Nursing (NCSBN) administers the National Council Licensure for Registered Nurses (NCLEX) exam to assess the minimally expected knowledge to practice safely. To obtain a license as an RN, you must pass this exam after completing three different pathways of education that are recognized as preparation to practice. NCSBN also administers this exam to internationally trained nurses. The pass rates between these two groups vary greatly. In 2013, 81% of the 53,735 United States educated nurses passed the exam, compared to 44% of the 277 internationally educated nurses (NCSBN, 2013). This variability is not necessarily related to the quality of education, but possibly the content and focus on the fundamentals of basic nursing knowledge and skills necessary to be called a nurse. It may also reflect a lack of familiarity with the English language (American style) and phrases used in the U.S. health care system, as well as familiarity with the testing system.

In Singapore, the Revised Nurse Practice Act of 2012 requires a nurse to have graduated from a recognized education program and to accumulate CE credits within a yearly qualifying period (Singapore Nursing Board, 2014). As of 2002, the Philippines have the only nurse practice act requiring that all nurses have a bachelor's degree in nursing (BSN) and successfully pass an examination to become an RN (Republic of the Philippines, 2014). However, with this revision, the requirement for CPD was removed. These examples represent the variation in how nursing ensures a well-educated and competent workforce. These variations also exemplify the need for standards for licensure, and CE and professional development.

CE AND PROFESSIONAL DEVELOPMENT

The profession of nursing depends on a foundation of education, licensure to practice, and a commitment to continuous knowledge development. Professions all have certain characteristics that define their practice (see Table 22.1). These defining elements include having a primary focus of interest and a code of ethics, and the need for continuous knowledge development and recognition by society as experts. Each of these are defined by a discipline and become the hallmark of professional practice. These attributes foster the identity of nurses regardless of their practice setting. For example, nurses have a distinct way of viewing their phenomenon of interest (the patient) and possess specialized knowledge that makes them competent to provide care. Nurses are guided by a code that mandates ethical comportment with patients and other professionals and they accept their social responsibility to regulate the profession. Finally, and of the utmost importance, nurses are dedicated to improving the quality of practice through lifelong learning These characteristics are universal and should be promoted through CE.

Nurses, like many health care providers, often learn from each other while practicing. Learning occurs best when nurses with skills work together collaboratively and learn from each other. This creates and supports a professional community of practice. Current evidence-based practice knowledge, however,

TABLE 22.1 Characteristics of a Profession

- Guided by a distinct way of viewing phenomena surrounding the knowledge base of the profession
- Recognizes specialized competencies and practitioners
- Members view education as a lifelong process and as a mechanism to advance within the profession
- Recognizes specialties with specific missions within the unified group
- Members are recognized by society as the authority in the discipline
- Guided by a code of ethics to regulate the relationships between professionals and society
- Has a commitment to self-regulation
- Recognizes a professional culture sustained by formal professional associations

Source: Matthews (2012).

is not always part of daily clinical experiences in global settings. Many clinical experiences perpetuate negative heuristics and bad habits in nursing practice (Thompson, 2003). Nurses must have current information to ensure they have the knowledge to practice in their local settings. The definition of CE overall is postbasic education aimed at engaging nurses in lifelong learning so as to improve nursing practice and the delivery of quality health care (Griscti & Jacono, 2006). The revised International Council of Nurses (ICN) Code of Ethics clearly states "the nurse carries personal responsibility and accountability for nursing practice and for maintaining competency for continued learning" (ICN, 2012b, p. 4). The use of personal in this statement is interesting; this implies it is not the health systems' responsibility to mandate education but the professional nurse's responsibility to seek it out and to participate. In describing the elements of how this is achieved, the ICN has made several suggestions of how leaders can establish, promote, and lobby to ensure nurses practice at the highest level. Table 22.2 depicts roles and suggested practices to ensure quality nursing practice. To accomplish these principles at each level of health care delivery requires a commitment from nursing across the continuum of the profession. For example, researchers have a responsibility not only to conduct nursing-focused studies but also to ensure that the findings are disseminated to colleagues closest to the patient. When findings are not disseminated and implemented, it is the researcher's role, in collaboration with colleagues in education and practice, to investigate the

TABLE 22.2 International Council of Nurses Code of Ethics Principal Elements: Roles and Practice

PRACTITIONERS AND MANAGERS	EDUCATORS AND RESEARCHERS	NATIONAL NURSES ASSOCIATIONS
Education		
Establish standards of care and a work setting that promotes quality care	Provide teaching/learning opportunities that foster lifelong learning and competence for practice	Provide access to continuing education (CE) through journals, conferences, distance education, and so on.
Assessment		
Establish systems for professional appraisal, CE and systematic renewal of licensure to practice	Conduct and disseminate research that shows links between continual learning and competence to practice	Lobby to ensure CE opportunities and quality care standards
Monitoring		
Monitor and promote the personal health of nursing staff in relation to their competence to practice	Promote the importance of personal health and illustrate its relation to other values	Promote healthy lifestyles for nursing professionals. Lobby for healthy workplaces and services for nurses

Source: International Council of Nurses (2012a).

reason for this lack of implementation. Of particular interest in the ICN code is the element to link continuous learning to competence to practice. Competence has been defined as a combination of knowledge, attitudes, skills, decision making, and values, each of which influence the other (Cowan, Norman, & Coopamah, 2005; Meretoja & Koponen, 2012; Numminen, Meretoja, Isoaho, & Leino-Kilpi, 2013).

With continued nurse migration internationally and within regions, particularly the European Union, the question of what the critical elements are that constitute competency to practice and how this is to be measured and demonstrated is an important issue for the nursing profession. Considerable work has focused on how to measure competency, with several studies utilizing the Nurse Competence Scale (NCS) (Meretoja, Isoaho, & Leino-Kilpi, 2004). Research has revealed that in the populations assessed, practicing nurse competency in general is perceived as good (Lejonqvist, Eriksson, & Meretoja, 2012; Meretoja & Koponen, 2012; Salonen, Kaunonen, Meretoja, & Tarkka, 2007). There is a gap though between the perceptions of nurses' competency and what experts believe is optimal nurse competency. The experts' definition of competency is higher than what nurses believe is competent (Meretoja & Koponen, 2012). Closing this gap is the role of CE.

The importance of having a competent nursing workforce is reflected in country statutes such as the American Nurses Association (ANA) policy statements; the United Kingdom's Nurse, Midwives, and Health Visitors Act of 1979; and the Canadian Nurses Association Policy Statements of 2004 (ANA, 2010; Canadian Nurses Association, 2004; Nursing and Midwifery Council, 2014). Each of these documents state that the practice of nursing should be monitored for continued competency. Monitored does not necessarily imply that CE credits must be mandatory for practice.

Yet how do we motivate nurses to participate in lifelong learning if it is not tied to their legal licensure to practice? It could be suggested that nurses who attend CE offerings are those who are engaged, competent, and continually challenging themselves with new knowledge (Callicutt, Norman, Smith, Nichols, & Kring, 2011). If that is true, then it can be inferred that those who do not attend such educational offerings may be the very nurses who need more education and, therefore, CE should be mandated. Lundgren and Houseman (2002) state that a pitfall of this logic is that mandating development will at a minimum ensure a minimum standard of practice. Only achieving the minimum standard of knowledge to practice may not be enough to address the needs of a population, especially nurses who care for those with a high burden of disease.

Nurses' motivation to participate in CE, regardless of mandates, varies related to practice settings. Lack of perceived motivation may be related to the environment in which nurses practice more than their personal disinterest. Many settings do not support learning as there are not enough nurses to care for the patients, let alone to take time off to attend a training program. Creating time in all settings for CE activities is essential. It does not have to be formal and time consuming. For example, nurses and midwives should have time to discuss what works well and what needs to be improved in their environment. From those conversations, education can be introduced to address identified needs at the same time and real time feedback can be garnered. This process of rapid cycle improvement with a focus on education can create a new level of commitment to learning.

Training activities are a way to build professional and community status in some health systems. Attendance is chosen based on rank in the system versus need, or is provided as a means of compensation. This has an unintended effect that those who are left behind to provide care in underresourced settings view training as a prize and may resent the person who is on leave. When they return, there may be limited sharing of new knowledge, which alters the intended effect of most training courses. Creating equal opportunity for all nurses to participate in training courses will improve morale and motivate nursing staff (Schoonbeek & Henderson, 2011).

CE has been identified as a target for interventions to entice professionals not to leave their home countries. In a Cochrane Database analysis of interventions to reduce emigration of professionals from low- and middle-income countries (LMIC) to high-income countries (HIC), no interventions were identified that were proven to reduce emigration (Penaloza, Pantoja, Bastias, Herrera, & Rada, 2011). Interventions that showed promise included financial rewards, career development and CE, improving hospital infrastructure, resource availability, better hospital management, and improved recognition of health professionals. These conditions mirror the findings of the World Health Organization report *Working Together for Health*, which notes the critical need of helping the existing workforce to perform more effectively (WHO, 2006).

Providing career development and CE in the workplace may also affect performance. Figure 22.1 describes three dimensions that influence health workforce performance: job-related factors, system support, and an enabling environment. Lifelong learning is a key component of the enabling environment that needs to be addressed. The effects of not tending to these key elements are seen as reasons why nurses migrate. Nurses who migrated to the United Kingdom from sub-Saharan Africa cited lack of professional development as a reason to migrate, as well as poor remuneration and poor health care systems (Likupe, 2012). Investment in nursing was seen as a key motivator to strengthening the nursing workforce. The Ugandan Nursing and Midwifery Board surveyed members and found that they were interested in counseling and training, research capacity building, improving professional relationships, and having the opportunity to share best practices (Zuyderduin, Obuni, & McQuide, 2010). The importance of creating an environment where nurses are motivated to learn is important to the practice of nursing globally regardless of whether it is mandated. Nurses have a social responsibility to engage in lifelong learning; as a profession, it is imperative that we create environments where learning is celebrated.

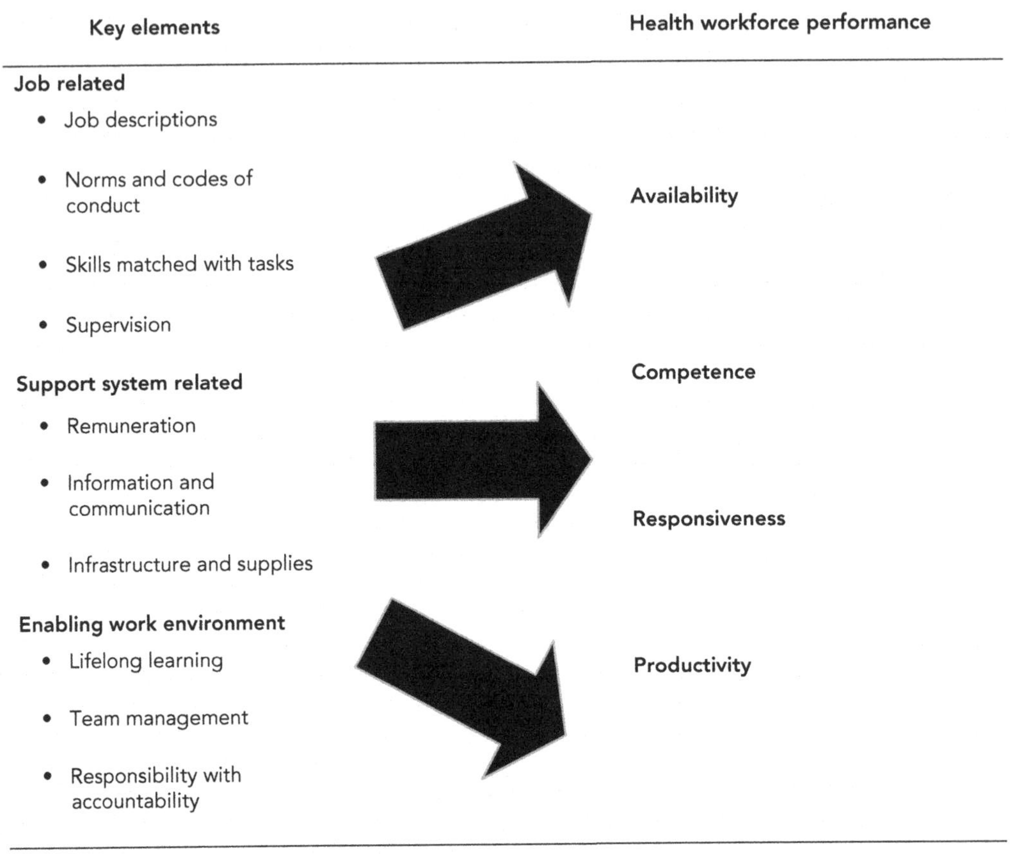

Key elements   Health workforce performance

Job related

- Job descriptions

- Norms and codes of
  conduct   Availability

- Skills matched with tasks

- Supervision

Support system related   Competence

- Remuneration

- Information and
  communication   Responsiveness

- Infrastructure and supplies

Enabling work environment

- Lifelong learning   Productivity

- Team management

- Responsibility with
  accountability

FIGURE 22.1 Key elements that influence all four dimensions of health workforce performance.
Source: WHO (2006, p. 71).

MODELS OF CE

The end goal of CE is to improve patient outcomes by enhancing the way nurses practice. Best practice is defined by the use of evidence that incorporates judgment, values, and individual factors that are population specific. Translating evidence into practice is supported by the model for action-based nursing (ICN, 2012a). Figure 22.2 depicts the ICN action model for best practices related to health systems, nursing practice, and evidence. This model suggests that evidence alone will not create good nursing care. It is creating the links between understanding evidence, the source of evidence, making a case for change, and nursing action. The critical elements of expertise, skills, and clinical judgment need to be continuously enhanced with education. This part of the model is also highly dependent on nurses having the confidence and authority to enact change. These two elements are often related to social and system attributes. Confidence is created when nurses are allowed to practice to the full scope of their education. The health system may not allow this and the social structure of a society may not accept it. For example, although well educated, many nurses who practice

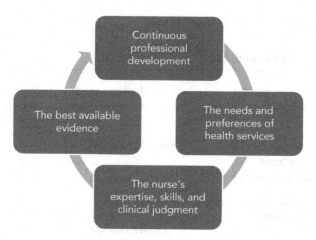

FIGURE 22.2 International Council of Nurses action model.
Source: ICN (2012a).

in predominantly Muslim countries continue to have their practice limited by the male-dominated society (Hadley et al., 2007). Assessing the impact of the practice environment on the scope of nursing practice will improve outcomes of educational offerings.

In any setting, knowledge transfer is rarely a linear process, depicted as educate then implement into practice. It requires assessment of what the desired change is first and then creation of a model of education to support the desired outcome with attention to local context. There are many informal and formal methods of CE such as train the trainer, group in-servicing, and focused-topic course work. Two other models that are promising are hybrid nurse residency models and accompaniment. Table 22.3 depicts the strengths and opportunities of each model. Success in improving care with evidence is dependent on choosing the right model (Forsetlund et al., 2009). Each model has a different level of sustainability and outcome metric. Key to each of these models is establishing if the purpose of education is general improved knowledge on a topic for competency or practice change. An outcome of all models should be improvement in patient outcomes. This is important when considering how to encourage nurses to participate. As a leadership model transferred to improving nursing knowledge, education should have a PACT: the program has to have a defined *purpose*, nurses have to be *accountable* to participate and apply knowledge, there needs to be good *communication* about how the education will improve nursing practice, and there needs to be a commitment of all participants to *teamwork* to ensure that the desired outcomes are obtained.

"Train the trainer" is a concept used globally to train medical personnel. It is based on the premise that knowledge transfer can occur between individuals when it is repeated in the context of care. This is an extension of the old phrase "see one do one," which is a large part of medical training in the United States. Nursing has tried to change this method by reinforcing the need to have a focal point of clinical knowledge with the presence of an expert in the form of a

TABLE 22.3 Continuing Education (CE) Methods

MODEL	KEY ELEMENTS	GOAL	OPPORTUNITIES TO IMPROVE
Train the trainer (TOT)	Standardized One skill	Individual knowledge transfer	With each transfer there can be deviations in practice
Group in-servicing	Standardized One topic System change	Group change	Assumption change will occur because all have heard the message
Focused-topic course	Standardized One topic Expert practice reinforced	Influence one population with large practice change	Can create gaps in other care and practice
Residency	Hybrid and highly dependent on the practice setting	Role modeling of newly acquired knowledge	Variation related to practice settings and leaderships support
Accompaniment	Bidirectional learning	Role modeling with equally engaged participants	Variation related to commitment of participants

clinical instructor. After formal training, train the trainer is an ideal way to focus learning on one topic. The success of "train the trainer" programs is having the trainer be viewed as an authority on the topic who has the capacity to communicate with the intended audience. A good example of this is the use of train the trainer to enhance teamwork to improve the rate of omitted nursing care (Kalisch, Xie, & Ronis, 2013).

Teamwork is a problem in many global care settings (Kalisch, Doumit, Lee, & Zein, 2013; Kalisch & Lee, 2011). To improve teamwork, the researchers employed a train the trainer method. This method was optimal as it used staff member talent and created an ongoing resource. These studies highlight the role of the trainer, who then becomes the internal mentor, change champion, and opinion leader to sustain change after the formal training (p. 411). The opportunity to improve when using this method requires use of a quality metric to assess if the knowledge being transferred remains the same and is not altered during translation. The concept of train the trainer can be applied in any care setting as it recognizes the expert local practitioner and, if focused, can be sustained.

Group in-servicing is widely used when a system change needs to occur. Sessions are usually short and intensive, with a structured approach focused on one topic, provided by internal or external experts, and seen as a "one and done" method. The success of in-service education is in the support rendered after education. The challenge is ensuring that change actually happens and that the knowledge is adopted. In line with diffusion of innovation theory, this method works best with early adopters as they have the capacity after introduction to move from the phase of knowledge and understanding, skipping the phase of persuasion and decision, and immediately moving into the phase of implementation (Rogers, 2003). Attention to the phases of adoption theory can improve the desired outcome of change in health professionals' practice.

In-service education has been applied globally by implementing recognized programs of excellence that strive to standardize approaches to common health care needs such as obstetrical care and neonatal resuscitation (Opiyo & English, 2010). These programs are designed with a standardized curriculum with focused teaching actions. The in-service model relies on everyone acquiring knowledge and agreeing to implement the actions. Neonatal resuscitation programs rely on this concept; if we teach people, they will commit to incorporating a skill into their practice. Yet there is often lack of assessment of the systematic application of the actions. Incorporating the known effect of decay of skills over time into the design of in-service education is vital (Opiyo & English, 2010). When planning in-service education it is imperative to consider the benefits of shorter versus longer training (longer has not been shown to improve results), the desired outcome (observed change in behavior as well as the desired patient outcome related to the behavior change), and the role of refresher training (Rowe et al., 2008). Successful in-service training relies on careful consideration of its long-term effects.

The focused-topic course is one step higher in content and structure than in-service training. It is a model of CE that is of greater length, has a multistaged approach, and often has expected outcomes over a longer period of time. The goal is to influence a target population with a large practice change. These CE programs are expensive and best adopted within a larger health system framework. The opportunity to improve the use of this method lies in ensuring that, with the shift in focus, there are not other unintended effects within the system. An excellent example of focused-topic training is the implementation of the Streamlining Tasks and Roles to Expand Treatment and Care for HIV (STRETCH) program (Uebel et al., 2011). Since 2004, nurses have played a vital role in assessing patients for initiation of antiretroviral therapy (ART) and implementation of nurse-led programs to improve respiratory disorders, tuberculosis, and HIV called PALSA PLUS (Practical Approach to Lung Health in South Africa Plus HIV Training; Schull et al., 2011). These programs were based on in-service education programs, clinical mentoring at the point of care, and continuous reassessment of the care provided. The outcomes were impressive, yet many people remained unable to access ART care. STRETCH would change the model from doctor-initiated to nurse-initiated therapy with the expansion of education (an additional four training sessions on HIV initiation) and careful monitoring of patient panel outcomes (Fairall et al., 2012). This task shifting initiative resulted in a change in national policy in South Africa in support of the nurse and thereby the patient.

Nurse residency programs in global health support a model that embraces learning in action. Recognizing that practicing nurses have limited opportunity in many settings to acquire CE unless they leave the practice setting, residency ensures that an investment in CE becomes part of daily operations. Nurses learn while in residence in their practice settings by applying knowledge learned in a dedicated learning environment. This is similar to academic service partnerships for higher education (Nabavi, Vanaki, & Mohammadi, 2012). Residency takes that model to the next level, the practicing nurse.

Residency requires that the host organization recognize that practicing nurses need continued professional development and extend a partnership to either an outside agency such as an NGO or develop an internal structure for education. The goal of residency is to improve skills with focused knowledge building and then applying new knowledge in daily practice. An example of this is the AK Khan Healthcare Trust partnership in Dhaka Bangladesh (Tyer-Viola et al., 2013). This residency program developed didactic education based on a needs assessment for each enrolled institution. Nurses participated in designated hospital-based education programs 1 day a week and implemented new knowledge within their respective practice settings. Most programs were at least 1 year in length and showed significant improvement in knowledge related to the fundamentals of nursing practice. The program has expanded with a public–private partnership between the Ministry of Health of Bangladesh, the Massachusetts General Hospital Center for Global Health, and Dhaka Medical College to implement a bone marrow transplant program using the nurse residency framework (A. Barron, personal communication, January 24, 2014). Nurse residency as a model for CE engages both the nurse and the health system in the need for continued professional development.

Continued education in the form of the practice of "accompaniment" is an extension of nurse residency and hybrid programs. Accompaniment is practiced in the form of bidirectional learning in the clinical setting. Education occurs *in situ* in patient care settings between a local nurse and a nurse expert, usually from another culture or setting. The focus is not on didactic knowledge but on learning in action using methods such as thinking aloud and critical reflection. Nurses learn from working with other nurses who have specific clinical knowledge that is needed with a specified population. Accompaniment values the nurse-to-nurse relationship. The goal is not for the expert to solve a local problem per se, but to exhibit partnership, teamwork, and respect for each person's knowledge. The nurse expert learns from the local nurse the local nursing care demands, their nursing structure, and how they solve problems and use clinical decision making, often in low-resourced settings. The local nurse learns from the expert nurse what the standard of care could be and how to practice that standard within the local setting. They have to identify how together they can improve patient outcomes with improved nursing care. Nurses around the world who work with Partners In Health (PIH) practice this model of CE (Davis, 2013; PIH, 2013). In several countries, nurses are deployed as volunteers to work side by side with local nurses, sharing knowledge while practicing as a team with the end goal of elevating the practice of nursing. This partnership, accompaniment, allows for both nurses to view their worlds from a position of equity. This model supports the local context of care as being of the utmost importance. Opportunities to improve require ensuring that partners are aligned with the same mission. When a focused practice change needs to occur, PIH has adopted the model of integrating a nurse educator.

This educator acts within the accompaniment model as an equal partner and in addition acts as a change agent. Nurse educators immerse themselves in the local care community and use daily care interactions as the method to educate about a clinical care topic.

In 2012 the Dana Farber Cancer Institute (DFCI) partnered with PIH to implement a nurse educator care model in Rwanda (Partners In Health, 2013). For 3-month deployments, expert nurses from DFCI functioned as staff nurses and educators to implement a chemotherapy transfusion education program. Education consisted of focused-topic courses in conjunction with interprofessional team training combined with daily care discussions as the program unfolded. The use of accompaniment and expert educators allowed for program implementation during patient care, with education following the implementation of the new program. This was enabled by the existence of a strong nursing system. Accompaniment is ideal in settings where a nursing structure exists and partnerships can be leveraged.

CONCLUSION

The practice of professional nursing requires a commitment to lifelong learning in all global settings. Whether it is in a high- or low-income setting, nursing practice must be guided by evidence-based knowledge. To be a competent and confident practitioner requires gaining new knowledge to support care for specific patient populations. There are many methods to obtain education and each has the ability to improve nursing care and ultimately achieve better patient outcomes. The responsibility of acquiring education to practice to one's full scope of practice lies with the nurse. Health care systems and government entities have the obligation to ensure that there are opportunities to acquire new knowledge. With these opportunities, together with professional organizations and governmental entities, nurses will be able to make a full commitment to the imperative of continued professional development to enhance the care of the populations served.

REFERENCES

American Nurses Association. (2010). *Nursing's social policy statement: The essence of the profession.* Retrieved from http://www.nursingworld.org/socialpolicystatement

Callicutt, D., Norman, K., Smith, L., Nichols, A., & Kring, D. (2011). Building an engaged and certified nursing workforce. *Nursing Clinics of North America, 46*(1), 81–87. doi:10.1016/j.cnur.2010.10.004

Canadian Nurses Association. (2004). *Promoting continued competence for nurses policy statement.* Retrieved from http://www.cna-aiic.ca/~/media/cna/page%20content/pdf%20en/2013/07/26/10/23/ps77_promoting_competence_e.pdf

Cowan, D., Norman, I., & Coopamah, V. (2005). Competence in nursing practice: A controversial concept—A focused literature review. *Nurse Education Today, 25,* 355–362. doi:10.1016/j.nedt.2005.03.002

Currie, E., & Carr-Hill, R. (2013). What is a nurse? Is there an international consensus? *International Nursing Review, 60*, 67–74. doi:10.1111/j.1466-7657-2012.00997.x

Davis, S. (2013). *From Boston to Haiti: A view from the window.* Retrieved from http://www.pih.org/blog/the-view-from-the-window

Fairall, L., Bachmann, M. O., Lombard, C., Timmerman, V., Uebel, K., Zwarenstein, M., . . . Bateman E. (2012). Task shifting of antiretroviral treatment from doctors to primary-care nurses in South Africa (STRETCH): A pragmatic, parallel, cluster-randomised trial. *The Lancet, 380*(9845), 889–898. doi:10.1016/S0140-6736(12)60730-2

Forsetlund, L., Bjorndal, A., Rashidian, A., Jamtvedt, G., O'Brien, M. A., Wolf, F., . . . Oxman, A. (2009). Continuing education meetings and workshops: Effects on professional practice and health care outcomes. Update of *Cochrane Database of Systematic Reviews.* 2001;(2):CD003030; PMID: 11406063. *Cochrane Database of Systematic Reviews, 2.* doi:10.1002/14651858.CD003030.pub2

Global Knowledge and Exchange Network. (2009). *An overview of education and training requirements for global health care professionals.* Retrieved from http://www.gken.org/Docs/Workforce/Nursing%20Educ%20Reqs_FINAL%20102609.pdf

Griscti, O., & Jacono, J. (2006). Effectiveness of continuing education programmes in nursing: Literature review. *Journal of Advanced Nursing, 55*(4), 449–456. doi:10.1111/j.1365-2648.2006.03940.x

Hadley, M., Blum, L., Mujaddid, S., Parveen, S., Nuremowla, S., Haque, M., & Ullah, M. (2007). Why Bangladeshi nurses avoid "nursing": Social and structural factors on the hospital wards in Bangladesh. *Social Science & Medicine, 64*(6), 1166–1177. doi:10.1016/j/socsciemed.2006.06.030

International Council of Nurses (ICN). (2012a). Closing the gap: From evidence to action (p. 58). Geneva, Switzerland: Author. Retrieved from http://www.icn.ch/publications/2012-closing-the-gap-from-evidence-to-action

Interntational Council of Nurses. (2012b). *Revised: The ICN code of ethics for nurses* (p. 8). Geneva, Switzerland: Author. Retrieved from http://www.icn.ch/about-icn/code-of-ethics-for-nurses

Kalisch, B. J., Doumit, M., Lee, K. H., & Zein, J. E. (2013). Missed nursing care, level of staffing, and job satisfaction: Lebanon versus the United States. *Journal of Nursing Administration, 43*(5), 274–279. doi:10.1097NNA.0b013e31828eebaa

Kalisch, B. J., & Lee, K. H. (2011). Nurse staffing levels and teamwork: A cross-sectional study of patient care units in acute care hospitals. *Journal of Nursing Scholarship, 43*(1), 82–88. doi:10.1111/j.1547-5069-2010.01375.x

Kalisch, B. J., Xie, B., & Ronis, D. L. (2013). Train-the-trainer intervention to increase nursing teamwork and decrease missed nursing care in acute care patient units. *Nursing Research, 62*(6), 405–413. doi:10.1097/NNR.0b013e3182a7a15d

Lejonqvist, G. B., Eriksson, K., & Meretoja, R. (2012). Evidence of clinical competence. *Scandinavian Journal of Caring Sciences, 26*(2), 340–348. doi:10.1111/j.1471–6712.2011.00939.x

Likupe, G. (2012). The skills and brain drain what nurses say. *Journal of Clinical Nursing, 22*(9–10), 1372–1381. doi:10.111/j.1365-2702.04242.x

Lundgren, B., & Houseman, C. (2002). Continuing competence in selected health care professions. *Journal of Allied Health, 31*(4), 232–240. Retrieved from http://www.asahp.org/publications/journal-of-allied-health

Matthews, J. (2012). Role of professional organizations in advocating for the nursing profession. *Online Journal of Issues in Nursing, 17*(1), Manuscript 3. doi:10.3912/OJIN.Vol17No01Man03

McCarthy, C. F., Voss, J., Verani, A. R., Vidot, P., Salmon, M. E., & Riley, P. L. (2013). Nursing and midwifery regulation and HIV scale-up: Establishing a baseline in east, central and southern Africa. *Journal of the International AIDS Society, 16,* 18051. doi:10.7448/IAS.16.1.18051

Meretoja, R., Isoaho, H., & Leino-Kilpi, H. (2004). Nurse competence scale: Development and psychometric testing. *Journal of Advanced Nursing, 47*(2), 124–133. doi:10.1111/j.1365-2648.2004.03071.x

Meretoja, R., & Koponen, L. (2012). A systematic model to compare nurses' optimal and actual competencies in the clinical setting. *Journal of Advanced Nursing, 68*(2), 414–422. doi:10.1111/j.1365-2648.2011.05754.x

Nabavi, F. H., Vanaki, Z., & Mohammadi, E. (2012). Systematic review: Process of forming academic service partnerships to reform clinical education. *Western Journal of Nursing Research, 34*(1), 118–141. doi:10.1177/0193945910394380

National Council of State Boards of Nursing (2013). *Pass rates for NCLEX 2013.* Retrieved from https://www.ncsbn.org/Table_of_Pass_Rates_2013.pdf

Numminen, O., Meretoja, R., Isoaho, H., & Leino-Kilpi, H. (2013). Professional competence of practising nurses. *Journal of Clinical Nursing, 22*(9–10), 1411–1423. doi:10.1111/j.1365-2702.2012.04334.x

Nursing and Midwifery Council. (2013). *Registry of nurses and midwives.* Retrieved from http://www.nmc-uk.org

Nursing and Midwifery Council. (2014). *The history of nursing and midwifery regulation.* Retrieved from http://www.nmc-uk.org/about-us/the-history-of-nursing-and-midwifery-regulation

Opiyo, N., & English, M. (2010). In-service training for health professionals to improve care of the seriously ill newborn or child in low- and middle-income countries. *Cochrane Database of Systematic Reviews, 4,* 1–34. doi:10.1002/14651858.CD007071.pub2

Partners In Health (PIH). (2013). *Rwanda trains a new generation of cancer nurses.* Retrieved from http://www.pih.org/blog/rwanda-trains-a-new-generation-of-cancer-nurses

Penaloza, B., Pantoja, T., Bastias, G., Herrera, C., & Rada, G. (2011). Interventions to reduce emigration of health care professionals from low- and middle-income countries. *Cochrane Database of Systematic Reviews, 9.* doi:10.1002/14651858.CD007673.pub2

Republic of the Philippines. (2014). *Philippine Nurse Practice Act 2002.* Retrieved from http://www.lawphil.net/statutes/repacts/ra2002/ra_9173_2002.html

Robinson, S., & Griffiths, P. (2007). *Nursing education and regulations: An international perspective.* National Research Unit. Retrieved from http://eprints.soton.ac.uk/348772/1/NurseEduProfiles.pdf

Rogers, E. (2003). *Diffusion of innovations* (5th ed.). New York, NY: Free Press.

Rowe, A., Rowe, S., Holloway, K., Ivanovska, I., Muhe, L., & Lanbrechts, T. (2008). *A systematic review of the effectiveness of shortening Integrated Management of Childhood Illness guidelines training: Final report.* Geneva, Switzerland: World Health Organization. Retrieved from http://whqlibdoc.who.int/publications/2008/9789241597210_eng.pdf

Salonen, A. H., Kaunonen, M., Meretoja, R., & Tarkka, M. T. (2007). Competence profiles of recently registered nurses working in intensive and emergency settings. *Journal of Nursing Management, 15*(8), 792–800. doi:10.1111/j.1365-2934.2007.00768.x

Schoonbeek, S., & Henderson, A. (2011). Shifting workplace behavior to inspire learning: A journey to building a learning culture. *Journal of Continuing Education in Nursing, 42*(1), 43–48. doi:10.3928.00220124-20101001-02

Schull, M. J., Cornick, R., Thompson, S., Faris, G., Fairall, L., Burciul, B., . . . Zwarenstein, M. (2011). From PALSA PLUS to PALM PLUS: Adapting and developing a South African guideline and training intervention to better integrate HIV/AIDS care with primary care in rural health centers in Malawi. *Implementation Science, 6*(82). doi:10.1186/1748-5908-6-82

Singapore Nursing Board. (2014). *Continuing education*. Retrieved from http://www .healthprofessionals.gov.sg/content/hprof/snb/en/leftnav/continuing_nursing_ education_cne.html

Thompson, C. (2003). Clinical experience as evidence in evidence-based practice. *Journal of Advanced Nursing, 43*(3), 230–237. doi:10.1046/j.1365-2648.2003.02705.x

Tyer-Viola, L. A., Timmreck, E., & Bhavani, G. (2013). Implementation of a continuing education model for nurses in Bangladesh. *Journal of Continuing Education in Nursing, 44*(10), 470–476. doi:10.3928/00220124-20130816-07

Uebel, K. E., Fairall, L. R., van Rensburg, D. H., Mollentze, W. F., Bachmann, M. O., . . . Bateman, E. D. (2011). Task shifting and integration of HIV care into primary care in South Africa: The development and content of the streamlining tasks and roles to expand treatment and care for HIV (STRETCH) intervention. *Implementation Science, 6*(86). doi:10.1186/1748-5908-6-86

World Health Organization (WHO). (2002). Nursing and midwifery: A guide to professional regulation. *WHO Technical Publications Series, 27*, 1–35. Retrieved from http:// applications.emro.who.int/dsaf/dsa189.pdf

World Health Organization. (2006). *World Health Report: Working together for health.* Retrieved from http://www.who.int/whr/2006/en

World Health Organization. (2009). *Global standards for the initial education of professional nurses and midwives (WHO/HRH/HPN/08.6)* (p. 40). Geneva, Switzerland: Author. Retrieved from http://www.who.int/hrh/nursing_midwifery/hrh_global_ standards_education.pdf

Zuyderduin, A., Obuni, J. D., & McQuide, P. A. (2010). Strengthening the Uganda nurses' and midwives' association for a motivated workforce. *International Nursing Review, 57*(4), 419–425. doi:10.1111/j.1466-7657.2010.00826.x

CHAPTER 23

Nursing Education and Practice in China and Thailand

Puangtip Chaiphibalsarisdi, Bridget E. Meedzan, Patrice K. Nicholas, and Nancy L. Meedzan

NURSING EDUCATION: AN OVERVIEW

This chapter focuses on an overview of nursing education and practice, especially the issues that impact nursing and health in China and Thailand. Nurses are in a unique situation to address the challenges of global health and share knowledge and resources, yet the profession is also impacted by the political and social factors within a country. An understanding of how nurse leaders navigate the political agenda to achieve health for all may inspire other countries to overcome burdens in the pursuit of health goals. Gennaro (2014) notes that if we understand the profession of nursing in a more global context, perhaps we can think about solutions that are generalizable to many settings rather than to our specific health care setting (p. 144).

This chapter reviews political landscapes in two countries and how policy and political climate influence the education and practice of nursing. This global perspective addresses the nursing profession's contribution to the health of the world's people. Thailand and China are two Asian countries that offer a lens on the past, current, and future contributions of the nursing profession.

NURSING IN CHINA

Following China's defeat in the Opium War of 1842, Western missionaries introduced modern nursing practices to the Qing dynasty (Smith & Tang, 2004). As missionary societies purchased land throughout China, these regions experienced a rapid emergence of Westernized hospitals and an influx of Western-educated nurses. With these establishments came the apparent need for trained hospital personnel. It was during this period that the traditional Chinese customs of medicinal practice, referred to as the *pei-ka* system, which granted all responsibility for the patient's basic health needs to family members (Chang, Green,

Wilson, & Hutchinson, 1983), were surpassed by the modern nursing education system developed by Florence Nightingale.

The first school for Chinese nurses was founded in 1888 through the efforts of the American nurse Ella Johnson (Smith & Tang, 2004). These early models of nursing education were 3-year "hospital-based" programs (Gao, Chan, & Cheng, 2012). For a decade, mission schools of nursing were established throughout China; however, the initial flow of students was extremely low due to social tradition that created cultural barriers for individuals, particularly women, pursuing the nursing profession. For example, the foundational concept of manual labor in modern nursing was condemned by Chinese tradition and the role of the female nurse in the care of a male patient was considered "indecent and immoral" (Hsu, 1956). With the gradual increase in primary and secondary education by the early 1910s, the nursing schools began to see larger portions of the female and male community entering its doors.

The Chinese Nursing Association (CNA) was established in 1909 with the goal of unifying and elevating the progress of nursing education to align China's progress with the development of nursing education globally (Smith & Tang, 2004). Initially titled the Chinese Nurses' Society, the CNA developed minimum educational standards, conducted national examinations, and acquired translated textual resources for the nursing students (Hsu, 1956). The first nurse training program was established in 1910; in 1915, the first examination for professional nursing certification was implemented (Gao et al., 2012). Nursing education at the tertiary level was introduced in 1920 with the induction of a 5-year baccalaureate program within Peking Union Medical College (Eddins, Hu, & Liu, 2011). Continuing the pattern of Western influence, the program was funded by the Rockefeller Foundation in the United States (Gao et al., 2012) and was introduced only a year after the first baccalaureate programs were launched in American and Canadian nursing education curricula (Eddins et al., 2011). As of 2004, the CNA has recruited over 330,000 members with 31 branches, seven working committees, and 13 academic committees (Smith & Tang, 2004). The CNA focuses on uniting, developing, and promoting nursing (Smith & Tang, 2004) throughout China. Presently, the CNA has focused efforts on protecting the rights of the national nursing community, circulating advanced nursing knowledge, cultivating academic exchange through national and international conferences, and publishing academic journals such as the *Chinese Journal of Nursing* (Smith & Tang, 2004).

By elevating the standards of nursing school system development and creating a college-level platform of education, the nursing profession began to adapt to the expectations of Chinese culture. By emphasizing the importance of higher learning within Chinese culture, the role of the nurse became one of the most attractive professions for female high school graduates. Between 1937 and 1949, the CNA had registered 183 nursing facilities and 6,000 members, and implemented 216 3- or 4-year nurse training programs (Hsu, 1956).

China's progress in nursing education was halted by the political climate of the 1950s under the communist leadership of Chairman Mao Zedong. The Cultural

Revolution reduced nursing education to a vocational training program with junior high school graduate admission (Gao et al., 2012). What initially began as a "soviet-modeled education reform program" (Smith & Tang, 2004) became an aggressive proletarian purge of capitalism and culture throughout China. Almost every nursing education facility was disbanded and formal education was declared unnecessary for the progress of the Republic (Chang et al., 1983). With limited trained health professionals, the *pei-ka* system reemerged as the primary method of health care and limited the patient to basic treatment by willing family and friends. The socialist economic mobilization that ensued did not end until Mao's death in 1977. It was not until 1983 that the baccalaureate degree was revived from the previously established nursing education system with the opening of the Tainjin Medical College nursing course (Smith & Tang, 2004). The Cultural Revolution formed a decade of incompetency, and nursing educators postrevolution were faced with the challenge of reeducating the entire nursing community.

Due to the substantial setback in nursing education development brought on by the Cultural Revolution, the progress of China's nursing schools and educational curriculum standards has only recently begun to make strides. At the end of 2012, there were more than 2.49 million nurses in China (English.people.cn, 2012). Estimates from China suggest that the nursing population will be 2.86 million by 2015.

Presently, there is a strict hierarchical system of education in place to promote advancement in the field of nursing practice. The lowest level of nursing education is in secondary "vocational" programs open to either junior high school or high school graduates. Junior high school admission entails 3 to 4 years of study while a high school graduate attends a 2- to 3-year program after completing 6 years of primary schooling (Gao et al., 2012). Vocational nursing programs of the second type provide the primary education for the majority of nurses in China, producing young professionals who will grapple with the increasing demands of contemporary health care (Gao et al., 2012). Although some of these "diploma" institutions are still active, the phase-out process began in 1999 with the goal of initiating nursing education at the university level (Eddins et al., 2011). In 1993, the Ministry of Health (MoH) regulated nursing practice with the Nurses Regulation Method, which required every secondary program graduate to be certified through the annual National Nurse Licensing Examination (NNLE) (Gao et al., 2012). All tertiary levels of nursing education, including associate, bachelor's, and master's degrees, are exempt from taking the NNLE and are automatically licensed upon program completion.

The associate degree nursing programs consist of a 3-year university enrollment and are open to high school and secondary program graduates. With more than 70,000 nurses graduating each year from nationwide associate programs, the curriculum focuses on the theory of nursing practice, clinical experience, and professional preparation (Gao et al., 2012). Although the system of nursing education in China has begun to build a solid foundation of competency among its graduates, the MoH further emphasized the imperative need for advanced nursing education with the Outline of the Development Plan of Nursing Services in P.R. China 2005–2010. Ling-Ling Gao et al. summarize this plan, stating:

> It addresses the need to modify the multi-level structure of the nursing education system; to promote the quality of nursing education; to restructure post-basic nursing education and continue nursing education; and design nursing education programs for meeting the specialty nursing practice and management and leadership in nursing. (Gao et al., 2012)

The baccalaureate nursing program, available in 200 universities, is a 4- or 5-year full-time commitment that grants graduates the knowledge and skills needed to administer high-quality health care (Eddins et al., 2011). Accelerated further by the efforts of the MoH, and following a disease-oriented curriculum, the baccalaureate focus is developed as a 3-year period of theoretical study followed by 1 or 2 years of clinical experience (Gao et al., 2012).

The master's degree in nursing was first offered in 1992 at the Beijing Medical University. There are now 50 universities across China, as well as multiple international institutions, that offer a 2- to 3-year master's degree for Chinese nurses. To gain admission into a master's program, however, the enrollee must have previously obtained a bachelor's degree (Eddins et al., 2011). An impressive addition to master's-level nursing education is the Program on Higher Education Development (1993–2000), which has increased the number of master's-prepared nursing faculty to accommodate enrollment numbers in baccalaureate programs (Gao et al., 2012). In comparison with the nursing education systems in other countries, the majority of China's nursing graduates opt to specialize in areas associated with education rather than service (Gao et al., 2012).

The highest achievement in nursing education is the doctoral degree. The emergence of doctoral education in China is in its infancy. First introduced in 2004, in collaboration with Johns Hopkins University School of Nursing, the doctoral nursing program is an advancement for nursing education. Throughout the country, 10 institutions offer enrollees full-time programs that are 3 years in length, and 3- to 7-year part-time programs (Gao et al., 2012).

It is interesting to note that the overall national nursing program of China has inherited two *novel strands* (Smith & Tang, 2004): the study of traditional Chinese medicine and the foreign language program. Nursing lectures are conducted in English and Japanese to increase fluency and allow students the ability to work internationally (Smith & Tang, 2004). Courses in traditional Chinese medicine are referred to as *Chinese nursing ethos* (Smith & Tang, 2004) and focus on the cultural understanding of health through the perspective of Chinese society. The curricula of these lectures are rooted in Confucian thought, fusing the practice of yin and yang with the theory of the five phases: wood, fire, earth, metal, and water. Illness, therefore, is thought to result from internal disharmony and disease is an unbalanced relationship between the body and its environment. The central tenets of traditional Chinese medicine challenge the nursing student to *restore the patient's balance* (Smith & Tang, 2004) while also attending to the treatable symptoms. With this as background, it is not surprising that Chinese healing is considered as 30% dependent on treatment and 70% dependent on the nursing care administered (Wong & Pang, 2000). The nurse is required to act in a most sincere form, carrying the moral obligation to treat the patient as if he or she was family. In accordance with the *pei-ka* system, the nurse may enter the patient's family *sphere* and may serve as a surrogate family member during the course of treatment (Smith & Tang, 2004). The cultural tradition is ingrained deeply in the mechanics of nursing practice within China, with sharing the nature of difficult diagnoses as variable in many settings.

At present, the strides in advancing the development of nursing education are more evident in the overall improvement of the health care system; however, a complex issue in this system is the physical stress on nurses. Occupational health issues have emerged due to the high nurse-to-patient ratio. Hospitals have very few rest areas for nurses and there is a pattern of overcrowdedness, poor ventilation, and excessive noise (Smith & Tang, 2004), thus creating an unsafe working environment.

The CNA rejoined the International Council of Nursing (ICN) in 2013 following a 66-year gap after the termination of their initial involvement, which began in 1922. Xiuhua Li expresses great optimism when stating:

> With the CNA rejoining the ICN in 2013, the dream of many generations of Chinese nurses comes true. [2014] This is a significant milestone for Chinese nursing in integrating back into the world's nursing family. It will bring new opportunities for the development of nursing in China. (Li, 2014)

The future of China's nursing education system lies in its ability to promote and enhance the bachelor's degree and postgraduate nursing programs. Advanced program enhancement must be considered in terms of not only the quality of the curriculum and the ability of the educators, but also in these preexisting institutions' ability to recruit enrollees and to prevent the brain drain—exits from the nursing profession—from occurring postcertification (Eddins et al., 2011). Gao et al. (2012) expands on this challenge when arguing that baccalaureate programs must compete with degree programs of other disciplines in recruiting talented high school students in the National University Admission Examination. The curriculum of these programs must transition from a *functional nursing model* to a *nursing process model* in order to establish solid nursing skills in clinical settings (Eddins et al., 2011).

Smith and Tang (2004) suggest that in elevating the requirements of nursing education, China's nursing system will expand the scientific research base of the profession and may gain understanding from an increased international focus, as well as developing a cooperative focus with nursing programs worldwide (Smith & Tang, 2004). As of 2004, of the 2.8 million nurses active in China, only 3% hold a postregistration bachelor's degree (Smith & Tang, 2004).

By advancing the academic rigor of the profession, nursing efforts will advance improved health outcomes of patients and the quality of nursing care overall. After the 2003 severe acute respiratory syndrome (SARS) outbreak, Smith and Tang (2004) noted that this epidemic highlighted the major challenges that the Chinese health care system has for patients, health care providers, and nurses (Smith & Tang, 2004). Through the efforts of the MoH and the progress of the nursing community postrevolution, it is evident that China is seeking to improve quality health care. With a working knowledge of the challenges and opportunities that China has, the development of nursing education may be poised to flourish, address the needs of a burgeoning country, and move from an acute-care, illness-focused approach to an overall curriculum of health and wellness promotion with a focus on the community (Gao et al., 2012).

NURSING IN THAILAND

Thailand covers an area of about 514,000 square kilometers. It is the third largest country among the 10 Southeast Asian nations, ranking after Indonesia and Myanmar. The borders around Thailand total about 8,031 km long, of which 5,326 km are inland and the other 2,705 km are coastlines (Wibulpolprasert, 2002, p. 16).

The population of Thailand in 2014 was 67,741,401 with the ratio of male to female 0.98 (Central Intelligence Agency, 2014). Life expectancy for males was 69.1 years in 2010 and is anticipated to rise to 71.1 years in 2020; and for females, the life expectancy will rise from 75.7 years to 77 years over the same period (Institute for Population and Social Research, Mahidol University, 2009).

Thai Economy and Global Health Nursing

Sufficiency Economy

Thailand is a middle-income country with impressive recent achievements in economic and social development (WHO, 2013). Since 1974, the sufficiency economy has been the highly respected, well-known philosophy of King Bhumibol Adulyadej of Thailand; this has guided all aspects of Thai life, including health care. The sufficiency economy has been recognized by the United Nations for its usefulness in sustainable development in Thailand and internationally.

Sufficiency economy philosophy guides economic development in Thailand and is based on the fundamental principles of Thai culture: moderation, prudence, and social immunity or risk management. It uses knowledge and virtue as guidelines in living and specifically states that intelligence and perseverance will lead to real happiness.

> Economic development must be done step by step. It should begin
> with the strengthening of our economic foundation, by assuring

> that the majority of our population has enough to live on. . . . Once
> reasonable progress has been achieved, we should then embark
> on the next steps, by pursuing more advanced levels of economic
> development. Being a tiger is not important. The important thing
> is for us to have a sufficient economy. A sufficient economy means
> to have enough to support ourselves . . . we have to take a careful
> step backward . . . each village or district must have relative self-
> sufficiency. (His Majesty King Bhumibol Adulyadej, Thailand, 1997;
> Chaipattana Foundation, 2015)

The first pillar of the sufficiency economy is *moderation*. This means that
sufficiency should be practiced at a level of not doing something too little or
too much at the expense of oneself or others, for example, producing and consuming at a moderate level. The second pillar is *prudence* or *reasonableness*.
This pillar states that the decision concerning the level of sufficiency must be
made rationally, with consideration of the factors involved and careful antici-
pation of the outcomes that may be expected from such action. The last pillar,
risk management, describes the preparation to cope with the likely impact and
changes in various aspects by considering the probability of future situations.
Furthermore, the philosophy of the sufficiency economy states that decisions
and activities must be carried out at a sufficient level based on the two conditions of *knowledge* and *virtue*. Knowledge is in-depth study in a given field and
prudence in using this knowledge to understand the relationships in any area.
Virtue is promoted through the awareness of honesty, patience, perseverance,
and intelligence in leading one's life.

> I may add that full sufficiency is impossible. If a family or even
> a village wants to employ a full sufficiency economy, it would
> be like returning to the Stone Age. . . . This sufficiency means to
> have enough to live on. Sufficiency means to lead a reasonably
> comfortable life, without excess, or overindulgence in luxury,
> but enough. Some things may seem to be extravagant, but if
> it brings happiness, it is permissible as long as it is within the
> means of the individual. (His Majesty King Bhumibol Adulyadej,
> Birthday Speech, December 4, 1998; Chaipattana Foundation, 2015)

The sufficiency economy can be applied to all levels, branches, and sectors of
the economy and is not necessarily limited to the agricultural or rural sectors.
By using similar principles of emphasizing moderation in performance, reasonableness, and creating immunity for oneself and society, the sufficiency economy can be used in the financial, real estate, international trade, and investment
sectors. Chaiphibalsarisdi et al. (2006) applied the sufficiency economy theory
to health and nursing in the flash flood and landslide survivors' project. The
goal of the study was to rehabilitate those who lost homes and livelihoods due
to the extensively damaged fruit crops during flash floods and landslides in a
province in northern Thailand. This project provided skills training coupled
with training in implementation of the Philosophy of Sufficiency Economy and

was found to support people in coping with external and internal stressors to live more comfortably.

Health Promotion in Thailand

Thailand has a long, successful history of health development and introduced universal health care for its citizens in 2002. In Thailand, the *Bangkok Charter for Health Promotion in a Globalized World* (Bangkok Charter for Health Promotion, 2005) makes the commitment to health for all and states that health professional associations have a responsibility to this charter. The Bangkok Charter affirms that policies and partnerships to empower communities and to improve the health and health equality of its people should be at the center of global and national development. Health promotion is the process of enabling people to increase control over their health and its determinants, and thereby improve their health. This includes the work of tackling communicable and noncommunicable diseases and other threats to health (Box 23.1). The four commitments to health for all include making the promotion of health central to the global development agenda; making the promotion of health a core responsibility for all of government; making the promotion of health a key focus of communities and civil society with a special contribution from health professional associations; and making the promotion of health a requirement for good corporate practice including the private sector.

To this end, nursing associations have been involved in a variety of projects to address the importance of a high-quality framework for the education of health personnel. The long-term plan is to continue to network locally and globally. In order to bring global health nursing in Thailand into the contemporary environment, it is necessary to have a vision of what can be achieved. Three essential elements of nursing, going into the future, are first, as described in Unit I of the text, that nurses should be ready and willing to work as part of multidisciplinary teams with other health professionals. Second, nurses must be ready to offer a range of choices for the client, with a variety of prices depending on the ability of the patient to pay. We see this concept emerging in most health care settings globally. Third, nurses must place more emphasis on care for women and the elderly, as these groups will become even more important to the development of society in the future. It is also important to note that in a developing society, women's health is a powerful indicator of the health of society as a whole, and that the difficulties associated with an unhealthy society are often linked with poorer women's and children's health. Several of the UN Millennium Development Goals (MDGs) address these key issues.

The Bangkok Charter is comparable to Healthy People 2020 in the United States (U.S. Department of Health and Human Services, 2012). Healthy People 2020 is an initiative developed with goals and objectives and 10-year health targets that are designed to guide national health promotion and disease prevention efforts to improve the health of all people in the United States, and offer a vision of a society focused on health for all.

BOX 23.1 APPLICATION OF THE SUFFICIENCY ECONOMY
PHILOSOPHY TO FUTURE HEALTH PROMOTION IN THAILAND:
"LIVING WITH DIABETES"

SUFFICIENCY ECONOMY PHILOSOPHY	APPLICATION OF THE PHILOSOPHY
Moderation	The patient with diabetes must practice moderation in choosing between high and low carbohydrate foods and also appropriate exercise to maintain a moderate blood sugar.
Prudence (Rationality)	The patient with diabetes must understand and be knowledgeable of the disease process and management of the disease, including medications, diet, and exercise. They must understand the interplay of all these aspects of one's life and be prudent in all areas.
Social immunity (Risk management)	The patient with diabetes will prevent risks or complications from the disease by following the above-mentioned criteria. Without practice of moderation and prudence, the patient will be at risk for developing long-term, chronic, secondary effects from the diabetes.

National Health Development Plans

The Ministry of Public Health (MoPH) in Thailand is the lead agency in developing the nation's health system, with the aim of advancing the health of all Thai people within the framework of the Green and Happiness Society. The Thailand Green and Happiness Index (GHI) is a tool developed in 2007 to evaluate the performance of national development and the happiness of all Thais (Ministry of Public Health, 2012a). The Green and Happiness Society was developed because of a shift from a focus on the Thai economy to a focus on human development; this paradigm shift occurred after the Eighth National Plan (1997–2001) to embrace a focus on social and environmental development. The GHI is aimed at "evaluating performance of national development and happiness of all Thais. The GHI is primarily based on the Philosophy of Sufficiency Economy, Human-Centered Development, and the Vision of the Tenth Plan, Green and Happiness Society "(Barameechai, 2007, p. 2). The GHI includes six components: health; warm and loving family; empowerment of community; economic strength and equity; good quality environment and ecological system; and democratic society and good government. The vision of the GHI and Green and Happiness Society is that

> Thai people uphold moral values, lead knowledge, can cope with all changes, and live in warm and loving families within empowered

communities and a peaceful society. Thailand has a sound, stable, and equity economy; good quality environment and sustainable natural resources; upholds good governance system for the administration at all levels under constitutional monarchy, and be able to live with dignity in the world community." (Barameechai, 2007, p. 5)

Notably, the GHI is a formal mechanism that has been used as a framework and benchmarking in Thai society.

Thailand's national health development plans are revised every 5 years to reflect areas of gain and areas needing improvement in the health of the nation. During the 10th National Health Development Plan, 2007–2011, Thailand invested in several health programs, "namely infrastructure for health services at various levels, human resources production and development, technical development, and knowledge creation for people's health development, especially for mothers and children and the underprivileged, all leading to the achievement of the MDGs related to health" (MoPH, 2012a). Thailand is regarded as one of the countries that has made progress toward the achievement of the MDGs; however, there are still some areas that need improvement. One area where achievement has not been met is in the incidence of poverty in rural areas, which is four to eight times higher when compared with Bangkok. Another area is noncommunicable diseases, which are major causes of death in Thailand—specifically, coronary heart disease, cancer, and diabetes. There is also a higher disease burden among migrant groups, and these groups remain vulnerable to public health hazards, exploitation, and human trafficking (WHO, 2013). In Chapter 14 of this text, Mary de Chesnay discusses the cultural aspects of sex trafficking, or sex tourism, with a focus on Thailand.

The 11th National Health Development Plan

The 11th National Health Development Plan (2012–2016), established under the 11th National Economic and Social Development Plan, emphasizes the importance of an integrated approach with public participation in all steps of the paradigm development process to achieve the health and happiness of the Thai people (MoPH, 2012a). The current plan focuses on development using the sufficiency economy philosophy, creating unity and good governance in the health system, giving importance to the participation of all sectors in society, creating health security and service delivery systems in a thorough and equitable manner, and valuing the creation of good provider-recipient relationships. The vision is for all Thai citizens to achieve optimal health and participate in creating a sufficiency health system with equity leading to social well-being. The sufficiency health system is the process of developing people's health toward physical, mental, social, and spiritual well-being through the use of a cost-effective health care system with quality standards, strengths, sufficiency, convenient accessibility, and responsiveness to people's health problems and needs.

Cost-effectiveness has not yet been achieved. Health spending in Thailand increased from 3.8% in 1980 to 6.4% in 2008. The rate of increase in health spending is greater than that for gross domestic product (GDP); that is, the health spending rose by 7.6% annually on average, but GDP growth was only 5.6% per annum (Health Expenditure in Thailand Health Profile, 2008–2010). The goals of the 11th National Health Development Plan (2012–2016) will provide the guidance for both national and global health initiatives, include five strategies that aim to strengthen health promotion, develop systems for monitoring and management of disasters, and increase the quality and standards of health care in Thailand.

WHO Country Cooperation Strategy 2012–2016 and Thailand

WHO is working in over 80 countries with host institutions to support WHO programs through Country Cooperation Strategies (CCS). The Southeast Asia Region (SEARO) has the second highest population among the six WHO regions and has the greatest burden of disease. The Royal Thai government and WHO are partnering on the fourth CCS, 2012 to 2016, which guides health planning, budgeting, resource allocation, and partnership. The key principles guiding WHO cooperation and on which the CCS is based are:

- Ownership of the development process by the country
- Alignment with national priorities and strengthening national systems in support of the national health strategies/plans
- Harmonization with the work of sister UN agencies
- Cooperation that fosters member states' contributions to the global health agenda (WHO, 2011)

Human resources for health are a much needed area of improvement. Thailand needs to develop policies and strategies specifically for the development of human resources for health so that health personnel are able to improve the quality of health care. In 2009, there were 35,789 doctors working in the country and the doctor/population ratio was 1 to 1,773. For the nursing workforce in 2010 (professionals or RNs), there were 138,710 RNs working at health care facilities: a nurse/population ratio of 1:458 (Ministry of Public Health, 2012b).

ASSOCIATION OF SOUTHEAST ASIAN NATIONS

Thailand belongs to the Association of Southeast Asian Nations (ASEAN). The objective of the ASEAN is to enhance cooperation among these countries in order to improve efficiency and competitiveness, diversify production capacity and supply, improve distribution of services, and the elimination of restrictions to trade in services among ASEAN member countries (ASEAN, 2014). The 10 ASEAN countries are Brunei Darussalam, Kingdom of Cambodia, Republic of Indonesia, the Lao People's Democratic Republic of Lao PDR, Malaysia, Republic of Philippines, Republic of Singapore, Kingdom of Thailand, the Socialist Republic of Vietnam, and Union of Myanmar. Nursing is one of the seven professions that can contribute to the knowledge and practice among the 10 ASEAN countries. This is challenging in the areas of education and practice in nursing. The objectives aim to facilitate mobility of nursing professionals within ASEAN, and include the following: exchange information and expertise on standards and qualification, promote adoption of best practices on professional nursing service, and provide opportunities for capacity building and training of nurses. In 2013, the Thai Cardio-Thoracic Nurses Association organized the first International Conference in Cardiovascular-Thoracic Nursing (ICCTN) and all ASEAN communities were invited to participate. Researchers from Cambodia presented on postoperative care of the pediatric cardiac surgery patient and Chaiphibalsarisdi (2013) presented in *Framework of Clinical Governance for Elderly With Cardiovascular Needs*. There were also nurse leaders participating from the Philippines, Singapore, and Japan. This collaboration will continue to strengthen the nursing profession in the ASEAN area for the health of the people.

Governance

Clinical governance is a systematic approach that calls for health organizations to become accountable for continuously improving the quality of services and maintaining high standards of care through innovations in policy and the clinical environment. Similar to the approach of the Joint Commission on Accreditation of Healthcare Organizations (The Joint Commission; TJC) in the United States, the goal is to promote excellence in clinical care. The seven elements of clinical governance are education and training, clinical audit and supervision, clinical effectiveness, research and development, openness, risk management, and information management. The approach to health management that may enhance clinical governance is a challenge that should be approached on a systematic basis. Innovative management in terms of shaping policy, budgeting, and other resources to support ongoing clinical and continuing education is a key issue. Additionally, clinical audits and research are important tools in improving clinical effectiveness. In terms of nursing education and nursing practice, nursing organizations have an important role in advancing professional nursing throughout Thailand. It is important for all clinicians to embrace continuing education and training, along with research and development, so as to create and sustain innovative care and services. There is also a role for expanding the nature and extent of advanced practice nursing in Thailand (Chaiphibalsarisdi, 2013).

In summary, there are numerous opportunities for nurses to contribute to the health of the Thai people. Nurses engage in caring for people across the life span and across community- and hospital-based care. Throughout the life cycle, people are influenced by the practice of nursing as well as the country's focus on engaging in the philosophy of the Green and Happiness Society. The nursing profession is poised to address health needs in the 21st century and advance the health outcomes of the people of Thailand.

CONCLUSION

Nursing, like all professions, functions within a broader context of the policies and philosophies of the geographical area in which it is practiced. Similarly, the historical and cultural underpinnings of the society impact the nursing profession and health care. This concept is portrayed so clearly in the exemplars presented here with their rich histories and backgrounds in Eastern medicine. These historical and cultural roots are so strong that they continue to be imbedded in 21st-century nursing education and practice. In both countries, Confucian thought fuses the Eastern practice of ying and yang with the theory of the five phases—wood, fire, earth, metal, and water (for China) and earth, water, wind, and fire (for Thailand). This cultural focus of balance is not only seen in the ying and yang principles, but also in the Green and Happiness Society in Thailand. Thailand's Green and Happiness Society openly acknowledges concern for the moral development and ability of its people to live with dignity. Possibly, these philosophical practices have enabled Thailand to realize gains in achieving the MDGs and providing universal health coverage for its citizens. To build on Gennaro's (2014) views, there are lessons to be learned from China and Thailand for nurses who practice in settings around the world that are complementary to Western approaches to nursing and medicine.

REFERENCES

Association of Southeast Asian Nations (ASEAN). (2014). *ASEAN mutual recognition arrangement on nursing services*. Retrieved from http://www.asean.org/communities/asean-economic-community/item/asean-mutual-recognition-arrangement-on-nursing-services

Bangkok Charter for Health Promotion. (2005). Retrieved from http://www.who.int/healthpromotion/conferences/6gchp/bangkok_charter/en/11 August 2005

Barameechai, J. (July, 2007). *The Green and Happiness Index*. Paper presented at the Office of the National Social and Economic Development Board International Conference on Happiness and Public Policy, Bangkok, Thailand. Retrieved from http://www.happysociety.org/ppdoconference/session_papers/session2/Juthamas-GHI.pdf

Central Intelligence Agency (CIA). (2014). *CIA world fact book*. Retrieved from https://www.cia.gov/library/publications/the-world-factbook/geos/th.html

Chaipattana Foundation. (2015). Philosophy of the Sufficiency Economy. Retrieved from http://www.chaipat.or.th/chaipat_english/index.php?option=com_content&view=article&id=4103&Itemid=293

Chaiphibalsarisdi, P. (2013). *Framework of clinical governance for elderly with cardiovascular needs*. Paper presented at the 1st international conference in cardiovascular-thoracic nursing (ICCVTN) 2013. "Seamless and participating in CVT care," August 10–12, 2013, at Hua Hin Grand Hotel & Plaza, Prachuap Khiri Khan, Thailand.

Chaiphibalsarisdi, P., Sopajaree, C., Nakwaree, K., Posri, A., Kasemsuk, P., & Chalyachet, M. (2006). Doing good deeds for His Majesty the King: Helping, rehabilitating/developing health for flash flood and landslide survivors, Uttaradit province, northern Thailand. *Asaihl-Thailand Journal, 9*(2), 112–138.

Chang, M. K., Green, N. K., Wilson, H. S., & Hutchinson, S. A. (1983). Nursing in China: Three perspectives. *The American Journal of Nursing, 83*(3), 389–395. Retrieved from http://www.jstor.org/stable/3470269

Department of Projects Management, Office of the Chaipattana Foundation, Dusit Palace, Sri Ayutthaya Road, Dusit, Bangkok 10300, Thailand. Retrieved from http://www.chaipat.or.th/chaipat_english/index.php?opiton=com_content&view=article&id=4103&Itemid=293

Eddins, E. E., Hu, J., & Liu, H. (2011). Baccalaureate nursing education in China: Issues and challenges. *Nursing Education Perspective, 32*(1), 30–33.

English.people.cn. (2012). *China's registered nurses near 2.5 mln.* Retrieved from http://english.peopledaily.com.cn/90882/8237285.html

Gao, L. L., Chan, S. W., & Cheng, B. S. (2012). The past, present and future of nursing education in the People's Republic of China: A discussion paper. *Journal of Advanced Nursing 68*(6), 1429–1438. doi:10.1111/j.1365-2648.2011.05828.x

Gennaro, S. (2014). Commentaries on the global state of nursing. *Journal of Nursing Scholarship, 46*(3), 144.

Government of Thailand, Public Relations Department. (2007). *Green and Happiness Index: Thailand's New Development Indicator.* Retrieved from http://thailand.prd.go.th/view_news.phpŒid=2154&a=2

Hsu, A. (1956). Nursing education in China. *American Journal of Nursing, 56*(8), 991–994. Retrieved from http://www.jstor.org/stable/3460982

Institute for Population and Social Research, Mahidol University. Thai Health Promotion Foundation and National Health Security Office. (2009). *ThaiHealth 2009.* Bangkok, Thailand: Amarin Printing and Publishing. Retrieved January 29, 2014, from th.wikipedia.org/wiki

Li, X. (2014). New opportunity for the development of nursing in China. *Journal of Nursing Scholarship, 46*(3), 145–146.

Ministry of Public Health. (2012a). *The 11th National Heath Development Plan under the National Economic and Social Development Plan B.E. 2555-2559 (2012–2016).* Nonthaburi, Thailand: Bureau of Policy and Strategy, Office of the Permanent Secretary, Ministry of Public Health, Thailand.

Ministry of Public Health. (2012b). The Nursing Council of Thailand. Retrieved from http://eng.moph.go.th/index.php/professional/97-the-nursing-council-of-thailand

Smith, D. R., & Tang, S. (2004). *Nursing in China: Historical development, current issues and future challenges.* Retrieved from http://www.oita-nhs.ac.jp/journal/PDF/5_2/5_2_1.pdf

U.S. Department of Health and Human Services, Office of Disease Prevention and Health Promotion. (2012). Healthy people 2020. Washington, DC. Retrieved from https://www.healthypeople.gov

Wibulpolprasert, S. (Ed.). (2002). *Thailand health profile 1999–2000.* Ministry of Public Health, Nonthaburi, Thailand: Express Transportation Organization.

Wong, F. N., & Pang, F. N. (2000). Holism and caring: Nursing in the Chinese health care culture. *Holistic Nursing Practice, 15,* 12–21.

World Health Organization (WHO). (2011). *WHO country cooperation strategy Thailand: 2012–2016.* New Delhi, India: WHO publication. Retrieved from www.geoba.se/population.pbp?OEpc=world&type=28; www.geoba.se/population.pbpOEpc=world&type-0012page1

World Health Organization. (2013). *County cooperation strategy at a glance: Thailand.* Retrieved from http://www.who.int/countryfocus/cooperation_strategy/ccsbrief_tha_en.pdf

CHAPTER 24

Professional Nursing Education in South Africa

Hester C. Klopper and Leana R. Uys

Professional nursing education in South Africa has a rich history and began formally in 1877 when Henrietta Stockdale started a training program at Carnarvon Hospital, Kimberley. Although South Africa was the first country in the world to have a register for professional nurses (from 1891), much development has taken place and nurses have become the drivers of change. To share the advancement of nursing education in South Africa, we are presenting this chapter in two sections; the first section addresses professional nursing education in South Africa, and the second section focuses on a specific organization, the Forum of University Nursing Deans of South Africa (FUNDISA), as a national driver of change in South Africa.

In order to make sense of the development of professional nursing education, understanding the context of South Africa is useful. South Africa is often called the "rainbow nation" due to the cultural diversity of the country, but this was not always the case. South Africa has experienced many years of racial divisiveness imposed by the apartheid policies. The decades 1950 to 1990 were specifically a dark time and major challenges were facing the country. On February 2, 1990, President F. W. de Klerk lifted restrictions on 33 opposition groups, including the African National Congress (ANC), the Pan-Africanist Congress (PAC), and the Communist Party. On February 11, 1990, Nelson Mandela, South African anti-apartheid revolutionary, politician, and philanthropist, was released after 27 years in prison. South Africa's story is one of hope and joy from the racial divide to a single nation whose dream of unity and common purpose is now capable of realization (South Africa.info, 2014).

PROFESSIONAL NURSING EDUCATION IN SOUTH AFRICA

The History of the Development of Nursing Education in South Africa

The history of the development of nursing education in South Africa follows the historical trends of the country, and in the 1900s was specifically linked to apartheid policies. In the 1700s local women were tested by doctors and then permitted to practice as midwives. The first midwife was Wilhelmina van Zyl in 1751. In the

1800s we saw the arrival of the Anglican sisters, who dramatically influenced the history of nursing education. Among these sisters was Henrietta Stockdale, who would in time play a major role in setting up nursing education in South Africa. Nursing education formally started in South Africa when Stockdale initiated the training program at Carnarvon Hospital, Kimberley, in 1877 (Bruce, Klopper, & Mellish, 2011). The first training course was over a period of 1 year, followed by a second year that the students had to spend in practice as staff nurses before being recognized as trained nurses. The success of the Kimberley-based training started spreading through the country; and by the end of the 19th century, 18 hospitals in South Africa conducted nursing training. In 1891 Sister Henrietta Stockdale's efforts led to the promulgation of an act that would enable state registration of health professionals, inclusive of nurses and midwives, making South Africa the first country in the world to list trained nurses and midwives on a register.

The next notable development was under the leadership of Miss Bella G. Alexander, matron of the Johannesburg General Hospital, who established the first preliminary training school for nurses in October 1921. The first nursing tutor, Miss M. Milne, trained in the United Kingdom, was appointed at the Johannesburg hospital. It became evident that training nursing tutors was important to ensure quality teaching, and in 1937 the University of the Witwatersrand and the University of Cape Town commenced to offer the diploma in nursing (tutor). In 1949 the University of Pretoria followed by instituting a 1-year diploma course for educators, and in 1956 the University of Natal initiated the first course for Black nurse educators.

In 1955 the University of Pretoria was the first to introduce a bachelor of nursing (for Whites only), after which it took 20 years before an undergraduate program for Black nurses was introduced at the University of the Western Cape in 1972 (Bruce et al., 2011). In 1966 the first professor of nursing was appointed as chair of nursing at the University of Pretoria. In 1969, the University of Pretoria also introduced postregistration baccalaureate degrees, that is, qualifications in nursing education, nursing administration, and community nursing. With the establishment of the Department of Nursing Science at the University of South Africa in 1975, Black nurses were given the opportunity to pursue graduate studies through distance education. In 1967, the first nursing students enrolled for a master's degree in nursing at the University of Pretoria. The first nurse to receive a doctorate was Charlotte Searle in 1964, and it was a PhD in sociology, followed by Joyce Mary Mellish, who received the first doctorate in nursing in 1976.

The Nursing Education System

The nursing education system in South Africa has been characterized by fragmentation for many years and we continue to see the aftermath. As the postapartheid democracy is closely linked to the issues of transformation and governance, consideration cannot be given to the governance of nursing education separate from South Africa's transformation agenda (Bruce et al., 2011). We have witnessed how the transformation agenda has impacted on nursing education. Nursing education has been offered in a dual system in South Africa for decades. Nursing colleges offer the diploma courses and university nursing schools the degree programs. Nursing colleges report to the National Department of Health and universities report to the Department of Higher Education and Training. This contributes to the fragmentation of the system. By 1994, the nursing programs were divided into pre- and postregistration programs (Mekwa, 2000). Preregistration programs included:

- A certificate program leading to a qualification as an enrolled auxiliary nurse (often referred to as the nursing assistant). This program was mainly offered through in-service training and the duration varied between 6 and 12 months, depending on the institution.
- A 2-year certificate program leading to a qualification as an enrolled nurse in accordance with the South African Nursing Council (SANC) Regulation R1664, as amended, and R2175. This program was offered by nursing colleges.
- A 2-year diploma in general nursing (referred to as the Bridging Program) leading to registration as a general or psychiatric nurse in accordance with SANC Regulation R683, as amended, offered by nursing colleges.
- An integrated 4-year diploma or degree qualification that included general, psychiatric and community health nursing and midwifery in accordance with SANC Regulation R425, as amended. This program was implemented in 1984 with the purpose to prepare a comprehensively trained nurse-midwife who could practice in primary health care as well as in hospital settings. The program furthermore intended to integrate psychiatric/mental health nursing as part of an entry-level RN program. The rationale was to prepare the professional nurse for the integration of psychiatric care in the general health system. The program also included community health nursing science in order to prepare the professional nurse to be able to practice in community health care settings.

The 4-year diploma course was offered by nursing colleges and the 4-year degree by university nursing schools. For a nursing college to be able to offer the comprehensive program, Regulation R425 included a requirement that nursing colleges, managed by a nursing college principal, had to be affiliated with a university to ensure standards and quality control. The Department of Health (DOH), as the controlling body of public nursing colleges, signed memoranda of understanding (MoUs) with the respective universities that entered into these agreements. With these MoUs in place, nursing education for professional nurses moved into the formal postsecondary education sector (Bezuidenhout, Human, & Lekhuleni, 2013). Notwithstanding these cooperation agreements, we continued to see the dual system enforce a diploma or a degree qualification, leading to the same registration with SANC. Postregistration programs that were offered included:

- Postbasic certificates (known as short courses and typically requiring 6 months for completion)
- Supplementary basic diplomas (e.g., midwifery for those RNs with a general nursing diploma—trained at nursing colleges prior to 1986 and typically offered over a 12-month period)

- Postbasic/postregistration diplomas were offered to RNs, that is, nursing education, nursing administration, community health nursing, pediatrics, orthopedic nursing, operating room nursing, critical care nursing, and so on
- Postbasic/postregistration bachelor degree programs leading to specialization in nursing education, nursing administration, and community health nursing, usually offered as combined qualifications in terms of these various disciplines; these programs were established to provide nondegree qualified RNs with the opportunity to obtain a bachelor's degree
- Honors, master's, and doctoral programs

As part of the transformation agenda, universities went through a restructuring and merging process between 2002 and 2004, resulting in some universities' nursing schools not being allowed to continue to offer the undergraduate degree program in nursing, for example, the University of Stellenbosch and University of Cape Town. It was also during this period that some nursing colleges were closed and others merged, resulting in retaining 12 public nursing colleges, several with multiple campuses. Although from a transformation perspective these decisions made sense, the impetus for the restructuring of higher education and nursing education was political rather than educational in nature. The main purpose of the transformation agenda was to increase accessibility to higher education opportunities for those who were previously disadvantaged and marginalized in terms of career progression (Bezuidenhout et al., 2013).

In an effort to align all nursing qualifications leading to the registration of a professional nurse with the SANC, a process of recurriculating was initiated in 2003. The underlying driving force was the changing focus of health care in South Africa, from hospital-centered care to a primary health care approach. Health services were decentralized to district and local levels to improve the delivery of health care in an attempt to make it more affordable, accessible, and acceptable to the total population (Bezuidenhout et al., 2013).

The National Qualifications Framework (NQF)

In 2000, a NQF of eight levels was developed (see Table 24.1). The rationale for the development was to ensure quality, formulate comparable standards, and provide an articulated structure to promote needs-driven education and training in South Africa. This implied that all qualifications offered in South Africa had to be aligned with the eight-level NQF and comply with the level requirements. The South African Qualifications Authority (SAQA) oversaw the implementation of the NQF.

In 2007, the NQF was amended to a 10-level framework as promulgated by the NQF Act, No. 67 of 2008. The amendment was made to guarantee equivalence and portability of qualifications. It was after implementation of the eight-level NQF that it became evident that it did not allow the necessary distinction between qualifications (see Table 24.1). Subsequently, the total SAQA Act No. 58 of 1995 was repealed by the Government Gazette No. 31909 of February 17, 2009, Section 37.

TABLE 24.1 The National Qualifications Framework (NQF) Levels of South Africa

LEVELS	EIGHT-LEVEL NQF (2000)	TEN-LEVEL NQF (2010)
5	National certificate—120 credits	Higher certificate—120 credits
	National diploma—240 credits	
6	National certificate—120 credits	Advanced certificate—120 credits
	National diploma—240 credits	Diploma—360 credits
	Bachelor's—360 credits	
7	National certificate—120 credits	
	National diploma—240 credits	
	Bachelor's (professional)—480 credits	
	Bachelor's (technical)—480 credits	
	Bachelor's/Honors—120 credits	
8	National certificate—120 credits	Bachelor's degree (professional)—480 credits
	National diploma—240 credits	Bachelor's/Honors degree—120 credits
	Master's—180 credits	Postgraduate diploma—120 credits
	Master's (technical)—180 credits	
	Doctoral—360 credits	
	Doctoral (technical)—360 credits	
	Post-doc	
9	Not applicable	Master's degree—180 credits
10	Not applicable	Doctoral degree—360 credits

Source: South African Qualifications Authority (2012).

However, SAQA as a juristic body continued to exist with changed functions and responsibilities in terms of Section 13 of the National Qualifications Act, 2008.

The New NQF

The establishment of the NQF provided an opportunity to align all nursing qualifications with the framework. Following a resolution by the SANC, all nursing qualifications (except for the nursing auxiliary category) will move to the higher education sector (see Table 24.2). These new qualifications were developed over the past 8 years and are now earmarked for implementation in 2016.

TABLE 24.2 Nursing Qualifications in Terms of the National Qualifications Framework (NQF)

NQF LEVEL	NURSING QUALIFICATION
10	Doctorate (360 credits)
9	Master's degree (180 credits)
8	Bachelor's degree (480 credits) (professional nurses and midwives) Postgraduate diploma (120 credits) (nurses specializing in specific disciplines such as nursing management, nursing education, theater technique, and others)
7	Advanced diploma (120 credits) (midwife)
6	Diploma (360 credits) (staff nurse)
5	Higher certificate (120 credits) (auxiliary nurse/auxiliary midwife)

- A 3-year diploma in nursing at NQF level 6 will be implemented to produce staff nurses. At this level, the staff nurses should have problem-solving skills and demonstrate an understanding of ethical implications and decisions, and they should also be able to apply well-developed processes of analysis, synthesis, and evaluation of the information that is accessed (Bezuidenhout et al., 2013).
- At NQF level 7 an advanced diploma (120 credits) implies that after the 3-year diploma a staff nurse can register for an advanced diploma in midwifery (120 credits). At this level, the student will be expected to demonstrate the ability to integrate knowledge within the main areas of nursing theory and practice.
- The NQF level 8 for the bachelor's degree for a professional nurse and midwife consists of 480 credits. The postgraduate diploma of 120 credits applies to specialization areas.
- The NQF level 9 applies to the master's degree and consists of 180 credits.
- NQF level 10 applies to the doctoral degree and comprises 360 credits. Evident from this qualification is the candidate's ability to develop new methods, techniques, processes, and systems; being original, creative, and innovative is also a primary goal.

The Council for Higher Education (CHE)

The amended Higher Education Act 101 of 1997 significantly impacted nursing regulation, specifically with regard to the regulation of education and training of professional nurses (Duma, 2012). The CHE, which has a statutory responsibility for assuring higher education through the Higher Education Act 101 of 1997, now also regulates nursing education programs offered by universities in South Africa. The main functions of the CHE, through the Higher Education Quality Committee (HEQC), are

- To promote quality assurance in higher education
- To audit the quality assurance mechanisms of higher education institutions
- To accredit providers of higher education institutions offering programs leading to particular NQF registered qualifications

All programs offered by higher education institutions, that is, universities, need to be approved by the CHE in South Africa. As indicated earlier, nursing education has been characterized by nursing programs offered in a dual system. However, with the new NQF, all nursing qualifications will be part of the higher education system. This has vast implications for nursing colleges, which will have to meet the criteria for approval by CHE. The HEQC, a permanent subcommittee of the CHE, has set criteria for program accreditation in higher education. These criteria (CHE, 2004) are a driver for the proposed new nursing qualifications set by the SANC (SANC, 2013). Quality-related criteria, such as the CHE input criteria for new programs, act as evaluative tools for accreditation activities and set broad benchmarks for quality management (Mulder & Uys, 2013). It is imperative that nursing colleges apply for accreditation of their various programs to the HEQC to safeguard continuation of their existence. The HEQC does not accredit institutions, but only the programs offered. All the new nursing qualifications (see Table 24.3) are aligned with the Higher Education Qualifications Sub-Framework (HEQSF) draft (CHE, 2013; FUNDISA, 2011; SANC, 2013; South Africa Ministry of Education, 2004) within the higher education sector as classified by the NQF Act 67 of 2008 (RSA, 2008a).

In order to be recognized and approved as a higher education institution that can legally offer programs, CHE (2004) uses a set of 18 criteria to evaluate a program, of which eight are input criteria, seven are process criteria, and the remaining three are output criteria. The first phase of the program accreditation process is called the candidacy phase (CHE, 2004). During this initial phase, an institution has to demonstrate that it meets the input criteria or that it has the potential or capability to meet these criteria in a stipulated period of time. The institution's

TABLE 24.3 Qualification Types on the Higher Education Qualifications Sub-Framework (HEQSF) and Correlating South African Nursing Council (SANC) Categories

	EXIT LEVEL	SANC CATEGORY
Undergraduate qualifications		
Higher certificate	5	Registered auxiliary nurse
Advanced certificate	6	
Diploma	6	Registered staff nurse
Advanced diploma	7	Registered midwife
Bachelor's degree	7 or 8	Registered professional nurse and midwife
Postgraduate qualifications		
Postgraduate diploma	8	Proposed specialist nurse
Bachelor's/Honors degree	8	
Master's degree	9	Proposed advanced specialist nurse
Doctoral degree	10	

Sources: CHE (2013); FUNDISA (2011).

application must be based on a critical self-evaluation of the new program against requirements of the HEQC program input criteria. The institution furthermore needs to submit a plan for the implementation of the new program specifying implementation steps including time frames, resources, and strategies to meet process, output, and impact criteria (Mulder & Uys, 2013).

It is evident from the information provided that South Africa higher education and nursing education continue to be in a transformation phase. With the focus of alignment of nursing education with higher education and the alignment of nursing programs with the HEQC, we can look forward to some exciting times in the advancement of professional nursing education in South Africa.

The Role of the Regulatory Body in Professional Nursing Education

The SANC, a professional body, regulates nursing and midwifery in South Africa. SANC is an autonomous statutory entity, established by the Nursing Act, No. 45 of 1944, amended by the Nursing Act, No. 50 of 1978, and the current Nursing Act, No. 33 of 2005. The SANC regulates the nursing and midwifery professions through the following functions:

• Development, maintenance, promotion, and control of standards in nursing education and training
• Registration of the different categories of nurses and midwives
• Monitoring the ethical and professional conduct of nurses and midwives

The professional council thus has the primary responsibility of determining who will practice and what competencies are needed (inclusive of knowledge, skills, and attributes). The licensure of nurses has remained an unchanged implement of the SANC in protecting the public through the Nursing Act, by ensuring that no persons may practice nursing or midwifery in the country unless they are registered to practice in the following categories: professional nurse, midwife, staff nurse, auxiliary nurse, or auxiliary midwife (South African Nursing Council, 2005).

In terms of the function of development, maintenance, promotion, and control of standards in nursing education and training, the SANC plays a significant role. As indicated earlier, the primary function of approval of programs lies with CHE; under the Higher Education Act 101 of 1997, the HEQC could take over this task from the SANC. We would then see SANC retaining the task of registration or enrollment of nurses and midwives. Correctly so, Duma (2012) states that, in principle, the separation of roles between the CHE–HEQC and SANC seems simple on paper, but in practice it has remained difficult as professional regulatory bodies have always been the main quality assurers.

SANC has been responsible for setting professional and educational standards and for evaluating the quality of their implementation. A solution to this problem came through the recognition of the professional regulatory bodies as Education and Training Quality Assurance (ETQA) bodies in terms of the South African Quality Authority Act of 1995 (Act No. 58 of 1995). SANC was formally accredited as an ETQA in November 2001 in terms of Section 5(1) (a) (ii) of the South African Qualification Authority Act No. 58 of 1995. This was regarded as an achievement and a complement to the SANC's original statutory functions of protecting the public through ensuring quality nursing education (Duma, 2012; Subedar, 2001). With this recognition, in addition to the SANC's original functions as an ETQA, the SANC was now accredited to

- Facilitate moderation among constituent providers
- Register assessors
- Cooperate with relevant moderating bodies
- Recommend new standards or qualifications to national standard bodies or modify existing standards and qualifications
- Submit reports to SAQA

Probably the biggest achievement of the SANC since 1994 is the unification of the nursing profession within one regulatory body within South Africa as it provides uniform national protection for the citizens of this country, irrespective of which province or area they reside (Duma, 2012). With obtaining the SAQA accreditation status as an ETQA, SANC retained the function of regulating nursing education and training in collaboration with the HEQC. Management of the ETQA status is crucial for the SANC to continue regulating the education and training of nurses and midwives in the country (Duma, 2012). In terms of regulation, nurses and midwives in both public and private health and education institutions have a critical role to play in assisting the SANC to regulate the nursing profession and protect the public.

FUNDISA AS A NATIONAL DRIVER FOR CHANGE IN NURSING IN SOUTH AFRICA

Globally, nursing organizations play a valuable role in the advancement of nursing and nursing education. Since 1994, FUNDISA has played an eminent role as the organization to assist in the transformation of nursing education in the higher education sector in South Africa.

Introduction

Historically, many people have tried to "change things" in Africa, some with spectacular success, others leaving almost no trace after much effort. Funding agencies often want to know, "How can the problem be solved?" Or a government asks, "How can this bad situation be changed?" Individuals and groups jump in "to help" but often little is changed after many years, large amounts of money spent, and many reports.

In the recent history of FUNDISA in South Africa, significant change was seen over a relatively short period of time. Between 2005 and 2014 concerted projects changed the climate and activities within the university nursing sector in South Africa in many ways (collaboration, research activity, clinical teaching, etc.).

In analyzing recent history, we have identified a few strategies that we believe made the difference without being seen as universal rules in any rational linear way (Saka, 2001). These changes in research development, policy involvement, educational development, and educational service provision seem to be the confluence of a range of factors that may provide an outline of a national change agent. To that end, we describe the four planned strategies the authors have identified as important in FUNDISA, as a national nursing professional organization, to act successfully as a national change agent.

In this section the usefulness of a national professional nursing organization as a change agent of the nursing profession in a country is explored. We accept that change in the broader nursing profession, by which we mean regulation, practice, education, policy, and research, is desirable and often essential. We also accept that any targeted change should be toward the greater good for the greater number in the long term for the profession and the health service users whom they serve, and not for a small parochial group often benefiting the powerful and privileged. However, unplanned change may take place too slowly, too discordant, and in the wrong directions for a good ultimate outcome to be reached by the profession. The lessons we have learned in the past decade of the work of one professional organization in one country may indicate how professional organizations can successfully act as a national sectoral change agent to initiate, harmonize, strengthen, direct, and target professional change.

Description of FUNDISA

FUNDISA is a registered not-for-profit organization that is the national voice for South Africa's baccalaureate and higher degree nursing education programs, and indirectly for all 4-year diploma and postbasic diploma qualifications provided by colleges. This is based on legal agreements between universities and provincial health departments. FUNDISA represents nursing education and nursing scholarship in South Africa and was constituted in 1994 by university nursing schools (UNS). The vision of FUNDISA is to be a unified platform to pursue excellence in nursing scholarship at universities in South Africa and its mission to provide strategic innovative leadership and expertise in nursing education, promote scholarship, and strengthen collaboration with stakeholders. The membership ascribes to the values of respect, integrity, commitment, cooperation, support, transparency, and equity. FUNDISA members are 22 university and university of technology nursing schools in the country.

FUNDISA offers the following services or products to its members and the broader nursing education community in South Africa:

• Support, coaching, mentoring, role preparation, and recognition of academic leaders for their academic and professional leadership roles
• Policy interrogation, development, advocacy, and evaluation with regard to nursing and health professional education

- Information and policy clearinghouse to inform nursing education stakeholders with regard to nursing education issues nationally and internationally
- Consultation and other professional services in the field of nursing education, such as external school reviews and external program reviews, and curriculum development for higher education institutions (FUNDISA, Monitoring and Evaluation Plan, 2011).

In 2009 FUNDISA obtained funding from the Atlantic Philanthropies (AP) to develop the organization, and in 2011 it contracted with the same funders and with the ELMA Foundation to do the project management for the University Nursing Education in South Africa (UNEDSA) Programme for 3 years. The UNEDSA Programme ran for a 5-year period ending in 2013. It was aimed at transforming nursing scholarship in selected South African university-based schools of nursing through grants made by two philanthropic organizations, the AP and the ELMA Foundation. Substantial grants totalling R70 million (6.6 million U.S. dollars) were allocated to six selected university-based nursing schools for the 5-year period. In November 2009, an anonymous donor boosted the program by an additional R29 million (US$2.7 million), bringing the total to nearly R100 million (about US$10 million). This is the largest single grant ever to nursing education in South Africa. Since the grantees of UNEDSA were also members of FUNDISA, the project management allowed FUNDISA to integrate the work of UNEDSA into the organizational initiatives. This greatly strengthened the work of FUNDISA.

Triggers of Change Between 2005 and 2013

Three triggers jointly allowed and stimulated the changes:

- A *general discomfort with the quality of nursing care* provided in the country, perhaps best illustrated by the process and content of the ministerial summit organized in 2011 by the National Department of Health (Nursing Summit Organizing Committee and Ministerial Task Team, 2012). The burden of disease and health indicators—nationally and compared with comparable countries internationally—also raised concern.
- The entry into South Africa of the *AP Foundation* with an interest in *focusing on nursing,* specifically for professional organizations. In an interview with Zola Madikizela of the AP Foundation, he explained these decisions as follows:

> Based on the investigative work done by a volunteer Board Member of the Foundation who spent time in the country, nursing was prioritized. The motivation was that they were interested in providing support for quality health care, especially in PHC [primary health care]. They found the contribution of the nurses in this component of health care a clear priority based on their distribution across the country and their ability to make PHC care accessible. The decision of where to focus within the profession led them to identify strengthening

NEIs, since the influence of these institutions will be felt long after the funding cycle. They also decided to include the 'voice, ears, and eyes of the nursing profession' by funding organizations working with nurses in practice (Democratic Nursing Organization of South Africa, DENOSA), the groups involved in preparing nurses (Nursing Education Association, NEA), FUNDISA and the statutory body (SANC). (Madikizela, personal communication, February 24, 2014)

The allocation decisions that were based on these choices were only made in 2008, but the crystallization of the focus happened over the preceding years.

- The presence simultaneously in the two major nursing education professional organizations, NEA and FUNDISA, of two exceptional leaders, Dr. Sharon Vasuthevan and Dr. Hester Klopper. They saw a greater and more formal role of professional education organizations and realized the unique opportunity for a great leap forward, rather than incremental change. With the capacity in and around the organizations they developed two acceptable proposals and were visionaries with an appetite of risk-taking to move nursing education forward in the country.

Change Strategies

Since 2005, FUNDISA has initiated a series of change strategies that were to shape the change happening inside the organization and the sector. The four major strategies are described here.

Structure, Focus, and Develop the Organization as an Arena of Social Exchange and Support to Be the Voice of Academic Nursing in the Country

In 2005, when Dr. A. S. vd Merwe took over as chair of FUNDISA, the organization followed the pattern of most professional nursing organizations in South Africa. It had an elected committee that managed the activities, which consisted almost exclusively of infrequent face-to-face meetings of representatives from all African nursing schools. The agendas did not always deal with the matters that were currently a priority to the members, and follow-up was sporadic and uncoordinated. It did not have a national identity outside the universities, and even there it had little influence. The status quo was challenged by an open letter written in April 2007 by Dr. Hester Klopper, and addressed to FUNDISA and all nursing academics, asking them to take up the leading role to be advocates for nursing education. The organization then decided to restructure and formalize its work to become "a real presence through its input" (Dr. A. S. vd Merwe, personal communication, March 5, 2014). The years of 2005 to 2007 involved many activities to create a clear identity for the organization and to fit the structure to that vision. Debates around issues such as who should be members (heads of schools or anybody) and who should represent the nursing schools at FUNDISA meetings became heated.

To give FUNDISA a reasonable chance of decisions being implemented, heads of schools were essential. But that was too exclusive and did not involve the rest of the academics. In the final instance, a system of the nursing school being represented at meetings by the head and a permanent secundus to ensure continuity was accepted. At the same time it was decided to have four meetings per year, hosted on a rotation basis by a nursing school. This rolling meeting schedule allowed all local academics to attend the meetings and led to much greater familiarity with other schools and their activities and strengths. The regular schedule also allowed for more appropriate agendas and better attendance. The organization worked not just on structure, but also on other documents about the organization, such as a position statement of their values, and a vision, mission, and logo for a corporate identity.

The relevance of the organization was immediately addressed by taking on projects of importance to the members. For instance, the academics were very concerned about the comparison between their own salaries and that of nurse educators in the public nursing college system, which was perceived to be much better, with lower expectations having to be met by incumbents. Recruitment and retention of academics for the university sector was very challenging. FUNDISA developed a document comparing salaries between these two sectors, which many heads of schools could use to negotiate improved scales for their own academics, rendering a major service to the sector. The result of this refocusing and reorganization was an organization much more in tune with its members and better organized and functioning.

When Dr. Hester Klopper took over as chair at the end of 2007 this process accelerated. She led the organization in an analysis of its income and increasing realization that the income sources had to be expanded. At that stage the AP call for proposals and their exploratory meetings had already taken place and FUNDISA had attended. This became its first venture into expanding its resource base. One of the activities that allowed for significant growth in the organization's understanding of itself and its context was the allocation to the AP of a planning grant for the development of a funding proposal. The task of developing the funding proposal fell mainly to the FUNDISA committee, but the regular membership was involved at meetings. In 2009 FUNDISA was successful in obtaining funding for 3 years "to develop its organization to play an emerging role as a significant champion of best-practices in nursing education and improved nursing scholarship in South Africa" (FUNDISA Organizational Development Project, 2009).

When FUNDISA members were asked in 2011 what they valued about the organization, the consensus was that FUNDISA managed to break the isolation within which most of the heads of schools had functioned up to that point. In many of the technology universities, as few as one permanent academic member worked with a group of contract academics to carry out the teaching and administration. In larger universities, the nursing schools were demanding, especially in terms of teaching/learning tasks and also their relationships with nursing colleges. Heads of both types of schools said they were poorly informed about many national issues and trends and they had no place to discuss their own problems with peers.

They did not know the other heads well enough to approach them on a person-to-person basis and did not get the opportunity at FUNDISA meetings to do this.

However, during the organizational development this changed. Dr. Martha Pinkoane (Vaal University of Technology) said of these changes: "FUNDISA has really fortified my position as a nurse educator in a University of Technology. I can negotiate from an informed and unified position. Truly this is very meaningful." Dr. Jermina Kgole (University of Limpopo, Turfloop Campus) also commented, "For me FUNDISA means networking and support. I will not miss a meeting if I can help it. Just discussing all the issues we have to deal with up to a point of seeing the way forward helps so much."

Publish Systematic, Scientific, Comprehensive Descriptions of Crucial Components of the Profession Over the Short Term

Since we started working within a strategic plan in FUNDISA, we have found that many studies describing problems in the profession were based on a single college, or a single survey, with no follow-up and no wider lens. It was too vague and too patchy to allow for planning and to direct and drive change. Research was being done but with no applicability.

The solution was the establishment of an annual *Trends in Nursing* publication in 2012 based on commissioned, targeted topics, and aiming for participation as close to nationally as possible in every aspect. The first *Trends in Nursing* focused on the academic nursing education sector (2011) and included chapters such as:

- Baseline measure of the implementation process of the proposed model for clinical nursing education and training in South African universities
- Status of research-related activities of South African university nursing schools
- The current status of the education and training of nurse educators in South Africa

Within months these substantive reports, together with the UNEDSA reviews, allowed us to identify research development nationally as a major limitation. This led to the planning of the program.

The second *Trends in Nursing* (2013) focused more strongly on the college sector, with chapters such as:

- Financing of public nursing colleges
- The evaluation of one public nursing college in terms of the program criteria of the HEQC
- The Nelson Mandela Metropolitan University and Lilitha College collaboration

The clear priority of the college sector in South Africa at this time was to get ready for their new position in the Health Education sector. Our substantive review of the needs of the KwaZulu-Natal College of Nursing provided the systematic data for this change (Mulder & Uys, in Klopper, 2013), while the example of a college where this change is already well underway provided an example to follow (van Rooyen et al., in Klopper, 2013).

This brings us to the major focus on publication. We have too many reports in developing countries that "belong" to nongovernment organizations (NGOs), community-based organizations (CBOs), and government departments. They are often difficult to obtain and to access, and it is very difficult to get up-to-date, systematic, in-depth data on an area such as nursing. We therefore created a publishing arena for nurses in the areas of the organized profession, nursing education, and health services. Authors find it difficult to obtain publishing opportunities in the readily accessible international nursing literature and it takes too long for such publications to reach readers. Open-source journals are less well-known to nurses and reach too few readers inside the country to make a difference to our local debates. The profession needed to get published material that is relevant to national debates and current affairs, and includes policy analysis, implementation, and evaluation. Publication should have a quick turnaround so that the profession and stakeholders can use the information.

FUNDISA started *Trends in Nursing* as a commissioned book in 2012, but by 2013 it was realized that for long-term sustainability the publication needed to fit into the funding framework for scientific publications in the country. The National Research Foundation (NRF) of South Africa pays universities a specific subsidy for every research article published in a research journal they recognize (www.nrf.ac.za). This also means that academics are encouraged to publish in such journals. FUNDISA also decided to move to an open access, web-based journal format. The move is currently underway for the 2013 *Trends in Nursing;* as of 2014, the journal will be published through the online system of the University of Stellenbosch.

Work Collaboratively in Partnerships

Before the changes in South Africa, university nursing schools and professional organizations often worked not only in isolation, but also in competition. With this change, the leadership decided to mine existing tentative relationships and build new ones (see Table 24.4). To do this, the organization used the relationships existing through its leaders and members, and relationships open to it as an organization. In identifying, strengthening, and using these partnerships, the effort was to identify the strengths of partners and to see what could be done to work together for the good of all. Most of the partnerships grew from the needs members identified, existing contacts, and the opportunities we saw when engaging with them. But the new focus on nursing schools partnering with each other should not be underemphasized. As the atmosphere inside the sector became more collegial and less competitive, and as the isolation of members was gradually reduced, informal and formal collaboration between member schools increased. Visibility of many nursing schools nationally and within their own organizations improved.

One good example of a national partnership is the work with the NRF and with SANTRUST (see Table 24.4). FUNDISA initiated discussions with the NRF in order to discuss the need for research development in nursing. The NRF had also identified nursing as a neglected field of science and was interested in collaboration. At the same time, the NRF had a relationship with SANTRUST,

TABLE 24.4 Major Partners of FUNDISA

PARTNER	CONTACT	AREA OF PARTNERSHIP
National Research Foundation (NRF)	FUNDISA	Research development and research capacity development
SANTRUST	Individual leaders	Research development
NEA	FUNDISA	Office sustainability
STTI	Chair and FUNDISA members	Organizational development
Nursing education stakeholders group, including SANC, DENOSA, public- and private-sector nursing education in schools and colleges	FUNDISA	Policy development
NEPI	Individual leaders	Educational service provision

DENOSA, Democratic Nursing Organization of South Africa; FUNDISA, Forum of University Nursing Deans of South Africa; NEA, Nursing Education Association; NRF, National Research Foundation; SANC, South African Nursing Council; STTI, Sigma Theta Tau International.

whose main objective is for African universities to sustain key capacities and competencies, raise their international profile, and tap the financial benefits that arise from high-quality human capacity and research outputs (www.santrust .org.za). Since 1997 they have developed an improved best practice model of the South Africa–Netherlands Research Programme on Alternatives in Development (SANPAD) Research Capacity Initiative, including a predoctoral program. Through open distance learning (ODL), e-learning, and a one-to-one consultation model, SANTRUST has prepared some 300 predoctoral candidates and 200 research supervisors for the successful completion of doctoral dissertations. Of the doctoral candidates, 93% graduated within 3 to 4 years as opposed to the South African average of 7 to 8 years. Clearly, the NRF, SANTRUST, and FUNDISA had to collaborate.

In 2012 SANTRUST offered a predoctoral program specifically for nurse-academics, while FUNDISA launched their departmental research development program aimed at academics who were already doctorally prepared and now needed to develop their own or school-based research programs. The FUNDISA postdoctoral program was aimed at developing lead researchers within each nursing department to lead a research program on a selected health topic (Uys & Klopper, 2014). The focus of the research platform was on the person as well as the department. The lead researchers were assisted in developing a research team for their program, in becoming part of an international network, in working with a research mentor in submitting proposals for external funding, and in preparing for NRF rating. This was done through a series of workshops and the appointment of a mentor for each lead researcher. The FUNDISA project was fully funded by the

NRF, and by 2013 there were 17 lead researchers from 14 universities registering. The NRF also funded successful peer-reviewed proposals from the lead researchers in this program in 2013.

The supplementary foci of SANTRUST and FUNDISA ensure that there is no competition between these two organizations, but it also drew them into closer collaboration about how, when, and what to do. Collaboration between these three partners is continuing and expanding.

Another example on a very different level was that with the NEA. The NEA is an organization of more than 1,000 nurse educator members in South Africa. Their vision is excellence in nursing education for practice (www.edunurse.co.za), and their focus is very strongly on professional development of the individual involved with nursing education in all nursing education sectors. Their professional development programs include such topics as simulation as a teaching approach, leadership development, and scientific writing skills.

While the NEA and FUNDISA worked together since 2005, it wasn't until both received grants from AP that this became a more explicit strategy. One of the activities they collaborated on was the purchase of an office building together and the launch of the Nursing Foundation of South Africa. The Nursing Foundation was created as a registered trust in June 2013 to build nursing and midwifery, targeting all nurses as opposed to only nursing education (www.nursingfoundation .co.za). The focus of this brief description of the NEA partnership focuses on the capital project.

Both organizations needed offices and they rented premises together. Both realized that this high monthly expense would be a barrier for future sustainability. Seeking a solution together seemed sensible. The two organizations started their funding cycle for AP at the same time and in the first year their spending was less than it should have been as it took time to get the office functioning and staff appointed. Funds were thus "saved" in their grants and together this amount would allow the purchase of an office building. In exploring this option, they decided to buy not only for their own need, but to be able to rent out some space, thus ensuring an income. AP was approached for permission to make an internal allocation shift in the grants to allow for the purchase with existing funds and they agreed. In 2011, in the second grant year, the two organizations bought a property together in the capital, Pretoria, centrally located and with easy access from trains and freeways. The property was extensively refurbished in order to make it as functional as possible, and facilities such as an Internet server were installed. The collaboration was based on a signed legal joint venture agreement about how the property will be managed, including how maintenance and income will be handled.

After the two organizations occupied what they needed, with many shared spaces such as the board room (used for meetings and smaller training sessions), the additional space was rented out. All of the renters proved to be organizations with which FUNDISA has a close link; for instance, UNEDSA, for whom FUNDISA did the project management, and the Africa office of Sigma Theta Tau International (STTI). With this rental income the two organizations currently cover their physical office cost fully. This has contributed to sustainability and also provides the partners with a major capital asset.

Deliver the Products of Planned Activities and Work to Build Capacity

Another strategy of FUNDISA was to ensure that project work was almost exclusively done by its own members in an effort to empower and capacitate people through being a participant in action. In this way members became familiar and involved with the current, real situation in their sector, and their understanding was shaped by working together, dialogue, and conversation. The system of having a person representing a portfolio on the FUNDISA committee, namely the research, practice, education, and marketing portfolios, was expanded. A working group was created for each portfolio and tasks were referred to these groups for action and report-back. Sometimes this involved total tasks, such as when the Practice Portfolio Group initiated and ran a survey about the community involvement of university nursing schools—an expectation within the higher education sector (Sibiya et al., 2013). This task led to a publication about this aspect, which acts as a baseline and example for other schools, not only about what to do (which most are doing), but also about how to classify and evaluate this kind of activity.

Members became part of field work teams that reviewed and analyzed findings and planned and implemented research projects. During all these efforts the values of integrity, equity, and respect were emphasized so that members did not feel threatened. The importance of producing quality products on time was also emphasized, and deadlines became serious work targets instead of a nice idea. Since there are so many "helpers" in the developing world, it is an art to involve them strategically and wisely. Otherwise they could become part of a disempowering, expert-dependent culture within the developing country. It must be remembered that the national nurses are the experts in the real world and they have to implement change. This demands that they own the change and they learn by doing. The philosophy works as well for nurse leaders as for student nurses.

Currently many member universities and/or individual academics are involved in capacity building efforts across the country and across the continent. One example is the work with the Nursing Education Partnership Initiative (NEPI), for which FUNDISA has become a service provider. NEPI funding is provided by the President's Emergency Fund for AIDS Relief (PEPFAR), which supports 120 countries in HIV/AIDS prevention, care, and treatment. In Malawi, Zambia, Lesotho, Ethiopia, and Democratic Republic of the Congo, the International Center for AIDS Care and Treatment Programs (ICAP) is partnering with the ministries of health and selected training institutions to implement NEPI, which supports innovative strategies and promising practices that will inform curricula development, faculty preparation and strategies for faculty retention, and educational models that prepare new nurses to practice in the diversity of medical and community settings where health needs are greatest. This is a great opportunity for further building the capacity of FUNDISA in a much wider arena, benefiting their hosts and partners, but also themselves.

In December 2013, FUNDISA received news of an additional grant from AP of ZAR 21.5 million (about US$2 million) for Connecting and Leading Research, Education and Practice through Support, and Capacity Building in Nursing (CLEARSCAN) (2014–2016). The aim of this program is to strengthen and transform nursing research, education, and practice by providing technical support and capacity building. CLEARSCAN will build capacity as knowledge, skills, and attitudes that will enable nurses to leverage their position and improve their status within the changing health care landscape in South Africa.

CONCLUSION

Looking back over almost 10 years of growth and development, two of our most crucial lessons have been the importance of leadership and the understanding of how long sustainable change takes. Emerging leaders have to establish themselves as trusted by the sector. Without this inherent trust, progress is not possible. This takes time and effort and selfless service. But this is not the only process that takes time. The opening of conversations, the building up of people so that they can take part productively in such discussions, building capacity to take matters forward, creating formal structures within the legal framework of the country, all takes much more time than one would expect.

FUNDISA is, of course, not perfect; neither has it arrived in terms of the objectives set for the organization. The greatest challenge it currently faces is to maintain the momentum of change. FUNDISA members have not become less busy; they actually have more activities than they had before. However, they are better capacitated and resourced to deal with their challenges. FUNDISA work has to be seamlessly integrated with the recognized expectations of university schools in order to not be seen as additional, but as part of their academic work. FUNDISA has also grown exponentially in its activities and keeping up organizationally with these changes is challenging. Change clearly is ongoing, and our past restructuring will not be appropriate forever. New thinking is again necessary.

REFERENCES

Bezuidenhout, M., Human, S. P., & Lekhuleni, M. (2013). The new nursing qualifications framework. In H. C. Klopper (Ed.), *Trends in nursing 2013*. Pretoria, South Africa: FUNDISA.

Bruce, J. C., Klopper, H. C., & Mellish, J. M. (2011). *Teaching and learning the practice of nursing*. Johannesburg, South Africa: Pearson Education.

Council on Higher Education (CHE). (2004). *Criteria for program accreditation*. Pretoria, South Africa: Author.

Council on Higher Education. (2013). *A framework for qualification standards in higher education*. Second Draft. Pretoria, South Africa: Author.

Duma, S. (2012). The state of nursing regulation. *Trends in Nursing, 1(1)*. Retrieved from http://fundisa.journals.ac.za/pub/article/view/20/12

Forum of University Nursing Deans in South Africa (FUNDISA). (2009). Grant application: Proposal for long-term funding of a professionalized FUNDISA. Retrieved from http://www.fundisaforum.org/docs/FUNDISAAtlanticGrantProposalFinal.pdf

Forum of University Nursing Deans in South Africa (FUNDISA). (2011). Preparation of nurse specialists by universities. *News November*. Retrieved from http://www.fundisaforum.org/archive.htm

Klopper, H. C. (Ed.). (2013). *Trends in nursing 2013*. Pretoria, South Africa: FUNDISA.

Mekwa, J. (2000). Transformation in nursing education. In A. Ntuli (Ed.), *South African Health Review, 2000* (pp. 271–284). South Africa: Health Systems Trust.

Mulder, M., & Uys, L. R. (2013). The evaluation of one public nursing college in terms of the program criteria of the Higher Education Quality Committee. In H. C. Klopper (Ed.), *Trends in nursing 2013*. Pretoria, South Africa: FUNDISA.

Nursing Summit Organizing Committee and Ministerial Task Team. (2012). The Nursing Summit of 2011. In L.R. Uys, & H. C. Klopper, H.C. (Eds.), *Trends in Nursing 2012* (pp. 33–48). Pretoria, South Africa: FUNDISA.

Republic of South Africa (RSA). (2008a). *Higher Education Amendment Act, No. 39 of 2008*. Pretoria, South Africa: Government Printer.

Republic of South Africa (RSA). (2008b). *National Qualifications Framework Act, No. 67 of 2008*. Pretoria, South Africa: Government Printer.

Saka, A. (2001) Internal change agents' view of the management of change problem. *Journal of Organizational Change Management, 16(5)*, 480–496.

Sibiya, N., Netshikweta, J., Kgole, J., Stellenberg, E., Seekoe, E., & Klopper, H. C. (2013). Community engagement by university nursing schools. In Klopper H. C. (Ed.), *Trends in nursing 2013 (*pp. 115–140). Pretoria, South Africa: FUNDISA.

South Africa. (2009). *National Qualifications Framework Act 67 of 2008*. Government Gazette No. 31909: Pretoria, South Africa.

South Africa.info. (2014). Retrieved from http://www.southafrica.info/about/history/521109.htm

South Africa Ministry of Education. (2004). *The higher education qualifications framework*. Pretoria, South Africa: Government Gazette No, 0000000.

South African Nursing Council (SANC). (2005). *Nursing Act No. 33 of 2005*. Pretoria, South Africa: SANC.

South African Nursing Council (SANC). (2013). *Details of new nursing qualifications*. Retrieved from http://www.sanc.co.za

South African Qualifications Authority. (2012). *The National Qualifications Framework*. Retrieved from http://www.SAQA.org.za

Subedar, H. (2001). *South African Nursing Council as an education and training quality authority*. Circular 13/2001. Retrieved from www.sanc.co.za/archive/2001/newsc.113.htm

Uys, L. R., & Klopper, H. C. (Eds.). (2012). *Trends in nursing 2012*. Pretoria, South Africa: FUNDISA.

Uys, L. R., & Klopper, H. C. (2014, January). Research development in university departments in South Africa. *South African Journal of Higher Education*. Retrieved from www.saqa.org.za

CHAPTER 25

Cultural Immersion Experiences in Nursing Education

Nancy L. Meedzan

Cultural competency is considered an important skill for nurses and will aid in the elimination of health disparities, with the goal of increased quality of care and improved patient outcomes. Cultural competence is a contemporary issue in health care today and educators are seeking the best practice for teaching cultural competence in nursing education. Therefore, this chapter discusses the problem and significance of cultural competence training for nursing students.

Accrediting agencies have made cultural competence an outcome requirement in all prelicensure baccalaureate nursing programs in the United States (Accreditation Commission for Education in Nursing [ACEN], 2013; American Association of Colleges of Nursing [AACN], 2008). This requirement is based on the changing demographics in the United States and the increase in health disparities among culturally diverse patients (Agency for Healthcare Research and Quality [AHRQ], 2012). Unfortunately, the most recent report from the AHRQ states, "Overall quality is improving, access is getting worse, and disparities are not changing" (2012). Nursing education accreditation agencies seem to be paying attention to these continued trends in American health care. The most recent update to the ACEN standards for baccalaureate education suggests incorporation of immersion experiences for undergraduate nursing students. ACEN Standard 4.5 states, "The curriculum includes cultural, ethnic, and socially diverse concepts and may also include experiences from regional, national, or global perspectives" (ACEN, 2013). It is thought that increased cultural competence among health care workers leads to the provision of patient-centered care, which has been shown to increase the quality of health care and lead to better patient outcomes (Institute of Medicine [IOM], 2001; IOM, 2002). In order to produce culturally competent nurses, nurse educators must incorporate cultural competence into the curriculum of nursing education. Cultural immersion, or an experience of living among a culture different from one's own, is a method of teaching cultural competence that appeals to the current generation of college students (Institute of International Education, 2013). There is evidence to suggest that cultural immersion experiences may contribute to the development of cultural competence while also providing an enriching travel opportunity previously unavailable in many nursing curricula (Amerson, 2010; Button, Green, Tengnah, Johansson, & Baker, 2005; Caffrey, Neander, Markle, & Stewart, 2005; Koskinen & Tossavairen, 2004; Larsen & Reif, 2011; Larson, Ott, & Miles, 2010; Maltby & Abrams, 2009; Ruddock & Turner, 2007; St. Clair & McKenry, 1999; Walsh & De Joseph, 2003).

BACKGROUND

Crossing the Quality Chasm (IOM, 2001) identified patient-centered care as one of the six quality pillars on which a 21st-century health care system should be built. Dr. Donald Berwick, former director of the Centers for Medicaid and Medicare Services and former president and chief executive officer of the Institute of Healthcare Improvement (IHI), defines patient-centered care as, "The experience (to the extent the informed, individual patient desires it) of transparency, individualization, recognition, respect, dignity, and choice in all matters, without exception, related to one's person, circumstances, and relationships in health care" (Berwick, 2009). Dr. Berwick is quick to state that the term "subject" in patient-centered care can be amended at any time to include the family and to read patient- and family-centered care.

To achieve patient-centered care, we must address the fact that American society, and the larger global society, is increasingly diverse in areas such as race, ethnicity, language, religion, gender, and sexual orientation. This diversity creates cultural gaps that must be bridged in order to provide quality health care. Looking just at the variable of race, we can see the shifts in U.S. population over the past 10 years. In 2013, the U.S. population was estimated at 316 million. The largest change from the year 2000 in percentage of total population according to race was seen in the Hispanic or Latino race. It is expected that the Hispanic population will more than double from 53.3 million, or 16.9% of the total population, in 2012 to 128.8 million in 2060. Similarly, Americans who classify their race as Asian have had a steady growth in the U.S. population. In 2012, 5.1% of the total population of the United States was Asian compared with 4.8% in 2010. This number is also expected to more than double from 15.9 million in 2012 to 34.4 million in 2060 (U.S. Census Bureau, 2012). Initiatives to improve patient-centered care include improving relationships between patient and provider as well as making systems more responsive to patients' needs and preferences (IOM, 2001).

The report, *Unequal Treatment: Confronting Racial and Ethnic Disparities in Healthcare* (IOM, 2002), addressed the changing demographics of the United States and how this is affecting the nation's health. This report identified concerns about racial and ethnic disparities throughout the health care system and the prevalence of their occurrence across a variety of illnesses. The most alarming data from this study revealed that, "[al]though myriad sources contribute to these disparities, some evidence suggests that bias, prejudice, and stereotyping on the part of health care providers may contribute to differences in care" (IOM, 2002). One would argue that prejudice is not part of a health care provider's values; moreover, nurses are morally obligated not to be prejudiced. In fact, *The Nursing Code of Ethics* reports, under Provision 1.2, "The need for health care is universal, [and] transcend[s] all individual differences. The nurse establishes relationships and delivers nursing services with respect for human needs and values, and without prejudice" (American Nurses Association [ANA], 2009).

The concept of health disparity is important to define in order to measure improved patient outcomes in this area. The American Academy of Nursing (AAN), which is considered the think tank of nursing, defines health disparity as, "differences in the incidence, prevalence, mortality, and burden of diseases and other adverse health conditions that exist among specific population groups in the United States" (Giger et al., 2007, p. 95). The common adage is that when America catches a cold, minority and other vulnerable groups get pneumonia. Tracking this data has been difficult in the past due to unstructured requirements for reporting health outcomes according to race or income. The Affordable Care Act requires that all federally funded health programs and population surveys collect and report data on race, ethnicity, sex, primary language, and disability and supports use of data to analyze and track health disparities (Andrulis et al., 2010). According to the National Healthcare Disparities Report (NHDR), "Racial and ethnic minorities and poor people often face more barriers to care and receive poorer quality of care when they can get it" (AHRQ, 2012). Three key themes emerged from the 2012 NHDR: "Health care quality and access are suboptimal, especially for minority and low-income groups; overall quality is improving yet access is getting worse; and disparities are not changing" (AHRQ, 2012).

Recommendations from the NHDR report to the AHRQ and the U.S. Department of Health and Human Services (HHS) were to increase the pace of improvement in the areas of diabetes care, maternal and child health care, and disparities in cancer care.

The health care system in the United States may be failing minorities because, as Washington (2006) suggests, "the original healthcare model was designed primarily to serve patients who spoke English, were able to read and write that language, typically had the resources to pay for care, believed in the germ theory of disease, valued biomedical preventative health practices, and acquiesced to the authoritarian model of the patient–healthcare provider relationship" (p. 45). The majority of patients today do not fit this description, and both health care and the education of health care providers need to change with the changing demographics of the United States. Van Ryn (2003) discusses social cognition, the study of how we make sense of other people, as a body of evidence that provides support for the hypothesis that providers contribute to a portion of racial/ethnic disparities in health care and outcomes. In time-limited encounters with patients, providers must rely on conscious and unconscious strategies to simplify massive amounts of complex information and make the world more manageable. One such strategy is categorizing, which ultimately leads to an unconscious stereotyping of individuals based on characteristics of a particular group applied to the individual. Van Ryn (2003) also suggests a reorganization of our service delivery and reimbursement systems "if providers are to have the time and cognitive resources needed to overcome unconscious bias" (p. 252).

Hospitals are now required to provide culturally competent care for all patients. The National Standards on Culturally and Linguistically Appropriate Services (CLAS) are 14 standards primarily directed at health care organizations that address how individual providers can provide culturally competent care (Office of Minority Health, 2005). For example, Standard 1 states, "Health care organizations should ensure that patients/consumers receive from all staff members effective, understandable, and respectful care that is provided in a manner compatible with their cultural health beliefs and practices and preferred language" (Office of Minority Health, 2005). In the recently released Healthy People 2020, the goal in regards to cultural competence for all Americans will be expanded to eliminate disparities, achieve health equity, and improve the health of all groups (U.S. Department of Health and Human Services [HHS], 2010).

Concept of Cultural Competency

An understanding of the theoretical components of cultural competence is imperative in designing teaching and learning methods for transforming nursing education. The lack of a standardized definition for culture or cultural competency leads to difficulty in measuring this important attribute. No standardization of terminology related to culture and ethnicity exists (Campesino, 2008; Purnell, 2002). Campesino (2008) states, "Culture is one of the two or three most complicated words in the English language."(p. 28). Several models have been proposed to describe the process of cultural competence (Jeffreys, 2010; Leininger, 2002; Purnell, 2002). Purnell's Model for Cultural Competence is a contemporary model and states, "an increase in consciousness of cultural diversity leads to increased culturally competent care and improved care" (Purnell, 2002, p. 8). Purnell describes this as a conscious process that moves the nurse through stages of knowing to the final stage of "unconsciously competent," which means "automatically providing culturally congruent care to clients of diverse cultures" (Purnell, 2002, p. 8).

Another contemporary grand theory on culture is Leininger's Culture Care Diversity and Universality theory (2002), which is based on the ideas that care is the essence of nursing and knowledge of cultural factors affects a nurse's ability to provide care. The model shows nursing care as integrating both the emic (the care system the patient believes is best) and etic (the professional care system) views. Deliberate planning and implementation of nursing strategies based on cultural assessment leads to the desired outcome of culturally congruent nursing care (Nelson, 2006). The Cultural Competence and Confidence Model (CCC) developed by Jeffreys (2010) provides an organizing framework for understanding the multidimensional process of cultural competence and confidence by illustrating major aspects of the learning process. This model is influenced by the work of Bandura (1986), who states that learning is directly influenced by self-efficacy perception or confidence.

There is much discourse over the terminology used to describe care for different cultures. Kleinman and Benson (2006) suggest that it is difficult to define the term *cultural competency* precisely enough to operationalize it in clinical training and best practice. The Explanatory Model Approach, developed by Kleinman, is widely used in U.S. medical school education today as an interview technique that tries to understand "how the social world affects and is affected by illness" (p. 1674). The Explanatory Model consists of asking the following questions: What do you call this problem? What do you believe is the cause of this problem? What course do you expect it to take? How serious is it? What do you think this problem does inside your body? How does it affect your body and your mind? What do you most fear about this condition? and What do you most fear about the treatment?

Tervalon and Murray-Garcia (1998) caution against using the term *competence* in any discussion of education because it implies mastery, which they argue is not possible when discussing cultural knowledge. They propose cultural humility or "a lifelong commitment to self-evaluation and self-critique. . ." as a path to improve patient–provider relations where differences of culture are involved" (p. 117). Nurses who exhibit cultural humility are aware of their inability to know everything about a particular culture, but they remain open and accepting to learning all they can from each patient's cultural perspective. When cultural humility is practiced, ethnocentrism is removed and the student can now understand the worldview of the patient. Another term used in the literature is *cultural sensitivity*, which has been described by Clinton (1996) as "knowledge of, respect for, and valuing of cultural diversity" (p. 5).

Nursing Education for Cultural Competence

Changes in health care education are needed to address the growing evidence that provider behaviors and attitudes can affect the health of different cultures (IOM, 2001, 2002; Massachusetts Department of Higher Education, 2006). To help future nurses achieve cultural competence, nurse educators will need to develop innovative instructional methods. The American Academy of Nursing Expert Panel Report (Giger et al., 2007) recommends that the elimination of health disparities must begin in educational settings and through "careful integration of content to develop sensitivity and competence in health care professional curricula" (p. 99).

Accrediting bodies for nursing education have addressed the need for cultural education in the undergraduate nursing program. *The Essentials for Baccalaureate Education for Professional Nursing Practice* (AACN, 2008) emphasizes cultural-sensitivity as a concept that must be addressed in nursing education due to the ever-changing and complex health care environment. The ACEN addresses cultural education of baccalaureate nurses under Standard 4.4, which states, "The curriculum includes cultural, ethnic, and socially diverse concepts and may also include experiences from regional, national, or global perspectives" (ACEN, 2013). However, most schools of nursing are not providing the required competencies in culturally relevant care to meet the changing health needs of the U.S. population (IOM, 2010; Jeffreys, 2010; Mareno & Hart, 2014). As far as the clinical component of teaching culture, the AACN (2008) further states, "The nursing program determines and assesses clinical sites to ensure the clinical experiences for students provide patients from diverse backgrounds, cultures, and of differing gender, religious, and spiritual practices" (p. 35). However, is this brief encounter on one or two clinical days enough to develop cultural competence in undergraduate nurses?

Benner, Sutphen, Leonard, and Day (2010) present recommendations to transform nursing education to meet the needs of today's nurses. The authors call for a radical transformation in nursing education through broadening of clinical experiences; "clinical time in school is spent on acute care hospital practice. However, more than 50 percent of nurses now work outside the hospital setting" (Benner et al., 2010, p. 219). A similar call for reform is presented by the IOM (2010) in the form of updated and adaptive curricula. "New models of care . . . as a result of health care reform will need to be introduced into students' experiences and will require competencies in [these areas]" (pp. 4–24). Community health care and home care are two areas that will need a larger focus as more of the population is either underinsured or uninsured. It is suggested that many of these models of care could be focused in alternative settings and will create "new student placement options that will need to be tested for scalability and compared for effectiveness with more traditional care settings" (IOM, 2010, pp. 4–25). Cultural immersion experiences may be an alternative to traditional clinical experiences for undergraduate nursing students as they add the cultural component to learning the health of a community.

A call for transformation of the education of health care professionals is not new. The Flexner Report of 1910 and the Goldmark Report of 1923 advocated for major changes in the education of physicians and nurses, respectively, citing the inadequacies of existing educational facilities and apprenticeship models for training these professionals. Frenk et al. (2010) marked the 100th anniversary of the Flexner Report with a comprehensive study of transforming health professions education for medicine, nursing, and public health. In regard to cultural education for health care providers, the researchers recognize that young professionals in both resource-poor and resource-rich countries have a desire to offer their services overseas. They suggest that this enthusiasm could be properly organized into a *Global Health Corps*—a program for sending young professionals for service abroad. "Active student exchange can strengthen the bonds of empathy and solidarity that an interdependent but highly inequitable world so greatly needs" (Frenk et al., 2010, p. 32).

Cultural Immersion Experiences for Nursing Students

There is very little data on the number of cultural immersion experiences offered as part of a nursing course or the number of nursing students who study abroad or on a service-learning trip. According to the Institute of International Education (2013), the total number of U.S. students studying abroad was 283,332 in 2011/2012. The trend in study abroad has been steadily increasing since the data has been tracked for the past 25 years. There have also been notable increases in the number of U.S. students going to study in less traditional destinations. According to the *Open Doors Report*, "campuses have noted that their students continue to show a strong interest in study abroad and study abroad providers have sought afford-able opportunities for these students to gain valuable international experience" (Institute of International Education, 2013). However, there are limited experi-ences available to students who are studying nursing.

Lipson and Desantis (2009) describe five types of curricular input to incorporate cultural competence knowledge, attitudes, and skills into nursing curricula. They have identified major strengths of cultural immersion programs, which include increased student self-awareness of their own health care preconceptions and how their own beliefs, values, practices, and behaviors affect care, interactions with patients, and health teaching; enhanced ability to deal with the situational, environmental, and sociocultural factors affecting their clients' health and living conditions; and ability to learn from patients and negotiate mutually satisfactory and culturally appropriate interventions (p. 17S). The researchers identified the major weaknesses of immersion programs, which they see as: (a) cost of travel and living expenses; (b) limited number of students who can participate; (c) lack of planned follow-up in the curriculum to build on increased cultural sensitivity and awareness; and (d) dependence of the experience on one faculty member, running the risk of the experience being discontinued if that faculty member leaves (Lipson & Desantis, 2009, p. 17S).

An integrative literature review by Button, Green, Tengnah, Johansson, and Baker (2005) searched the literature from 1980 to 2003 and examined the impact of international placement programs on the lives and practice of nurses. Of the 54 papers retrieved, 43 papers using qualitative and/or quantitative approaches were inspected for recurring themes. The literature review identified three prominent areas when examining the effects of international placement programs on the lives and practice of nurses: benefits, program differences, and transcultural adaptation. Major benefits of international placement programs were learning cultural differences, comparing health care systems and nursing practice, and personal development. According to Button et al. (2005), "despite the increasing emphasis on cultural education in nursing worldwide, culturally-based problems persist. There is a continuing need for academic institutions throughout Europe and the United States to offer international placement opportunities to foster cultural sensitivity and global awareness in nursing students" (p. 317). In the area of personal development, the literature supported the fact that international placement programs can have a profound and influential impact, helping the students to mature personally and professionally. Gains in the area of personal development included increased self-confidence, self-awareness, coping, and self-reliance. Cognitive development was the area with the greatest gains from international experience.

Button et al. (2005) presented research literature on differences in program components and their impact on the lives and practices of nurses. Program components that were discussed included the length of placement (short term of

1 to 4 weeks versus long term of 4 or more weeks); location, such as developed versus developing country; preparation of students; and support or mentoring for students while abroad. This paper provided support for the benefits of international placement programs. The literature also showed that although short-term placements are valuable, long-term placements may have more impact. Regarding program components, there is disagreement in the literature regarding programs in developed versus developing host countries. Reasons for choosing developing countries for international experiences for nursing students have been the existence of historical ties, intense cultural differences, and the preconception that they have a poorer health care system. Developed host countries have been chosen for international placement programs because of cost, similarities in language, and alternative health care systems.

According to Button et al. (2005), the literature shows that orientation programs minimize culture shock by promoting insight into key cultural differences. These orientation programs have consisted of language courses, lectures, assignments, and readings about the host destination prior to departure. Social support in the form of mentoring from academic staff or through communication with fellow students, which occurred throughout the immersion experience, was effective in alleviating feelings of culture shock as well. Button et al. (2005) conclude that preplacement preparation/orientation and support in the form of mentoring for students while abroad are important components of the program to promote maximum benefit. The researchers concluded that few researchers have conducted collaborative studies with other institutions to supply more participant data, and also to provide a more in-depth analysis of the placement program. Among the limitations to this study, the search was limited to papers published before 2003, and the researchers rejected papers that lacked an educational theme that may have included papers on service learning, as this was not one of the researcher's search terms.

Beach et al. (2005) conducted a systematic literature review and analysis of 34 studies that evaluated interventions to improve cultural competence of health professionals. The researchers abstracted and synthesized data from studies that had both a before- and after-intervention evaluation or had a control group for comparison. Using a tool developed by the researchers, they graded the strength of the evidence as excellent, good, fair, or poor. The grading showed there was excellent evidence (Beach et al., 2005) that cultural competence training improves knowledge of health professionals. There was also good evidence (Beach et al., 2005) that cultural competence training improves attitudes and skills of health professionals. When evaluating outcomes associated with specific features of cultural competence training, Beach et al. (2005) found that "both shorter and longer duration interventions appeared effective, as do methods using experiential learning. The researchers were unable to conclude which types of training interventions are most effective on which types of outcomes due to the "heterogeneity and intermingling of cultural content and methods" (p. 366). They note that, "there were no two studies that evaluated the exact same educational experience" (p. 366). The authors recommend that future research compare interventions varied by either curricular content or training methods; that future research should include data about the resources and costs of training; and that future researchers should use objective and standardized evaluation methods. The systematic review of nonrandomized trials conducted by Beach et al. (2005) provides evidence that cultural competence training improves attitudes and skills of health professionals.

In their systematic review of quantitative measures of cultural competence, Kumas-Tan, Beagan, Loppie, MacLeod, and Frank (2007) critically examined the quantitative measures of cultural competence most commonly used in medicine and in the health professions to examine the understandings of cultural competence that these measures embody. The researchers identified 54 distinct instruments and noted that few were cited more than once in the literature. The most common focus of the instruments was evaluation of students' or practitioners' competence. In their review of the literature, the researchers found evidence to suggest that increased confidence may not be a measure of increased competence. For example, one instrument measured awareness and skills subscales and found that "awareness of differences would lead to acknowledging one's lack of skills to deal with the cross-cultural barriers" (Kumas-Tan et al., 2007, p. 554). The researchers suggest that existing quantitative measures of cultural competence "ignore the power relations of social inequality and assume that individual knowledge and self-confidence are sufficient for change" (Kumas-Tan et al., 2007, p. 548). The researchers also question if confidence and comfort are valid indicators of cultural competence and if higher levels of confidence and comfort may, in fact, be indicative of lower insight and awareness. They recommend the development of measures that assess cultural humility or actual practice are needed to inform future educational needs and advocate for the use of mixed methods research to achieve this goal.

Other researchers have also found the cultural immersion teaching method to be an effective and enjoyable instructional method to teach cultural competence (Amerson, 2010; Button et al., 2005; Caffrey et al., 2005; Koskinen & Tossavairen, 2004; Larsen & Reif, 2011; Larson et al., 2010; Maltby & Abrams, 2009; Ruddock & Turner, 2007; St. Clair & McKenry, 1999; Walsh & De Joseph, 2003). Some studies have used quantitative instruments to measure cultural self-efficacy (Amerson, 2010; Caffrey et al., 2005; Larsen & Reif, 2011; St. Clair & McKenry, 1999), however, most studies have used a qualitative methodology (Koskinen & Tossavairen, 2004; Larson, Ott, & Miles, 2010; Maltby & Abrams, 2009; Ruddock & Turner, 2007; Walsh & DeJoseph, 2003). In studies that used a quantitative instrument to measure changes in self-efficacy scores, the largest increase in scores was in the cognitive domain (Amerson, 2010; Button et al., 2005; Larsen & Reif, 2011). Researchers have integrated the immersion experience as part of a service-learning experience (Amerson, 2010; Walsh & DeJoseph, 2003) or as a study abroad (Koskinen & Tossavairen, 2004; Ruddock & Turner, 2007). The countries that students have visited for the cultural immersion experiences have varied and include Bangladesh (Maltby & Abrams, 2009), Guatemala (Amerson, 2010; Caffrey et al., 2005; Larson et al., 2010; Walsh & DeJoseph, 2003), and Mexico (Larsen & Reif, 2011).

CONCLUSION

There is support in the literature for the use of cultural immersion as a worthwhile teaching method to improve cultural competency and these programs should be implemented in nursing curricula. The program components of duration, destination, preparation, mentoring and debriefing are important aspects of a cultural immersion program. More research should be conducted to create a model of an effective cultural immersion program. Most importantly, research has shown that cultural immersion experiences appeal to the current generation of undergraduate nursing students. Effective teaching methods that are appealing to students and that successfully meet the educational needs of this generation should be adopted by nurse faculty and supported by college administrators.

REFERENCES

Accreditation Commission for Education in Nursing (ACEN). (2013). *ACEN 2013 standards and criteria baccalaureate degree programs in nursing*. Retrieved from http://acenursing.org/accreditation-manual

Agency for Healthcare Research and Quality (AHRQ), U.S. Department of Health and Human Services. (2012). *National Healthcare Disparities Report*. AHRQ Publication No. #13-0003. Retrieved from http://www.ahrq.gov/research/findings/nhqrdr/nhdr12/index.html

American Association of Colleges of Nursing (AACN). (2008). *The essentials of baccalaureate education for professional nursing practice*. Washington, DC: Author.

American Nurses Association. (2009). *Code of ethics for nurses*. Retrieved from http://www.nursingworld.org/MainMenuCategories/EthicsStandards/CodeofEthicsforNurses

Amerson, R. (2010). The impact of service-learning on cultural competence. *Nursing Education Perspectives, 31*(1), 18–22.

Andrulis, D. P., Siddiqui, N. J., Purtle, J. P., and Duchon, L. (2010). *Patient Protection and Affordable Care Act of 2010: Advancing health equity for racially and ethnically diverse populations*. Supported and released by the Joint Center for Political and Economic Studies. Texas Health Institute. Retrieved from http://www.texashealthinstitute.org

Bandura, A. (1986). *Social foundations of thought and action: A social cognitive theory*. Englewood Cliffs, NJ: Prentice-Hall.

Beach, C. M., Price, G. E., Gary, T. L., Robinson, K. A., Gozu, A., Palacio, A., & Cooper, L.A. (2005). Cultural competence: A systematic review of health care provider educational interventions. *Medical Care, 43*(4), 356–373. Retrieved from http://www.jstor.org/stable/3768438

Benner, P., Sutphen, M., Leonard, V., & Day, L. (2010). *Educating nurses: A call for radical transformation*. San Francisco, CA: Jossey-Bass.

Berwick, D. M. (2009). What "patient-centered" should mean: Confessions of an extremist. *Health Affairs, 28*(4), w555–w565. Retrieved from http://content.healthaffairs.org/content/28/4/w555.full.pdf+html?sid=2d6824fe-abaa-41b0-ac5e-fbf05962f004

Button, L., Green, B., Tengnah, C., Johannson, I., & Baker, C. (2005). The impact of international placements on nurses' personal and professional lives: Literature review. *Journal of Advanced Nursing, 50*(3), 315–324.

Caffrey, R.A., Neander, W., Markle, D., & Stewart, B. (2005). Improving the cultural competence of nursing students: Results of integrating cultural content in the curriculum and an international immersion experience. *Journal of Nursing Education, 44*(5), 234–240.

Campesino, M. (2008). Beyond transculturalism: Critiques of cultural education in nursing. *Journal of Nursing Education, 47*(7), 298–304.

Clinton, J. F. (1996). Cultural diversity and health care in America: Knowledge fundamental to cultural competence in baccalaureate nursing students. *Journal of Cultural Diversity, 3*(1), 4–8.

Frenk, J., Chen, L., Bhutta, Z. A., Cohen, J., Crisp, N., Evans, T., & Zurayk, H. (2010). Health professionals for a new century: Transforming education to strengthen health systems in an interdependent world. *The Lancet*. doi:10.1016/S0140-6736(10)61854-5

Giger, J., Davidhizar, R. E., Purnell, L., Harden, J. T., Phillips, J., & Strickland, O. (2007). American Academy of Nursing Expert Panel Report: Developing cultural competence to eliminate health disparities in ethnic minorities and other vulnerable populations. *Journal of Transcultural Nursing, 18*(2), 95–102. doi:10.1177/1043659606298618

Institute of International Education. (2013). *Open doors report on international education exchange*. Retrieved from http://www.iie.org/Who-We-Are/News-and-Events/Press-Center/Press-releases/2013/2013-11-11-Open-Doors-Data

Institute of Medicine (IOM). (2000). *To err is human*. Washington, DC: National Academy of Sciences.

Institute of Medicine. (2001). *Crossing the quality chasm*. Washington, DC: The National Academies Press.

Institute of Medicine. (2002). *Unequal treatment: Confronting racial and ethnic disparities in healthcare*. Retrieved from http://www.nap.edu/catalog/10260.html

Institute of Medicine. (2010). *The future of nursing: Leading change, advancing health*. Washington, DC: The National Academies Press.

Jeffreys, M. R. (2010). *Teaching cultural competence in nursing and health care: Inquiry, action and innovation*. (2nd ed.). New York, NY: Springer Publishing Company.

Kleinman, A., & Benson, P. (2006). Anthropology in the clinic: The problem of cultural competency and how to fix it. *PLoS Medicine, 3*(10), 1673–1676. Retrieved from http://www.plosmedicine.org/article/info%3Adoi%2F10.1371%2Fjournal.pmed.0030294

Koskinen, L., & Tossavainen, K. (2004). Study abroad as a process of learning intercultural competence in nursing. *International Journal of Nursing Practice, 10*, 111–120.

Kumas-Tan, Z., Beagan, B., Loppie, C., MacLeod, A., & Frank, B. (2007). Measures of cultural competence: Examining hidden assumptions. *Academic Medicine, 82* (6), 548–557.

Larsen, R., & Reif, L. (2011). Effectiveness of cultural immersion and culture classes for enhancing nursing students' transcultural self-efficacy. *Journal of Nursing Education, 50*(6), 350–354. doi:10.3928/,01484834-20110214-04

Larson, K. L., Ott, M., & Miles, J. M. (2010). International cultural immersion: En vivo reflections in cultural competence. *Journal of Cultural Diversity, 17*(2), 44–50.

Leininger, M. (2002). Culture care theory: A major contribution to advance transcultural nursing knowledge and practices. *Journal of Transcultural Nursing, 13*(3), 189–192. doi:10.1177/10459602013003005

Lipson, J. G., & Desantis, L. A. (2009). Current approaches to integrating elements of cultural competence in nursing education. *Journal of Transcultural Nursing, 18*(1), 10S–20S.

Maltby, H. J., & Abrams, S. (2009). Seeing with new eyes: The meaning of an immersion experience in Bangladesh for undergraduate senior nursing students. *International Journal of Nursing Education Scholarship, 6*(1). doi:10.2202/1548-923X.1858

Mareno, N., & Hart, P. L. (2014). Cultural competency among nurses with undergraduate and graduate degrees: Implications for nursing education. *Nursing Education Perspectives, 35*(2), 83–88.

Massachusetts Department of Higher Education; Massachusetts Organization of Nurse Executives. (2006). *Creativity and connections: Building the framework for the future of nursing education and practice.* Retrieved from http://www.mass.edu/currentinit/documents/NursingCreativityAndConnections.pdf

Nelson, J. (2006). Madeleine Leininger's culture care theory: The theory of culture care diversity and universality. *International Journal for Human Caring, 10*(4), 50–54.

Office of Minority Health. (2001). *National standards for culturally and linguistically appropriate services in health care, executive summary.* Washington, DC: U.S. Department of Health and Human Services. Government Printing Office. Retrieved from at http://minorityhealth.hhs.gov/templates/browse.aspx?lvl=2&lvlID=15

Purnell, L. (2002). The Purnell model for cultural competence. *Journal of Transcultural Nursing, 13*(3), 193–196.

Ruddock, H. C., & Turner, D. S. (2007). Developing cultural sensitivity: Nursing students' experiences of a study abroad program. *Journal of Advanced Nursing, 59*(4), 361–369. doi:10.1111/j.1365-2648.2007.04312.x

St. Clair, A., & McKenry, L. (1999). Preparing culturally competent practitioners. *Journal of Nursing Education, 38*(5), 228–234.

Tervalon, M., & Murray-Garcia, J. (1998). Cultural humility versus cultural competence: A critical distinction in defining physician training outcomes in multicultural education. *Journal of Health Care for the Poor and Underserved,* (9)2, 117–125.

U.S. Census Bureau. (2012). Retrieved from http://www.census.gov/en.html

U.S. Department of Health and Human Services. (2010). *Healthy People 2020* (2nd ed.). Washington, DC: Government Printing Office; 2000. Retrieved from http://www.healthypeople.gov/2020/about/default.aspx

U.S. Department of Health and Human Services. Office of Minority Health. (2005). *National standards for culturally and linguistically appropriate services in health care, executive summary.* Washington, DC: Government Printing Office. Retrieved from http://minorityhealth.hhs.gov/Assets/pdf/Checked/HC-LSIG-ExecutiveSummary.pdf

Van Ryn, M. (2003). Paved with good intentions: Do public health and human service providers contribute to racial/ethnic disparities in health? *American Journal of Public Health, 93*(2), 248–255.

Walsh, L. V., & DeJoseph, J. (2003) "I saw it in a different light": International learning experiences in baccalaureate nursing education. *Journal of Nursing Education, 42*(6), 266–272.

Washington, D. (2006). Moving toward a culturally competent profession. In L. C. Andrist, P. K. Nicholas, & K. A. Wolf (Eds.), *A history of nursing ideas* (pp. 45–54). Boston, MA: Jones and Bartlett.

CHAPTER 26

Working Globally With Faith-Based Organizations

Teri Lindgren, Sally Rankin, and Ellen Schell

The recent report of *The Lancet* Commission on Investing in Health proposes an ambitious new framework to achieve a "grand convergence" to close the gaps in health achievements between developed and developing countries (Jamison et al., 2014). Faith-based organizations (FBOs) are of particular interest in realizing this goal, especially in many parts of the developing world, since they often provide the only infrastructure reaching rural areas (World Health Organization [WHO] 2008; Widmer, Betran, Merialdi, Requejo, & Karpf, 2011). Religion has long been recognized as wielding a significant impact on the health and well-being of individuals, families, and communities across the globe. Historically, church, temple, and mosque members were often the first-line providers of health care, and many health care delivery systems today continue to be funded through FBOs. This is especially true in much of Africa, where missionaries from several faiths, primarily monotheistic faiths (Christianity and Islam), came with traders, explorers, business developers, and ultimately colonizers to convert the local populations. Through this process, FBOs built and staffed churches and mosques, schools, and hospitals that reflected the faith, values, and health practices of missionaries. These systems have evolved over time and have been incorporated into the health infrastructure of many African countries. In sub-Saharan Africa, for example, approximately 40% of formal health care is delivered by hospitals and clinics funded and run by FBOs (WHO, 2008; Widmer et al., 2011). However, this reflects only part of the influence that FBOs exert on the health of their members.

At the community level, especially in rural areas of the developing world, FBOs provide basic social structures and resources that directly and indirectly impact the lives of congregations. With increased discourse on health promotion and disease prevention as a means to reduce health care costs and improve people's lives both nationally and internationally, health care providers look to FBOs as a means to extend the reach and effectiveness of their health messages (Widmer et al., 2011). Indeed, nurses and public health providers are actively seeking ways to collaborate with and utilize the resources of FBOs to provide screening, health promotion programs, and home care support to community members (Seboni et al., 2013). Therefore, it is critical for health care providers seeking to impact the health of individuals and populations worldwide to understand the role of FBOs in both health promotion and delivery of care globally, and how to effectively harness the power and resources of FBOs. This chapter discusses the lessons learned by the authors based on their experiences of working with FBOs in Malawi, an impoverished country in southern Africa, to address the HIV/AIDS crisis that has claimed nearly 1 million lives in the past 30 years and produced 770,000 orphans (UNAIDS, 2012).

BACKGROUND AND CONTEXT

Religion plays an important role in both the lives and identities of people worldwide, but especially in Africa. Indeed, Africans are more likely to ask you about your religious affiliation before they ask about your livelihood. FBOs provide critical infrastructure, particularly in rural African communities from both a leadership perspective and social support. Religious leaders are frequently accorded respect as opinion leaders in their communities (Rankin, Lindgren, Kools, & Schell, 2008). And whether in urban or rural settings, religious bodies tend to be the custodians of values influencing behaviors—paramount among these are compassion, community service, and care for the whole person. The role of FBOs in health matters is of critical importance in encouraging health-promoting behavior as well as care-seeking and caregiving behavior when members fall ill. Moreover, religious bodies can play an important role in providing moral leadership. For example, in religious ceremonies, leaders have a public platform from which to challenge destructive prejudices that plague certain conditions such as HIV. Religious leaders can use the pulpit to confront stigma, call for compassion, exhort people to care for themselves and each other, and even use this forum to convey important health information (Otolok-Tanga, Atuyambe, Murphy, Ringheim, & Woldehanna, 2007). Subgroups typically found in FBOs, such as women's, youth, Bible study, and service groups, are logical affinity gatherings for health interventions and are well-placed to solve "the last mile" problem, ensuring that the end users receive and correctly utilize health inputs (USAID, 2011).

However, religious groups also have engaged in harmful teaching and practices that promulgate stigma, inaccurate information, and other judgmental attitudes and behaviors. This is especially true for highly stigmatized diseases such as HIV. While much progress has been made in the past decade, the stigma remains a major barrier to the success of programs to prevent, diagnose, and treat HIV infection (Mahajan et al., 2008; Mukolo et. al., 2013; W. W. Rankin et al., 2005; Tsai, Bangsberg, & Weise, 2013; Wolfe et al., 2008). Fear of stigmatization and subsequent abandonment and rejection continues to deter subjects from being tested and treated for HIV. FBO members continue to be reluctant to disclose their HIV status to their local leaders (pastors, priests, imams) and are even more reluctant to openly disclose their status to FBO members (Lindgren et al., 2013). Widespread programs to prevent mother-to-child-transmission (PMTCT) have made testing more routine for women who encounter the opportunity to be tested when they become pregnant; however, some women still refuse testing because they lack permission from their husbands to be tested (Van Lettow et al., 2012).

The situation for men is even more problematic. Men do not have such a naturally placed life cycle event to bring them in for testing. Some recent studies have shown that fear of stigmatization, loss of employment, and abandonment by partners prevent men from getting tested, or delay testing until they become ill (Mageda, Leyna, & Mmbaga, 2012; Skovdal et al., 2011). As a result, men have poorer outcomes once they are tested and are started on antiretroviral therapy (ART). African religious organizations, both formally and informally, deliver much of the care and support reaching into African communities (WHO, 2008; Widmer et al., 2011). Within the formal health care systems of many African countries, FBOs provide economic, material, and human capital to run clinics and hospitals. As noted, many of these facilities were originally started and staffed by missionary groups from various parts of the developed world; however, they tend now to be run, and in many cases partially supported, by local FBO populations and/or negotiated service agreements from the national government that focus on key health issues, particularly maternal and child care. However, nursing care and medical care provided by these entities, as in public hospitals, remains limited due to lack of resources and severe staff shortages across health cadres. Because of the lack of staff, family members are expected to provide much of what would be considered basic nursing care in the West. For example, families bathe patients, provide and serve food, and provide linen and clean clothing; in fact, every patient admitted to a hospital or clinic needs to come with a designated "guardian" to carry out these responsibilities. FBOs have informally helped in this process by providing food and other support for both the patients and their guardians.

At the community level, FBOs have a history of providing assistance to the ill in the home setting. Members routinely visit and provide informal care for fellow members. This care includes companionship and spiritual care (praying with an ill member) as well as practical care such as cleaning their abode, providing food, cooking meals, and bringing water or firewood. FBO-based women's group leaders often coordinate and monitor this type of care. However, the AIDS crisis significantly impacted both the informal care of FBOs and the formal care the religious organizations provided.

The advent of AIDS stressed the informal care network through the increasing numbers of ill members and orphans left behind. At the same time, it also brought into African communities funding opportunities from national and international entities. FBOs responded in various ways. Some readily ramped up their already existing care networks and clinics to reach out to ill community members while others hid their heads in the sand. The coming of widely available ART has changed the mission of care for HIV-positive people. Increasingly, community-based groups, including FBOs that originally focused on care for the dying, are helping people return to health by providing the support needed to maintain adherence to ART, nutritional supplementation (a critical component for successful ART), and the household supports (child care, assistance with household chores) needed while the person's health is restored.

Religions contain many of the psychological and spiritual resources associated with the renewal of life, the prospect of hope, and the recovery of human dignity, while their regular meetings provide a forum for the continuous reinforcement of such messages. Religion is a coping strategy used by women found to be HIV positive (Olley et al., 2003). On the other hand, prior to the rollout of ART, Rankin, Lindgren, Rankin, and Ng'Oma (2005) found religion to be one of three factors (burden and sexual relationships being the others) that influenced Malawi women's risk-taking behaviors. The women found the FBOs provided little support to them in their caregiving work, did not encourage HIV prevention education, and reinforced stigma.

Religious organizations have been effectively used to buttress health promotion messages. For example, FBOs in Uganda were important to the success of reducing HIV incidence in the years prior to the ART rollout (Byamugisha, 2000; Hogle, 2002). On the other hand, investigators have found that missionary religious organizations reinforced customs that precluded frank or open discussions of issues that impact health, such as risky sexual behaviors (Caldwell, Orubuloye, & Caldwell, 1992; Lindgren et al., 2013). Moreover, harmful traditional practices that place members at risk of HIV infection (such as initiation ceremonies and widow cleansing) have been identified as important factors in the spread of HIV, and religious organizations have mobilized against these practices (Chakanza, 1995; Lindgren et al., 2013; Phiri, Haddad, & Masenya, 2003). Yet they have done so without always being fully sensitive to the importance and attraction of these rituals to the society, and so their efforts have not always been successful (Fiedler, 2005).

Religious beliefs can provide important support for scientifically proven prevention strategies. For example, abstinence and faithfulness, commonly held sexual values in both Islam and Christianity, supported the first two messages of the ABC (Abstinence, Be Faithful, or Use Condoms) HIV prevention campaign that was broadly used throughout Africa in the first decade of this century. As will be discussed later, the "C" aspect of that campaign was extensively rejected by both Islamic and Christian leaders (Rankin et al., 2008).

At the same time, what has been described as a "theology of blame" has sometimes fueled the Christian responses to the suffering caused by disease, especially in the case of HIV/AIDS. This understanding sees suffering as the just desserts of sinful behavior. Bible verses such as "the wages of sin is death" (Romans 6:23) are quoted to support this view, and especially early in the epidemic, hampered an effective response by silencing those who were HIV positive through fear of being judged by their FBO communities (Lindgren et al., 2013; Morris, Schell, Schell, & Rankin, 2008–2009). The theology of blame fueled stigma and discrimination and hindered open discussion. It was easier for the church to respond to the plight of orphans, who were seen as the blameless victims of the epidemic, than to encourage care for those who were sick due to behavior that was (sometimes hypocritically) viewed as sinful.

A similar mixed dynamic is apparent in the Muslim community as research from the past decade has resulted in a better understanding of the Muslim response to HIV. Prohibitions on extramarital and premarital sex and the widespread adoption of religiously mandated male circumcision (associated with decreased risk of HIV transmission) have helped to maintain lower HIV prevalence in Muslim communities in Northern Africa (Drain, Halperin, Hughes, Klausner, & Bailey, 2006). However, recently, there has been an increase in HIV incidence in Islamic countries among intravenous drug users (IDUs), female sex workers (FSWs), and men who have sex with men (MSM). Malaysia, a predominantly Muslim country, has faced a particularly alarming rise in rates in the IDU population. It responded by boldly addressing the issue with harm reduction programs. However, there has been a reluctance to confront the epidemic in FSWs and MSM, resulting from the fact that sex work and homosexual sex are forbidden by Islam, and many health care providers have a deeply rooted reluctance to address the issue in these population groups (Kamarulzaman, 2013).

THE AUTHORS' EXPERIENCES, OR "WHO ARE WE TO BE TALKING ABOUT THIS TOPIC?"

The authors have worked together to develop, implement, and evaluate health-related service projects and to conduct health research in Malawi. The following describes how we have garnered the experience of working with FBOs in Malawi over the past 10 years and what that experience has taught us.

Country Background

Sub-Saharan Africa remains the epicenter of the global HIV and AIDS epidemic with 25 million people presently living with HIV (UNAIDS, 2013). Malawi, where our programs are implemented and our research was conducted, is a small, landlocked country about the size of Pennsylvania, with a population of 15 million. It is a densely populated country, but overwhelmingly rural, with 80% of the population living in rural villages and sustained by subsistence farming. The economy is agricultural with tobacco being the main revenue-producing export. One of the poorest nations, the gross national income per capita is under $320 (World Bank, 2012), and only 9% of the population has access to electricity (Index Mundi, 2010; Kandiero, 2014).

Just over one million people are living with HIV, and in 2011 approximately 46,000 Malawi adults and children died of AIDS-related illnesses (UNAIDS, 2012). The HIV epidemic places great stress on already impoverished rural communities. Villages are remote, located far from doctors, nurses, and hospitals, and lack of transportation makes it difficult to access care. The country has one of the world's most formidable orphan problems with at least 770,000 orphaned children under the age of 18 orphaned by AIDS (UNAIDS, 2012). In addition to HIV, other infectious diseases, chiefly malaria, claim thousands of lives each year. While Malawi has made progress on key maternal and child health indicators, its maternal death rate remains one of the highest in the world with 460 deaths per 100,000 live births (World Bank, 2010). Due to the HIV epidemic, life expectancy from birth has fallen to 53 years (CIA, 2013).

Malawi's health care is delivered through three levels: four central referral hospitals (located in major cities), district hospitals, and rural health clinics. There is a mix of government (Ministry of Health [MoH]) and mission or church-related health facilities, organized under the Christian Health Association of Malawi (CHAM). The MoH provides free health care, but government facilities are extremely underresourced. There is an acute shortage of health care personnel, and one nurse commonly cares for 50 or more hospitalized patients. The CHAM hospitals are estimated to provide about 40% of Malawi's health care. These serve patients for a modest—though for many rural villagers, unaffordable—fee, with the exception of certain services such as maternity and a limited number of under-5 services that are paid for under government contracts. Care in the CHAM facilities suffers from the same constraints as those that limit the government hospitals.

Program Development Through an Interfaith Nongovernmental Organization (NGO)

Global AIDS Interfaith Alliance (GAIA) is an international NGO working to address HIV/AIDS and other health issues in Malawi. In 2000, the Rev. Dr. William Rankin, an Episcopal priest, collaborated with Dr. Charles Wilson, professor emeritus and chairman of Neurological Surgery at the University of California San Francisco, to respond to the devastating sub-Saharan AIDS epidemic. Initially, Dr. Rankin utilized religious networks he had access to in Africa to begin work. Recognizing that religious leaders had insufficient knowledge of HIV and, in some cases, were contributing to stigma, and also understanding that religious institutions were often the only infrastructure in remote rural areas, Dr. Rankin chose to work through these institutions and networks.

Dr. Rankin's long career in social justice work and his training as an ethicist led him to reflect critically on what it meant to take on international work and to develop a bilateral organization that raised funding from U.S. sources but implemented programs in a developing African nation half a planet away. We have excerpted a section from his writings about this process:

> At the outset I must devote a bit of space to myself, because I was greatly concerned about who I was and how I would come across to African people. I had read and been disturbed by horrifying accounts of the West African slave trade to the Americas and Caribbean islands, then by the Portuguese and Arab slave trade in East Africa. Though all this had happened considerably before my time, I had a clear sense of being privileged as a White male and likely as a beneficiary of the slave system, of capitalist modernity, of patriarchy, and of colonialism in general. I had a corresponding sense of how the African people

whom I would meet were perhaps greatly disadvantaged by all that had benefitted me and my kind. I knew that feeling guilty was no help, but neither could I be oblivious to this sordid and outrageous history and how my sex and my color and even the language I spoke were vividly emblematic of it in Africa. I also knew how easy it was for a person of privilege in terms of money and political power to be appallingly unaware of one's own entitlement, unconscious of unexamined feelings of superiority, of condescension, and even unconscious of "disempowering" impoverished people, particularly women, by seeing only squalor and missing the remarkable resourcefulness and agency that enables survival and even flourishing in a tough context. Perhaps one of the trickiest of dynamics that might afflict someone in this role was what D.H. Lawrence in *The Man Who Died* called "the greed of giving." This phrase describes the way that our own "needs" to be appreciated, approved, and possibly loved, could cause us selfishly to feed off the gratitude or admiration (whether sincere or tactical) of others. I decided to trust Africans, and in particular, GAIA's country director, to be my, and our, guide in the Malawi work, and later when we had numerous Malawi women employees we all learned a lot from them as well. All these staff people, and later the women and men of the GAIA-Malawi trustees, detailed what issues should be addressed, and how programs should be designed, implemented, monitored, and followed up in Malawi. (William Rankin, personal communication, n.d.)

Dr. Rankin's philosophy has guided the way GAIA has implemented its programs and shaped the interactions of the United States and Malawi sides of the organization. We believe that Westerners who seek to involve themselves in international work do well to engage in this kind of reflection.

GAIA's first intervention was a conference to educate Anglican clergy in Tanzania about HIV. Subsequently, a similar conference was held in Malawi with leaders from across religious denominations, including Muslims. That conference allowed GAIA to develop important networks across FBOs throughout Malawi. Dr. Sally Rankin utilized this conference to begin a program of research to develop interventions to help stem the tide of HIV in Malawi.

For the first few years of its existence, GAIA provided small grants to community-based organizations across Malawi, many based out of churches or mosques. In 2003, with funding from the Bill and Melinda Gates Foundation, GAIA began implementing its own community-based programs that provided service directly. Since that time, GAIA has continued to develop its own programs, including a mobile clinic program (Lindgren et al., 2011) and a nurse workforce scholarship and professional development program (Schell, Rankin, Chipungu, Rankin, & Weiller, 2011). However, the interface with the religious community continues to be an important resource in program development and implementation. Most recently, the nursing scholarship program, which receives funding from the U.S. Agency for International Development (USAID), was expanded to include the nurse-midwife technician (NMT) cadre of health workers. NMTs are educated at 10 colleges of nursing associated with mission-based hospitals run by churches (Anglican, Roman Catholic, Church of Central Africa Presbyterian, and Seventh Day Adventist) under the umbrella of the Christian Health Association of Malawi. We are working with one of the Roman Catholic schools in a remote rural district where we are sponsoring a cohort of 84 students. We work with the principal of the college, a dynamic and committed Malawi Roman Catholic nun. Understanding the organization, dynamics, and motivations of the religious organizations we work with helps us to be more effective.

Research With Religious Leaders and Their Members From 2006–2009

In 2006, Dr. Sally Rankin (principal investigator), Dr. Ellen Schell (coinvestigator), and Dr. Teri Lindgren (project director) embarked on an ambitious 4-year National Institutes of Health (NIH)-funded research project (RO1 HD050147) with religious leaders from five FBOs in Malawi, four Christian and one Muslim. The primary aims of the study were to: (1) explore the strategies being used by religious leaders to address HIV prevention and care; (2) identify the knowledge, attitudes, and behaviors of religious leaders and their members related to HIV prevention and care; and (3) test the power and influence of local (congregational) leaders on the HIV risk and care behaviors of their members. Using GAIA's connections with religious leaders as an entrée to FBOs situated in southern Malawi, we qualitatively interviewed 305 FBO leaders (central and local) and members and quantitatively surveyed 75 local leaders and 667 members. Central leaders were those in authority within the FBO—for example, general secretaries, bishops, and central administrators of the different FBOs. Local leaders were those who managed their own congregation—the church (typically a pastor or priest) or mosque leader (typically an imam). We began by interviewing 44 central leaders and then progressed to interviewing and surveying 15 local leaders from each FBO and at least eight members from each local leader's congregation. We finished by interviewing 49 people living with HIV who self-identified as members of the FBOs being studied; a total of 791 participants comprised the study. To complete this study, we spent approximately 6 months living and working in Malawi over the course of 3 years.

The five FBOs we studied included three missionary-based Christian organizations (Catholic, Anglican, and Baptist), one indigenous Pentecostal organization, and one Islamic organization. For each of these, we had a consultant who identified appropriate central FBO leaders to interview and those who could facilitate access to local FBO leaders and members. In the process of conducting the research we came to understand how these organizations function, how information diffuses through the system from top to bottom and bottom to top, the importance of a FBO hierarchical structure, and how these FBOs mobilize their members.

During data collection it became evident that the various FBOs had differing hierarchical structures through which the local congregations were connected to the national organization. Certain FBOs had a well-defined hierarchical structure with a clear line of authority that had to be addressed if anyone wanted to work with a church in this organization. In other words, if you wanted to work with a specific local church, you needed permission from someone of higher authority than the local priest or pastor. Within these organizations, the national administrators had the power to appoint or remove a local leader; because these organizations had a clearly defined structure, communication between central leaders, local leaders, and members diffused more easily from top to bottom and bottom to top. Once we had permission from a central administrator of the FBO, we were able to send out information about our study and recruit local leaders. Conversely, several of the FBOs under study had a very diffuse structure, where the central leaders had little or no direct authority over the local leaders, as it was the church or mosque members who could call the leader to that role and only the members could dismiss a local leader. Within this type of structure, communication between the central FBO and the local churches/mosques was more difficult.

It became clear early in the research that many of these FBOs did not function in the same way that similar FBOs do in the United States. For example, we thought we could easily get a list from central leaders of all of their local leaders' names, contact numbers, church/mosque locations, and so on. While the most hierarchical organizations, such as the Catholics and Anglicans, did have lists of local priests and some catechists, the data were rarely current. In FBOs with the most diffuse hierarchy, such as the Baptists and the Muslims, no such list existed; indeed, the heads of these organizations did not necessarily know how many or where all of the churches or mosques existed. We had also planned to utilize church/mosque registries to sample members, but these too either did not exist (mosques have no such registry), or what existed had not been updated for a number of years. However, despite the lack of such information on members, all of the churches and mosques were able to mobilize their members as needed. This was due to the administrative structures situated within each individual church or mosque.

Among the larger churches and mosques, the local leaders described a structure, generally referred to as a cell or a zone, where members were allocated to a particular group, usually geographically defined, and each group had a designated leader. The leaders' duties included communicating with members; conducting Bible, Qur'an, and prayer meetings; organizing group members to provide services to the church or mosque, such as cleaning; and repairing the buildings; and visiting ill members. Additionally, every FBO had other groups within the church or mosque that cut across the geographically defined groups; all of the FBOs identified having a women's group, a youth group, and many had a men's group. Each group had its own leadership and these leaders reported to and were supported by the local leader.

Understanding these diverse structures was critical to working effectively with the FBOs at both the central and local levels. These structures were used by the churches and mosques to do the pastoral and outreach work of the FBO and therefore could be utilized to assist in promulgating health-related messages. In some of the most organized FBOs, funding was garnered to develop effective home-based care programs using these church structures; however, once the funding ceased, these programs struggled to continue to help ill members due to lack of money to buy the needed supplies and food to take when making home visits.

Regardless of the FBO, the messages related to HIV were very much the same: abstinence, be faithful, and *no* condoms. For all, these messages were embedded in their religious beliefs that pre- and extramarital sex was immoral and against the word of God and/or Allah, and that condoms promoted promiscuity. In essence, FBOs were behind only the AB part of the Abstinence, Be Faithful, or Use Condoms campaign.

Activities of HIV care were supported in both Muslim and Christian traditions. Muslims noted the importance of caring for orphans, noting the Prophet himself was an orphan, and Christians similarly pointed to biblical proscriptions of the importance of caring for widows and orphans. However, the activities of the FBOs with regards to HIV care were somewhat different. This difference was partially due to the level of hierarchy evident in the organization such that the FBOs with the most hierarchical structure tended to provide the most care to members with HIV. A more structured hierarchy allowed the FBO to mobilize responses more quickly with infrastructure and experienced groups already in place with clear chains of command and supply structures. For example a Roman Catholic parish had a storage building where members contributed excess maize that was stored and given to parishioners in need. This program had been in place for years, so it was readily adapted to the needs of the increasing number of AIDS orphans requiring help.

Although local religious leaders believed that they had a great deal of power over the behaviors of their members, in actuality, our data showed that they positively influenced their members' risk behaviors only through dissemination of concrete knowledge about HIV transmission, not through messages preached about the morality of certain behaviors (Lindgren et al., 2013) On the other hand, local leaders' stigmatizing attitude translated into fewer care behaviors on the part of their members—in effect, members were less motivated to care for ill members of their community if stigmatizing messages were coming from the pulpit. Stigma continues to be a significant problem within religious communities as well as the community at large.

Despite the FBO's stated position on condoms, we also uncovered a level of pragmatism within individual leaders that was surprising, as the following examples demonstrate: One pastor's wife discussed, at length, the messages around abstinence and discouragement of condom use that she delivers to her husband's congregation and indeed her own children. However, she also admitted that she keeps a bowl of condoms in her house for her children to use, which she has to periodically refill. Although they do not talk about it, she knows on the one hand, that her young unmarried adult sons are using condoms (so are engaging in premarital sex, a sin) but that they are also being protected from contracting HIV. The second example was a nun who taught nursing students. She stated that although the Pope was against condoms even for discordant couples, she teaches students and patients what all the options are to protect the nonpositive spouse and then tells them to decide for themselves.

Additionally, we learned that nurses in congregations were often the ones charged with delivering the HIV messages and coordinating FBO outreach for community care of those living with HIV. Weekly religious services, a critical part of the fabric of Malawian life, are regularly attended by the vast majority of Malawians and provide an excellent way to reach large numbers of people. In addition to serving worship needs, Sunday morning church is a major social event each week for many Malawians. Services typically last 2 to 3 hours, and people stay to socialize after the formal service is over. One nurse took advantage of this opportunity to serve her large congregation by instituting quarterly health fairs on Sunday mornings after church in which HIV testing and blood pressure measurements were made available to congregational members.

LESSONS LEARNED

Working with FBOs is both rewarding and challenging. First, FBOs can be good partners in promoting health, disseminating health education messages, and delivering care. Their individual church-/mosque-based structures can be mobilized to assist in health outreach to communities. Indeed, it is in their best interest to have a healthy congregation because without healthy members to do the work of the FBO, the "church does not develop." We heard repeatedly from central leaders, local leaders, and members that FBO members needed to be healthy for the church/mosque and the country to "develop" and grow. Therefore, FBO leaders are willing and indeed are actually delivering health-related messages to their members. However, one must also remember that FBO leaders tend to focus on the spiritual health of their members as they see this as their primary charge, to prepare members for the next life, and they will not deliver messages that contradict religious teachings. As such, they exhort their members to be good Christians and Muslims, and God/Allah will take care of them. FBO leaders relegate the "body" to the hospital or the traditional village authority.

Cultural taboos are also woven into the religious framework and can restrict the messages and modes of delivery by FBO leaders. For example, a distinction is made between what is acceptable to discuss in public (from the pulpit) and what they might discuss in small group teaching or counseling. Additionally, discussion of sexual behavior beyond exhorting members to abstain and/or be faithful to their spouses and even pregnancy is difficult, so messages are often vague in nature. Although, as one participant noted, the Qur'an "talks about everything," it remains difficult for imams (and priests, pastors) to discuss sex and reproduction in public settings.

Second, it is important to know what one should expect when seeking to work with FBOs in countries like Malawi. It is difficult to overstate the way religion is woven through the fabric of Malawian life and it may be startling to Westerners, especially those coming from more secularized parts of the developed world and with a heightened sensitivity to respecting religious diversity, that the United States leads in avoiding making explicitly religious statements in the workplace or secular gatherings. In Malawi, it is common to open meetings of any kind with prayer, often explicitly Christian in nature, including meetings in settings that in the United States would be entirely secular, such as gatherings with government officials. Do not be surprised if you are called on to deliver the prayer yourself. If you are not comfortable doing so, let the leader know ahead of time. Groups and organizations may hold weekly prayer meetings to which all the staff are invited, and there is an expectation that all will participate. This doesn't mean that religious diversity isn't tolerated or respected, but reflects a different worldview in which acknowledgement of a divine force is considered as normal and necessary as acknowledging the weather. Similarly, you can expect to hear references to the Bible or Qur'an sprinkled throughout conversations of all types, and the scriptures are commonly referred to for advice and wisdom. You may see Bibles or Qur'ans in the workplace.

While Christianity and Islam are the major world religions represented over 90% of the population in Malawi, religious syncretism is also present. Aspects of ancient animist indigenous religion persist, even in devout Christian and Muslim communities. Across socioeconomic classes, there is a belief in the power of witchcraft and the power of evil spells. Some indigenous Pentecostal-type churches support this belief through a cosmological understanding holding that forces of evil bring illness into communities. We have heard highly educated Malawians speak authoritatively of ancestral and village spirits, both good and evil. And especially in village settings, belief in supernatural forces is evident. Traditional healers (sometimes referred to as "witch doctors") are thought to have special healing gifts. One of our colleagues conducted research on traditional healers and found that many had sound knowledge of herbal remedies for symptomatic treatment, were educated about HIV, and referred clients suspected of having HIV for testing and treatment to government facilities (Youmans, Rankin, Phiri, Mguntha, & Chihana, 2010). There is a national association of traditional healers that works to assure ethical practice. Some traditional healers are also participants in mainstream religions. On the other hand, other traditional healers take advantage of ill people, charging money for ineffective "cures." Community health education programs such as village dramas attempt to educate people about avoiding these.

Third, we have learned the importance of persevering in the work for the long haul. One church-related, home-based care leader told us that her group had done good work when financial aid from the international body of the organization provided the inputs for the group. Members visited those who were ill, provided companionship, and helped with chores. But when they were told that they needed, in the name of "sustainability," to become completely self-sufficient, and outside help was cut off, the group began to flounder. It was hard to continue visiting people who were ill and needed food when the visitors had nothing to bring and these caregivers had no resources to share except their time.

While developing the capacity of groups of people to help themselves is an important goal, the process takes time and the context of extreme poverty cannot be overlooked in chasing sustainability. GAIA's village intervention is an intensive 3-year intervention that works to develop a sustainable infrastructure of knowledge and expertise, and contact is maintained with villages for years afterward, with some supports, such as school fees for orphans, continuing for years after the initial 3-year intervention.

In contrast to organizations that build capacity, there are also "helicopter" groups that fly in and leave after having been on the ground for very limited periods of time. Their nonnative understanding of the local cultural folkways can lead to major misunderstandings. Thus, we recommend that anyone working globally be well aware of the culture in which they work and bring cultural humility to every venture. Building trust in low- and middle-income countries (LMIC) takes a long time, and although most medical missions are well intended they may not offer sustainable services. Indeed, they may instead require a great deal of the religious organization's time and expertise to mount a health care program. Therefore, anyone seeking to work with FBOs in poor countries should spend time reflecting on what they are bringing to the project, why they are doing it in the first place, and what they will leave behind.

Yet another important consideration is design of the contemplated project. Well-meaning Western health care providers think they know what is needed but it is the people from LMICs, the recipients of such projects, who really know their problems, are able to prioritize their difficulties, and know what will work in their contexts. We need to ask ourselves if the project we are proposing may inadvertently "disempower" (by casting them into a condition of dependency and subservience) the very people we are trying to assist.

This brings us to a fourth lesson learned, which is that international religious leaders and organizations must be held accountable for managing funds given to them, and for producing evidence that program outcomes have truly been achieved. The accountability principle operates from the beginning when funds are first delivered and continues through the project's duration. A culture of poverty and scarcity sometimes causes well-meaning NGO leaders and academics to ignore irresponsible behavior related to funding and/or program implementation, but the disruption caused in the community by corrupt and/or incompetent behavior puts into question the FBO leaders' ability to lead their organizations and usually results, over time, in feelings of anger and betrayal among the funders, as well as the discontinuation of funding to the communities. It was clear from our data that a great deal of distrust can be generated around funding opportunities that increase access to resources, especially money. People living with HIV spoke of money disappearing into funding recipients' pockets and not reaching those who should be receiving this assistance. Whether this is true or not, the lack of transparent accountability fosters this distrust. Altogether, competent and honest personnel must be in place to account for all funds and to demonstrate that research or program goals have been met.

Likewise, the precedent set many years ago to encourage academics and health care professionals to become involved in research and to reimburse them for the expenses accrued by such consultation has led to an unhealthy system of "sitting fees," where everyone expects to be paid for participating in research and, related, paid for participating in education and professional development workshops.

Professionals pick and choose the projects in which they want to be involved based on the size of the "consultation fees" promised. Such systems are difficult to change since most LMIC implicitly support such policies and ministries of health perpetuate them by setting up fee structures that result in employees "double dipping," that is, receiving a salary that is then supplemented by the payment of consultation fees, as well as reimbursement for travel, lodging, and meals. Such payment systems are as ingrained in religious organizations as in any other structures within LMIC, including universities and health care systems. The dangers of such systems include governmental entities (universities and health care systems) limiting the pay of employees, expecting them to make up the difference through sitting and/or consulting fees and, at the community or FBO level, leaders and members unwilling to participate in community-based programs unless they get "compensation." This increases the difficulties NGOs face in mobilizing community members to develop, test, and sustain interventions that could improve the health and lives of everyone.

Finally, FBOs have many excellent leaders who have either been appointed or have grown into their leadership positions over time and have been recognized by the FBO members for their outstanding qualities. We have found that FBOs enhance leadership abilities in women through their dependence on the organizations' women's groups, and that this opportunity encourages women to assume leadership positions in other societal venues. Likewise, in Malawi and in other LMIC, religious leaders have been responsible for bringing about political change through the steadfast support of human rights and peaceful attempts to unseat unscrupulous leaders. International NGO leaders could learn important lessons from these religious leaders, who have brought about policy change for the good.

In conclusion, our experiences working with FBOs in Africa have led us to continue to develop networks and establish relationships with FBO leaders, both nationally and internationally. FBOs and their members can be a great resource in reaching large numbers of people with health promotion and disease prevention messages. We recommend health care providers continue to explore ways to utilize the potential mobilization and leadership resources that reside in FBOs, even in the most rural settings. Our lessons learned have been varied and far ranging, but we believe that it is important to fully understand a country in which one plans to work. Our experiences in Malawi, the "warm heart of Africa," have been largely positive, and we are grateful to the many FBO leaders who have helped us build programs of service and research and to implement useful programs arising from our combined work in Africa. We are aware that there is much we do not understand about customs and folkways when working internationally, and we are grateful to our Malawi friends and cultural guides for their patient teaching.

We believe that people seeking to work with FBOs should be self-reflective, collaborative, patient, and committed to sustaining engagement for the long haul. Religion plays a critical role in the lives of people living in LMICs, and religious organizations in these countries tend to be more conservative than in the West. One needs to be prepared for the role that faith and FBOs play in members' lives and be ready to engage in openly religious behaviors in order to earn the trust and collaboration of FBOs. However, building these relationships can be rewarding, practical, and altogether powerful.

REFERENCES

Byamugisha, G. (2000). *Breaking the silence on HIV/AIDS in Africa: How can religious institutions talk about sexual matters in their communities?* Kampala, Uganda: Tricolour.

Caldwell, J. C., Orubuloye, I. O., & Caldwell, P. (1992). Underreaction to AIDS in sub-Saharan Africa. *Social Science & Medicine, 34*, 1169–1182. doi:10.1016/0277-9536(92)90310-M

Chakanza, J. C. (1995). The unfinished agenda: Puberty rites and the response of the Roman Catholic Church in southern Malawi, 1901–1994. *Religion in Malawi, 5*, 3–7.

Drain, P. K., Halperin, D. T., Hughes, J. P., Klausner, J. D., & Bailey, R. C. (2006). Male circumcision, religion, and infectious diseases: An ecologic analysis of 118 developing countries. *BMC Infectious Disease, 6*, 172–182. doi:10.1186/1471-2334-6-172

Fiedler, R. N. (2005). *Coming of age: A Christianized initiation among women of Southern Malawi, Zomba.* Kachere Series.

Hogle, J. A. (2002). *What happened in Uganda? Declining HIV prevalence, behavior change, and the national response.* Washington, DC: The Synergy Project.

Index Mundi. (2010). *Malawi-access to electricity.* Retrieved from http://www.indexmundi.com/facts/malawi/access-to-electricity

Jamison, D. T., Summers L. H., Alleyne G., Arrow K. J., Berkley S., Binagwaho A., . . . Yamey G. (2014). Global health 2035: A world converging within a generation. *The Lancet, 372*(9648), 1473–1483. doi:10.1016/S0140-6736(08)61345-8

Kamarulzaman, A. (2013). Fighting the HIV epidemic in the Islamic world. *The Lancet, 381*(9883), 2058–2060, doi:10.1016/S0140-6736(13)61033-8

Kandiero, C. (2014). Malawi electrification rate the lowest in Africa. *BNL Times.* Retrieved from http://timesmediamw.com/malawi-electrification-rate-the-lowest-in-africa

Lindgren, T. G., Deutsch K., Schell E., Bvumbwe A., Hart K. B., Laviwa J., & Rankin S. H. (2011). Using mobile clinics to deliver HIV testing and other basic health services in rural Malawi. *Rural and Remote Health, 11*(2), 1682.

Lindgren, T., Schell, E., Rankin, S., Phiri, J., Fiedler, R., & Chakanza, J. (2013). A response to Edzi (AIDS): Malawi faith-based organizations' impact on HIV prevention and care. *Journal of the Association of Nurses in AIDS Care, 24*(3), 227–241.

Mageda, K., Leyna, G. H., & Mmbaga, E. J. (2012). High initial HIV/AIDS-related mortality and its predictors among patients on antiretroviral therapy in the Kagera region of Tanzania: A five- year retrospective cohort study. *AIDS Research and Treatment,* Retrieved from http://dx.doi.org/10.1155/2012/843598. http://www.hindawi.com/journals/art/2012/843598

Mahajan, A. P., Sayles, J. N., Patel, V. A., Remien, R. H., Ortiz, D., Szekeres, G., & Coates, T. J. (2008). Stigma in the HIV/AIDS epidemic: A review of the literature and recommendations for the way forward. *AIDS. 22*(Suppl 2), S67–S79. doi:10.1097/01.aids.0000327438.13291.62

Morris, L. M., Schell, E., Schell, D., & Rankin, S. H. (Nov 2008–Nov 2009). Theologies of blame and compassion in the response of religious organizations to the AIDS crisis in Malawi, Central Africa. *Journal of Religion in Malawi, 15*, 3–10.

Mukolo, A., Blevins, M., Victor, B., Paulin, H. N., Vaz, L. M., Sidat, M., & Vergara, A. E. (2013). Community stigma endorsement and voluntary counseling and testing behavior and attitudes among female heads of household in Zambézia Province, Mozambique. *BMC Public Health, 13*, 1155. doi:10.1186/1471-2458-13-1155

Olley, B. O., Gxamza, F., Seedat, S., Theron, H., Taljaard, J., Reid, E., . . . Stein, D. J. (2003). Psychopathology and coping in recently diagnosed HIV/AIDS patients the role of gender. *South African Medical Journal*, (93)12: 928–931.

Otolok-Tanga, E., Atuyambe, L., Murphy, C. K., Ringheim, K. E., & Woldehanna, S. (2007). Examining the actions of faith-based organizations and their influence on HIV/AIDS-related stigma: A case study of Uganda. *African Health Sciences*, 7(1), 55–60.

Phiri, I. A., Haddad, B., & Masenya, M. (Eds.). (2003). *African women, HIV/AIDS, and faith communities*. Pietermaritzburg, South Africa: Cluster Publications.

Rankin, S., Lindgren, T., Kools, S., & Schell, E. (2008). The condom divide: Disenfranchisement of Malawi women by church and state. *Journal of Obstetric, Gynecologic, and Neonatal Nursing*, 37, 596–606.

Rankin, S. H., Lindgren, T., Rankin, W. W., & Ng'Oma, J. (2005). Donkey work: Women, religion, and HIV/AIDs in Malawi. *Health Care for Women International*, 26(1), 4–16.

Rankin, W. W., Brennan, S., Schell E., Laviwa J., & Rankin S. H. (2005). The stigma of being HIV positive in Africa. *PLoS Medicine*. 2(8), e247. Retrieved from http://www.ncbi.nlm.nih.gov/pmc/articles/PMC1176240

Schell, E. S., Rankin, W. W., Chipungu, G., Rankin, S., & Weiller, R. (2011). Building the nursing workforce in Malawi: Helping a developing African country solve its nursing shortage. *American Journal of Nursing*, 111(6), 65–67.

Seboni, N., Magowe, M. K. M., Uys, L. R., Suh, M. B., Djeko, K. N., & Moumouni, H. (2013). Shaping the role of sub-Saharan African nurses and midwives: Stakeholder's perceptions of the nurses' and midwives' tasks and roles. *Health SA Gesonheid*, 18(1), 1–11. Retrieved from http://www.hsag.co.za/index.php/HSAG/article/view/688/846

Skovdal, M., Campbell, C., Madanhire, C., Mupambireyi, Z., Nyamukapa, C., & Gregson, S. (2011). Masculinity as a barrier to men's use of HIV services in Zimbabwe. *Globalization and Health*, 7, 1–14. Retrieved from http://www.globalizationandhealth.com/content/7/1/13

Tsai, A. C., Bangsberg, D. R., & Weise, S. D. (2013). Harnessing poverty alleviation to reduce the stigma of HIV in sub-Saharan Africa. *PLoS Medicine*, 10(11), e1001557. doi:10.1371/journal.pmed.1001557

UNAIDS. (2012). *HIV and AIDS estimates*. Retrieved from http://www.unaids.org/en/regionscountries/countries/malawi

UNAIDS. (2013). *HIV estimates with uncertainty bounds*. Retrieved from http://www.unaids.org/en/dataanalysis/knowyourepidemic

USAID. (2011). *Using last mile distribution to increase access to health commodities*. Retrieved from http://deliver.jsi.com/dlvr_content/resources/allpubs/guidelines/UsinLastMileDist.pdf

Van Lettow, M., Kapito-Tembo, A., Kaunda-Khangamwa, B., Kanike, E., Maosa, S., Semba, M., . . . Cataldo, F. (2012). *Increasing the uptake of HIV testing in maternal health in Malawi*, (Discussion Paper No. 5). AI Research. Retrieved from http://www.africaportal.org/articles/2012/07/27/increasing-uptake-hiv-testing-maternal-health-malawi

Widmer, M., Betran, A. P., Merialdi, M., Requejo, J., & Karpf, T. (2011). The role of faith-based organizations in maternal and newborn health care in Africa. *International Journal of Gynecology and Obstetrics*, 114, 218–222.

Wolfe, W. R., Weiser, S. D., Leiter, K., Steward, W. T., Percy-de Korte, F., Phaladze, N., . . . Heisler, M. (2008). The impact of universal access to anti-retroviral therapy on HIV stigma in Botswana. *American Journal of Public Health, 98*(10), 1865–1871.

World Bank. (2010). *Malawi*. Retrieved from http://search.worldbank.org/data?qterm= maternal_20mortality_20Malawi&language=EN

World Bank. (2012). *Malawi*. Retrieved from http://data.worldbank.org/country/malawi

World Health Organization (WHO). (2008). *Faith-based organizations play a major role in HIV/AIDS care and treatment in sub-Saharan Africa*. Retrieved from http://www.who .int/mediacentre/news/notes/2007/np05/en

Youmans, S., Rankin, S., Phiri, J., Mguntha, A., & Chihana E. (2010). *Traditional healers of Malawi: Their role in HIV/AIDS prevention and treatment*. AIDS 2010 - XVIII International AIDS Conference. Abstract no. THPE0670.

CHAPTER 27

Global Nursing Issues in China: A Partnership of Boston Children's Hospital and Shanghai Children's Medical Center

Patricia A. Hickey, Jianhua Lou, and Lily Hsu

*B*oston Children's Hospital has a long history of supporting pediatric health care in Shanghai. The history of the relationship began in 1983 when Dr. William Norwood and Dr. Stephen Sanders travelled to Shanghai to conduct an assessment of Xin Hua Hospital's capacity to develop a pediatric cardiac surgery program. In 1986 and 1987, Drs. Richard Jonas and Patricia Hickey led the first interdisciplinary teams to Xin Hua Hospital, including many individuals from Boston Children's. For nearly 20 years semiannual or annual trips of pediatric cardiac teams from Boston Children's Hospital to Shanghai were supported by Project HOPE of Milwood, Virginia, under the leadership of Drs. Robert Crone, Lesley Mancuso, and the current chief executive officer, Dr. John Howe. In 1998 the pediatric cardiac surgery program transitioned from Xin Hua Hospital to the new Shanghai Children's Medical Center (SCMC) in Pudong. Following rapid expansion of the program, in 2007, a Heart Institute was built at SCMC, with the creation of an entire tower to house the cardiovascular program. The pediatric cardiovascular program at SCMC is now the largest in the world, with more than 3,500 open heart procedures performed annually.

The SCMC in Pudong is the result of more than 25 years of close collaboration between Project Hope; the Shanghai Second Medical University, now known as Jiao Tong University; and the Shanghai municipal government. Today, SCMC is a major teaching facility for all of Asia. Nurses and physicians from SCMC travel not only throughout China but also as far as Bangladesh and other developing countries to support new programs and educate clinicians in a collaborative fashion. The success of this endeavor is a tribute to the vision and leadership of Dr. Richard Jonas and Dr. Ding Wen Xiang and their commitment to an interdisciplinary practice model for achieving optimal outcomes for pediatric cardiovascular patients and their families.

Throughout our decades-long relationship, pediatric cardiovascular nurses have been viewed as full partners in the development of the SCMC cardiovascular program with Drs. Jonas and Ding. Dr. Patricia Hickey has been privileged to be a leader in the development of this program for 26 years. Her nursing partners in this process are Ms. Lily Hsu, program director for Project HOPE, and Ms. Lou, chief nurse of SCMC. Together, over a 26-year period, they have developed the largest pediatric cardiovascular nursing program in the world. This chapter is written through the lens of three experienced nurse leaders.

THE EARLY DAYS, 1984–1998

For any global health initiative to be successful, it is important to have the support of the local government. We were very fortunate to be supported by the Shanghai municipal government from the beginning of our collaboration. It is, however, important to note that during the Cultural Revolution in China from 1966 to 1976, pediatric cardiac surgery was rare and the babies and children with congenital heart disease did not receive adequate, if any, surgical care during those years. We learned that not only had teachers in the universities and schools been targeted, but advanced technical specialties such as cardiac surgery were singled out as elitist in many hospitals and closed down (Jonas, 2007). So there was an enormous need for pediatric cardiovascular care with training and education of clinicians by 1986.

Before attempting to establish the cardiovascular program, a preliminary team visit was made to Xin Hua Hospital in old Shanghai, where we worked for the first 10 years. A small group of cardiovascular nurses and physicians, along with perfusionists, biomedical engineers, and respiratory therapists, identified the equipment and personnel requirements to establish a pediatric cardiac surgery program. The advice to us in 1984 was to bring everything that would be needed from Boston. However, understanding that our goal was to establish a full-service program, including a pediatric cardiology diagnostic program, cardiac intensive care, and operating rooms, as well as a pediatric cardiac ward, it was clear that we would need a reliable partner in this endeavor. Fortunately, with Project Hope's background in developing the Krakow Children's Hospital in Poland, they had important experience in understanding the equipment needs and American and European companies that would be willing to donate equipment. By late 1985, Project Hope had coordinated donations of more than $500,000 (Jonas, 2007). Bioengineers were critically important to this project as the equipment not only had to be shipped from the United States, but the infrastructure to support the ongoing maintenance needed to be established at the Xin Hua Hospital.

By 1986, we had established a dedicated group of 15 volunteers from Boston Children's, including four intensive care nurses who would be able to care for patients and teach the Chinese nurses around the clock, a cardiac operating room nurse, a respiratory therapist, a catheterization lab technician, a catheterization laboratory cardiologist, an echocardiographer, a cardiac radiologist, a cardiac anesthesiologist, and a cardiac surgeon. The first working team visit occurred in March 1986. The Boston team stayed for 3 weeks at a time and were accommodated in the famous Peace Hotel on the Bund, which had been a grand institution in the past. However, during these initial visits to China, it was in dire need of renovation. The Boston team considered the Peace Hotel a "home away from home" during visits to Shanghai in the middle and late 1980s. One of the most striking memories of the early days was hosting a good-bye party for the Chinese nurses at the Peace Hotel after our first visit. There was a wonderful celebration with orange soda pop and peanut M&M candies. This was the beginning of a positive and inspired relationship between the United States and China and emblematic of the importance of nursing in the creation and execution of this new pediatric cardiovascular program.

In the early time period, the lack of adequate facilities and equipment was not trivial. For example, there were no transport oxygen cylinders, so the oxygen was stored in large inflatable pillows that provided very limited time for transport to the intensive care unit. Because the operating rooms were in a different building from the cardiac ward and early intensive care unit, patients had to be carried upstairs on a stretcher from the operating room across to the cardiac ward. Despite these and many other incredible challenges, the teams continued to work together to achieve a number of small wins that evolved into major successes for the patients and the program being developed in Shanghai. Our first surgical patient had a large secundum atrial septal defect (ASD) repaired. The entire team was thrilled to see the first patient do well and it was quite a shock and surprise for our Chinese hosts, who were accustomed to patients with ASDs being in the intensive care unit for 1 week and in the hospital for 1 month. This first patient was extubated on postoperative day one, and when the Chinese nurse was asked to help the boy get out of bed the request was greeted with a gasp by all of the Chinese physicians and nurses, who insisted that the patient should stay in bed for 1 week. At that time, "bed rest" was considered requisite in the Chinese culture for disease recovery, and it was a major change to encourage early mobilization for patients. When the patient was ready to go home a few days later, there was a wonderful celebration of this significant milestone.

UNDERSTANDING THE CULTURE

Many lessons have been learned over the past 25 years, and the Chinese and American nurses have grown personally and professionally in the process. One of the most important strategies to achieve success in any international exchange is to respect the culture and honor the preferences of each society. Learning about the host country, its people, culture, and history, will always facilitate the international experience. As Westerners during the first decade of visits, it was important to not assume anything and be open to all the possibilities. It was critical for the Americans to appreciate learning from the Chinese, not only teaching them. Being interested and humble are attributes that foster relationships of mutual respect, especially at the beginning of the international experience, when each group is assessing the other.

Another successful strategy in this American and Chinese international exchange was to celebrate small wins and milestones of achievement. This concept may be applied to any global health endeavor. After the first 10 years of this collaboration, Sino-American international conferences were jointly conducted every couple of years, with Chinese and American nurses and physicians presenting their work together. These conferences attracted clinicians from throughout China and other Asian countries. Of course, such achievements followed hundreds of collaborative clinical rounds, case conferences, in-service education sessions, and other educational forums that were held on a daily basis during the visits. Each time the Boston team returned to Shanghai, the Chinese nurses and physicians were demonstrating incremental growth in knowledge, confidence, and ability to sustain a world-class cardiovascular program.

Understanding the government and politics of each nation, and being politically sensitive, are requisite skills for anyone engaged in an international collaboration. Failure to understand the politics can lead to a variety of unfortunate outcomes from personal or public embarrassment of the host institution to much worse. Clinicians engaged in an international collaboration need to understand that they are guests, as well as collaborative partners in the foreign country. There are behavioral norms and expectations in those roles. Knowledge of the Chinese society, history, and culture is needed to engage in a productive working relationship. Knowledge of the status of nursing and its educational preparation in Chinese society is also important for successful collaboration (Giger, 2013).

Cultivating Relationships—Nurse Observership Program

In today's globalized world, there are enormous opportunities for free exchanges of ideas in person and through the digitized Internet and other forms of communication. As a result, nursing and medical knowledge and skill acquisition are always possible, and the opportunity to make a global impact is real. Although language may be perceived as a barrier to communication and education, the Chinese nurses and physicians have been committed to learning English. It is actually a mandatory part of the national educational curriculum across China, beginning in elementary school. Needless to say, the Chinese nurses have learned English but the American nurses have not learned Chinese.

For the past 20 years, there has been an ongoing exchange of physicians and nurses between SCMC and Boston Children's Hospital. Over the past decade, most of the visits have been Shanghai nurses visiting Boston. Each fall, a group of 4 to 6 staff nurses and nurse leaders travel to Boston for an observership experience of 6 weeks. The Chinese nurses are selected by the chief nursing officer and chief executive officer of SCMC, and Boston Children's Hospital requires a list of their professional goals to tailor an experience that will be valuable to share when they return to Shanghai.

The Boston Children's Hospital observership program involves significant effort from the host institution. Senior staff nurses and nurse leaders from Boston serve as preceptors for the Chinese nurses and assume responsibility for providing a rich educational experience. Table 27.1 illustrates a 6-week observership at

TABLE 27.1 Observership Experience for Nurses From Shanghai Children's Medical Center at Boston Children's Hospital

MONDAY	TUESDAY	WEDNESDAY	THURSDAY	FRIDAY
8:00–2:30 Welcome • Introductions • Review goals • Review schedule • Tour of unit • Tour of hospital • Meet leadership staff	8:00–3:30 Precepted shift in the CICU	8:00–3:30 Precepted shift in the CICU 12:00–3:00 Meet with CNS, review role, shadow	7:30–3:30 CICU Education Day Conference 1:00–2:00 Unit-based, Interdisciplinary Quality Improvement meeting	8:00–3:30 Precepted shift in the CICU 2:30–3:30 Meet with educator to review the week and evaluate goals
8:00–3:30 Precepted shift in the CICU 12:00–3:00 Meet with NP, review role, shadow	8:00–3:30 Precepted shift in the CICU 2:00–3:00 Journal club	8:00–3:30 Precepted shift in the CICU 6:00–8:00 Dinner with vice president and staff	8:00–3:30 Precepted shift in the CICU 8:30–9:00 Unit-based staff meeting	8:00–3:30 Precepted shift in the CICU 2:30–3:30 Meet with educator to review the week and evaluate goals
08:00–12:00 CICU Crisis Resource Management Course High-fidelity, interdisciplinary simulation course	8:00–3:30 Precepted shift in the CICU	7:30–3:30 Unit-based nursing orientation classes and high-fidelity simulation	8:00–3:30 Precepted shift in the CICU	8:00–3:30 Precepted shift in the CICU
1:00–3:00 Meet with simulator program coordinator	1:00–2:00 Education Council meeting		1:00–2:00 Nursing grand rounds	2:30–3:30 Meet with educator to review the week and evaluate goals
8:00–3:30 Precepted shift in the CICU 1:00–2:00 Unit based Interdisciplinary practice meeting	8:00–3:30 Precepted shift in the CICU 9:00–11:00 Meet with infection-control coordinator, review role, shadow 1:00–2:00 Bereavement rounds	7:30–3:30 Unit-based nursing orientation classes and high-fidelity simulation	8:00–3:30 Precepted shift in the CICU 2:30–3:30 Meet with educator to review the week and evaluate goals	8:00–12:30 Precepted shift in the CICU 8:00–9:00 Farewell breakfast with slide presentation

CICU, cardiac intensive care unit; CNS, clinical nurse specialist; NP, nurse practitioner.

Boston Children's Hospital based on the educational goals submitted by a Chinese cardiovascular critical care nurse. The Chinese nurse is paired with a senior nurse preceptor and the experience includes observing in-patient care areas and participating in simulated experiences, including crisis resource management and emergency response training. Additionally, the Chinese nurses receive didactic lectures and debriefing sessions as they work to achieve their observership goals. In each instance, a wonderful friendship evolves that lasts for many years after the nurse returns home to Shanghai. A framed certificate of observership from Boston Children's is presented to each of the Chinese nurses and physicians at the end of their Boston experience. This small gesture has been extremely meaningful to our Chinese colleagues. In this age of Internet and cloud-based technology, the Boston nurses continue to serve as coaches and collaborators to the nurses in China. The observership program serves as a wonderful exemplar for cultivating relationships, knowledge exchange, and a way to enhance understanding among the two cultures and societies.

QUALITY IMPROVEMENT STRATEGIES FOR NURSING EDUCATION

While visiting SCMC, the Boston team has shared the importance of improvement science, quality measurement, and rapid cycle change with performance improvement results. These initiatives have demonstrated the impact of quality improvement tools such as key driver diagrams in improving clinical quality and performance. The concepts of improvement science and interprofessional collaboration have been successfully integrated into the practice in SCMC's cardiovascular program. Chinese nurses have embraced new practices including evidence-based bundles to prevent patient harm, an early warning sign assessment tool to prevent deterioration of the patient's condition, pain and sedative management, and the Nightingale metrics for improving nurse-sensitive outcomes. An exciting part of this work has been the sharing of quality data between the cardiovascular intensive care units in Boston and Shanghai for learning and improving clinical practice in both units. The nursing staff in both units are equally committed to optimizing outcomes for cardiovascular patients and their families.

LEVERAGING TECHNOLOGY FOR NURSING EDUCATION IN CHINA: OPENPEDIATRICS

Despite significant medical advancements in the 21st century, dramatic inequalities in health care currently persist across the globe, particularly in nursing education. The teaching hospital apprenticeship model, which once revolutionized medical and nursing education, now fails to keep up with an increasingly interconnected world. As a result, expert knowledge is bottlenecked within the walls of academic institutions. Such deficiencies in the nursing education system have culminated in a global shortage of effective pediatric care. Over the past decade, however, innovative Internet-based technology has emerged that effectively scales knowledge exchange across the world. The rise of this technology has led to the opportunity for a fundamental revision of methods for nursing learning and knowledge exchange.

For the past 2 years, the Boston team has utilized OPENPediatrics to enhance the education experience for clinical nurses in many countries, including China. OPENPediatrics is a social learning platform designed to promote the exchange of knowledge between clinicians caring for critically ill children around the world. The platform offers rigorous, peer-reviewed educational content free of charge to clinicians worldwide.

By fusing world-class nursing and medical expertise with the power of the Internet, OPENPediatrics has created an interactive virtual training and knowledge exchange platform to enhance the quality of pediatric critical care and transform the existing nursing and medical education models. Designed by experienced clinicians at Boston Children's Hospital, in collaboration with IBM Interactive, OPENPediatrics is the first global health initiative to utilize innovations in cloud-based technology for advancements in nursing education. Currently, it is being used in five large children's hospitals in China, including SCMC, and in many other countries. OPENPediatrics is changing the existing nursing education paradigm by offering asynchronous interactive learning and various avenues for knowledge sharing outside the walls of select institutions. Those accessing the online platform are offered free access to academically rigorous and peer-reviewed lectures, simulators, and protocols. Using these materials to encourage active learning and information exchange, this platform has already begun to create a global community of pediatric critical care practitioners. Consequently, Chinese nurses and physicians are able to collaborate with experts around the world through the OPENPediatrics web-based platform.

The OPENPediatrics content was developed based on David Kolb's theory of adult education, which suggests learning is more effective when content is presented in four distinct learning steps: concrete experience, reflective observation, abstract conceptualization, and active experimentation (Kolb & Kolb, 2005). Chinese nurses experience this educational model through three main features of the OPENPediatrics Platform: World Shared Practices Forum, Guided Learning Pathways, and the Content Library (Wolbrink, Kissoon, & Burns, 2014).

The World Shared Practices Forum is a monthly video lecture delivered by a nurse or other clinician on a critical issue in pediatric care. This forum connects a global community of care, allowing health care teams from around the world to communicate via a discussion forum, comment on and ask questions of the video, and gain knowledge of international best practices. This function facilitates asynchronous learning and knowledge exchange across geographic borders and time zones by allowing users to add comments at anytime, anywhere, throughout the life of the video.

The Guided Learning Pathways offer an opportunity for users to expand their knowledge of topics relevant to their practice in critical care. The learning pathways comprise 15 to 20 short lessons, which each begin with a pretest followed by a video, summary, and, if applicable, a simulator, and conclude with a posttest.

The Content Library includes the full extent of the platform's content, which includes medical lectures and demonstrations by experts, protocols, medical calculators, and a virtual ventilator simulation.

OPENPediatrics has been and continues to be an innovative and highly successful solution for ongoing competency development and education of pediatric nurses in China and across the globe.

LEVERAGING TECHNOLOGY FOR NURSING EDUCATION IN CHINA: THE INTERNATIONAL QUALITY IMPROVEMENT COLLABORATIVE FOR CONGENITAL HEART SURGERY

Another highly successful education program for pediatric cardiovascular nurses is the International Quality Improvement Collaborative for Congenital Heart Surgery (IQIC) across 27 congenital heart centers in 16 developing world countries. The IQIC utilizes collaborative learning strategies to guide local quality improvement efforts targeted at three key drivers for reducing mortality from congenital heart surgery. These key drivers are safe perioperative practices, infection reduction, and team-based practice. The key driver diagram, a known quality improvement tool, is illustrated in Figure 27.1.

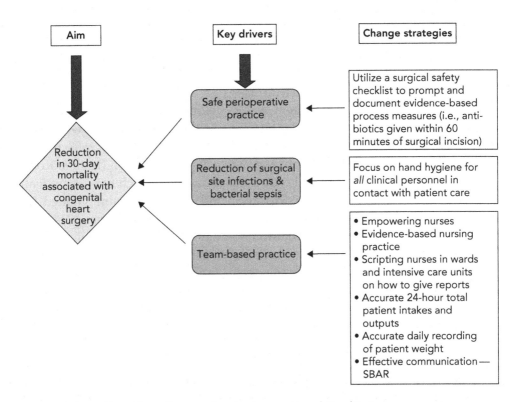

FIGURE 27.1 Key driver diagram for the International Quality Improvement Collaborative for Congenital Heart Surgery (IQIC).

One important feature of quality improvement is the need to monitor clinical outcomes and benchmark performance. A major challenge faced by health care professionals in the developing world is the lack of benchmarking data for purposes of evaluating performance of their congenital heart surgery programs and guiding efforts to make improvements. To address these gaps and strengthen health care systems across the world, the IQIC was conceived in 2007 by Dr. Kathy Jenkins et al. from Boston Children's Hospital, along with international colleagues and nongovernmental organizations (NGOs). A web-based data entry tool was devised to collect data, and physician-nurse teams from each hospital oversee the data collection and project management. The hospitals submit diagnostic, procedural, and clinical information for all congenital heart surgeries on patients into the web-based entry tool. Hospitals report de-identified patient data only. SCMC performs more pediatric heart surgery than any other institution in the world and is the major contributor to the IQIC database.

Safe Perioperative Practice

Risk management is an important component of patient safety. The IQIC is a way to leverage technology for sharing information, education, and procedures to address safe perioperative practices. Using design principles outlined by the World Health Organization's (WHO) Safe Surgery Saves Lives (Weiser et al., 2010) campaign and a previously published pediatric surgical safety checklist as a conceptual framework (Norton & Rangel, 2010), a checklist was designed specifically to meet the needs of children undergoing congenital heart surgery. The checklist was disseminated to all IQIC hospitals, and they were encouraged to make further modifications as necessary to meet unique needs of their institutions. Members of perioperative care teams at each hospital were trained on effective checklist utilization through interactive webinars and one-on-one site mentoring. SCMC has implemented this checklist in their cardiovascular operating rooms.

Infection Reduction

Learning modules were developed to introduce the concept of evidence-based "practice bundles" and teach specific components of infection reduction. A bundle is defined as a set of evidence-based practices that improve patient outcomes when implemented by every member of the health care team (Institute for Healthcare Improvement [IHI], 2006). The Chinese nurses have embraced the concept of evidence-based bundles and have successfully implemented bundled care for prevention of ventilator-associated events, deep vein thrombosis, and also environmental hazards. They meticulously track their unit-based data and work to improve performance through rapid cycle change processes and other improvement science tools. An initial IQIC education module focused on developing a hand hygiene program and included strategies to improve hand-washing compliance, recognizing that hands of health care workers are responsible for the transmission of the majority of pathogens in hospitals (Boyce & Pittet, 2002). Additional modules focused on practice bundles to improve sterility with respect to central venous catheter insertion, central line access, and central line dressings based on evidence (Jeffries et al., 2009); to reduce surgical site infections, emphasizing correct antibiotic timing, hair removal with clippers, preoperative skin disinfection, and postoperative wound management; and to reduce urinary tract infections and ventilator-associated pneumonia. The importance of standardizing care, auditing practice, and the feedback of practice audit results and infection rates were common themes across all of the IQIC education modules.

Team-Based Practice Through Nurse Empowerment

To optimally meet the complex health care needs of pediatric cardiovascular patients, an interprofessional model of collaborative practice was introduced in the 1980s and continually reinforced in the Boston and Shanghai partnership. Thus, the SCMC nurses are able to experience a professional environment. Opportunities for professional advancement, beginning with a well-designed, competency-based education program and a career ladder, are in place as they advance their practice from novice to expert. Through consistent modeling of a collaborative team approach, the confidence of the Chinese nurses has grown in tandem with their professional practice environment.

A major goal of the IQIC is to achieve team-based practice through nurse empowerment, and the Chinese nurses were well ahead of most institutions in this domain when the IQIC began in 2007. Numerous tools were provided for empowering nurses, including high-fidelity, case-based teaching videos; standardized scripts for nurses to give comprehensive patient reports in the intensive care unit and ward; and behavioral techniques of assertion, closed loop communication, and a structured situation briefing framework with four components: Situation, Background, Assessment, and Recommendation (SBAR). SBAR, a communication model adopted from U.S. Nuclear Navy (Kosnik, Brown, & Maund, 2007), has been found to be beneficial in health care settings. An example of assertion training, which reinforces infection reduction strategies, includes empowering nurses to speak up in a professional manner when sterility is compromised or when practice bundles are not followed. Detailed demonstrations of fundamental and advanced competencies for pediatric cardiovascular nurses are also presented in the IQIC educational webinars.

Strategies for preventing hospital-acquired infections are significantly less robust in the developing world (Crawford, Skeath, & Whippy, 2013; Haynes et al., 2009). Therefore, empowering nurses and creating a collaborative team to take charge in preventing hospital-acquired infection are keys to building staff competency and competence in infection prevention and surveillance. Hospital-acquired infections that are associated with increased morbidity, mortality, and hospital costs require a team effort for proper prevention everywhere in the world (de Vries et al., 2010). The occurrence of these infections in countries with limited resources imposes a significant burden on the health care system, and results in resources being directed away from care of additional patients (Neily et al., 2010). In recent years, hospitals that have introduced evidence-based practice bundles to prevent occurrence of device-associated and surgical site infections have successfully decreased occurrence of these infections (Allegranzi et al., 2011; Haynes et al., 2009; Semel et al., 2010; Leonard, 2004; WHO, 2015a, 2015b, n.d). Hand hygiene is the cornerstone of every bundle to reduce device-associated and surgical site infections. These and other practices were incorporated into IQIC learning modules in order to reduce hospital-acquired infections.

It is widely recognized that effective communication and teamwork are essential for the delivery of high quality and safe patient care. Ineffective communication has been linked to inadvertent patient harm (Allegranzi et al., 2011). Nurses need to feel empowered to confidently communicate patient concerns. Educational and cultural barriers that preclude nurses from speaking freely are prevalent among developing world countries (World Health Organization, 2013). Thus, team-based practice through nurse empowerment and effective communication was included as a major key driver for reducing mortality. Fortunately, effective communication and team collaboration were already addressed over many years in the Boston Shanghai partnership so the SCMC nurses were well poised to continue and reinforce their success through the IQIC learning modules.

FUTURE PLANS

The partnership between Boston Children's Hospital and SCMC has evolved over several decades and will continue to be sustained due to the long history of collaboration and respectful exchange. The bilateral exchange of nurses and physicians is ongoing and the two hospitals have built increased capacity for caring for pediatric cardiovascular patients in both countries. Not only is SCMC the major teaching institution for all of Asia, recently their nurses and physicians also started to travel to underresourced institutions in Bangladesh and other developing world sites to help build self-sustaining programs. The next phase of the collaboration will strengthen and expand the clinical research currently being conducted in the IQIC to more projects. Planning for Chinese nurses to lead lectures on OPENPediatrics is also in progress so nurses across the globe can gain value from this long-standing collaboration. The nurses from Boston Children's and Shanghai are working together to elevate nursing knowledge and improve the lives of young patients with cardiovascular disease across the globe. Table 27.2 lists a summary of lessons learned over 25 years in the partnership between Boston Children's Hospital and SCMC. These lessons are based on our success in building capacity for pediatric cardiac surgery and cardiovascular nursing.

TABLE 27.2 Summary of Lessons Learned

When building capacity for pediatric cardiac surgery and cardiovascular nursing, a number of considerations are critical.

1. Identification of a nurse and physician leader and interdisciplinary team that is committed to building a self-sufficient program in collaboration with the foreign institution and it's clinicians
2. Support from institution executives in the American and Chinese hospitals
3. Support from the Chinese government
4. Support from a nongovernmental organization that can raise money for expensive equipment and facilities
5. Recognition that more similarities than differences exist; honor preferences and respect cultural norms and behaviors; be culturally and politically sensitive
6. Create mutually supported goals and objectives and clarify ongoing timeline for goal achievement
7. Build trust through transparent sharing of quality and safety data for performance improvement
8. Celebrate small wins and achievement of collaborative milestones
9. Effectively communicate via Internet, telephone, fax, and in person with interpreters if needed
10. Be available throughout the year for ongoing coaching, mentorship, and consultation

REFERENCES

Allegranzi, B., Bagheri Nejad, S., Combescure, C., Graafmans, W., Attar, H., Donaldson L., & Pillet, D. (2011). Burden of endemic health-care-associated infection in developing countries: Systematic review and meta-analysis. *Lancet, 377*(9761), 228–241.

Boyce, J. M., & Pittet, D. (2002). Guideline for hand hygiene in health-care settings. Recommendations of the Healthcare Infection Control Practices Advisory Committee and the HICPAC/SHEA/APIC/IDSA Hand Hygiene Task Force. *MMWR Recommendations and Reports, 51*(RR-16), 1–45.

Crawford, B., Skeath, M., & Whippy, A. (2013). Multifocal clinical performance improvement across 21 hospitals. *Journal for Healthcare Quality.* doi:10.1111/jhq.12039

de Vries, E. N., Prins, H. A., Crolla, R. M., den Outer. A. J., van Andel, G, van Helden, S. H., . . . SURPASS Collaborative Group. (2010). Effect of a comprehensive surgical safety system on patient outcomes. *New England Journal of Medicine, 363*(20), 1928–1937.

Giger, J. N. (2013). *Transcultural nursing: Assessment and intervention* (6th ed.) St. Louis, MO: Elsevier/Mosby.

Haynes, A. B., Weiser, T. G., Berry, W. R., Lipsitz, S. R., Breizat, A. H., Dellinger, E. P., . . . Safe Surgery Saves Lives Study Group. (2009). A surgical safety checklist to reduce morbidity and mortality in a global population. *New England Journal of Medicine, 360*(5), 491–499.

Institute for Healthcare Improvement. (2006). *Protecting 5 million lives from harm.* Retrived from http://ihi.org/IHI/Programs/Campaign

Jeffries, H. E., Mason, W., Brewer, M., Oakes, K. L., Munoz, E. I., Gornick, W., . . . Jarvis, W. R. (2009). Prevention of central venous catheter-associated bloodstream infections in pediatric intensive care units: A performance improvement collaborative. *Infection Control and Hospital Epidemiology, 30*(7), 645–651.

Jonas, R. (2007). Pediatric cardiovascular surgery: Porject Hope and the Shanghai Children's Medical Center. *Pediatric Cardiovascular Surgery, 1,* 427–438.

Kolb, A., & Kolb, D. (2005). Learning styles and learning spaces: Enhancing experiential learning in higher education. In *Academy of Management Learning & Education* (pp. 193–212). Briarclliff Manor, NY: Academy of Management.

Kosnik, L. K., Brown, J., & Maund, T. (2007). Patient safety: Learning from the aviation industry. *Nursing Management, 38*(1), 25–30.

Leonard, M. (2004). The human factor: The critical importance of effective teamwork and communication in providing safe care. *Quality and Safety in Health Care, 13*, i85–i90.

Neily, J., Mills, P. D., Young-Xu, Y., Carney, B.T., West, P., Berger, D.H., . . . Bagian, J.P. (2010). Association between implementation of a medical team training program and surgical mortality. *Journal of the American Medical Association, 304*(15), 1693–1700.

Norton, E. K., & Rangel, S. J. (2010). Implementing a pediatric surgical safety checklist in the OR and beyond. *AORN Journal, 92*(1), 61–71.

Semel, M. E., Resch, S., Haynes, A. B., Funk, L. M., Bader, A., Berry, W. R., . . . Gawande, A. A. (2010). Adopting a surgical safety checklist could save money and improve the quality of care in U.S. hospitals. *Health affairs (Millwood), 29*(9), 1593–1599.

Weiser, T. G., Haynes A. B., Dziekan G., Berry W. R., Lipsitz S. R., Gawande A. A., & Safe Surgery Saves Lives Investigators and Study Group. (2010). Effect of a 19-item surgical safety checklist during urgent operations in a global patient population. *Annals of Surgery, 251*(5), 976–980.

Weiser, T. G., Haynes, A. B., Lashoher, A., Dziekan, G., Boorman, D. J., Berry, W. R., Gawande, A. A. Perspectives in quality: Designing the WHO surgical safety checklist. (2010). *International Journal for Quality in Health Care, 22*(5), 365–370.

Wolbrink, T., Kissoon, N., & Burns, J. (2014). The development of an Internet-based Knowledge exchange platform for pediatric critical care clinicans worldwide. *Pediatric Critical Care Medicine, 15*(3), 1–9.

World Health Organization. (n.d.). *Health care-associated infections (fact sheet).* Retrieved from http://www.who.int/gpsc/country_work/gpsc_ccisc_fact_sheet_en.pdf

World Health Organization (WHO). (2005a). *New scientific evidence supports WHO findings: A surgical safety checklist could save hundreds of thousands of lives.* Retrieved from http://www.who.int/patientsafety/safesurgery/checklist_saves_lives/en/index.html

World Health Organization. (2005b). *Global patient safety challenge.* Retrieved from http://www.who.int/patient safety/challenge/en

CHAPTER 28

Developing a Sustainable Model for Cardiovascular Care in Rwanda

Ceeya Patton-Bolman, Noella Bigirimana, and Julie Carragher

*I*n developing countries, severe resource limitations and competing priorities impede even the most basic health care services. Consequently, low- and middle-income countries (LMICs) leverage local and global partnerships in addressing health gaps. These strategic collaborations play a key role in tackling unmet health needs and systemic issues such as inadequate infrastructure, shortage of health workforce, and inequity of access to care (Little, 2012).

Health partnerships can be particularly beneficial in addressing the growing disease burden of major noncommunicable diseases (NCDs)—cardiovascular diseases, cancer, diabetes, chronic respiratory diseases, and mental illnesses—in LMICs, where 80% of NCD-related deaths occur (World Health Organization, 2011a). These conditions put further pressure on often fragile health systems. Current projections by the World Health Organization (WHO) suggest NCDs will be the leading causes of mortality by 2030, with a significant share of this increase found in developing countries. Beyond impacting health outcomes, NCDs hinder development and can perpetuate poverty, with an estimated cumulative output loss of $47 trillion within the next two decades (Bloom et al., 2011). The scale and growing impact of NCDs require strong collaborative efforts to address these challenges in less developed countries.

This chapter discusses several partnerships that focus on tackling cardiovascular diseases, under the umbrella of NCD programs, in Rwanda. We introduce an integrated approach to preventing and managing rheumatic heart disease (RHD), one of the most common acquired cardiac diseases among children and young adults in developing countries. The collaborative approach combines disease-specific programs and health system strengthening in areas such as health service delivery and the health workforce. Rwanda is used as context due to our affiliation with a long-standing partnership between the Ministry of Health (MoH), the Rwanda Heart Foundation, and Team Heart, Inc.—a Boston-based nongovernmental organization. In addition to the local context, regional and global implications are mentioned with regard to other low-income countries facing similar challenges.

This chapter explores selected strategies in six main sections. In the first two sections, we briefly discuss the health system and current status of NCDs in Rwanda, with a particular focus on rheumatic heart disease. The third section introduces two partnerships established to promote specialty care, including a country-led cardiac surgery program. The next section examines Team Heart's approach to addressing RHD and strengthening the health system in Rwanda. Priority strategies include providing cardiac surgery education and in-service training for local clinical teams, designing a national curriculum in cardiology, developing postsurgery care pathways, supporting outreach clinics, and facilitating procurement of essential medications. In the fifth section, a partnership is discussed to illustrate a more regional component of cardiovascular care in Rwanda. In the last section, upcoming initiatives are presented, including plans to build the first national center of excellence in cardiovascular care.

As the impact of these collaborative efforts is discussed, we show how the interventions align with the national health priorities and promote country ownership. We hope the strategies discussed will provide insights into a framework to promote health and development outcomes in resource-limited settings.

HEALTH SYSTEM IN RWANDA

Low-income countries face major barriers to improving health service delivery, such as human resources, financing, infrastructure, and equipment. Identifying and addressing these common barriers is crucial in achieving health and development priorities (Travis et al., 2004). The context of Rwanda, although unique in some aspects, is highly similar to other resource-limited settings.

According to the MoH of Rwanda (2012b), the country has nearly 12 million inhabitants, 80% of whom live in a rural setting. The 1994 genocide resulted in major human, social, and economic devastation, including a distressed health system (Binagwaho et al., 2013a). Twenty years later, the country is following a national development plan with a strong focus on health care. The health sector performance and indicators reflect this priority, as the country is on track to reach health-related Millennium Development Goals (MDGs) by 2015 (MoH of Rwanda, 2013). Table 28.1 provides some context on the local health system by introducing key health and demographic indicators. Many of these estimates represent significant progress from previous years, including life expectancy, health insurance coverage, and child mortality. Despite this progress, several gaps remain and are integrated into the national health priority areas.

The MoH plays a central role in managing interventions in the health sector, and provides national guidelines for health-related interventions through the Health Sector Strategic Plan (HSSP) (MoH of Rwanda, 2012a). The HSSP includes key priority areas for addressing challenges such as geographical and financial access to health services, inadequate human resources, and poor infrastructure.

TABLE 28.1 Key Health and Demographic Indicators, Rwanda (2012)

Total population (2013)	12 million
Population living in rural areas	81%
Life expectancy	58
Total fertility rate	4.6
Infant mortality rate	50/1,000 live births
Maternal mortality ratio	487/100,000 live births
HIV prevalence	3%
Health insurance coverage	91% to 96%
Physicians	1/15,428
Nurses	1/1,200
Midwives	1/23,364
Community health workers	1/266
Major health facilities	
Referral hospitals	5
District hospitals	41
Health centers	451
Health posts	60
Dispensaries	130

Source: MoH of Rwanda (2013).

Similar to other low-income countries, Rwanda relies significantly on external donor contributions for an estimated 43% of the health budget (MoH of Rwanda, 2012a). In this context, external partners, such as multilateral funders and nongovernmental organizations, contribute to an influx of resources and expertise to address growing health needs. A successful collaboration requires partner organizations to align with the national health strategies and system-wide frameworks.

Rwanda has focused on country-led strategies, including an effective decentralization model and community-based health insurance (Logie, Rowson, & Ndagije, 2008). A multiphased decentralization framework launched in 2000 led to the aggregation of provinces and districts. This national decentralization policy made the district a central unit in poverty reduction and economic development plans, including in the health sector. The health system is organized in several levels of service delivery with increasing complexity: community-based care, health posts, health centers, district hospitals and referral hospitals (MoH of Rwanda, 2012a). Under this model, specialty care is found mostly at the referral level, where trained physicians and nurses provide most of these health services. The majority of the 42 district hospitals are equipped to provide some specialty care through general practitioners and nurses. At the sector level, the nursing staff at 450 health centers works closely with colleagues at 60 health posts to ensure that basic health services are available to communities. Table 28.1 shows the number of physicians, nurses, and midwives in Rwanda. The table also lists the number of major health facilities by type.

The main health insurance scheme in Rwanda, *Mutuelle de Santé*, is community based and allows even the poorest citizens to access a package of basic health services (Binagwaho et al., 2013a; Logie, Rowson, & Ndagije, 2008). This community-based health insurance (CBHI) is almost universal with more than 90% of population covered (see Table 28.1), and it has contributed to an overall increase in the utilization rate for health services nationwide. Under the CBHI, members receive basic services such as antenatal care, family planning, generic drugs, and some tertiary care. Other health insurance schemes include the employment scheme for the civil servant (RAMA) and the Military Medical Insurance plan for the armed forces (Logie et al., 2008).

Despite significant progress with interventions targeting infectious diseases and health-related MDGs, further attention is required to address noncommunicable diseases. Although NCD control is part of the health sector strategic plan, implementing prevention and management strategies within local capacity presents major constraints (MoH of Rwanda, 2012a).

NCDs: THE RWANDA CONTEXT

The major contributors to the global burden of NCDs include cardiovascular diseases, cancer, diabetes, chronic respiratory diseases, and mental illness (WHO, 2011a). In Rwanda, the limited data suggest that NCDs account for nearly 30% of total deaths (WHO, 2011b). This evaluation might represent a significant underestimate given the high potential for misdiagnosis. In 2009, the country began to integrate NCDs into the national chronic care plans, and a special division was put in place to coordinate the planning and implementation of related interventions (MoH of Rwanda, 2012a). Moreover, Rwanda has established collaborations with development partners and nonprofit organizations to address critical gaps in NCD management and care.

Burden of Cardiovascular Diseases in Rwanda

Cardiovascular diseases are the leading cause of NCD-related mortality worldwide, including in the most vulnerable populations (WHO, 2011a). Similarly, heart diseases represent an increasing public health concern in Rwanda. Data collected at district hospitals and health centers suggest that cardiovascular diseases were the third leading cause of mortality in 2011 and 2012 (MoH of Rwanda, 2012b, 2013). Moreover, a survey showed that nearly 65% of NCD-related consultations and hospitalizations are due to heart failure (MoH of Rwanda, 2013).

It is important, however, to note the type of heart diseases facing communities in Rwanda. Although affluent countries encounter mostly ischemic and nonrheumatic valvular diseases, the majority of developing nations are disproportionately affected by congenital heart disease (CHD), RHD, and other acquired conditions (Zühlke, Mirabel, & Marijon, 2013).

The diagnosis and treatment of heart diseases are particularly problematic in resource-limited settings. Rwanda, a predominantly rural country, faces tremendous challenges in identifying and addressing congenital or acquired cardiovascular diseases. For instance, there is no catheterization facility countrywide and only six functioning echocardiographic machines, two of which were procured through our partnership with Rwanda. The data available suggest that the primary conditions responsible for heart failure admission are cardiomyopathies, RHD, and untreated hypertension (Bukhman & Kidder, 2011). Among them, RHD creates serious strain for the health system as the leading cause of acquired heart disease (Ngirabega, 2013).

RHD is a cardiovascular condition linked to several socioeconomic and environmental factors such as poverty, overcrowding, and poor nutrition and sanitation (WHO, 2004). This disease disproportionately affects children and young adults in developing countries. It results from complications of rheumatic fever (RF), which stems from a reaction to group A streptococcal (GAS) infection. RF is largely found in school-age children and, if untreated, results in heart valve damage. Although easily preventable and treatable in the early stage, RHD can develop with complications leading to valvular lesions that require surgical interventions to avoid premature death (WHO, 2004).

Addressing the burden of RHD is a challenge throughout developing countries, beginning with the lack of data to assess its impact in these settings. The current global prevalence estimate for RHD is 15 million people, which is projected to be higher given the increasing data on subclinical RHD (Zühlke et al., 2013). A handful of population-level studies have been conducted to measure the incidence, with many countries relying on extrapolations from studies in North Africa or the Middle East. According to several WHO reports, it is suggested that RHD accounts for 300,000 deaths and 500,000 new cases annually. A report by WHO Expert Consultations estimates that 770,000 disability-adjusted life years (DALYs) are lost due to RHD in Africa (World Health Organization, 2004). This increasing burden further weakens an already limited health care system with inadequate prevention and treatment services. In addition to deaths and disabilities, this disease has major economic implications as it affects individuals at a peak age of productivity.

Most low-income countries lack local resources to tackle RHD independently. In Rwanda, a program for the control of RHD was introduced through a long-standing collaboration between Team Heart, Inc, the MoH, the Rwanda Heart Foundation, and other key organizations. Box 28.1 outlines a national prevalence survey introduced through this partnership that estimates the national prevalence of RHD at 6.8 per 1,000 (Mucumbitsi et al., 2013). The implications of this survey will be discussed later in this chapter. The next sections outline collaborative efforts providing cardiovascular care and clinical training in Rwanda.

BOX 28.1 NATIONAL PREVALENCE SURVEY OF RHEUMATIC HEART DISEASE IN RWANDA

In 2011, an echocardiography screening study was performed among 2,800 school-age children in Gasabo district, which represented the first school age survey of RHD in Rwanda. The initiative was developed by Team Heart, Inc., in partnership with key collaborators: in-country cardiologists, the Rwanda Biomedical Center, the Rwanda Ethics Board, the MoH, the Ministry of Education, and the Rwanda Heart Foundation.

After the study was approved by the Rwanda Ethics Board, participants were identified and selected by the Rwanda Biomedical Center through a randomized process of lists of students provided by the Minister of Education to represent both urban and rural populations. Alternates were listed in the case of absence on the screening day. The parents and students completed an informational session in the native language, French, and English. Parental permission was obtained and each student was interviewed to complete a demographic survey.

Using the World Heart Federation (WHF) guidelines for echocardiographic diagnosis, the images were obtained by echocardiography. Twelve highly skilled sonographers from the United States were selected using a competitive application, and the echo machines were provided by Sonosite. The local health staff was trained during screening, thus establishing a structure that will be used subsequently to train a larger group of clinicians. The images were read and graded by sonographers. In the event of a positive finding by echo, or unrelated medical finding, an onsite pediatric cardiologist evaluated and confirmed findings. All images were recorded and downloaded daily to a server. Studies were read blindly and evaluated based on preidentified WHF international guidelines. Data from demographics and echo findings was collated and analyzed by the Rwanda Biomedical Center.

The study showed that the RHD prevalence among school-age children was around 6.8 per 1,000, of which 100% were new diagnoses. The study results were presented at the 11th Pan-African Society of Cardiology (PASCAR) congress and will be part of an upcoming manuscript (Mucumbitsi et al., 2013). This initial study focused on an at-risk population with relative access to care, and might not have accounted for other epidemiologic and geographic profiles. A follow-up study is in the planning stage to document these findings in a defined population, as well as provide data from more remote settings in the country.

Data from this study also found undiagnosed CHD cases, thus underscoring the high likelihood that these estimates are largely underrepresentative. This prevalence estimate is within the range of findings in other regions of Africa, which are from 2.3 to 30/1,000 (Zühlke et al., 2013).

BUILDING SPECIALTY CARE PROGRAMS THROUGH GLOBAL PARTNERSHIPS

The Rwanda Cardiovascular Care Consortium

Since 2009, Rwanda has increased access to cardiovascular care through doubling the availability of cardiologists and acquiring echocardiographic machines, among other efforts. A major issue, however, remains the lack of in-country cardiac surgeons. Recognizing the pressing and increasing need for cardiac surgery, the government of Rwanda is invested in establishing a national self-sustaining cardiac surgery program. The initial step was to develop collaborations with four expert teams to provide cardiac surgery in-country by leveraging their expertise and financial resources. With a shared vision, these visiting teams established the Rwanda Cardiovascular Care Consortium (RCCC), comprised of the Rwandan MoH, four Rwandan cardiologists, the Rwanda Heart Foundation, Team Heart, Inc. (the United States), Open Heart International (Australia), Healing Hearts Northwest (the United States), and Chain of Hope (Belgium). While global partnerships encounter major issues related to fragmentation and duplication of resources, the RCCC is committed to fostering synergy in participation and capacity building. For instance, RCCC members participated in the design of a customized surgical pack available in Rwanda. This customized pack was successfully debuted in 2014.

Under the collaborative leadership of the MoH, each team operates on acute and complex cases at King Faisal Hospital, a leading national referral center in Rwanda. At the time of this publication, RCCC members have performed 453 cardiac surgery procedures in Rwanda (Swain, Mucumbitsi, Rusingiza, Bolman, & Binagwaho, 2014). Figure 28.1 shows that in the period between 2006 and 2014 more than 70% of Rwandan patients that received cardiac surgery were treated by RCCC teams. Prior to this collaboration, the bulk of patients requiring cardiac surgery were sent abroad or added to an extensive waitlist.

Currently, it is estimated that nearly 2,000 patients with advanced RHD and CHD are awaiting surgery. This estimate far exceeds the ability of the country to send patients abroad for surgery. Only a small number of critically ill patients are

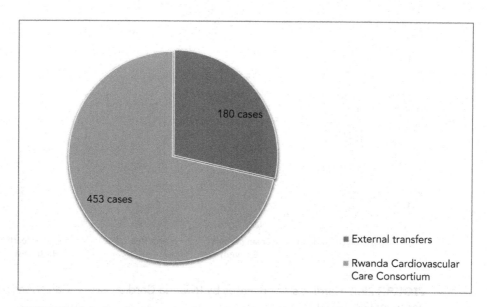

FIGURE 28.1 Cardiac surgery experience in Rwanda (2006–2014).
Adapted from Swain, Mucumbitsi et al. (2014). Adapted with permission.

transferred abroad with government support or private funding. The exact number of external transfers is unknown, but it is estimated that nearly 30 patients are sent to India, and 10 children are sent to Sudan to undergo surgical intervention at Salaam Hospital annually. However, several challenges make these out-of country transfers unsustainable. First, many patients die while awaiting transfer to external sites. Moreover, the costs associated with medical care and airfare can average $10,000 per person, requiring either the family or a donor to sponsor the patient and the accompanying care provider. Additionally, postsurgery outcomes can be affected as patients treated out of country might not access adequate follow-up care in case of complications.

Beyond critical challenges for patients, out-of-country transfers also result in missed opportunities, including training for the local health staff and strengthening the national health system. Rwanda has committed to establish an in-country solution by bringing together various stakeholders.

Each year, surgical development programs led by each visiting team provide surgery for 15 to 20 patients, with the majority of teams having operated on more than 100 patients since 2006 (see Figure 28.2). These teams are multidisciplinary and include surgeons, anesthesiologists, nurses, perfusionists, nurse practitioners, support staff, and volunteers (Swain, Mucumbitsi et al., 2014). The surgical development trips also present an important platform to raise awareness about the importance of prevention and early treatment, and sharing best practices in cardiovascular care. The impact of these procedures is being evaluated as part of a study on the cost-effectiveness of cardiac surgery interventions in resource-limited settings. This study will be mentioned further later in the chapter.

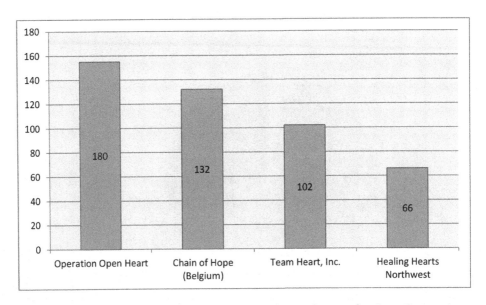

FIGURE 28.2 Cardiac surgery cases by Rwanda Cardiovascular Care Consortium per team (2006–2014).

Adapted from Swain, Mucumbitsi et al. (2014).

We believe the RCCC members have succeeded in streamlining innovative health care delivery infrastructures and helping to transition temporary measures into self-sustaining health care delivery that can be integrated into existing chronic-care delivery systems. In 2013, representatives of RCCC teams organized a special international session during the 9th Global Forum on Humanitarian Medicine in Cardiology and Cardiac Surgery held in Geneva, Switzerland. At the end of the special session, recommendations were shared by representatives of RCCC teams and a proposal was presented to the Rwandan MoH. This proposal will be a key document in developing the national cardiovascular care program. Such a program will ultimately be staffed by Rwandan physicians, nurses, and health staff trained in up-to-date care delivery skills. The benefit of a strong commitment to academic, research initiatives and collaboration will continue over time.

To maximize impact, Team Heart, Inc., a RCCC founding member, has expanded its contribution to the Rwandan health system by focusing on developing local capacity in various areas like supply chain management, health care workforce, and nursing care. We will discuss this comprehensive approach in a later section.

Human Resources for Health in Rwanda

In Rwanda, improving local capacity in human resources is among the national priority strategies (MoH of Rwanda, 2012a). In this section, we highlight two capacity-building programs addressing human resources challenges in specialty care: Human Resources for Health (HRH) and a Team Heart–led initiative.

Human Resources for Health

The HRH program is a 7-year partnership comprised of leading U.S.-based academic centers working to strengthen the education of nursing and medicine programs in Rwanda. HRH is the result of collaboration between the Rwandan MoH, USAID, and the Clinton Health Access Initiative. One of the main objectives of the HRH program is to create a strong foundation in the delivery and accessibility of health services. This initiative uses a "twinning" model for identified Rwandan teaching faculty and faculty from the U.S. academic centers. The targeted specialty areas include internal medicine, pediatrics, surgery, cardiology, critical care, health care management, and dental care (MoH of Rwanda, 2012a).

Team Heart Initiative in Human Resource Training

Since 2008, Team Heart has engaged nursing faculty in Kigali Health Institute, as well as faculty in medicine and surgery, to facilitate didactic and point-of-care learning opportunities. Team Heart and its partner organizations have mentored a core group of Rwandan health professionals through education, advising, and providing scholarships for specialized training abroad. However, many clinics and hospitals are severely short staffed, making it difficult to increase time for health professionals to learn specialized skills such as the basics of echocardiogram. As a bridge for improved care, expatriate nurses and part-time positions are incorporated to provide a temporary solution.

In 2013, an overall restructuring took place as part of a national effort to improve the quality of education and the number of graduates. The University of Rwanda, the only medical school in the country, reorganized several departments under new leadership to meet identified challenges in training the health workforce. It is anticipated that this major restructuring will impact chronic care for heart diseases and other NCDs. Thus, an initiative involving the national medical school was established to develop a 2-year certificate program with a comprehensive cardiology curriculum for internal medicine physicians and nurses (Come, 2012). This Team Heart–led effort was implemented in close collaboration with the MoH, local cardiologists, and the national College of Medicine and Health Sciences. The curriculum has been approved and a cohort from various district hospitals was selected.

Rwanda has sponsored the training of two anesthesiologists, in cardiac surgery and intensive care, who have since returned and work closely with the visiting teams. In 2012, a postgraduate surgical resident, and a former Team Heart mentee, was selected to go to South Africa for general and cardiovascular surgery training. He will most likely be among the first Rwandan cardiac surgeons in-country. Another collaborative capacity-building focus is perfusion, an area where trained individuals are scarce, yet in high demand locally and regionally. RCCC visiting teams work closely with two Rwandan perfusionists who received training in India but often work in other services. These perfusionists rely on the visiting teams to refresh and improve their skills.

Team Heart continues to work closely with the MoH and local key institutions listed in Box 28.2 to improve the capacity of human resources and to address the medical and surgical burden of rheumatic heart disease. The focus remains

BOX 28.2 LIST OF RWANDAN ORGANIZATIONS AFFILIATED WITH TEAM HEART, INC., THROUGH COLLABORATORS AND PATIENTS

Kanombe Military Hospital
Kigali Health Institute
King Faisal Hospital, Kigali
Ministry of Education, Rwanda
Ministry of Health, Rwanda
Rwanda Biomedical Center
Rwanda Heart Foundation
Rwanda Patient Care Network
University of Rwanda, College of Medicine and Health Sciences
University of Rwanda, School of Public Health
University Teaching Hospital of Butare
University Teaching Hospital of Kigali

on strategic interventions in line with national priorities, using a comprehensive approach detailed in the next section.

BUILDING A CARDIOVASCULAR CARE PROGRAM—THE TEAM HEART APPROACH

Over the past 8 years, Team Heart–supported projects have addressed gaps in cardiovascular care while strengthening the national capacity for the prevention and management of RHD in Rwanda. Although Team Heart's involvement began as a short-term mission, it has evolved into an implementing partner participating in a range of activities across Rwanda (Swain, Pugliese, et al., 2014). The evidence-based approach combines disease-specific and system-wide strategies to improve the access to cardiac care.

Cardiac Surgery

In resource-limited settings, the lack of access to basic health services results in patients presenting with illnesses in advanced clinical stages. A number of these patients become surgery candidates. We believe that providing specialty care such as cardiac surgery should be an ethical priority, regardless of individual or national income levels. Since 2008, Team Heart has performed more than 100 surgical operations at the King Faisal Hospital in Kigali, including on patients suffering from stage III and IV heart failure due to RHD (Swain, Pugliese, et al., 2014b). These high-risk surgical candidates would otherwise face premature death.

Preoperative surgical screening is organized annually, and occurs at least a week prior to the surgical schedule. The patients identified by local cardiologists are referred to major hospitals in Kigali for evaluation, including physical exams and echocardiography. The number of patients received during preop screening week varies, but has averaged 70 to 80 patients each year. Once the screening evaluations are completed, patient cases are prioritized by severity of illness and postoperative survival risk–benefit ratio. A patient selection meeting is held with all medical and surgical clinicians to finalize the surgical patient schedule. The case selection requires a close collaboration involving local and visiting specialists, and takes into account several factors (Swain, Pugliese, et al., 2014b).

Following patient selection, the clinical team and the patient determine the type of surgical intervention necessary. This process requires a thorough discussion regarding the appropriate valve type—mechanical or bioprosthetic—for each patient. Mechanical valves are the best option for durability but require a lifelong commitment to anticoagulant and international normalized ratio (INR) monitoring due to a high susceptibility to blood clotting. Female patients of childbearing age who receive mechanical valves are strongly advised to use birth control given potential major complications during pregnancy and childbirth. Another set of patients elects to receive bioprosthetic valves, particularly female patients who plan to have children. The bioprosthetic valves, however, are less durable than mechanical valves and may require subsequent replacement.

Access to surgical interventions is often a crucial limiting factor impeding health outcomes in resource-limited settings. However, high-risk surgical candidates with advanced RHD can receive triple valve operations in Rwanda with a high success rate (Swain, Pugliese, et al., 2014b). This Team Heart–led program has performed one of every four cardiac surgery procedures in the country (see Figure 28.2), and provided screening for nearly 4,000 patients. The surgical procedures performed involve single and multiple valve replacement for increasingly complex surgical cases. Through providing state-of-the-art patient care in Rwanda, visiting specialists contribute to the government of Rwanda's priority of decreasing external transfers, often unsustainable due to associated prohibitive costs. Furthermore, this effort promotes the ultimate national goal of developing a country-led cardiac surgery program. It also contributes to retaining and incentivizing physicians aspiring to practice surgical specialties.

Education and Training

Mentorship and in-service training are crucial components of our program. In Rwanda, a large number of district clinics are run by nurses (MoH of Rwanda, 2012a). Thus, investing in the advanced skills transfer can impact the system at large. For the past 7 years, Team Heart has facilitated skill acquisition and inpatient management by key operating room personnel, nurses, and medical residents at major referral hospitals. Ultimately, the trained staff transitioned from supervised clinical tasks to fully assuming patient care responsibilities. In addition to in-service training, a formal training program will be introduced to supplement the national efforts in training and retaining skilled nurses and health professionals (MoH of Rwanda, 2012a).

The minister of health requested the development of a comprehensive internal medicine curriculum for physicians across the country. A cardiology curriculum emerged from a needs assessment to examine the cause of complications and fatalities in postoperative cardiac surgery patients (Come, 2012). As mentioned earlier, this comprehensive curriculum was developed by cardiologists working in Rwanda, including members of Team Heart, Inc. and Healing Hearts Northwest. The curriculum was approved by the national medical school and the national senate. Twelve cohorts were selected for the program in 2014. The teaching team includes local cardiologists, HRH faculty, and scheduled visiting cardiologists. The curriculum allows general practitioners to graduate with fundamental knowledge in diagnosis and management of various heart conditions. Since general practitioners are rotated to health facilities countrywide, this curriculum will largely strengthen cardiovascular care both at the central and district levels.

Follow-Up Care

A major challenge following cardiac surgery operations is ensuring adequate follow-up care, particularly for patients in remote settings. Once patients are discharged postsurgery, they require routine and critical lifelong follow-up for treatment adherence and surveillance. An essential part of our program focuses on facilitating adequate and constant monitoring for postoperative patients.

Patients with mechanical valves require constant anticoagulation, including warfarin. The degree of anticoagulation is monitored closely through the INR test. At discharge, patients are provided with a booklet used to record their INR values, medication lists, and other comprehensive information. Patients are asked to bring this booklet at each subsequent visit to ensure optimal care and promote continuity of care from inpatient to outpatient management. Postcardiac surgery patients are particularly vulnerable to infections and require thorough monitoring. Patients traveling from remote sites are at risk to develop complications due to limited access to follow-up care. Our program identifies vulnerable patients that require additional support to meet follow-up appointments and receive medication.

As patients may require long-term anticoagulation regimens known to increase the risk of birth defects, it is critical to offer close follow-up care and educate postcardiac surgery female patients regarding pregnancy and childbirth. Female patients of childbearing age receive counseling on family planning and reproductive rights. In our experience, the most effective approach to minimizing postoperative risks has been to combine strong clinical care and patient education. Our team has developed patient education modules on pre- and postoperative care, with a special section on pregnancy. We introduce these discussions during preoperative patient education and the teaching is reinforced in a unified teaching plan until discharge from the hospital. The information is reiterated during follow-up visits. Currently, these tools are only available at referral hospitals but they will be widely distributed across the district sites.

A model of community-based intervention is being explored to further ensure continuity of care. This year, our program collaborated with health care providers at the district hospitals and health centers to reinforce education components including the types of heart valves, anticoagulation, and physical exam techniques. An effort that has resulted from the need to establish high-quality standardized care is the creation of postsurgery care pathways.

Postsurgery Care Pathways

Clinicians need clear guidelines to map clinic visits and assess progress during recovery. Our program has developed clinical pathways for valve replacement that were introduced during a recent cardiac surgery development visit. These care pathways ensure an effective model of care for postsurgery management, including an approach to heart failure and anticoagulation (see Figures 28.3 and 28.4). These pathways outline a comprehensive care protocol for patients with mechanical and bioprosthetic valves. Using an integrated care pathway provides guidelines to clinicians in the management of postsurgery follow-up care.

The potential for errors increases during the transfer of patient care responsibilities from central to district and eventually to the health center level. As discussed in a previous section, it is extremely important for patients of childbearing

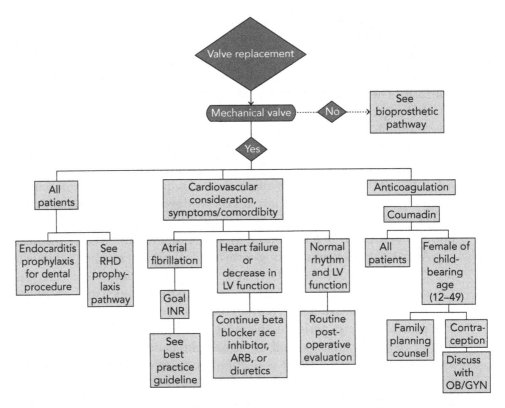

ARB, angiotensin receptor blocker; LV, left ventricle; RHD, rheumatic heart disease.
FIGURE 28.3 Mechanical valve replacement postoperative care pathway in Rwanda.
©Team Heart, Inc. (2014).

age (12 to 49 years) receiving warfarin to explore birth control options to prevent the high risk of birth defects and maternal health complications. Other postsurgical complications can also occur without an effective mechanism for continuity of care. Thus, tools and guidelines such as these pathways can facilitate the integration of postsurgery follow-up care. These care pathways will be distributed to clinicians at several levels of care, with an initial focus placed on the central and district facilities given the availability of trained personnel. Additional tools are being developed, including the best practice framework for postsurgical follow-up and a warfarin dosage protocol for further detailed guidelines.

National Nurse Coordinator

In 2010, Team Heart, Inc., in partnership with other RCCC teams, proposed a national nurse coordinator position created to coordinate postoperative care. Discussions regarding objectives, perceived needs, and supervisory oversight of the position created the opportunity to explore advanced nursing roles and the necessary partnerships for training. The position was developed over a few months with input from all partners, including the local team creating a new role of independent nursing practice.

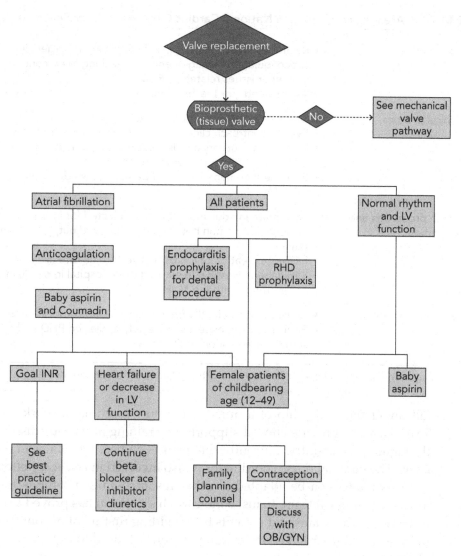

LV, left ventricle.

FIGURE 28.4 Bioprosthetic valve replacement postoperative care pathway, Rwanda.

©Team Heart, Inc. (2014).

Following two early deaths from preventable complications, the nurse clinical coordinator moved to the top of the task force agenda and was subsequently assigned to a Rwandan nurse. Team Heart and Healing Hearts Northwest provide financial support for this position while new funding and care priorities are being explored. Oversight, supervision, and monitoring are provided in close collaboration with the MoH. Four focus areas for the national nurse coordinator are included in Table 28.2.

In addition to improving access to cardiac surgery, the nurse coordinator works with health providers to address barriers to care. This approach acknowledges and addresses the fact that the majority of patients are received at health centers, which

TABLE 28.2 Areas of Focus for the National Cardiac Care Nurse Coordinator in Rwanda

Education	• Reinforce patient teaching, including cardiac surgery information, anticoagulation management and teaching (diet, conception, etc.), and other issues related to RHD • Assess needs for teaching tools utilization and improvement
Clinical practice	• Document existing system and identify strengths and weaknesses • Evaluate outreach clinic facilities and resources for follow-up care • Identify postsurgery needs and promote patient outcomes to monitoring INR and medication supply • Evaluate diet management of patients on warfarin and reinforce teaching
Health promotion and prevention	• Participate in education of nurses selected for screening project • Promote interaction between inpatient and outpatient clinical teams • Facilitate creation of a prospective chronic care clinic at Kibagabaga Hospital (a major district hospital in Kigali) in collaboration with the MoH
Research	• Collaborate to identify preliminary key indicators in improving care • Participate in prospective research studies on RHD and cardiac surgery interventions in Rwanda

INR, international normalized ratio; MoH, Ministry of Health; RHD, rheumatic heart disease.

fall under the leadership of a nurse. The nurse coordinator works closely with Team Heart to provide clinical support and training at various district hospitals throughout the country. Currently, the focus is on health facilities in remote rural areas. The national nurse coordinator is also involved in advocacy efforts.

This model can be adapted in other resource-limited settings that have no in-country surgical team. In just 6 months, this position has proved to be valuable in assisting physicians and patients by providing first point of contact for follow-up care. This important coordination position will need to expand as the number of cardiac surgery patients increases.

Outreach Clinical Services

In addition to providing surgical services, a continued focus is the promotion of early diagnosis and treatment of rheumatic heart surgery. This approach acknowledges the importance of addressing RHD primary and secondary prevention strategies. Our program coordinates and supports several outreach clinical services with in-country cardiologists and nurses. It is estimated that more than 90% of patients are received at the health center and district levels (MoH of Rwanda, 2012b). Thus, the main goal is to bridge the gap in diagnostic and therapeutic services between the central level, district centers, and remote areas in Rwanda.

In addition to confirming new diagnoses, trained staff and Team Heart specialists are developing further training, including instruction on basic echocardiography. We have facilitated the procurement of two portable echocardiographic machines used for outreach diagnosis and teaching tools. The local team will be able to significantly contribute to care management and education of onsite staff utilizing these resources.

A next step will be increased leadership by the MoH in securing a long-term budget and providing training to health care workers in areas removed from district health posts. Such a program is important, as it promotes disease prevention, case finding, and management. The growing and changing health needs will require providing access to diagnosis in remote areas, often high-risk areas for RHD, and target the most vulnerable individuals in society. We see outreach clinics as an important step in the management of acute rheumatic fever and rheumatic heart disease. Team Heart–led initiatives will continue to support outreach efforts to communities across Rwanda and improve the skills of clinicians involved.

Advocacy and Patient Support

Postsurgery, advocacy and support also play a key role as patients confront major challenges. Forced to interrupt work or education due to critical heart disease, patients may have been perceived as unable to function normally. An important part of the return to productive life is overcoming constraints due to prior physical limitations and potential stigmatization associated with heart disease.

Although it is beyond the current budget of the program to support all patients, some temporary assistance has been provided to help with urgent financial needs for medication, postoperative clinical visits, and nutritional support. A more sustainable solution currently being explored is facilitating income-generating activities and vocational education for postcardiac surgery patients, with local advocacy groups as stakeholders.

The Rwanda Patient Care Network (RPCN) was established to promote advocacy and patient support at the national level. The RPCN is an initiative that includes patients who received cardiac surgical care in-country by expatriate teams and those who received surgery abroad. Initially, this network provided an environment in which patients could access and receive support as they recovered. Subsequently, patient peers began to promote self-management efforts, an ideal approach given the chronic nature of their medical needs. This component of the program promotes mutual encouragement and support, reinforces health progress, and fosters community awareness and primary prevention. The RPCN also collaborates with Team Heart in developing long-term strategies that impact the socioeconomic background of patients, including income-generating activities.

We believe patient-centered organizations like the RPCN can be a driving force for patient support and advocacy locally and regionally. The RPCN is in the early stages of developing a potential partnership with a new RHD support group in Kenya to promote regional collaboration. The RPCN has become a key local implementation partner, and ensures that our approach remains context-specific and equitable.

National Registry

For many years, Rwandan cardiologists have maintained basic registries of the RHD patients they follow. However, there is currently no nationally maintained list that meets the guidelines for ASAP—awareness, surveillance, advocacy, and prevention—a regional model for RHD control (Robertson, Volmink, & Mayosi, 2006). Our program is part of a national strategy to create a reliable database to promote efficient chronic care systems, a priority for the MoH (Binagwaho et al., 2013b). Among other benefits, the registry would enhance patient follow-up, track critical resources for medication, and monitoring progress. We are collaborating with local colleagues to design the initial stages of organizing an electronic system to record patient information for RHD and other cardiovascular conditions. We hope to finalize this record-keeping system as an integrated component with the national medical record system.

National Prevalence Survey

As outlined in Box 28.1, a prevalence survey introduced a platform for early detection of RHD and other cardiovascular conditions among school-aged children. These participants are part of a high-risk group given their demographic profile. Team Heart and its partners engaged in this effort following projections that RHD was endemic in certain parts of the country (Ngirabega, 2013).

These efforts also aim to strengthen primary care by enabling structures for early diagnosis and surveillance of RHD that could be adapted to other disease clusters. The involvement of multiple local partners ensures that the tracking issues and trends are evaluated at various levels, and inform policy at the national level.

Procurement

The costs of medication can be prohibitively high for patients. Special consideration must be given to the distribution of cardiovascular medications, which can cause catastrophic outcomes if interrupted or overprescribed. We have found it extremely beneficial to distribute INR strips for self-monitoring to patients on warfarin, particularly those who live in remote settings. However, it is not a broad solution to addressing the countrywide need for all patients requiring INR management. The necessary equipment should be available for patients at various levels of care for adequate follow-up care.

Since 2010, our program participates in coordinating the implementation of warfarin distribution at the district and health center levels. While Team Heart-supported facilities subsidize warfarin for individual patients, national level strategies have to be developed to address shortages on a larger scale. In 2012, warfarin was added to the national list of essential medications in response to post–cardiac surgery patients facing complications due to limited access to anticoagulation.

Advanced medical interventions like specialty surgery require meticulous management of equipment and consumables. Typically, these are acquired and transported from external sources at large costs, which in turn increases the cost of procedures at the local level. Thus, a successful procurement program requires coordinated local participation and involves obtaining equipment and pharmaceuticals needed at an efficient price, while concurrently developing processes for tracking and safe storage. Rwanda has integrated supply chain strategies in response to procurement challenges. A growing number of medications including equipment are delivered by local providers. Our program is working closely with pharmacists and other procurement professionals to implement warfarin distribution, avoid stock-outs, and strengthen supply chain management for cardiac care. Another component discussed earlier is the design of a customized national surgical pack—a procurement and coordination strategy by the RCCC teams. Table 28.3 outlines the approach to RHD used by Team Heart.

TABLE 28.3 Overview of Team Heart's Approach in Addressing Rheumatic Heart Disease in Rwanda

PROGRAMS	OBJECTIVES
Cardiac surgery	• Provide lifesaving heart surgery to adolescents and young adults affected by critical RHD, who would otherwise face premature death • Reduce out-of-country patient transfers for cardiac surgical procedures • Provide collaborative leadership in establishing a country-led, sustainable cardiac surgery program
Education and training	• Provide in-service training and education to medical and nursing staff (medical residents, OR, ICU, and step-down nurses, perfusionists, medical students) • Participate in the national capacity-building efforts for nursing and medical education and facilitate the retention of trained clinicians • Organize seminars and guest speaker series to promote best-practice sharing among health workers, policy makers, and other stakeholders
Follow-up care	• Provide follow-up care in inpatient setting • Facilitate follow-up care and management in outpatient setting • Develop and distribute patient education modules to improve patient outcomes and self-management of INR
Postsurgery care pathways	• Introduce tools to promote a standardized process of care • Ensure that clinical outcomes are achieved and maintained • Enhance continuity of care for postcardiac surgery patients at the district and health care levels
National nurse coordinator for cardiac care	• Facilitate cooperative efforts in clinical care, health promotion, training, and research (see Table 28.2)

(continued)

TABLE 28.3 Overview of Team Heart's Approach in Addressing Rheumatic Heart Disease in Rwanda (*continued*)

PROGRAMS	OBJECTIVES
Outreach clinical services	• Promote early diagnosis, case finding, and disease management • Bridge the gap in diagnostic and therapeutic services between the central level and district centers • Provide training in basic echocardiography and procure necessary equipment
Advocacy and patient education	• Reduce stigma and promote patient compliance • Promote community awareness and primary prevention • Support and collaborate with the Rwanda Patient Care Network
National prevalence survey	• Strengthen strategies for early diagnosis and surveillance of RHD • Involve multiple local partners at various levels to ensure that implementation, and build foundation for subsequent national prevalence survey • Inform policy at the national level
National Registry	• Assist in establishing reliable national database for RHD and other heart conditions to be integrated in the national medical record system • Facilitate compliance with regional models for RHD control like ASAP program • Enhance patient follow-up, track critical resources for medication and monitoring progress
Procurement	• Facilitate provision and distribution of cardiovascular medication • Distribute INR strips for self-monitoring to patients receiving warfarin, with a particular focus on those who live in remote settings • Collaborate with procurement professionals to implement warfarin distribution, avoid stock-outs, and develop a strong supply chain process for cardiac care • Assist in the design and procurement of a customized surgical pack for cardiac surgery procedures in Rwanda

ASAP, awareness, surveillance, advocacy, and prevention; ICU, intensive care unit; INR, international normalized ratio; OR, operating room; RHD, rheumatic heart disease.

The partnership between Team Heart and Rwanda is also generating strong collaborations regionally and globally. The recognition that cooperative efforts must move the agenda forward led to the involvement of internationally renowned clinicians like Sir Magdi Yacoub, founder of Chain of Hope (CoH) UK,—in a forthcoming project to improve cardiovascular disease outcomes in the region. Team Heart was also invited to participate in the NCD Synergies Initiative discussed in the next section.

NCD SYNERGIES INITIATIVE

Currently, only a few countries in sub-Saharan Africa and other resource-limited settings have integrated NCDs into their national health plan. Team

Heart-sponsored projects have been credited with significant contributions in the area of cardiovascular care in Rwanda. In 2013, Team Heart representatives were invited to join the NCD Synergies Initiative as implementing partners during the inaugural meeting in Kigali, Rwanda. The NCD Synergies Initiative is a driving force behind the recent global health movement "80×40×20" (Binagwaho, Muhimpundu, & Bukhman, 2014). Currently, the ministries of health in 12 sub-Saharan African countries have pledged support to this initiative. This coalition will identify and promote a global community focused on planning and implementation of services for NCDs in the identified high-risk areas.

The organization is establishing a platform for partner organizations and individuals to convene around a common agenda, share good practices, and coordinate initiatives in the region. The ultimate goal is to integrate the NCD program in the country's health system, and improve effectiveness by encouraging local ownership. This goal will be facilitated by support and planning for new integrated NCD services, identification of people living with NCDs, and provision for their long-term care.

LOOKING AHEAD

A sustainable partnership requires a strong multidisciplinary team with clear and collaboratively defined goals. Team Heart, the Rwanda MoH, and other key partners continue to design a sustainable and integrated model for RHD care with local and regional implications. Our program will continue to follow and advance the evidence base on cardiovascular care in resource-limited settings.

Ongoing assessment of various projects is used to identify and address major gaps. It is clear that providing cardiac surgery through visiting teams four times a year is a temporary solution, especially given the expanding waiting list of nearly 2,000 individuals in need of cardiac surgery. Moreover, integrating visiting teams into the surgical schedule of existing referral hospitals is a limiting factor, as these high-volume health facilities have to manage other types of surgeries using the same operating rooms. As a result, elective surgery is curtailed and emergency care must take priority. A permanent solution is required in order to improve long-term health and development outcomes.

National Cardiovascular Care Center

Although referral hospitals are the major sites of specialty care, there is no health facility that offers advanced cardiovascular care year-round. As discussed earlier, cardiac surgery is provided periodically by visiting teams. Recognizing the need for a permanent health facility, the government of Rwanda and Team Heart, Inc. are planning to build the first national center of excellence for cardiovascular care. The hospital will be dedicated to the diagnosis and medical and surgical management of cardiac diseases in Rwanda and East Africa. Beyond impacting health outcomes countrywide, the cardiac center will also serve as a training site for clinicians from district hospitals. This joint venture will ultimately develop local and regional capacity.

While establishing the country-led cardiac care center, our ongoing collaboration with the faculty of the medicine and nursing programs at the University of Rwanda will be key in ensuring effective strategies in strengthening the national health workforce.

Cost-Effectiveness Study

Our program is committed to an evidence-based approach. Currently, Team Heart is a principal collaborator on a study looking at the cost-effectiveness of cardiovascular interventions in resource-limited settings. Two major outcomes will be evaluated: the utility and cost-effectiveness of surgery and the improvement in the quality of life gained from surgical intervention. The study will provide instrumental data and inform evidence-based interventions in Rwanda. It is anticipated that this study will also have regional implications as other low-income countries consider the need and feasibility of establishing a national cardiac surgery program.

Team Heart affiliates are also contributing to biomedical research in the country. A study is being developed to identify the genetic etiologies of RHD in Rwanda. The study population will include Team Heart patients. Results from this study can have a significant impact given the extremely limited data on genetic determinants of rheumatic fever and rheumatic heart disease.

CONCLUSION

The partnerships presented demonstrate the important role of collaborative efforts in tackling complex and changing health issues. In this chapter, the discussions focused on partnerships that are integrated within the national program to promote a long-term impact on health outcomes. As our experience shows, effective disease management and control require evidence-based interventions. While Team Heart and partner organizations have supported projects specific to rheumatic heart disease, these efforts have been integrated into the HSSP and the NCD strategic plan, thus ensuring a system-wide impact. By creating scalable programs of RHD outreach and detection, and designing clear pathways for long-term follow-up care, our program has prepared a platform to ensure that building a cardiac center would be a sustainable solution to the growing cardiovascular care needs.

We recognize that there are many complex issues beyond the scope of this chapter, such as addressing risk factors for heart diseases. For instance, the impact of social determinants should be considered in order to achieve optimal health outcomes for RHD. Often, the sociocultural context of patients and their families deeply influences delivery of care. An extensive program of social support for patients would tackle some of these factors.

Although it is outside the scope of this chapter to discuss medical comorbidities like mental illness, sexual reproduction, and malaria, these challenges add to the complexity of patient cases. An effective method to address these challenges has been to refer affected patients to appropriate care providers and facilitate follow-up care whenever possible. The need remains to build capacity and facilitate other specialty care partnerships for these complex patients.

A country-led approach is needed to ensure significant progress is achieved and maintained. Although regional and global partnerships can play an important role in providing health interventions, local leadership should ensure that it fits within national priorities.

REFERENCES

Binagwaho, A. N., Farmer, P. E., Nsanzimana, S., Karema, C., Gasana, M., Ngirabega, J. D., . . . Drobac, P. (2013a). Rwanda 20 years on: Investing in life. *The Lancet, 14.* doi:10.1016/S0140-6736(14)60574-2

Binagwaho, A., Rusingiza, E. K., Mucumbitsi, J., Wagner, C. M., Swain, J. D., Nutt, C. T., . . . Bolman, R.M. (2013b). Uniting to address pediatric heart disease in Africa: Advocacy from Rwanda: Commentary. *South Africa Heart, 10,* 440–446.

Binagwaho, A. N., Muhimpundu, M. A., & Bukhman, G. (2014). 80 Under 40 by 2020: An equity agenda for NCD's and injuries. *The Lancet, 383,* 3–4. doi:10.1016/S0140-6736(13) 62423-X

Bloom, D. E., Cafiero, E. T., Jané-Llopis, E., Abrahams-Gessel, S., Bloom, L. R., Fathima, S., Feigl, A. B., . . .Weinstein, C. (2011). *The global economic burden of noncommunicable diseases.* Geneva, Switzerland: World Economic Forum.

Bukhman, G., & Kidder, A. (2011). *The PIH guide to chronic care integration for endemic noncommunicable diseases.* Boston, MA: Partners In Health.

Come, P. C. (2012). *Curriuculum for diploma program for general practitioners in cardiology and care of postoperative cardiac surgery patients.* Unpublished manuscript, University of Rwanda, Kigali, Rwanda.

Little, M. (2012). *Working toward transformational health partnerships in low- and middle-income countries.* Retrieved from https://www.bsr.org/en/our-insights/report-view/working-toward-transformational-health-partnerships

Logie, D. E., Rowson, M., & Ndagije, F. (2008). Innovations in Rwanda's health system: Looking to the future. *Lancet, 372*(9634), 256–261. doi:10.1016/S0140-6736(08)60962-9

Ministry of Health of Rwanda. (2012a). *Health sector strategic plan III 2012–2018.* Kigali, Rwanda.

Ministry of Health of Rwanda. (2012b). *Rwanda annual health statistics booklet 2011.* Retrieved from http://www.moh.gov.rw/fileadmin/templates/HMIS_Docs/MOH_Annual_booklet-2011.pdf

Ministry of Health of Rwanda. (2013). *Rwanda annual health statistics booklet 2012.* Retrieved from http://www.moh.gov.rw/fileadmin/templates/MOH-Reports/MOH_Booklet_2012_final_September_2013.pdf

Mucumbitsi, J., Rusingiza, E. K., Bulwer, B., Puneeta, A., Breakey, S., Bolman, C. P., . . . Kaplan E. L. (2013, May). *Echocardiography prevalence study for rheumatic heart disease in school children in Rwanda.* Abstract presented at the Pan-African Society of Cardiology (PASCAR) conference, Dakar, Senegal.

Ngirabega, J. (2013, May). *Integrating rheumatic heart disease in Rwanda's national NCD plan.* Presentation at the World Heart Federation, Geneva, Switzerland.

Robertson, K. A., Volmink, J. A., & Mayosi, B. M. (2006). Toward a uniform plan for the control of rheumatic fever and rheumatic heart disease in Africa—the Awareness, Surveillance, Advocacy, and Prevention (A.S.A.P.) Program. *South African Medical Journal, 96*, 241–245.

Swain, J. D., Mucumbitsi, J., Rusingiza, E., Bolman, R. M., & Binagwaho, A. (2014). Cardiac surgery for advanced rheumatic heart disease in Rwanda. *Lancet Global Health, 3.* doi:10.1016/S2214-109X(14)70022-1

Swain, J., Pugliese, D. N., Mucumbitsi, J., Rusingiza, E. K., Ruhamya, N., Kagame, A., & Bolman, R. M. (2014). Partnership for sustainability in cardiac surgery to address critical rheumatic heart disease in sub-Saharan Africa: The experience from Rwanda. *World Journal of Surgery.* Retrieved from http://www.biomedsearch.com/nih/Partnership-Sustainability-in-Cardiac-Surgery/24728579.html

Travis, P., Bennett, S., Haines, A., Pang, T., Bhutta, Z., Hyder, A. A., . . . Evans, T. (2004). Overcoming health-systems constraints to achieve the Millennium Development Goals. *The Lancet, 364*, 900–906.

World Health Organization. (2004). *Rheumatic heart disease and rheumatic fever.* (Technical Report Series 923). Geneva, Switzerland: World Health Organization.

World Health Organization. (2011a). *Global status report on non-communicable diseases 2010.* Geneva, Switzerland: World Health Organization.

World Health Organization. (2011b). *Non-communicable diseases country profiles.* Geneva, Switzerland: World Health Organization.

Zühlke, L., Mirabel, M., & Marijon, E. (2013). Congenital heart disease and rheumatic heart disease in Africa: Recent advances and current priorities. *Heart BMJ, 99*, 1554–1561. doi:10.1136/heartjnl-2013-303896

CHAPTER 29

Dreyfus Health Foundation: Advancing the Future of Global Health Nursing

Pamela Hoyt-Hudson, Hsin-Ling Tsai, Joyce J. Fitzpatrick, and Barry H. Smith

THE GLOBAL BURDEN OF DISEASE AND THE GLOBAL HEALTH IMPERATIVE

Assessing the global burden of disease (GBD) is a critical but challenging endeavor. If health systems and interventions around the world are to be effective and measurably reduce this burden, accurate information about the true burden must be available. To address this need for data, the World Bank and the World Health Organization (WHO) launched the GBD Study in 1991 (World Bank, 1993). The most recent GBD assessment is the 2010 study, which provides data for 1990, 2005, and 2010 (Murray & Lopez, 2013). The report represents the herculean efforts of several hundred investigators examining data from 187 countries covering 291 diseases and injuries, with additional data on 1,160 sequelae of these causes, as well as assessment of the mortality and disease burden attributable to 67 risk factors or clusters of risk factors.

The report makes several critical points relevant to this chapter. First of all, despite the relative stability of the disability-adjusted life years (DALYs) figure between 1990 and 2010 (2,497 million DALYs in 1990 versus 2,482 million DALYs in 2010) and the good news that that stability implies,[1] it is clear that the burden of disease remains unacceptably high. Tables 29.1 and 29.2 present a comparative look at the DALYs' ranking of the 25 leading diseases and injuries, as well as for the 25 leading risk factors, for 1990 and 2010. Among the 25 top diseases and injuries (Table 29.1), there have been some dramatic positive changes, with diarrhea having moved from a rank of 2 to 4; preterm birth complications from 3 to 8; tuberculosis from 8 to 13; protein-energy malnutrition from nine to 20; and meningitis, from 18 to 25. On the negative side, ischemic heart disease has moved from a rank of 4 to 1 in 2010; stroke from 5 to 3; HIV from 33 to 5; diabetes from 21 to 14; and major depressive disorder from 15 to 11. Over the 20-year period, malaria moved from a rank of 7 to 6, indicating that we have not made anywhere near the progress we should have made with this debilitating communicable parasitic disease.

TABLE 29.1 Ranking of Disability-Adjusted Life Years (DALYs) by Disease

CAUSE	2010		1990	
	RANK	DALYs (95% UI) IN THOUSANDS	RANK	DALYs (95% UI) IN THOUSANDS
Ischemic heart disease	1	129,795 (119,218–117,398)	4	100,455 (96,669–108,702)
Lower respiratory tract infections	2	115,227 (102,255–126,972)	1	206,461 (183,354–222,979)
Stroke	3	102,239 (90,472–108,003)	5	86,012 (81,033–94,802)
Diarrhea	4	89,524 (77,595–99,193)	2	183,543 (168,791–197,655)
HIV/AIDS	5	81,549 (74,694–88,371)	33	18,118 (14,996–22,269)
Malaria	6	82,689 (63,465–109,846)	7	69,141 (54,547–85,589)
Low back pain	7	80,667 (56,066–108,723)	12	56,384 (38,773–76,233)
Preterm birth compilations	8	76,980 (66,210–88,132)	3	105,965 (88,144–120,894)
Chronic obstructive pulmonary disease	9	76,779 (66,000–89,147)	6	78,298 (70,407–86,849)
Road-traffic injury	10	75,487 (61,555–94,777)	11	56,651 (49,633–68,046)
Major depressive disorder	11	63,239 (47,894–80,784)	15	46,177 (34,524–58,436)
Neonatal encephalopathy	12	50,163 (40,351–59,810)	10	60,604 (50,209–74,826)
Tuberculosis	13	49,399 (40,027–56,009)	8	61,256 (55,465–71,083)
Diabetes mellitus	14	46,857 (40,212–55,252)	21	27,719 (21,668–32,925)
Iron-deficiency anemia	15	45,350 (31,046–64,616)	14	46,803 (32,604–66,097)
Sepsis and other infectious disorders in newborns	16	44,236 (27,349–72,418)	17	46,029 (25,147–70,357)
Congenital anomalies	17	38,890 (31,891–45,739)	13	54,245 (45,491–69,057)
Self-harm	18	36,655 (26,894–44,652)	19	29,605 (23,039–37,333)
Falls	19	35,406 (28,583–44,052)	22	25,900 (21,252–31,656)
Protein-energy malnutrition	20	34,874 (27,957–41,662)	9	60,542 (50,378–71,619)
Neck pain	21	32,651 (22,783–44,857)	25	23,107 (16,031–31,890)

(continued)

TABLE 29.1 Ranking of Disability-Adjusted Life Years (DALYs) by Disease (continued)

CAUSE	2010		1990	
	RANK	DALYs (95% UI) IN THOUSANDS	RANK	DALYs (95% UI) IN THOUSANDS
Cancer of the trachea, bronchus, or lung	22	32,405 (24,401–38,327)	24	23,850 (18,839–29,837)
Other musculoskeletal disorders	23	30,877 (25,858–34,650)	29	20,596 (17,025–23,262)
Cirrhosis of the liver	24	31,026 (25,951–34,629)	23	24,325 (20,653–27,184)
Meningitis	25	29,407 (25,578–33,442)	18	37,822 (33,817–44,962)

Source: Murray and Lopez (2013). Copyright Massachusetts Medical Society. Reprinted with permission from Massachusetts Medical Society.

Table 29.2 reports the 25 leading risk factors for DALYs in 1990 and 2010. High blood pressure, as can be seen, has moved from a rank of 4 to 1, consistent with the change in ischemic heart disease over the same period. Tobacco smoking increased its rank from 7 to 2; diet low in fruit from 7 to 4 and suboptimal diet in several categories increased ranking; high-fasting plasma glucose level, from 9 to 7; lead exposure from 31 to 25; alcohol use from 8 to 5; and drug use from 25 to 19. On the positive side, childhood underweight moved from 1 to 8; iron deficiency from 11 to 13; suboptimal breastfeeding from 5 to 14; and exposure to ambient particulate matter pollution, from 6 to 9. Physical activity and intimate partner violence were not examined in 1990, but it seems likely that the former has decreased and the latter has increased over this period. As with the disease and injury categories, there has been significant progress in some areas and none or even worsening in others.

Clear from the data in Tables 29.1 and 29.2, as well as the additional analyses of the GBD Study (Murray & Lopez, 2013), is the fact that the global health situation has changed dramatically and will continue to do so. The first major change is in the demographics, with both an increase in the global population and the increasing average age of that population. The second shift is in the age- and sex-specific rates of death associated with diseases and injuries. DALYs associated with communicable, maternal, neonatal, and nutritional diseases decreased by 52.1% because of decreases in the corresponding rates of death, while decreases in DALYs associated with noncommunicable diseases (NCDs) were much smaller. These data indicate that despite the global increase in life expectancy from 1990 to 2010 (62.8–67.5 years for men and 68.1–73.3 years for women), the burden of noncommunicable disease continues to grow and will mean that globally, although people are living longer, more of those years will be spent living with the consequences of chronic illness and, consequently, the DALYs associated with them. This is, in fact, the key to the third major

TABLE 29.2 Ranking of Disability-Adjusted Life Years (DALYs) by Risk Factor

RISK FACTOR	2010		1990	
	RANK	DALYs (95% UI) IN THOUSANDS	RANK	DALYs (95% UI) IN THOUSANDS
High blood pressure	1	173,556 (155,939–189,025)	4	137,017 (124,360–149,366)
Tobacco smoking, including exposure to secondhand smoke	2	156,838 (136,543–173,057)	3	151,766 (136,367–169,522)
Household air pollution from solid fuels	3	108,084 (84,891–132,983)	2	170,693 (139,087–199,504)
Diet low in fruit	4	104,095 (81,833–124,169)	7	80,453 (63,298–95,763)
Alcohol use	5	97,237 (87,087–107,658)	8	73,715 (66,090–82,089)
High body mass index	6	93,609 (77,107–110,600)	10	51,565 (40,786–62,557)
High-fasting plasma glucose level	7	89,012 (77,743–101,390)	9	56,358 (48,720–65,030)
Childhood underweight	8	77,316 (64,497–91,943)	1	197,741 (169,224–238,276)
Exposure to ambient particulate–matter pollution	9	76,163 (68,086–85,171)	6	81,699 (71,012–92,859)
Physical inactivity or low level of activity	10	69,318 (58,646–80,182)	—	—
Diet high in sodium	11	61,231 (40,124–80,342)	12	46,183 (30,363–60,604)
Diet low in nuts and seeds	12	51,289 (33,482–65,959)	13	40,525 (26,308–51,741)
Iron deficiency	13	48,225 (33,769–67,592)	11	51,841 (37,477–71,202)
Suboptimal breastfeeding	14	47,537 (29,868–67,518)	5	110,261 (69,615–153,539)
High total cholesterol level	15	40,900 (31,662–50,484)	14	39,526 (32,704–47,202)
Diet low in whole grains	16	40,762 (32,112–48,486)	18	29,404 (23,097–35,134)

(continued)

TABLE 29.2 Ranking of Disability-Adjusted Life Years (DALYs) by Risk Factor (*continued*)

RISK FACTOR	2010		1990	
	RANK	DALYs (95% UI) IN THOUSANDS	RANK	DALYs (95% UI) IN THOUSANDS
Diet low in vegetables	17	38,559 (26,006–51,658)	16	31,558 (21,349–41,921)
Diet low in seafood n-3 fatty acids	18	28,199 (20,624–35,974)	20	21,740 (15,869–27,537)
Drug use	19	23,810 (18,780–29,246)	25	15,171 (11,714–19,369)
Occupational risk factors for injuries	20	23,444 (17,736–30,904)	21	21,265 (16,644–26,702)
Occupation-related low back pain	21	21,750 (14,492–30,533)	23	17,841 (11,846–24,945)
Diet high in processed meat	22	20,939 (6,982–33,468)	24	17,359 (5,137–27,949)
Intimate-partner violence	23	16,794 (11,373–23,087)	—	—
Diet low in fiber	24	16,452 (7,401–25,783)	26	13,347 (5,970–20,751)
Lead exposure	25	13,936 (11,750–16,327)	31	5,365 (4,534–6,279)

Source: Murray and Lopez (2013). Copyright Massachusetts Medical Society. Reprinted with permission from Massachusetts Medical Society.

trend, which is that disability, rather than premature death, is becoming the predominant feature of the burden of disease in both the highly developed and still developing regions of the world. Disability is costly both in terms of quality of life and the health systems required to manage or mitigate them (see, e.g., Coyte, Asche, Croxford, & Chan, 1998; Honeycutt et al., 2013; United States Renal Data System [USRDS], 2013;[2] Yelin & Callahan, 1995).

One must be careful not to overuse the global picture in relation to specific countries or regions and/or communities within them. While the broad trends remain valid, approaches to reducing both premature death and DALYs must be specific to local situations. Nonetheless, if one looks at the risk factors correlated with the leading cause of attributable DALYs, the list includes alcohol use (22 countries), high body mass index (32 countries), high fasting plasma glucose level (three countries), household air pollution (14 countries), high blood pressure (59 countries), smoking tobacco (24 countries), and low childhood weight (31 countries) (Murray & Lopez, 2013). In other words, there are both differences and commonalities. The bottom line, however, is that a substantial portion, if not the majority of, the major risk factors have strong elements of human behavior. This, coupled with the fact that NCDs, and chronic illness more generally, develop over time with a host of modifiable risk factors responsible, suggests an important imperative regarding approaches to the reduction of global and local disease burdens, as well as their quality of life and economic costs in the years ahead. That clearly is the urgent imperative for all the health professions.

MEETING THE CHALLENGES

Achieving better health outcomes and better quality of life for all people, while making our health care systems sustainable from an economic point of view, are the three critical elements of the challenges outlined by the data collected and analyzed by the GBD study over the past 20 years. The challenge of communicable diseases, with HIV and malaria prominent among them, as well as maternal mortality and low birth weight and childhood underweight remain, but noncommunicable disease and/or chronic illness present new and costly challenges both in regard to quality of life and economic cost (productivity and care) to society. Medical and nursing care in the traditional sense must continue to improve through new efficiencies and new treatments derived from basic and clinical research. However, the elements of health promotion, disease prevention, earlier detection, and better disease management must have far greater emphasis in the overall model of health and health care delivery. Beyond this, the public at large must be engaged as active participants in their own health care. They must be made members of the health care and promotion team. This approach means a revolutionary change in our concept of the health workforce and the way we think about health. Health must be both a right and responsibility if we are to achieve better "health for all."

There will never be enough nurses, physicians, and other health professionals to meet the health care needs of today or tomorrow. The traditional health care workforce can never be everyplace it needs to be, nor can it be fully effective in these same places. Health care cannot remain behind the walls of clinics or hospitals, but must rather move out into the community, where the most positive and cost-effective benefits can be achieved. This is where the greatest good can be done (Smith, 2013). Individuals and communities must be mobilized and encouraged to do what needs to be done to make the world a healthier place.

THE CRITICAL PLACE OF NURSING IN THE NEW HEALTH MODEL

It is one thing to consider the new model of achieving health in the abstract, but it is not enough. How are we to implement this sea change? We need to start with some basic principles. They include:

1. There is far too much unnecessary disease, suffering, and lost human potential and this cannot be tolerated. A correlate of this is that every human life is of tremendous value both intrinsically and in relation to its ability to contribute to the common good.

2. A significant percentage of the disease burden of individuals and communities is secondary to human behavior and therefore is subject to preventive and healthy lifestyle measures.

3. Individuals and communities, given the proper education and tools, are going to be the most effective means of addressing the behaviors that lead to specific disease problems. Put another way, the people with the problems are not the problem. Rather, they are the solution, and their capacity to make the required changes must be unleashed.

4. Nurses and nursing are in the ideal position to act in the capacity of the unleashers of the potential of individuals and communities to take far more responsibility for their own health. In effect, the individuals and communities become an integral, active part of the health care system, rather than its (passive) objects.

The reason that nurses and nursing are so critical in the respect described above, as well as in health reform more generally, is that they are at the crucial interface between the complex, often highly technological, health care system and individuals and communities. Acting in a wide range of roles, they have the ability to interact directly with individuals, families, and communities, as well as with the myriad of health care providers and payers, regulatory bodies, bureaucracies, and policy makers/legislators that are part of health care today. Whether as a school, clinic, home-visit, hospital, community, research, or administrative, supervisory nurse, he/she is the critical nexus between the professional side of the health system and the widest possible implementation of good health practices in society as a whole. The nurse supervising individuals who may be serving their communities as community health workers of one sort or another is also their anchor, while the community people serve as his/her extension in the community to be certain that everyone is getting the best care possible and experiencing the highest quality of life attainable, given the particular circumstances. Nurses and nursing can, and must, seize the opportunity being presented for the good of the people as well as the system. Nursing as a discipline is what will hold the new system together and make it function well.

To seize the opportunity, indeed the imperative facing the health system, nursing must take on an increasing leadership responsibility. To do so is not a simple matter. It means that nursing can and must be the organizing principle for any health system. That has not been the traditional view. Rather, it has been the physician who has been presumed to be the center of the health care universe. The level and rigor of education provided to, and/or required of, nurses, and the historical domination of health care by males (physicians and administrators) in both the developed and developing worlds, have conspired to constrain the practice of nursing. However, the new organizational and economic structure of health care, as well as the demands placed on that structure, mandates a change. Nursing can, and must, take a new and very central role in the new structure.

How is nursing to meet the challenges and take its role in the new model of health? The answer to this question must be multifactorial. Improved education, leadership training and opportunities, support from physicians as individuals and professional organizations, and governmental legislators and regulators, among others, are important. This chapter details one approach to enhancing the role of nursing and nurses as leaders and innovators in achieving sustainable change for the betterment of health. The approach is that of the Dreyfus Health Foundation (DHF) and its Problem Solving for Better Health®(PSBH) model, which has been developed over 25 years and implemented in 32 countries. Focused initially on community mobilization, it has increasingly evolved to emphasize nursing because of the critical role it holds in the entire health model.

THE DHF MODEL FOR IMPROVING GLOBAL HEALTH

The DHF is a division of the Rogosin Institute (RI), a not-for-profit (501)(c)(3) medical care and research organization affiliated with New York-Presbyterian Hospital (NYPH) and Weill Cornell Medical College. DHF seeks to improve health throughout the world by leveraging the capabilities of people through two programmatic models tied together by the common theme of strengthening the world's workforce. What makes DHF unique is the emphasis on drawing upon the innate potential of all people . . . the world's most important resource—and, of course, nursing as the way to maximize realization of that potential.

By mobilizing members of the general population as part of the workforce, PSBH is introduced at the grassroots level to involve the community in developing ways to solve their own health challenges. PSBH workshops have been implemented in more than 30 countries with more than 60,000 participants, inspiring 40,000 individual projects to improve health (Smith, 2011).

The result is an increase in the ownership and acceptability of approaches related to prevention, treatment, and the social determinants of health. By applying the PSBH approach, health professionals, including students and practitioners, and community members develop solutions to local health care problems, improve health care delivery, and work together to support and maximize each other's strengths.

The success of the PSBH program replicated worldwide demonstrates how even very poor communities can organize themselves in collective, participatory, and constructive ways to solve immediate problems, influence public policy, and strive for better life conditions no matter where they live. PSBH is about creating systemic change at the local level through civic engagement, continuous community health improvement, and an emphasis on improving quality of life for individuals and families.

THE PSBH MODEL

The history of the PSBH model is described in detail in Smith (2011). The founders shared a frustration with the lack of impact of the standard approaches to better health projects around the world. They saw a clear need for a program that encouraged people to:

1. Think more critically about the problems they face
2. Take more responsibility for solving those problems in order to create better health and a better quality of life

3. Develop confidence in their abilities to solve the problems without waiting for someone else, from within or outside the country, to do it
4. Make use of available resources to solve the problem. (Instead of saying "Give us some money and we'll solve the problem," the PSBH approach teaches "Let us solve the problem first and then see what is really needed to implement the solution proposed" (Smith, 2011, p. 18)

The first PSBH program was launched in August 1989 at West China University of Medical Sciences (WCUMS) (now part of Sichuan University) in Chengdu, Sichuan Province, China. The program engages individuals and communities in the following action-oriented five-step process to solve local health problems (Smith, 2011, p. 19).

Step One: Define the problem
Step Two: Prioritize the problem
Step Three: Define a solution
Step Four: Create an action plan
Step Five: Take action

The five-step framework is introduced over the course of an initial 2- to 3-day PSBH workshop held in community-based settings, academic institutions, or health care facilities. During the initial workshop, each participant devises an action plan to address a relevant health problem that he or she wants to solve. After the workshop training, the participant executes the project in his or her work environment or home community. Each project requires an evaluation tool so that impact and outcomes can be measured (Hoyt, 2007; Smith, 2011).

DHF created a global network to decentralize the operating and management structure of the program. National coordinators organize the local PSBH workshop trainings, including the selection and recruitment of the target audiences. These coordinators, together with their local PSBH teams, work with the participants during project implementation to assist with follow-up and monitoring. A follow-up workshop is conducted approximately 3 to 6 months after the initial PSBH training. The follow-up workshop provides a venue for participants to share their project results, discuss project challenges, and identify potential projects for expansion or replication (Smith, 2011).

THE RATIONALE FOR A GLOBAL NURSING FOCUS THROUGH PSBH

As the PSBH program expanded to more than 30 countries, it became evident that nurses were critical to the success of these community-based initiatives. Nurse consultants were invited to join the DHF team, leading workshops and participating in implementation and evaluation of PSBH projects in several countries. Based on experiences with PSBH around the globe, a program was designed specifically for nurses, and in 2002, the Problem Solving for Better Health Nursing™ (PSBHN) program was officially launched. DHF believed that bringing nurses together in a workshop setting (separate from participants from other disciplines or community members) would provide more opportunities for nurses to assume leadership roles, and potentially serve as key facilitators for the community-based PSBH programs (Hoyt-Hudson, 2011a).

The PSBH framework is similar to the nursing process: assess, plan, implement, and evaluate. The PSBH five-step process is an easy-to-follow tool, yet it is radical in its approach. Program participants undergo a personal transformation in the ability to think critically, creatively, and practically. Participants learn that problems cannot be solved before they are adequately "defined" or clearly understood. The initial step of "defining the problem" is crucial to the future success and impact of each health project. If a nurse chooses a realistic problem within a targeted population and geographic region, the probability of achieving measurable effective results increases significantly. Each nurse experiences the "transformation" at different stages of participation with PSBHN. Once the nurse recognizes his or her potential to significantly impact many peoples' lives, the fruitful efforts of the PSBHN program begin to unfold within the individual. First and foremost, it is vital for each nurse to truly understand his or her value first and foremost before he or she can act as effective agents of change for the betterment of others.

Nurses often understand and appreciate the essence and meaning of "health." According to WHO, "health is a state of complete physical, mental and social well-being, not simply the absence of disease or infirmity" (WHO, 2006). Nurses have the privilege as well as the responsibility to function as catalysts to improve people's quality of health. Imagine if each and every nurse around the world took personal responsibility and action to raise the capacity of others, thereby improving their quality of life; the world would likely be a healthier and more harmonious place. PSBHN strives to unlock this potential among nurses so they ultimately assume a more responsible and active role in the global effort toward "Health for All."

Once the potential of these nurses is "unlocked" the work truly begins. PSBHN follows its participants through the implementation phase of actualizing their projects and, on a deeper level, helping them to achieve their professional mission. Inevitably, nurses meet challenges in the project implementation phase and require ongoing support from DHF facilitators. The local facilitators offer assistance to the workshop participants throughout the PSBHN experience, so that project challenges are overcome and the nurses ultimately achieve their desired objectives as well as a deep sense of personal accomplishment.

On another level, PSBHN aims to influence the profession of nursing from an educational perspective. If we expect professional impact, we must have a plan to reach nurses from students to senior level nursing administrators. If we start by introducing the PSBHN process to nurse educators and student nurses we can influence the educational process. PSBHN has piloted this approach to target nurse faculty and student audiences in the following countries: Bulgaria, China, Dominican Republic, Ghana, India, Indonesia, Jordan, Kenya, Lesotho, Lithuania, Poland, Romania, United States, Vietnam, and Zambia. Each participating student is expected to put his or her "better health project" into action, thereby generating positive outcomes for the student and the target population addressed within the project. Importantly, it is not the number of projects that have been generated around the world that make the difference but the inner transformation within each PSBHN participant that is our valued goal. If this process touches a greater number of individuals, the outcomes and benefits will reach beyond these individuals and communities will be noticeably and positively transformed.

PSBHN is a cost-effective and practical approach to achieving nursing and health care goals for targeted populations. Many of the nurse-led projects implemented in hospital and community settings have been sustained, expanded, and replicated in other hospitals and communities, resulting in policy impact. Preliminary data from the DHF global nursing initiative indicates that the problem-solving process has increased the skill set and professional confidence of the nurses, and enhanced their leadership potential (Hoyt, 2007).

Consider the example of a successful PSBHN project titled You Can Save Our Lives, implemented in Lithuania by a nurse, Ugne Shakuniene. She created a website to encourage people throughout the country to become organ donors. This project had an even greater effect when Mrs. Shakuniene wrote to the president of the country asking him to support the organ donor idea. He not only announced the website at an important speech but also signed a donor card himself, and encouraged other government and military officials to do the same (Donauskaite-Tang, 2011). This nurse made a difference in her community. She had wanted to create organ donor awareness for some time; the PSBHN model gave her the structure, the tools, and, more importantly, the confidence to act to solve this problem.

In Hue, Vietnam, PSBHN was implemented within the community health nursing courses at Hue University. Students have implemented several projects, including those focused on improving nutrition of children younger than 5 years of age, implementing an immunization program for children, and improving garbage management. The immunization project placed an emphasis on educating mothers about the importance of immunizations. Their interventions consisted of brochures, posters, and recorded messages throughout the village for a period of 6 months. Based on their interventions there was both an increase in the vaccination rate and in knowledge about vaccinations. This project has been sustained by the local health workers at the Nam Dong Health Center (Thai, Ha, & Derstine, 2011).

In the following section, several PSBHN projects are described in more detail. These exemplars are models that will be used for future program expansion.

Mississippi Delta: "New Pathways to Health"

The Delta region of northwest Mississippi is plagued by high poverty, low educational attainment, and high rates of diseases including diabetes, heart disease, hypertension, obesity, and asthma (Green & Phillips, 2011). While demand for health care is expected to grow as further aspects of the Affordable Care Act (ACA) are implemented in the coming months and years, the state of

Mississippi is already experiencing a health care provider shortage. According to the Association of American Medical Colleges, in 2010, Mississippi had the fewest number of active physicians for its population out of all 50 states and the District of Columbia. Whereas nationally there were 258.7 active physicians per 100,000 people, in Mississippi there were only 176.4 per 100,000 (Jones & Danish, 2011). Similarly, the state faces a nursing shortage; hospitals and long-term care facilities have expressed difficulty in recruiting RNs (Jones, 2007). Many rural communities have a particularly difficult time recruiting and retaining qualified health care providers. As a result of these difficulties, the Health Resources and Service Administration (HRSA) has designated much of the state as a health professional shortage area (U.S. Department of Health and Human Services, 2012).

Despite the many health-related challenges in the Mississippi Delta, there is substantial energy among a number of organizations to tackle these problems and increase opportunities for people in the Delta. There are also many treasures in the region, including the unique culture, a strong sense of identity, and, most importantly, the people who reside there. DHF was invited to launch its PSBH program in the Delta's Coahoma County in 2003. Over the years, PSBH participants have achieved significant success in identifying solutions to health problems that affect the well-being of individuals living in the region. Several projects have been implemented over the years and many of these have become an integral part of community life.

In 2006, DHF was awarded funding from the Robert Wood Johnson Foundation through the Partners Investing in Nursing's Future Program (PIN) to develop tailored solutions to nursing workforce issues in the Mississippi Delta. The PIN program funded the DHF, in partnership with Delta State University (DSU) School of Nursing, and Coahoma Community College School of Nursing, to improve the retention and progression of minority nursing students in the Delta area, where attrition in the baccalaureate program had been as high as 54%. Through this project, members of the Eliza Pillars Registered Nurses of Mississippi, a professional organization for African American nurses, mentored students in achieving their personal and professional goals, and nurses and students were engaged in developing solutions to local health and social problems using the PSBHN model (Hoyt-Hudson, 2011b; Woodruff, 2011). This PIN nursing initiative led to additional partnerships with the Institute for Community-Based Research, the Mississippi Hospital Association Foundation, the Mississippi Office of Nursing Workforce, as well as other partners beyond the borders of the State of Mississippi.

These partnerships have now resulted in a diverse coalition of organizations committed to the development of better health and economic opportunity for vulnerable populations in the region and are known as New Pathways to Health. The collaborative work, catalyzed by DHF, has also led to several grant awards from the W.K. Kellogg Foundation. Core partners in this interdisciplinary health coalition include the Aaron E. Henry Community Health Services Center, the Mississippi Office of Nursing Workforce, the Tri-County Workforce Alliance, and the University of Mississippi Center for Population Studies. Other collaborating organizations and entities include two community health centers, three schools of nursing, three community-based organizations, three local hospitals, six health care providers, four business enterprises, several elementary schools, three middle schools, and eight high schools.

DHF and its collaborative network have successfully implemented several program strategies as part of the New Pathways to Health initiative to address the following project goals: (1) increase enrollment and retention of minority students in pathway programs for health care professions, (2) improve academic skills, (3) increase dual enrollment of high school students in college courses that lead to nursing and other health care fields, (4) target prominent health disparities and children's health issues in Mississippi, and (5) increase access to care. Engaging the youth in the PSBH program has led to two large-scale community-based projects, and increased awareness of healthy behaviors.

Overall, this initiative is designed to continue and generate broader and longer term outcomes. The collaborative program participant reach continues to expand, which will help us to achieve the longer term health, education, and workforce outcomes. Thus far, as a result of this collaborative, daily exercise routines have been incorporated into local elementary schools; a fitness and nutrition summer camp for kids of all ages has become an annual program in the community; student test scores have increased, opening the door to health professional college courses; and a youth-run school health council has formed. This past year, 10 recent high school graduates were trained as certified nursing assistants, and four are now employed in nursing homes while pursuing college degrees. Nursing students have received more hands-on training and, as a result of their increased exposure to local hospitals, are seeing the Delta region as a more promising place to work. Additionally, a community health worker curriculum was developed, and the first cohort completed the training. DHF/RI, together with its lead partners on the ground in Mississippi, continue to work to develop a collaborative assessment, monitoring, and evaluation framework to inform their efforts and advocate for broader programmatic and policy changes. With funding from the W.K. Kellogg Foundation, the collaborative is currently in the implementation phase of a 3-year initiative to further expand New Pathways to Health on behalf of vulnerable populations in the Mississippi Delta.

U.S.-Affiliated Pacific Islands Nursing Initiative

DHF/RI's work in Mississippi led to additional partnerships in the U.S.-Affiliated Pacific Islands (USAPI) as a result of national networking opportunities through the PIN program platform. While attending an annual PIN meeting, DHF/RI engaged with project partners based in the USAPI and began to explore the possibility of a collaborative relationship. The Pacific Island Network of Nursing Education Directors (PINNED) was intrigued by the PSBH model and DHF's global work.

Building on these conversations, in 2011, DHF/RI was awarded a "synergy grant" to strengthen professional nursing capacity and address local public health needs in the USAPI in partnership with Nursing Education Program Directors from the following collegiate nursing programs: American Samoa Community College, University of Guam, Guam Community College, Northern Marianas College, College of the Marshall Islands, College of Micronesia-FSM, and Palau Community College.

This project encompassed *the* nursing workforce needs of the seven member nations in the USAPI jurisdictions—U.S. Territories of Guam and American Samoa, the Commonwealth of the Northern Mariana Islands (CNMI), and the three former trust territories of the United States: the Freely Associated States (FAS) of the Republic of Palau, the Republic of the Marshall Islands, and the Federated States of the Micronesia. These island jurisdictions, with over 104 inhabited islands and low-lying atolls, cover a geographic expanse greater than that of the continental United States. In addition to English, 19 languages are used in the various nations. The synergy grant initiative additionally involved key partners including WHO, the American Pacific Nurse Leaders Council, the Pacific Islands Health Officers Association, the Micronesian Area Health Education Center, the University of Hawaii School of Nursing and Dental Hygiene, the U.S. Department of Health and Human Services, Region IX Office of the Regional Health Administrator, and the Center for Population Studies at the University of Mississippi.

All PINNED members were trained in the PSBH methodology in December 2011. This provided each of the participants with a framework and set of process strategies for creative approaches to problem solving, and it provided a forum for sharing other approaches between the USAPI and the mainland. Participants representing each of the participating Pacific jurisdictions developed an individual PSBH plan for managing a local situation. This helped the participants to make real life applications of the PSBH concepts.

Additionally, elements of the PSBH project plans developed during the training were later implemented. For example, a project in American Samoa focused on engaging nursing students in community outreach and education activities to serve the broader public, to provide students with public health experience, and to increase the visibility of local nurses. This project was ultimately integrated into the nursing student course requirements and will therefore continue into the future.

Another illustrative example comes from the CNMI. The proposed PSBH project was to increase clinical sites for placement of nursing students for their clinical experience, and to include this in the fiscal year 2012 operational plan for the nursing program. This goal was placed under the college's strategic goal to optimize financial resources and leverage current resources. The expected outcome was to officially establish partnerships with health care agencies for clinical site experiences in the CNMI. To date, action steps have included the drafting of several memorandum of understanding (MOU) documents for four clinical sites to submit to the dean for review.

One major success from this collaborative work is that PINNED is now recognized as a group with an identity and the ability to be at the table with leaders from government, education, and the private sector. Plans are in progress to disseminate additional outcomes from this project in future publications.

United States: PSBHN

In 2009, PSBHN was introduced in three university schools of nursing in the United States. The university programs included a 4-year generic bachelor of science nursing (BSN) program, an accelerated BSN program, and a clinical nurse leader program (Fitzpatrick & Hoyt-Hudson, 2013). Students in all of the programs worked in groups to launch community-based projects using the PSBHN model. Successful outcomes included the introduction of a hand-hygiene program for elementary school children (Lotas, Hardee, Hovancsek, & Fitzpatrick, 2013); a childhood obesity class for middle school children, and a mobility and exercise class for seniors (Grobbel, 2013); and a medication administration program in Honduras and several other global projects (Rigney & Baernholdt, 2013). Across all programs students and faculty evaluations were positive. This work continues and plans for expansion are being discussed.

China as an Exemplar

Emerging Health Challenges

With a population of over 1.3 billion, China is the most populous country in the world and has experienced remarkable economic growth over the past three decades. China is now the second biggest economy in the world and has been successful in combating communicable diseases. NCDs, however, have become a severe threat, and it is estimated that 82% of all deaths in China are from NCDs: cancer, heart attacks, strokes, asthma, chronic obstructive pulmonary disease, diabetes, and mental health disorders. For example, more than 92 million adults in China have diabetes, and nearly 150 million more are on their way to developing it (Yang et al., 2010).

Meanwhile, due to the "one family, one child" policy and an increase in life expectancy, with life expectancy at birth for women and men reaching 76 and 72, respectively, by 2011, China's population is aging rapidly (National Health and Family Planning Commission of the People's Republic of China, 2011). In 2011, about 170 million Chinese citizens (more than 12% of the total population) were aged 60 and older (National Health and Family Planning Commission of the People's Republic of China, 2011) and the number of the aging population is estimated to double to more than 345 million by 2030 (United Nations Department of Economic and Social Affairs, 2012). The rapid shift to an older society, combined with the prevalence of NCDs, is generating a profound impact on the Chinese health care system.

Nursing Workforce in China

Crucial to the health of the people, nurses are at the interface between the health care system and the patients they serve. However, China is one of the few countries that has more doctors than nurses. As of 2011, there were 2.24 million RNs and 2.49 million physicians (the ratio of nurses to physicians is 0/9) in China (National Health and Family Planning Commission of the People's Republic of China, 2011). As there is a shortage of nurse educators, a master's program in nursing was not established in China until 1990. The majority of Chinese nurses receive the three years of training after graduating from either junior or high schools. Only 9.5% of RNs hold a bachelor's degree, and 0.1% hold a master's degree. Currently, about 70% of RNs work in hospitals. (National Health and Family Planning Commission of the People's Republic of China, 2011). If they are integrated within the health care team, Chinese nurses have the potential to ensure patient safety and improve health.

Solution—Introduction to PSBHN (History)

Recognizing the potential of Chinese nursing professionals and the rising demand for higher quality of care and prevention and control of NCDs, DHF/RI launched the PSBH program and established a strategic partnership with Peking Union Medical College School of Nursing (PUMCSON). Thus, the PSBHN program was officially launched in China in 1996 (Liang, Liu, & Liu, 2011). The overarching goal of PSBHN is to empower nurses to assume a more active role in health care and to significantly improve the health of more people through collective efforts with other health care professionals and community partners. PSBHN in China targets nurses and nursing students as "agents of change" and introduces the five-step process that enables them to lead problem-solving and quality-improvement efforts. DHF/RI then monitors and evaluates the results of the program and shares China's best practices with its partners from other countries in the world.

Results and Impact

Since PSBHN was launched in 1996, it has been applied in communities, academic institutions, and hospitals in 14 cities throughout China. To date, more than 6,000 nurses and nursing students have participated in the PSBHN program and generated approximately 4,000 better health projects that tackle local health problems of concern. In addition to PUMC SON, additional partners include Xi'an Jiatong University School of Nursing, Kiang Wu Nursing College (KWNC) of Macau, Fujian Provincial Hospital (FPH), First Affiliated Hospital of Kunming Medical College, and Community Health Alliance in Shanghai, among others. DHF/RI, in partnership with these institutions, has been instrumental in utilizing the PSBHN process to elevate nursing professionals. Moreover, both PUMCSON and KWNC have incorporated PSBHN into the curriculum for nursing students from the bachelor of science program.

Of the 4,000 PSBH projects initiated by nurses or nursing students, approximately half of the projects are implemented to address improvements in quality and patient safety in the hospital setting, whereas 40% of the projects are implemented to fulfill the needs for health promotion and disease prevention in the community setting. The remaining 10% of the projects were implemented to address health issues (i.e., physical inactivity, obesity, etc.) among students on campus. Some of these projects have received government support to sustain and expand the efforts, and several of these initiatives have become national models to address targeted health care issues. The PSBHN program has effectively empowered Chinese nurses and nursing students to be agents of change and positively influenced their attitudes toward the nursing profession. More importantly, it has led to an improvement in quality of care and better health of the people.

A Success Story: The PSBHN Program at FPH

In 2003, with the leadership support from the PUMCSON, DHF/RI first introduced the PSBHN program to FPH, a 1,800-bed tertiary hospital in Fuzhou. The hospital's vice president, Ms. Hong Lee, soon embraced the concepts of the PSBHN program and became an active promoter to involve nursing leaders from different departments in the PSBHN process. Since its initial launch, all of the nursing leaders (including head nurses and nurse supervisors) have participated in the PSBHN program. The program has not only transformed individual nurses who have been part of the process but also created transformational change at the institutional level. At the individual level, one of the PSBHN program participants, Ms. Juan Lin, head nurse of the endocrinology department, applied the PSBHN method to a common problem, poor glycemic control among patients seen in her department. The PSBHN process enabled Ms. Lin to think creatively about the resources that are often neglected and take actions to improve her patients' health. She actively approached other health professionals and developed an 8-month health promotion and support program (offering participants a variety of activities once every week) for about 140 patients whose glycemic control was suboptimal. Ms. Lin shared PSBHN's belief that people are part of the solution and engaged her patients in identifying barriers to maintaining healthy lifestyles. As a result, this health promotion and support program led to a significant improvement in the target patients' knowledge of healthy eating and physical activity as well as their self-care practices. One of the unanticipated benefits of this program was the improved relationship between health professionals and patients. Both health professionals and patients showed high levels of satisfaction with the program. The program was so successful that the FPH decided to incorporate it into its community outreach effort and offer it on a yearly basis. Since 2004, the 8-month program has benefited more than

1,500 people. In addition, this Patient-Centered Diabetics Health Promotion and Support Program was selected by Fujian Provincial Health Bureau as one of the model programs to be replicated in the rural and urban communities of Fujian Province. To date, Ms. Lin and her team have helped 100 community health workers from seven different communities implement this model to reach more diabetic patients and improve their health (Lee, Lin, & Zhang, 2011).

PSBHN not only catalyzed Ms. Lin's personal transformation, but it also helped the FPH develop a culture of continuous quality improvement. PSBHN became the backbone of FPH's continuous quality improvement effort and FPH's 1,200 nurses have continuously applied key PSBHN concepts and methodology to quality and safety problems. The accumulated positive outcomes led FPH Department of Nursing to be appointed by the Health Department of Fujian Province as the Nursing Quality Control Center to provide advanced training for nursing leaders from other hospitals across Fujian Province. Between 2008 and 2012, nursing departments at FPH received 16 provincial and national awards for outstanding clinical performance, and FPH nurses published 431 quality-improvement papers in provincial and national journals (Lee et al., 2011).

Future Directions for PSBHN in China

DHF/RI is actively exploring partnerships with global and national organizations and corporations to scale up the existing program success to benefit more Chinese nurses, nursing students, and citizens. In the meantime, DHF/ RI continues to build relationships with local governments and organizations as their support is critical to PSBHN program sustainability. A web-based platform is currently in development to provide a mechanism to more easily share best PSBHN practices and maintain an engaged network of empowered nurses and nursing students. The PSBHN network from different regions throughout China is poised to develop large-scale initiatives to address national health care challenges. Ultimately, DHF/RI aims to develop 200,000 PSBHN nurses who are change-makers and collaborators to lead better health initiatives for more people in China.

OPPORTUNITIES AND FUTURE DIRECTIONS

We have consistently shown our methodology for educating, training, and inspiring local nurses in a multitude of cultures around the globe to make an impact on their community's health with relatively simple projects and limited budgets is extremely effective. However, before applying this program systematically to achieve targeted health care goals, we need rigorous monitoring and evaluation to generate direct and indirect health outcomes. Data collection is necessary to validate our conclusions about the PSBHN model. To date, the evaluations have been localized case studies, primarily providing in-depth information on processes and outputs. We now turn our attention toward the development of broader metrics to provide the basis for monitoring outcomes and impacts between places and over the course of time. Further evaluation is also necessary to identify barriers to successful program implementation and delivery. We must demonstrate with a degree of statistical certainty that we have made a difference in public health as a result of nursing outreach and mobilization in underserved communities.

We will proceed by taking PSBHN's successful approach and engaging in the following:

1. Codifying our methodology
2. Improving communications between local leaders with both PSBHN staff and other local leaders, we will be more able to effectively share lessons learned and experiences as well as prior mistakes, and keep better managerial control if problems arise
3. Implementing and leveraging statistical and clinical resources as projects are *developed* and before full implementation, we will improve our ability to make valid claims as to successful outcomes, and publish articles in peer-reviewed journals (e.g., questions that could be addressed include what confounding factors are present? How can we adjust for any such factors? Can we locate similar communities with the same demographic profile and track their outcomes without our program in place as a control? Are we asking the right questions? Are we following the right data points and outcomes? etc.)
4. Improving data collection, ensuring its validity, and storing the data for further statistical analysis and modeling

PSBHN has the ability to dramatically impact the health of the world's people, reducing the GBD, improving their quality of life, and producing a sustainable, cost-effective system. With these enhancements, it can do so, achieving its full potential as a tool. More important is the fact that it can contribute to nursing's realization of its own potential and its fulfillment of its evident responsibilities within the new health system. Nursing is the critical element in the new model of health and we believe that PSBHN is one tool that can help nursing fulfill both its responsibilities and full potential.

CONCLUSION

We are at a critical point in time with regard to the GBD and the opportunity we have to create a new health system that will not only reduce the disease burden and its cost, but also contribute meaningfully to the relief of human suffering and the betterment of quality of life for all the world's people. Much has already been accomplished, but much more remains to be done, and the challenges facing us now and in the future are greater and not less than they have been in the past. Nursing and nurses around the world are critical to seizing the opportunity we have and meeting the health and quality of life challenges we face as a global community. They are vital because they are the critical nexus between the people and the knowledge and skills of the health professions. Nursing can bring individuals and the community on to the health team in a meaningful way.

The view of nursing put forward here is not the usual one. Traditionally, medicine has been considered to be the essence of health care. Nurses and nursing have been playing a supportive role. As important as medical care remains, however, health today must be seen in the far broader context of the total society. In fact, the vast majority of "health" is a product of the functioning or malfunctioning of that society. Economics, education, the availability of jobs, recreation, faith, and a host of other things, such as the need for compassion and respect, that make up people's lives and contribute to their total well-being are important as well. Nursing is well positioned to bring all of these elements together to serve the best interests of the people and enable them to do more for themselves. We believe that PSBHN is a tool for nursing to use to fulfill its true potential and meet the world's need for better health and life for everyone.

NOTES

1. On the basis of population increases alone, DALYs could have been expected to increase by 37.9% from 1990 to 2010, The 0.6% decrease in DALYs over this time means that progress was made in reducing the DALYs associated with the causative diseases (Murray & Lopez, 2013).
2. The data reported here have been supplied by the United States Renal Data System (USRDS). The interpretation and reporting of these data are the responsibility of the author(s) and in no way should be seen as an official policy or interpretation of the U.S. government (USRDS, 2013).

REFERENCES

Coyte, P. C., Asche, C. V., Croxford, R., & Chan, E. (1998). The economic cost of musculoskeletal disorders in Canada. *Arthritis Care Research, 11,* 315–325.

Donauskaite-Tang, G. (2011). Lithuania. In B. H. Smith, J. J. Fitzpatrick, & P. Hoyt-Hudson (Eds.), *Problem solving for better health: A global perspective* (pp. 119–122). New York, NY: Springer Publishing Company.

Fitzpatrick, J. J., & Hoyt-Hudson, P. (2013). Problem solving for better health nursing: Application of an internationally tested model to nursing schools in the United States. *Journal of Professional Nursing, 29* (1), e1–e2.

Green, J. J., & Phillips, M. (2011). Building the capacity of schools to confront asthma in the Delta: Report from an action research and participatory planning project to improve population health. *Working paper for the Center for Community and Economic Development School-based Asthma Management program.* University of Mississippi: Institute for Community-Based Research.

Grobbel, C. (2013). Problem solving for better health in nursing: Application in an accelerated bachelor of science in nursing program. *Journal of Professional Nursing, 29*(1), e6–e9.

Honeycutt, A. A., Segel, J. E., Zhuo, X., Hoerger, T. J., Imai, K., & Williams, D. (2013). Medical costs of CKD in the Medicare population. *Journal of the American Association of Nephrology, 24,* 1478–1483.

Hoyt, P. (2007). An international approach to Problem Solving for Better Health Nursing™ (PSBHN). *International Nursing Review, 54,* 101–106.

Hoyt-Hudson, P. (2011a). Problem solving for better health nursing. In B. H. Smith, J. J. Fitzpatrick, & P. Hoyt-Hudson (Eds.), *Problem solving for better health: A global perspective* (pp. 20–21). New York, NY: Springer Publishing Company.

Hoyt-Hudson, P. (2011b). Problem solving for better health nursing in Mississippi. In B. H. Smith, J. J. Fitzpatrick, & P. Hoyt-Hudson (Eds.), *Problem solving for better health: A global perspective* (pp. 209–210). New York, NY: Springer Publishing Company.

Jones, K., & Danish, S. (2011). Association of American Medical Colleges. *2011 State Physician Workforce Data Book.* Retrieved from http://www.aamc.org

Jones, W. (2007). *Mississippi Office of Nursing Workforce, Mississippi state health plan fiscal year 2008.* Retrieved from http://www.monw.org/publications

Lee, H., Lin, J., & Zhang, X. (2011). Fuzhou-Fujian Provincial Hospital. In B. H. Smith, J. J. Fitzpatrick, & P. Hoyt-Hudson (Eds.), *Problem solving for better health: A global perspective* (pp. 74–76). New York, NY: Springer Publishing Company.

Liang, X., Liu, J., & Liu, H. (2011). Beijing-Peking Union Medical College School of Nursing. In B. H. Smith, J. J. Fitzpatrick, & P. Hoyt-Hudson (Eds.), *Problem solving for better health: A global perspective* (p. 74). New York, NY: Springer Publishing Company.

Lotas, M., Hardee, E., Hovancsek, M., & Fitzpatrick, J. (2013). Implementation of the PSBH model in a 4-year baccalaureate nursing program. *Journal of Professional Nursing, 29*(1), e3–e5.

Murray, C. J., & Lopez, A. D. (2013). Measuring the global burden of disease. *The New England Journal of Medicine, 369*(5), 448–457.

National Health and Family Planning Commission of the People's Republic of China. (2011). *Chinese Health Statistical Digest.* Retrieved from http://www.nhfpc.gov.cn/zwgkzt/pwstj/list.shtml

Rigney, D. B., & Baernholdt, M. (2013). Using problem solving for better health nursing in a clinical nurse leader program. PSBHN Model. *Journal of Professional Nursing, 29*(1), e10–e13.

Smith, B. H. (2011). The Dreyfus Health Foundation and problem solving for better health. In B. H. Smith, J. J. Fitzpatrick, & P. Hoyt-Hudson (Eds.), *Problem solving for better health: A global perspective* (pp. 17–22). New York, NY: Springer Publishing Company.

Smith, B. H. (2013). Nursing, health reform, and the achievement of better health for all people. In G. Glazer & J. Fitzpatrick (Eds.), *Nursing leadership from the outside in* (pp. 213–226). New York, NY: Springer Publishing Company.

Thai, T. D., Ha, L. T. L., & Derstine, J. B. (2011). Vietnam. In B. H. Smith, J. J. Fitzpatrick, & P. Hoyt-Hudson (Eds.), *Problem solving for better health: A global perspective* (pp. 109–113). New York, NY: Springer Publishing Company.

United Nations Department of Economic and Social Affairs: Population Division, Population Estimates and Projections Section. (2012). *World Population Prospects: The 2012 Revision.* Retrieved from http://esa.un.org/unpd/wpp/index.htm

U.S. Department of Health and Human Services. (2012). *Designated health professional shortage areas (HPSAs) statistics, health resources and service administration (HRSA).* Retrieved from www.hrsa.gov

U.S. Renal Data System. (2013). *Annual data report: Atlas of chronic kidney disease and end-stage renal disease in the United States.* Bethesda, MD: National Institutes of Health, National Institute of Diabetes and Digestive and Kidney Diseases.

Woodruff, J. (2011). Partners investing in nursing's future. In B. H. Smith, J. J. Fitzpatrick, & P. Hoyt-Hudson (Eds.), *Problem solving for better health: A global perspective* (pp. 209–210). New York, NY: Springer Publishing Company.

World Bank. (1993). *Investing in health: World development indicators*. Oxford, UK: Oxford University Press.

World Health Organization. (2006). *Constitution of the World Health Organization* (45th ed.). Retrieved from http://who.int/governance/eb.constitution/en//index.html

Yang, W., Lu, J., Weng, J., Jia, W., Ji, L., Xiao, J., . . . He, J. (2010). Prevalence of diabetes among men and women in China. *New England Journal of Medicine, 362*(12), 1090–1091.

Yelin, E., & Callahan L. F. (1995). The economic cost and social and psychological impact of musculoskeletal condition. *Arthritis Rheumatology, 38*, 1351–1362.

CHAPTER 30

The Fulbright Scholar Program and Nursing in Southern Africa

R. Kevin Mallinson

The African continent is infinitely diverse; it boasts a range of dramatic landscapes, exotic flora and fauna, and human cultures that embody the ages and still continuously adapt to contemporary issues. There are serious challenges for African nurses that force their cultures and traditions to be altered. Southern Africa, the sub-Saharan region, bears 24% of the global burden of disease, particularly HIV, tuberculosis, and malaria, but is home to fewer than 3% of the world's health care workers (Anyangwe & Mtonga, 2007). Numerous countries are experiencing an unparalleled shortage of health care workers that threatens the stability of their societies and severely shortens the life expectancy of its people. The World Health Organization (WHO) has identified 57 countries as having a crisis-level shortage of health care workers; 35 of these are on the African continent and six of them—Mozambique, Malawi, Zambia, Zimbabwe, Lesotho, and Swaziland—are in Southern Africa (USAID, 2013). To close the gaps in the health care workforce, a major goal for the President's Emergency Plan for AIDS Relief (PEPFAR) has been to prepare an additional 145,000 health care workers to strengthen the health systems in Southern Africa (PEPFAR, 2013).

Many factors undermine efforts to build an adequate health care workforce in sub-Saharan Africa. Stilwell (2011) encapsulated the problem to be the production, retention, and distribution of adequately trained personnel. This chapter describes how one nurse has aimed to address nursing production and retention issues to strengthen the health care workforce while serving as a Fulbright Scholar in the Kingdom of Swaziland. Through an overview of my journey in cultural immersion, I highlight relevant "lessons learned" that may be useful to nurses seeking a global nursing exchange as a Fulbright Scholar.

The Health Care Workforce Crisis in Swaziland

The Kingdom of Swaziland is a small country in southern Africa; it is landlocked by Mozambique on its eastern border and South Africa on its northern, western, and southern borders. The country's population of approximately 1.1 million people (Ministry of Health [MoH], 2011) is cared for by too few practitioners; the MoH employs an estimated 173 generalist and specialist physicians and 1,164 nursing professionals (WHO, 2009). Data are unavailable to ascertain the additional health providers who serve through nongovernmental agencies or faith-based organizations.

The Kingdom of Swaziland has the highest rate of HIV infections in the world; recent surveys show that 26% of the country's population is HIV infected (WHO, 2009). In parallel with the HIV epidemic, the MoH reported that the annual cases of tuberculosis quadrupled during the period 2006 to 2010 (MoH, 2012). An estimated 69% of the population lives in poverty and 39% do not have access to safe drinking water (WHO, 2009). The life expectancy at birth for a Swazi is now estimated to be 48.7 years, one of the lowest in the world (World Bank, 2013).

In 2006, with funding from PEPFAR, I developed and implemented a nursing capacity-building program for the countries of Lesotho, South Africa, and Swaziland. The Nurses SOAR! [Strengthening Our AIDS Response] program was administered by the U.S. Health Resources and Services Administration (HRSA). Over a 3-year period, the Nurses SOAR! program activities in Swaziland were based at the Wellness Center for Health Care Workers and two faith-based entities: the Raleigh Fitkin Memorial Hospital and the Nazarene College of Nursing, both situated on the Nazarene Mission campus in the city of Manzini.

I designed the Nurses SOAR! activities to align with the WHO (2006) model to "treat, train, and retain" health workers in an effort to strengthen the workforce. In collaboration with the Wellness Center, the Nurses SOAR! program encouraged health care workers to access voluntary counseling and testing (VCT) for HIV; those who tested positive were referred for follow-up and initiated on antiretroviral therapy (ART) when medically eligible. Additional activities were designed to strengthen training programs (particularly the College of Nursing's diploma program), enhance nurses' clinical knowledge and skills, and reduce the impact of personal stressors and workplace conditions that led to job dissatisfaction, frequent absences, and attrition.

As the principal investigator for the Nurses SOAR! program, I visited Swaziland often and developed an appreciation for the severe lack of infrastructure, resources, and human capital that threatens the country's health care workforce and its ability to achieve any of the Millennium Development Goals. It became apparent that a "capacity building" initiative for nurses would require concentrated efforts over an extended period of time to assure the adequate transfer of knowledge and the sustainability of new processes. My commitment to the Swazi people led me to apply for a Fulbright Scholar award.

FULBRIGHT SCHOLAR PROGRAM

The U.S. Department of State, Bureau of Educational and Cultural Affairs, collaborates with governments around the world to support an exchange of expertise and culture through the Fulbright Scholar program. Since 1948, Americans have been traveling abroad as Fulbright Scholars to promote mutual understanding and goodwill (Council for International Exchanged of Scholars [CIES], 2013). The Fulbright Scholar living in a foreign country receives support from the State Department staff at the U.S. Embassy to enhance his or her ability to accomplish the goals or the mission. Every Fulbright experience is different; each is designed to meet the needs of the host institution and the expertise and objectives of the participating scholar.

My Fulbright Scholar Plan

During the months that I was writing my Fulbright application, I was asked by colleagues why I would want to live in sub-Saharan Africa for an entire year. My heartfelt response was, "I have a lot to learn." Perhaps those words best summarize the core of my experience; I *did* have a lot to learn, personally and professionally. There also was a lot for me to teach, a lot to share.

Teaching

I was awarded a year-long Fulbright Scholar position as a research professor in the Faculty of Health Sciences at the Southern Africa Nazarene University (SANU) in Manzini, the second largest city in the Kingdom of Swaziland. The faith-based institution was granted university status in 2010 when its three long-standing academic components—the colleges of nursing, education, and theology—merged and upgraded their programs to the baccalaureate level. In writing the intended plan of action in the Fulbright application, I responded to the needs of the university for building their capacity for teaching and conducting research.

When I arrived in the country and settled into my flat (rental housing on the Nazarene Mission property), I met with the vice chancellor and representatives from the faculty of Health Sciences and the faculty of Theology to confirm my teaching assignments for the year. As expected, I was assigned to teach Nursing Research to the upper-level nursing students in Manzini. In an effort to strengthen their capacity for teaching research, a young lecturer in the nursing department was assigned to coteach with me. I was to mentor him and demonstrate a variety of pedagogical strategies to effectively teach our large undergraduate class (a total of 91 senior nursing students).

The students were initially intrigued by having an American professor for their class. It became obvious almost immediately that they were taken aback by my style of teaching and expectations for timeliness. My interactive, engaging style of teaching did not allow for the students to be unprepared for classroom lectures; they were unable to be "anonymous" in the large classroom as I called on individual students to provide opinions, insights, or examples to supplement the lecture. Worse yet, in a culture that has a vastly different appreciation for time, I expected that students be punctual, and in their seats at 8:00 a.m. for the start of class. As much as half the class was more than 30 minutes late to class the first week. As a Fulbright, I reasoned that I was expected to encourage the exchange of cultural beliefs and traditions. Hence, the students would have to learn that this American professor shut the door at 8:05 a.m. Needless to say, the students learned quickly to arrive to class on time.

For my second teaching assignment, I was surprised to learn that I was being asked to teach an Introduction to Study and Research course for theology students each Monday at the Siteki campus (nearly 1.5-hour drive to the east, near the border with Mozambique). An initial lesson I have learned in Africa is to be flexible. So, despite being a non-Christian, I prepared to engage students in the faculty of theology at an evangelical Christian university. Throughout the course, I was able to challenge the theology students (most were assistant pastors in local Nazarene churches) to identify issues relevant to their congregations, conduct a review of the literature, and compose a position paper that integrated various opinions and perspectives. For each of the selected topics—poverty, malnutrition, HIV/AIDS, sexuality, child abuse—I was able to help them identify resources and experts (especially nurses) to address the problems. It was one of the most rewarding teaching experiences I have had in my career.

Both courses allowed me to demonstrate the integration of interactive teaching methods, critical thinking exercises, and student-centered approaches to learning. My colleagues learned about utilizing online resources, integrating audiovisual materials into lectures, and using small group exercises to promote learning in a large class of students. In context, it is easy to focus on the lack of educational materials, adequate seating, or Internet access. Therefore, I endeavored to communicate that the most valuable outcome would be for the students to maximize their ability to think critically, act with intent, and envision more creatively.

Although English is the second official language of Swaziland, and the preferred language in the health care environment, it was exhausting for students to listen to an American speaking at a rapid pace for long periods of time. Therefore, I learned to speak more slowly and distinctly; I removed the usual idioms from my vocabulary; and I lectured for shorter periods of time and integrated small group learning activities into the classroom so students could discuss their projects in siSwati. I often highlighted specific English terms for them to master.

Research

My Fulbright plan of action included conducting an outcomes evaluation for a nurse-managed clinic in Swaziland: the Wellness Center for Health Care Workers. Health care workers in Swaziland were reluctant to seek HIV-related services at their place of employment for fear of stigmatization and a lack of privacy (Baleta, 2008). Opened by the Swaziland Nurses Association in 2006, the Wellness Center provides free primary care services for health care workers and up to four of their immediate family members. In an accessible, though private, location in the community, the Wellness Center provides health care workers with HIV counseling and testing, prevention education, and antiretroviral medications in a confidential and stigma-free environment. The outcomes evaluation study could demonstrate the effectiveness of the center's innovative approach to the MoH and a variety of international donors.

There were challenges in conducting the research study. Although I submitted the study to the country's scientific and ethics committee for human protections approval before arriving in Swaziland, it was a full 7 months before I received the approval to initiate the research. While compiling the quantitative data (medical records), I was impeded by poor documentation, filing discrepancies, and an unstable database software package. As my Swazi colleagues experienced these barriers with me, they began to understand how an evaluative process can inform their plans for improving processes for documentation and the maintenance of medical records.

The qualitative data collection encountered very few problems. I had trained two Swazi research assistants to conduct individual interviews with health care worker clients in their native language, siSwati. Both of the men (one nurse and one HIV specialist) had collected qualitative data as part of their graduate theses. Additional interviews were conducted with the staff of the Wellness Center. Subsequently, the audiotaped interviews were translated into English and transcribed by the two research assistants. The qualitative data have clarified what the clients value about the Wellness Center and its provision of services to health care workers. Interview data from the staff members are being used to develop a strategic plan for development.

Collegial Mentoring

An expectation of my position as a research professor on the SANU campus was that I would mentor my colleagues in research-related activities. Throughout the year, this included 11 mentees with projects ranging from abstracts for research conferences to the completion of master's theses. I provided guidance on research designs, sampling strategies, and qualitative research methods. The enthusiasm for conducting research was invigorating.

Currently, there are no requirements for nurses in Swaziland to earn continuing education credits as a condition of continued licensure. As a result, there are many nurses who may not have received structured clinical updates since graduation from their basic program. The SANU faculty of health sciences established a Continuing Professional Development (CPD) Committee to explore how the university could provide appropriate educational opportunities for health care workers. Though the provision of updates on clinical procedures, policy initiatives, or contemporary issues would be considered valuable, some faculty were reluctant to having required programs for which they would not be paid. As a member of this fledgling new committee, I facilitated the identification of objectives and the development of CPD processes that would be appropriate in the Swazi context.

Additional Capacity-Building Activities

One of the benefits of having implemented the Nurses SOAR! program in Swaziland was that I had already established relationships across numerous sectors of the community. During my year as a Fulbright Scholar, I engaged in many capacity-building activities that were not specifically a part of my Fulbright award. These activities were designed to strengthen the skills of clinicians, educators, and administrators across a variety of acute care, community, and academic settings.

Wellness Center Programs

One of the more valuable activities in the Nurses SOAR! program was facilitating a loss and grief intervention for health care workers. The director of the Wellness Center requested that I conduct the intervention for his staff in conjunction with the staff of the "sister" Wellness Center for Health Care Workers in the neighboring country of Lesotho. Once in Maseru, the capital city, I elucidated the importance of managing grief symptoms in health care workers in a presentation before a MoH committee. The next day, I facilitated the 24-hour grief intervention for the combined Wellness Center staff cohort in a rural, pastoral setting in Roma.

The Wellness Center has been spearheading a new initiative by the MoH to screen all health care workers in the country for tuberculosis (TB). As TB has long been endemic to Swaziland, the use of a skin test is not indicated; workers would need to be screened for symptoms and provide sputum smears, as indicated. It was anticipated that there would be significant resistance to widespread screening, as workers may feel that their job could be threatened by a positive screen. To address such concerns, I engaged a Swazi theatre troupe to develop a short, engaging skit to allay the health care workers' fears. At the official launching of the screening program at the National TB Referral Hospital, the minister of health, local health officials, and nearly 100 health care workers in the audience witnessed the theater presentation. Using a mix of humor and relevant factual information about TB, the group was able to communicate how a TB screening program would be beneficial to maintaining the health and well-being of health care workers and their family members.

Ministry of Health Technical Working Group

Another ad hoc activity was to serve as a representative for the university on a technical working group (TWG) for the MoH in Swaziland. The ministry was establishing an office for research that would support the scientific and ethics committee (i.e., the human protections committee), survey the current health research being implemented in the country, and assist future applicants in submitting proposals for health research in the country. As a TWG, we served as advisors on the development of policies and procedures, the implementation of specific guidelines, and the maintenance of collaborative relationships with numerous governmental, parastatal, and nongovernmental partners who might be involved in research activities. One of the goals of the MoH is to have enough evidence to identify its own health research priorities and issue its own health research agenda on a regular basis.

Customer Care Program

The reputation of nurses and health care workers as compassionate and caring professionals has been deteriorating in Swaziland. Noting widespread incidents of health care workers being rude, dismissive, or abusive to patients and family members, the MoH has created a "customer care" initiative. The nurse charged with instituting the program at the campus hospital engage my assistance in developing creative and effective strategies for delivering the program content. With the help of several young volunteers from Scandinavia, we were able to develop a faith-based set of posters that communicated central tenets of customer care in a way that was most appropriate for the Nazarene Mission hospital. I also introduced the Swazi theater troupe to the customer care coordinator so they could create skits to communicate the importance of being caring, compassionate, and respectful to those who came to the hospital.

American Nursing Student Immersion Program

Over the years, I have organized trips to South Africa and Swaziland for approximately 70 undergraduate and graduate students in nursing or pharmacy. During my time in Swaziland, a colleague in the United States came with six nursing students; they engaged with other nursing students at the university on various wards throughout the hospital. On a rotating basis, students also accompanied the Wellness Center staff to the rural homesteads to provide a variety of homecare services. The students learned about poverty, nursing in a resource-limited setting, and cultural influences on health behaviors. They also helped to build capacity among the Swazi nurses. The students demonstrated physical assessment skills, role modeled caring behaviors and enhanced nurse–physician communications, and assisted the Swazi nurses in solving clinical problems. The two-way exchange of skills and knowledge was highly valued by all.

CULTURAL CHALLENGES

I expected that there would be unique challenges to face while living in Swaziland for a year. In preparation for my time in Africa, I spent a considerable amount of time in personal reflection; I wanted to have a firm "philosophy" to guide my behavior while in Swaziland. Rather than having "knee-jerk responses," it was important to me to respond *intentionally*, with respect and humility, when confronting the inevitable cultural differences that would evoke emotional responses. The following section describes a few such cultural challenges and my responses.

Homogeneity

The Swazi culture is very homogenous. Nearly 97% of the population identifies as ethnic Swazi (CIA, 2014). To paraphrase a young nurse who was decrying the lack of diversity, "The greatest *strength* of my country is that we are one people, one culture, with one language. The greatest *weakness* of my country is that we are one people, one culture, with one language!" As a consequence, it is quite obvious when an individual stands out from the crowd with a different perspective, a divergent opinion. Depending upon the situation, that person can be perceived as simply odd, a threat to the status quo, or a danger to the well-being of the culture. I was keenly aware of such perceptions during my year in Swaziland for several reasons.

Religion

Generally, anyone in Swaziland who is not easily identified as a Muslim is assumed to be a Christian. There was considerable pressure put on me by colleagues to attend prayer meetings and church services. Though I initially attended some church services—more out of curiosity—it was a cause for concern when I began to respectfully decline. When I would explain that I was not a Christian, reactions ranged from disbelief to disgust. I was prepared for the confrontations; I respectfully reminded my colleagues that there were many other religions in the world and that approximately two thirds of the world's people do not identify as Christian. Eventually, I stopped receiving invitations to attend church.

For many of my Swazi colleagues and students, their faith was a source of strength and comfort. I appreciated how faith allowed one to forge ahead in the midst of poverty, hunger, or traumatic life events. There were times, however, when the quick answer to a conundrum was to decide on *inaction* and to "leave it up to God." The challenge for me was to encourage positive actions that might resolve the issue without devaluing their religious beliefs or questioning the wisdom of the Almighty. My most successful approach was to suggest they consciously decide to act because "God helps those who help themselves."

Heteronormativity

Similarly, adults in Swaziland are assumed to be heterosexual to have children of their own. I was quite aware, however, that Swazi culture was not only characterized by common heteronormativity, it was blatantly homophobic. In professional situations, I would respond in the affirmative that I was married; many times, the ensuing conversation led to me talking about my husband of 20 years. Frequently, I would be told that homosexuality was "contrary" to Black African culture and could not be accepted. At this point, I would note that South Africa (the next door neighbor to Swaziland) had legalized marriage equality in 2006; since that time, many Black Africans had married their partners. It was frequently an uncomfortable discussion, not unlike discussions about the oppression of women, arranged marriages for children, or the legality of abortion. In the rural settings, there was less expectation of an "academic" discourse and more danger of a violent reaction to my being gay; I would refrain from talking about my marriage in detail.

My usual approach in these situations was to remind my Swazi colleagues that they had *elected* to engage with Americans (or other outsiders) to build their capacity. Therefore, they should expect to encounter differing cultural perspectives on religious freedoms, political expression, and human rights related to sex, sexual orientation, or health choices (e.g., abortion). Then I would suggest that engaging as members of the "global community" meant there was an expectation of tolerance for other cultures. In effect, cultural sensitivity should be a two-way street and not a unilateral expectation of the Americans.

Language and Ceremonies

I endeavored to learn as much siSwati as possible. Knowing how to pronounce names of individuals or select towns and locales proved valuable. It was mentioned more than once that "Americans never try" to learn siSwati and that my attempts were valiant. There were times when my mispronunciations were fodder for a good laugh. Similarly, my enthusiastic willingness to attend traditional Swazi events (e.g., engagement ceremonies in which the men pay 15 cows as *lobola* to the woman's family) was noted and appreciated. At such ceremonies, I ate the traditional foods and drank whatever was being served. Surely, I had to occasionally tend to the gastrointestinal consequences as they arose.

Acquiescence to the Monarchy

The Kingdom of Swaziland is the last absolute monarchy on the African continent and there are tensions between those who swear loyalty to King Mswati III and those who wish to have a full democratic government (Swaziland's election, 2013). Knowing the sensitivity surrounding the king and the symbolic role he holds in the tribal culture of the Swazi people, it was never my intent to question his authority. However, in a country that has unprecedented levels of morbidity and mortality, my work often focuses on the management of grief. During my year in Swaziland, King Mswati III made a formal pronouncement before a group of pastors that they should not be discussing death with their congregants as death was deemed "an abomination" before God.

My students in the faculty of theology were eager to wrangle over the king's statement as they were frequently responsible for ministering to congregants in distress over the impending death of a loved one. To avoid appearing to contradict the ruling monarch—and spiritual leader of the Swazi tribe—I relied on eliciting the students' feelings about what was best for their ministry. So, through playing "devil's advocate," I facilitated debates concerning the pros and cons of taking specific actions. For me, the act of building capacity is not about providing an answer, but rather about helping the Swazis to develop the skills for arriving at their own answers.

CHALLENGES TO BUILDING NURSING CAPACITY

Building and sustaining an adequate nursing workforce in the Kingdom of Swaziland. or across the sub-Saharan region, is a formidable task. The challenge will require significant funds and an extraordinary effort from all interested parties. While one should be optimistic, it is also reasonable to be a realist; there are challenges that must be addressed if capacity is to be built.

Inadequate Resources

The nursing programs lack up-to-date textbooks and reliable access to electronic library resources. Frequently, the Internet access is unreliable or the bandwidth is insufficient to view and download materials. In Swaziland, there is a significant cost associated with downloading files from the Internet. As a benefit of my Fulbright Scholar award, I was able to ship 50 new, or nearly new, textbooks to Swaziland to support their library.

It is not so easy to address the lack of appropriate materials in the clinical laboratories at the training institutions. My university's clinical lab in Swaziland had two outdated, dilapidated mannequins that were missing limbs. The cost to update to modern mannequins would break their budget. It would be too expensive for the university to supply the labs with the basic materials needed to conduct effective demonstrations, such as latex gloves, IV bags, and supply lines, or mock medication containers.

Professional Mentoring

The lecturers in the nursing institutions need additional mentoring to develop innovative teaching/learning activities designed to develop critical thinking skills, professional ethics, and improved nurse–physician communication. The faculty would benefit from mentors or coaches who could help them advance their educational or research activities. The Fulbright program is an ideal opportunity for nurses to contribute their expertise and mentorship.

Advancing Professionalism

There is a need to provide support for nurses who wish to improve their professional reputation. The general expectation for professional accountability in the Swazi culture is quite low. It is not uncommon to encounter a professional who is unwilling to accept responsibility for his or her actions—or inactions; it is unlikely that personnel would be subject to reprimand or provided remedial training on professional behavior. I witnessed situations in which individuals with personal drive and motivation wanted to initiate an innovative program but encountered resistance from colleagues who were either suspicious, envious, or strategizing to undermine the success of the project. Even when a Swazi nurse wants to make progress, he or she may be constricted by the dominant culture that may perceive no urgency or provide few options for achieving success.

Similarly, nurses can be observed publicly "chastising" patients for their behaviors; it is not uncommon to hear nurses blaming, shaming, and demeaning patients. Patients are, at times, also the target of stigmatization and discrimination at the whim of the nurse with authority. While the official position at most institutions is that such behavior is unacceptable, there are few standards to which health care professionals are held. It is uncommon to conduct annual job performance appraisals with employees. It is understandable why "professional accountability" is a central theme in the MoH's initiative for improving customer care.

Promoting Confidentiality in Health Care

In Swaziland, there is little expectation from the public that their health care information will be kept confidential; therefore, there are few guidelines for maintaining the privacy of patient information. Breaking a patient's right to privacy can have untoward consequences; for example, it may undermine nurse–client rapport and trust, potentially resulting in an unwillingness by patients to adhere to prescribed plans of care.

PERSONAL CHALLENGES AND LESSONS LEARNED

Throughout my career, I have traveled extensively. The Fulbright program provided me with an extraordinary opportunity to live in—not simply visit—the Kingdom of Swaziland. The experience challenged me in ways I could not have expected. I left the country a different man, a more reflective human being, a better nurse. An overview of two of my personal struggles, and the lessons learned, may prove helpful to others who would pursue global nursing.

The Best-Laid Plans . . .

Before coming to Swaziland for the year, I reflected upon how I would respond when poor persons approached me to ask for money. The majority of Swazis live in poverty. I was aware that White persons, particularly Americans, are often perceived as being "rich" and are, therefore, approachable for donations. Surely, by comparison, my standard of living is vastly different than the average Swazi. My decision to not provide handouts was based upon sound reasoning: I would be walking the same dirt roads each day from my Swazi flat to the university. If I gave money to anyone out of sympathy for his or her situation, I would be an easy mark each day thereafter. Soon, others would approach me for support and, quickly, the situation would not only be unmanageable, but unsafe. So, my plan was to quietly, respectfully acknowledge that they were in dire straits, but note that I was unable to help out. At least I had a plan ready.

My plan was good, in theory. The challenge came one day when I was walking in town. A young woman, perhaps in her late 20s, approached me and asked for 10 rand (~$1.00) so that she could get food for her baby. Dressed in worn, tattered clothes, the woman was emaciated; her face exhibited such extreme wasting that it was difficult to discern if she suffered from HIV disease, malnutrition, or a combination of both. The small child in her arms was, obviously, suffering the same fate in my estimation. I struggled . . . my plan to deny her didn't seem so good anymore. How could I walk away from someone asking for so little?

I asked her name. *Nosipho* [meaning mother who brings a gift]. I noted that she did have, indeed, a gift in her arms. She explained that her father had been a Zulu from South Africa and her mother was a Swazi from Hlatikulu (a rural town in the south). Almost by instinct, I walked over to a woman sitting on the sidewalk selling fruits and bought some bananas. I sat with the young woman for nearly 30 minutes, conversing about her life circumstances, struggles, and options. She occasionally gave small amounts of the ripest banana to her baby. She came to the conclusion that going back to her mother's homestead, seeking care from the clinic, and staying healthy to care for her child was the best plan of action. Staying in town exposed her to men who wanted to take advantage of her vulnerability. I walked her over to the taxi rank and paid the driver the fare to Hlatikulu. Once in her seat, I gave her the remaining fruits and wished her well. Though I never saw her again, I often wonder if she is alive—if her baby survived. Often, I count my blessings and never take for granted the resources at my fingertips. I imagine, at times, that Nosipho brought me a gift, a chance to reflect on my place in this world and to be thankful.

Not All Capacity Building Is "Professional"

There is no doubt that the Fulbright Scholar program provided me with opportunities to build the capacity of nurses and other health care workers to deliver quality services with caring and compassion. Yet, there was so much "capacity building" that occurred unexpectedly during my off-times. I came to appreciate how my nonprofessional activities contributed significantly to the goals of mutual understanding and cultural exchange inherent to the Fulbright mission.

Often, my weekends were spent at rural Swazi homesteads of friends I had come to know and love. To the outside observer, I was helping to build a latrine (i.e., outhouse), plant a garden, construct a chicken house, or devise a rainwater collection system. However, in the minutes, hours, and days spent on these activities, I engaged in meaningful conversations about poverty, resourcefulness, and personal resilience. My friends and I debated the rights of women to full engagement in society and politics; we deconstructed the roles of males in traditional culture and potential ways to be better fathers, brothers, or lovers; and we explored practical ways by which Swazis could recapture the value of "communality" by "practicing random acts of kindness" for those who were less fortunate. These everyday activities, relatively unremarkable for many, were building capacity in ways I had not imagined. If these men and women were able to envision a different future for their children—or better prepared to make their current situation safer or more stimulating—then I made an impact. I treasure the relationships I built on the homesteads.

Sacrifice and Patience

It is only fair to mention that living on the African continent for a year meant that I would be away from my husband and family in times of need. Indeed, there were deaths of family members, storm damage to my house, and other minor calamities for which I could only be virtually present through the phone or online videochats. This was a sacrifice that I knew I had to bear; I only hoped that my family understood that there is never, really, a good time to be away. It was my hope that friends, family, and colleagues back home would respect my decision.

It took considerable introspection, however, to acquire the patience needed to live in a culture so different from one's own. Compared with American culture, almost everything moves more slowly, or through a more circuitous route, in Swaziland. A scheduled meeting may start 2 hours late because attendees had not yet arrived; timely requests may be answered within days to weeks; obtaining signatures on important documents may take months. At times, the wait was laughable. Sometimes, the time spent waiting was irritating. The worst situations were when I perceived the delays to be purposeful or disrespectful of my time and effort. Ever so slowly, the lack of attention to timeliness became expected; I developed a peaceful acquiescence to its ubiquitous nature. Be assured, though, it was a personal struggle that tested my resolve.

CONCLUSION

Building an adequate and sustainable health care workforce in Southern Africa is truly a formidable task. The goal is more than admirable; it is a moral imperative for those who have the knowledge, skills, and ability to act. Over the year, the U.S. Fulbright Scholar program provided me with extraordinary opportunities to contribute, meaningfully, to the health and well-being of the Swazi people. Moreso, the experience opened my eyes, expanded my perspective, and deepened my commitment to my family, my work, and my African colleagues.

Nurses have a unique knowledge base, the requisite clinical skills, and a humanistic philosophy to make a significant contribution as Fulbright Scholars. One can apply for periods that range from several weeks to a year in a country or region; the Fulbright program is flexible. The impact that nurses can make by taking the time to share their professional expertise and engaging as full partners in cultural exchange is immeasurable. It is, surely, meaningful.

In this chapter, I have provided glimpses into my experience in Swaziland. Each nurse who ventures into global nursing will have a unique experience and be changed in ways that one cannot predict. There is a lot of work to do in partnership with the global community and many nurses are ready for the challenge. Plan, engage, and enjoy!

ACKNOWLEDGMENT

The author claims ownership and responsibility for all of the comments, opinions, and insights in this chapter. In no way should this material be construed as representative of the U.S. Fulbright Program, the CIES, or the U.S. Department of State.

NOTES

For more information, please visit the following websites:

- Fulbright Scholar Program, visit http://www.cies.org
- Nurses SOAR! program, visit the U.S. Department of State report at http://iipdigital.usembassy.gov/st/english/article/2008/12/20081229094029abretnuh0.5824396.html#axzz2s5AzgFjQ
- Wellness Center for Health Care Workers: http://www.icn.ch/projects/wellness-centres-for-health-care-workers

REFERENCES

Anyangwe, S. C., & Mtonga, C. (2007). Inequities in the global health workforce: The greatest impediment to health in Sub-Saharan Africa. *International Journal of Environmental Research and Public Health, 4*(2), 93–100.

Baleta, A. (2008). World report: Swaziland nurses the wellbeing of its health workers. *The Lancet, 371,* 1901–1902.

Council for International Exchange of Scholars (CIES). (2013). *The Fulbright Scholar program.* Washington, DC: Council for International Exchange of Scholars, the Institute of International Education. Retrieved from http://www.cies.org/about-us/what-fulbright

Ministry of Health. (2011). *Annual health statistics report 2011.* Mbabane, Swaziland: Government of the Kingdom of Swaziland. Retrieved from http://www.gov.sz/index.php?option=com_content&view=article&id=751&Itemid=599

Ministry of Health. (2012). *Human resources for health strategic plan 2012–2017.* Mbabane, Swaziland: Government of the Kingdom of Swaziland. Retrieved from http://www.gov.sz/index.php?option=com_content&view=article&id=751&Itemid=599

President's Emergency Plan for AIDS Relief (PEPFAR). (2013). *Nursing Education Partnership Initiative* (NEPI). Washington, DC. Retrieved from http://www.pepfar.gov/partnerships/initiatives/nepi

Stilwell, B. (2011). Will they stay or will they go? Putting theory into practice to guide effective workforce retention mechanisms. *World Health & Population, 13*(2), 34–40.

Swaziland's election: Africa's last absolute monarch may not keep his lavish lifestyle for long. (2013, September 14). *The Economist*. Retrieved from http://www.economist .com/news/middle-east-and-africa/21586354-africas-last-absolute-monarch-may-not-keep-his-lavish-lifestyle-long-royal/comments

U.S. Agency for International Development (USAID). (2013). *Human resources in health toolkit. Knowledge for health (K4Health)*. Retrieved from http://www.k4health.org/toolkits/hrh

World Bank. (2013). *Swaziland overview*. Washington, DC: The World Bank. Retrieved from http://www.worldbank.org/en/country/swaziland/overview

World Health Organization (WHO). (2006). *Treat, train, retain: The AIDS and health work-force plan. Report on the consultation on AIDS and human resources for health*. Geneva, Switzerland: World Health Organization. Retrieved from http://www.who.int/hiv/pub/meetingreports/ttr/en

World Health Organization. (2009). *Africa Health Workforce Observatory: Human Resources for Health (HRH) country profile: Swaziland*. Geneva, Switzerland: World Health Organization. Retrieved from http://www.hrh-observatory.afro.who.int/images/Document_Centre/Country_profile_Swaziland.pdf

CHAPTER 31

Interdisciplinary Collaborations in Global Health Research

Ann Kurth, Allison Squires, Michele Shedlin, and James Kiarie

Global health problems are complex, requiring approaches and solutions that engage the insights of multiple disciplines and professions. There is a growing recognition of the need for more interprofessionalism in designing, conducting, and implementing research, along with translating scientific findings into practice. Outmoded dichotomizations of "biological versus behavioral" or "basic versus applied" research are becoming less relevant. Newer ideas about "systems," "team," and "implementation" science illustrate the opportunity for multidisciplinary research groups to address problems holistically and create evidence-based approaches. At many universities, however, truly interdisciplinary and interprofessional research is lacking or is just beginning. In this chapter we review frameworks for interdisciplinary research, follow them with specific case studies outlining some of the challenges and opportunities of such work, and close with principles of interprofessional research in the global context, with lessons for nursing in particular. We concentrate on interprofessional research capacity-building issues and examples, rather than interprofessional education or clinical practice. Although those are related and integral elements are needed to achieve optimal health for individuals, communities, and populations, we emphasize research because of its role in creating the evidence that helps improve health.

BACKGROUND

When trying to cull lessons learned from research experiences and published studies, it becomes clear that health researchers in a variety of disciplines have begun to respond in creative ways to the critical and constantly changing challenges of global health. This is happening because of a growing awareness that single method studies and uni-professional perspectives do not always provide the knowledge needed to confront these challenges and inform effective responses. Openness to new approaches is also supported by the urgency to address not only infectious diseases, such as the HIV pandemic, but also the surge in chronic diseases, global aging, ongoing reproductive health challenges, substance abuse, trauma and violence, mental health, and health systems issues.

The advantages of a multidisciplinary or interprofessional approach to research are many. A diverse toolkit helps facilitate understanding of the context of the health problem and seek more viable solutions. The literature demonstrates, for example, how social science theories and perspectives can provide a crucial bridge between epidemiological surveys, clinical research, and program development. More frequently, study designs and global health program evaluations incorporate multimethod or mixed-method approaches (Institute of Medicine [IOM], 2014) that provide not only the "how many" and the "where," but also the "why" and the realities of the environments and context in which research is conducted.

If nursing is to continue to be key in responding to new needs and opportunities in global health research, interdisciplinary and interprofessional collaboration is critical. Now more than ever, nurse researchers recognize the social and health imperatives that require theories from multiple disciplines and more diverse analytic approaches. This means collaboration not only by nurse, midwife, and physician investigators, but with colleagues from public health, the humanities, law, business, engineering, and the social sciences, among others.

All of this said, there are historical, practical, and resource obstacles to achieving a collaborative approach to research. As professionals with different training, experience, and points of view, each discipline may have different priorities, theoretical perspectives, and skills—all those *strengths* within each profession that may become *barriers* in an interprofessional collaboration. Even the language of research may vary between professions and disciplines. There also may be competing demands by institutions and funders. Stakeholders to whom researchers must respond as individuals and as teams add complexity to this work. When teams of researchers have access to different levels of resources, as is often the case in global health research efforts where team members come from both high- as well as low-income-country settings, power differentials can be an underlying reality. Researchers need to be mindful of avoiding "extractive" science: the case where only some team members receive professional benefits of the work, often at the expense of low- and middle-income-country (LMIC) collaborators.

Donor priorities also can hinder the natural technical and infrastructure capacity building that can and should accompany international research collaborations. The very questions examined by research teams may be influenced more by donor than by local country priorities, in the least optimal situations. Supporting development of grants administration and ethical review board procedures, for example, are critical for effective global health research practice and important for sustaining research capacity in LMICs. These activities, however, may not always be explicitly supported by research funders or be seen as a priority by some team members' home universities (Chu, Jayaraman, Kyamanywa, & Ntakiyiruta, 2014).

What are some of the lessons learned so far to overcome these barriers to needed collaborations? As nurses, physicians, public health practitioners, social scientists, and others involved in interprofessional global research, it is helpful to identify pitfalls to avoid and characteristics of successful collaborations.

Interprofessional Research Frameworks

Interprofessional research frameworks have received less emphasis than interprofessional education frameworks that have been developed by different groups, including the World Health Organization (WHO). Nonetheless, other disciplines provide useful tools researchers can draw from to shape their collaborations.

For example, "team science" has a history of investigation in the business world (Gully, Incalcaterra, Joshi, & Beauien, 2002; Guzzo & Dickson, 1996; Wang, Waldman, & Zhang, 2014) as measured by publications and patents, as noted in a seminal 2007 review (Wuchty, Jones, & Uzzi, 2007). It is increasingly the norm in scientific discovery and production. Research also shows that team-based, interprofessional care improves clinical outcomes (Reeves et al., 2008). Canada has been a leader in funding interprofessional health research and "team science" approaches. The National Academy of Sciences (NAS) in the United States has published a report on the "science of team science" outlining successful principles and recommending best approaches to optimizing collaborative research (NAS, 2014). A team-based approach can help facilitate productive research collaborations. Though there are acknowledged and anticipated strong benefits of interdisciplinary and interprofessional research, the evidence base delineating the specific impact in the global health context has been slower to accrue. There are a growing number of publications in implementation science and open access journals that describe how interprofessional research takes place, as well as analytic studies documenting the impact of interprofessional research on key indices such as health measures, economic efficiencies, and health system operations.

Governance also plays a role in international research, especially when it concerns the complex ethics of human subjects' protection in low resource settings. In 2013 the WHO called for strengthening research capacities worldwide. Then in early 2014, a consortium that includes the International Alliance of Patients' Organizations (IAPO), International Council of Nurses (ICN), International Federation of Pharmaceutical Manufacturers and Associations (IFPMA), International Pharmaceutical Federation (FIP), and the World Medical Association (WMA) established a Consensus Framework for Ethical Collaboration in Research. This framework was derived from the individual codes of ethical practice and health policy positions of each of the supporting organizations, and promulgates four overarching principles: putting patients first; supporting ethical research and innovation; ensuring independence and ethical conduct; and promoting transparency and accountability (IFPMA, 2014).

Research Challenges—History and Funding

Nursing's contribution to global research has been at multiple levels—via involvement in clinical trials (often for pharmacologic agents), as researchers on clinical and behavioral interventions, conducting qualitative research and program evaluations, and other topical areas. Barriers to conducting interprofessional research include different histories of research training and variations in resources available to different professions in different regions of the world. Nursing, for example, has had doctoral programs since the mid-20th century in high-income countries (HICs) such as the United States and a federal nursing-research funding agency (the National Institute of Nursing Research [NINR], www.ninr.nih.gov/aboutninr) only since 1986. Yet a similarly well-resourced nation (Germany) did not have nursing PhD programs until the year 2000; the first government-funded nursing research project there was not until 1988 (Cassier-Woidasky, 2013). While nurse faculty in LMICs may still need to seek their doctoral training outside of their home country, there are increasing south-south exchanges and capacity-building efforts, such as PhD programs in Brazil attended by nurses throughout Latin America, or nursing doctoral programs in Thailand attended by nurses throughout Asia.

The level of funding available to individual professions and disciplines for doctoral preparation, postdoctoral work, and for a sustainable research career also vary tremendously by discipline and region. It is difficult to promote interprofessional research teams when one profession (historically, in most countries, medicine) has such different access to preparation in research methods and funding. Layered on top of these fundamental constraints are the additional practical issues of differing communication patterns and terminology and acronyms, as well as more subtle variations in the language of research that each discipline brings to a research question or study team.

Within nursing, the ability to attain significant external funding as principal investigator (PI) of a multiprofessional research team arguably has been a less common experience. In the United States, National Institutes of Health (NIH) Fogarty funds provide support for international scholars to receive graduate and advanced research methods training. Only a handful of these trainees, however, have been nurses. Even those few nurses who receive Fogarty or other research training return to home country settings where there are not designated nursing research funding entities, and their ability to conduct independent, funded research is limited. This is in addition to the fact that many nursing faculty in LMICs with advanced education, including doctoral degrees, are often assigned heavy administrative, teaching, and clinical loads that makes carving out time for research difficult. Despite these obstacles, nurses around the world conduct research that advances patient and community health. An impressive example of nurse-led research that has successfully undertaken research resulting in dozens of multiauthored publications is the International HIV Nurse Research Network, which has successfully conducted six study protocols in multiple countries on a comparatively small budget (Holzemer, 2007).

Some resources that are relevant for nurses and others engaged in research globally are summarized in Table 31.1. In the following pages we provide case examples of interdisciplinary and interprofessional research and program delivery collaborations that cover major geographical regions. We will illustrate some of the various ways that interprofessional research collaborations can occur to produce evidence, improve evidence-based practice (EBP), and build research capacity.

TABLE 31.1 Global Health Research Resources

Consortium of Universities for Global Health http://www.cugh.org	Global Health Council http://www.globalhealth.org
ICN http://www.icn.ch	Kaiser Family Foundation http://www.globalhealthfacts.org
PAHO http://new.paho.org	WHO http://www.who.int/en
Global Health Research Nurses http://globalresearchnurses.tghn.org http://globalresearchmethods.tghn.org	Global Health Hub http://www.globalhealthhub.org
International Resource Center/NACUBO http://irc.nacubo.org	Joanna Briggs Institute http://www.joannabriggs.edu.au

NACUBO, National Association of College and University Business Officers; PAHO, Pan American Health Organization; WHO, World Health Organization.

CASE STUDY: REPUBLIC OF GEORGIA RESEARCH CAPACITY-BUILDING PROJECT

U.S. State Department Funding, NYU College of Nursing, PI Dr. Deborah Chyun, co-PI Dr. Allison Squires

In LMICs, research capacity building often needs to take two forms: developing research consumers and research producers. An interprofessional team from New York University (NYU) and a consortium of Georgian universities developed a U.S. State Department–funded project in the country of Georgia aimed at developing research capacity among health care professionals in the country. The unique aspect of the project was that it conceived research capacity building as not only mentoring PhD students in the health professions, but also as building capacity for EBP among frontline health care providers. With the dual approach, the project had the potential to impact patient outcomes in the short term while developing domestic health research capacity for the long term.

Good quality working relationships are key to any research study and also are essential for international research collaborations and capacity building. A NYU team member's long-established professional relationships in the country helped to facilitate grant development and project implementation. The team could capitalize on the basic networks and then expand relationships because of a positive prior history. With that foundation to work from, the following sections describe project implementation and offer considerations for similar partnerships.

Needs Assessment

An interprofessional team initiated the project with a formal needs assessment. The team included a PhD-prepared nurse with extensive experience working in LMICs and a master's degree in public health (MPH) with extensive experience

(continued)

CASE STUDY: REPUBLIC OF GEORGIA RESEARCH CAPACITY-BUILDING PROJECT (*continued*)

working in the region on international development projects. Focus groups with faculty, students, and front-line health care professionals comprised the needs assessment. Meeting with local Ministry of Health (MoH) officials also occurred to ensure that the government perspective was incorporated into program planning and to ensure political support during implementation.

The team anticipated that English language skills, library resources, and technology (e.g., availability of computers, reliability of Internet access, etc.) would affect student participation in both programs. The team did not anticipate the lack of training by librarians on Internet searching methods and open access journals. This issue occurred even in the top research universities and informed program design. Research resources, as expected, were limited, although a domestic general science research fund was available.

During the needs assessment, it was important to separate students from professors, as well as frontline workers from supervisors, during interviews. That move generated much more open dialogue about the key issues around research capacity building. Students, for example, felt freer to discuss the issues that arise around mentoring and supervision. They also raised concerns about themselves eventually passing their advisors in terms of research skill and the political implications that could have in the future.

The EBP Training Program

EBP is the incorporation of research findings with provider experiences and patient perspective (Polit & Beck, 2014). EBP requires frontline health care professionals to have the skills to read and critique research studies so they can determine if they should apply them to practice. Building clinical research capacity in any country, therefore, should include this component.

The NYU team designed a 1-week, 20-hour intensive, interprofessional, EBP training course for front-line health care providers. Among the 97 attendees at the two sites where the workshop was offered, there were physicians, administrators, nurses, researchers, insurance industry representatives, pharmacists, and public health professionals working for nongovernmental organizations (NGOs). Offering the workshop outside of the main capital city offered the potential for greater national impact of the project.

The EBP workshop was well received overall and the practicing clinicians rapidly grasped the concepts. Translation was provided as necessary by in-country partners. Online follow-up after workshop implementation was able to (1) capture whether the participants had been able to apply the concepts to their work, (2) assess the barriers and facilitators to implementing EBP in the local context, and (3) provide the binational research team with data to develop the next collaboration opportunity.

Building the Next Generation of Health Researchers

Through a selective process, 18 PhD student participants from Georgian universities were selected from 150 applicants to be in an intensive mentoring program that was the second part of the project. Competence in reading, writing, and speaking English was the minimum language requirement. Over a 2-year period, in-country and online mentoring occurred with NYU faculty matched based on student interest. A week-long research methods intensive course started the program to ensure that everyone was at the same level. As with PhD students in the United States, goals were set for each visit. Students focused the development of their research based on those individual goals. Most students had a public health background, but the cohort included a laboratory services director, pharmacist, one nurse, and a lawyer with a health and human rights interest.

The majority of participants made rapid progress in the development of their proposals, study implementation, or finalization of their research project. As expected, some students had more difficulty progressing than others. Intensive editing of English language writing by the students was required of all participating faculty members, but their writing improved with the mentoring.

The program finished with a conference where the top students presented their work to a local health care and MoH audience. The final event allowed all the partners to highlight how the project had impacted students and clinical practice. It also generated the necessary political support among all the stakeholders to move ahead with pursuing funding opportunities to continue the work and attract additional funding sources.

Dissemination

All publications resulting from the project include a local author. Inclusion of local partners on all publications and dissemination activities is important. It documents true intercountry collaboration. It also appropriately helps to advance the careers of local partners in terms of first or senior authorships. Mutual recognition in dissemination activities helps reinforce the relationships that are essential for building collaborative research opportunities, establishing research capacity, and fostering EBP in places where the research culture is more nascent.

CASE STUDY: THE HEALTH VULNERABILITY OF COLOMBIAN REFUGEES IN ECUADOR

NIH/NIDA Funding, PI Dr. Michele Shedlin

Background/Context

War, illegal drug operations, violence generated by guerrilla and paramilitary groups, and lack of viable economic alternatives are all factors that are increasingly disrupting communities and generating worldwide population mobility and migration. Population displacement, especially when involuntary and at a large

(continued)

CASE STUDY: THE HEALTH VULNERABILITY OF COLOMBIAN REFUGEES IN ECUADOR (continued)

scale, contributes to the spread of disease and influences the health vulnerability of individuals and communities alike. Latin America is not an exception, and migrant and refugee men and women in South and Central America have become increasingly vulnerable. Longstanding international relationships were fundamental in establishing an interdisciplinary team to carry out an investigation of the health vulnerability of Colombian refugees in Ecuador.

The study brought together extensive research experience with national and international Hispanic communities, including the prior development of instruments and strategies for studies of at-risk groups and "hidden populations" in Latin America and the United States. The U.S. research team that designed the application included anthropologists and a physician/immunologist. The Ecuadorian NGO staff that worked on modifying the instruments and coordinated the data collection was led by physicians with master's degrees in public and environmental health with extensive experience in community-based initiatives among vulnerable populations.

There were three objectives of the study. This included identifying the sociodemographic characteristics and migratory trajectories of recent Colombian refugees in Ecuador; exploring the individual and contextual factors that influence health risks, including cultural factors and structural violence associated with the sending country's drug wars and receiving country stigma and discrimination; and developing institutional capacity, especially in the NGO sector, to conduct immigrant health research in Ecuador focusing on drug use and sexually transmitted infection (STI)/HIV risk.

Research Collaboration

After the award of the grant, U.S. investigators traveled to Quito to work with the Ecuadorian in-country team to review the instruments and to plan research activities. During this trip, discussions were initiated with the organizations in direct contact with the refugee population, and it was agreed that they would assist with recruitment for the study. Follow-up was made in subsequent meetings by the NGO staff. However, during the initial meeting with the NGOs, it became clear that there was a great deal of political sensitivity regarding the refugee population as well as the topics of drug use and HIV, two of the priorities of the research. The major obstacle at that point was the title of the study, which included mention of those health issues. Thus, the in-country title of the project was modified, and in Ecuador, the study was called Health Vulnerability: The Colombian Population in Ecuador in Need of International Protection (Vulnerabilidad de La Salud: La Población Colombiana en El Ecuador con Necesidades de Protección Internacional; James, 2013).

In addition to concerns about the project title, the Ecuadorian colleagues were also involved in a detailed review of the research instruments, their content, and language/terminology. This discussion began during an initial visit and lasted for a number of months via e-mails and phone conversations.

The revised, politically modified instruments did not omit questions concerning HIV and drug use, but rather embedded these sensitive topics within more general health-oriented sections. Subtleties of language were also discussed and incorporated. The revised instruments were then submitted to the institutional IRBs in Ecuador and the United States, and were approved.

The NGO staff, all experienced scholars and activists, was also aware of the lack of knowledge about HIV and substance abuse research in the country, especially among NGOs working with at-risk populations. As part of the grant, the U.S. investigators provided expert training in these areas, in Spanish, by means of a workshop for government, NGO, and university representatives, not only those immediately involved in the study. By inviting many professional groups involved in any way with the refugee population, the study team assured not only a wider understanding of the research methods involved, but also clarity of the objectives of the study and the commitment of the investigators toward contributing to a better understanding of the needs of the refugee population.

Interviews were carried out in confidential spaces where the refugee men and women felt safe and welcome. The PI and NGO team carried out individual interviews and focus group discussions, building relationships and rapport with the refugee-serving agencies that were understandably protective of their constituents.

While the majority of the interview data were analyzed in the United States (content analysis of 1 year of media reports of the refugee situation was carried out in-country), all data collected also remained in secure files in Ecuador. This was important for many reasons, above all to counter any possible concerns that data would be taken out of the country and not shared with Ecuadorian institutions. Unfortunately, this concern has a very real basis, historically, and at no point in the study was there a gap in data sharing.

Dissemination

A number of papers have resulted from this study, published in U.S. peer-reviewed journals with coauthorship of the entire team. Meetings in Ecuador to present results of the study have been held with university, NGO, and government leadership. The study was also published in Spanish, in book form, and is being distributed by a well-known and respected Latin American publisher (Shedlin et al., 2014). These results include powerful accounts of the Colombian refugees' experience of drug war violence and discrimination in their new environments, and the critical needs of this population for basic health care and prevention services.

Aside from the contribution of the study to the knowledge base of the impact of forced migration on individuals and families in the Latin American context, the project illustrated lessons learned regarding how international collaborations can be enriched by interdisciplinary, inter-institutional relationships at the national, institutional, and individual levels. Communication and understanding were enhanced by the bilingual abilities and cultural sensitivities of the U.S. investigators. Political pitfalls were avoided and validity addressed by genuine collaboration on the presentation of the study and the instruments. The many health, and social service disciplines represented by the U.S. and Ecuadorian research teams contributed in important ways to the successful implementation of the study and dissemination of the results. Finally, incorporation of government and health and social service individuals and agencies ultimately support the possibility that the study results will actually contribute to the program, and perhaps even policy change.

CASE STUDY: MEDICAL EDUCATION PARTNERSHIP INITIATIVE IN KENYA

NIH and PEPFAR Funding, NIH Grant 1R24 TW008889, PI James Kiarie

With funding from the President's Emergency Plan for AIDS Relief (PEPFAR) and the NIH, through the Medical Education Partnership Initiative (MEPI),[1] the University of Nairobi, University of Washington, and University of Maryland Baltimore initiated the Partnership in Innovative Medical Education for Kenya (PRIME-K) project. A description of the overall MEPI program has pointed out that some, but not all, of the programs funded by MEPI have reached "beyond the medical school to involve other faculties, such as nursing, public health, and dentistry" (Mullan, Chen, & Steinmetz, 2013). This latter approach is the path chosen by the PRIME-K project with joint activities in the School of Medicine, School of Nursing Sciences, School of Dental Sciences, School of Public Health, and School of Pharmacy.

Background

The University of Nairobi is the largest university in Kenya, offering approximately 200 programs of study to 62,000 students in six colleges spanning seven campuses across the capital city. Although officially established in 1970, its roots extend to 1956. The College of Health Sciences offers both undergraduate and postgraduate programs for health workers with the School of Medicine training over half of the medical doctors entering the country's workforce each year.

The mission of PRIME-K is to improve health outcomes in Kenya through medical education and clinical research. To achieve its mission, PRIME-K promotes innovative teaching methods, decentralized training, institutional research support designed to attract and retain highly qualified faculty, and capacity building for research administration. The PRIME-K program has strong partnerships with the MoH, Kenyatta National Hospital, Kenyatta University, and Maseno University, extending the impact of the training beyond the University of Nairobi.

The program has several specific aims. The first is to increase the quantity and quality of health professionals. This is achieved by development of a multidisciplinary skills lab, provision of e-learning resources, faculty training on innovative teaching methods, and development of new training initiatives. The second aim is to improve retention of health care workers. This is achieved by training health professionals in decentralized training sites whose capacity is built by improving data systems and capacity building of adjunct faculty. A third aim is to improve faculty retention by investing in regionally relevant research. This aim is achieved through Implementation Science Fellowships training, mentored seed projects, and career development projects. A final aim is to build capacity for research administration and oversight. This is achieved by training on responsible conduct of research, bioethics, critical appraisal of research proposals, proposal development, manuscript writing, and mentorship. Further institutional capacity building has been supported by also developing strategic plans for the University of Nairobi Grants Management Office and the University of Nairobi–Kenyatta National Hospital Ethics Review Committee.

PRIME-K has a linked project on Maternal Neonatal and Child Health (MNCH) that builds upon the programmatic award's activities by establishing a Collaborative Center of Excellence in MNCH. This Center of Excellence is building research capacity and providing training in implementation science and applied research, evaluation, and program leadership relevant to achieving Kenya's health development goals. Specifically, this project aims to: (1) build capacity to conduct multidisciplinary implementation science research that translates into policy and practice by conducting training for medical faculty and postgraduates in Pediatrics, Obstetrics/Gynecology, Nursing, Pharmacy, and Public Health; (2) promote implementation science research that strengthens MNCH efforts at the community level in collaboration with the MoH, by providing opportunities for teams of medical faculty and/or postgraduates from at least two different disciplines to compete for MNCH projects based at decentralized clinical training sites; (3) enhance MNCH program leadership capacity and build bridges between the University of Nairobi and the Kenya MoH programs in MNC. To accomplish this, the University of Nairobi will collaborate with the Afya Bora Consortium (afyaboraconsortium.org) to offer a 9-month fellowship and a short course in leadership and teamwork in MNCH.

Notable achievements in interprofessional research by PRIME-K have been attained and are outlined in the following text.

Research Training

PRIME-K conducted two phases of implementation science research training of medical doctors, nurses, pharmacists, dentists, and health informaticians. The first phase was 3 days at the health facility for 30 to 60 staff covering developing research questions, research proposal writing, and data collection. The second phase was 2 days for three to five staff (adjunct faculty) from the pool of those trained in the first phase, who developed a research proposal based on research questions identified in phase one. The adjunct faculty will be mentored by University of Nairobi faculty to submit the proposals for ethics review, collect and analyze data, and disseminate results. Adjunct faculty at nine health facilities have developed draft research proposals covering various areas including impact of national health financing policies, staff retention, and quality of services.

(continued)

CASE STUDY: MEDICAL EDUCATION PARTNERSHIP INITIATIVE IN KENYA (continued)

The linked MNCH project partnered with the Kenyan MoH to identify priority research questions. Teams of postgraduate students from the University of Nairobi Schools of Medicine, Nursing, Pharmacy, and Public Health submitted proposals to study the prioritized MNCH questions in public facilities. Successful applicants were funded and paired with mentors from the University of Nairobi and MoH. The research studies were conducted over 3- to 6-month periods. Seven of the nine applications (total of 51 students) were funded over the first 2 years. Funded research projects focused on malnutrition in mothers and children, perinatal morbidity and mortality, prevention of mother-to-child transmission of HIV, and guideline utilization for common maternal and childhood morbidities.

PRIME-K has supported an Implementation Science Fellowship program aimed at training academic and health care system leaders who can translate evidence-based interventions into health care practice and policy. The key strengths of the fellowship program lie in its multidisciplinary approaches, which offer diverse experiences, perspectives, and linkages to the trainees; innovative use of information technology; and a team model for mentorship and supervision. The minimum qualification for entry is a master's degree in the health sciences, including pharmacy, nursing, medicine, dentistry, and public health. The criteria for admission are not restricted only to candidates with qualifications in health sciences. Persons with master's degrees in biomedical sciences or social sciences are also eligible. In the first cohort of fellows admitted to the program, six individuals who received letters of offer had qualifications in the following disciplines: public health (2), pharmacy (2), medicine (1), and nursing (1). Of the five participants who started the program, two were female. The second cohort has five trainees, with professional qualifications in public health (1), pharmacy (2), dental sciences (1), and nursing (1).

Dissemination

The MEPI teams have presented project findings at national, regional, and international conferences and are publishing in journals that target medical, nursing, and other health-related profession audiences. Peer-reviewed journal articles also are forthcoming. A key component of dissemination has been presentation of research findings to local health facility staff. These meetings are usually well attended by staff from all professions that provide health care.

A challenge of interprofessional education that was experienced in this MEPI project is that many professionals are fairly set in their ways and were initially skeptical about working with others. However, as they worked together and developed joint proposals there was increased appreciation of the value added by each profession. For postgraduate student research, the schools of medicine, pharmacy, nursing, and public health also have set expectations with which the scientific team had to work in order to ensure that the students could conduct joint research yet still each be able to satisfy their school requirements. These kinds of institutional negotiations should help facilitate more interprofessional research in the future.

DISCUSSION

Common themes in the case studies illustrate some general principles to address what Masiello (2009) has summarized as communication, culture, commitment, and challenges (Thistlethwaite & Grin Working Group, 2013) for effective inter-professional research in global health. These principles can be applied throughout the research process. The WHO has outlined principles to consider when conducting global health research (Table 31.2). We endorse these and elaborate further here to highlight considerations around the conduct of interprofessional global health research.

Communication

As noted, the business world has refined the science of teams and there is a body of literature focused on what makes for an effective team—balancing personalities, managing cultural differences, and communicating effectively. Researchers, both novice and established, may consult this literature prior to creating a new team because communication is a critical component of a successful research collaboration.

For global health research teams, several factors may affect communication. Differing expertise may generate communication challenges. Furthermore, professional hierarchies that may exist in clinical and other settings may introduce attitudes and behaviors counterproductive to research collaborations. Power imbalances based on titles, professions, and funding are often obstacles to

TABLE 31.2 Principles of Global Health Research

Further details of these 11 principles can be found in *Guidelines for Research in Partnership With Developing Countries*, prepared by the Swiss Commission for Research Partnership with Developing Countries (64). The 11 principles (with minor adaptation) are as follows.

1. Decide on bidirectional research objectives among both international and local stakeholders that are mutually beneficial.
2. Build mutual trust, stimulating honest and open research collaboration.
3. Share information and develop networks for coordination.
4. Share responsibility and ownership.
5. Created transparency in financial and other transactions.
6. Monitor and evaluate collaboration, judging performance through regular internal and 1. external evaluations.
7. Disseminate the results through joint publications and other means, with adequate communication to those who will finally use them.
8. Apply the results as far as is possible, recognizing the obligation to ensure that results are used to benefit the target group.
9. Share the benefits of research equitably, including profit, publications, and patents.
10. Increase research capacity at individual and institutional levels.
11. Build on the achievements of research—especially new knowledge, sustainable development, and research capacity.

Source: WHO (2013).

successful collaborations because of the communication issues they produce. Even in this digital age, researchers should not undervalue the importance of in-person meetings for establishing fruitful working relationships. "Live" connections are still important in many countries around the world and can help avoid misunderstandings that can occur via digital communication. Prior to final decisions, potential team members need to meet in a way that balances cultural expectations around relationship building to discuss ideas, explore communication styles, and have clarity regarding future roles.

Once the team is formed, it is helpful to establish a common research language within the team. Different professions have different communication styles, "languages," and expectations. It is important for a collaborative research team to address linguistic and disciplinary worldviews, which may or may not differ. Jargon often varies widely since each profession develops its own memes, acronyms, and other codes that are easily understood internally but can be arcane to other groups. An e-mail communication protocol can also be helpful when English is not the first language of collaborators to minimize the risk for miscommunication issues resulting from "text message" style writing. Standards for good and effective e-mail communication should apply to everyone.

With relationships, communication rules, and the common language established, the team then proceeds with working through who actually sets the research agenda and the questions to be explored. This is a critical step, and one in which all disciplines and players, including study participants and patients/clients, should be involved. Data access and "ownership" during and after the study should be discussed early on. A team should collectively navigate the competing demands of research funders, donors, and country representatives including Ministries of Health as well as NGOs. With these factors in mind, feasible and answerable research questions should be developed collaboratively and reflect local priorities, not just those of the higher-resourced partners in a scientific team.

PIs from *both* the host and the funding nations (if they differ) should lead the research project. Each will bring different strengths, resources, and attention to an international research project. This arrangement ensures an ethical grounding for the study along with a pragmatic foundation from which the work will be managed. The U.S. NIH has allowed such a "multiple PI" model for several years. Authorship, including who will be coauthors, who will take the lead authorship, and consensus on fair rules for transferring authorships if needed, is best discussed at the outset of a study rather than at the end.

Philosophical and theoretical differences need to be addressed early on, especially in clarifying research goals and methods. How theory and methods of different professions are integrated and triangulated must reflect the research questions and research goals, not the investigator hierarchy or other interests.

Once a study design emerges, research tools, such as survey instruments, ideally will be cross-culturally relevant and also capture key domains relevant to multiple disciplines. In-country colleagues need to lead regarding cultural nuances and political sensitivities, not only about research topics (e.g., HIV, sexual behavior, violence) but about the appropriateness of specific field methods and research instruments. Analyses should be conducted as a group since there is enrichment gained by the different methodologies and explanatory power of involving more than one discipline. Equity of access to and determination of resources in a research project, hierarchy and power differentials between and across disciplines on the team, and other potentially uncomfortable issues can and should be addressed throughout the life cycle of the research project.

As this section demonstrates, communication is a fundamental part of the entire research process, especially in the context of multidisciplinary work. Its power and influence over a study's success should not be underestimated.

Capacity Building

International research collaborations have the potential to contribute significantly to research capacity building. Educational initiatives and other in-country trainings to develop institutional capacity for collaborating agencies and colleagues must be respectful of positions and other demands on time and space, as well as resources. Educational efforts focused on building research skills should incorporate as wide a range of agency personnel as appropriate, and budgets need to reflect this attention to inclusiveness.

PhD students conducting international research are a special category. There are two types: LMIC students obtaining degrees internationally, and HIC students seeking to build a global research career in their specific topic area. Research collaborations that involve students outside of the student's country either should involve preexisting relationships or occur with a mentor with well-established networks of collaboration in the country. A lack of either puts the student at risk for failing to complete a dissertation within a required time period. Additionally, doctoral committees should be interdisciplinary wherever possible and have at least one representative with national or regional expertise.

Research Prioritization and Dissemination

At the outset of any collaborative interprofessional research, including proposal writing, the fit of the research with the MoH and host country priorities must take precedence over home institution or funder's priorities. With an eye toward the end stage of collaborative research, there should be clarity in advance regarding dissemination objectives, journals, and authorship. This may be less of an obstacle with interdisciplinary teams as primary authorships for articles and professional presentations could reflect different and multiple professional journals of the disciplines involved.

As a general rule, it is important to acknowledge that professions have protective loyalties that must be respected and negotiated, especially when they may bias or interfere with roles and responsibilities. Nonetheless, we believe that professional diversity enriches the research and supports rigor. This is a challenge for team leaders who need to identify and address potential conflicts and differences of opinion continually.

APPLICATION TO NURSING AND INTERPROFESSIONAL PRACTICE

In this chapter we reviewed some of the challenges, approaches, and benefits to be gained by engaging in multidisciplinary global health research. Nursing is a profession that is rightly proud of its hard-won founding as a respected science, yet we, as a group, have long understood the richness that comes from working as a team with other disciplines' engagement. Following core principles for such interprofessional research can contribute to improved insights and application to better health for the clients and communities that we serve.

NOTE

1. There is also a Nursing Education Partnership Initiative (NEPI) whose goal is to "strengthen the quality and capacity of nursing and midwifery education institutions, increase the number of highly skilled nurses and midwives, and support innovative nursing retention strategies in African countries" (see http://www.pepfar.gov/partnerships/initiatives/nepi).

REFERENCES

Cassier-Woidasky, A. (2013). *PowerPoint: Nursing education in Germany—challenges and obstacles in professionalization.* Retrieved from http://www.klinikum.uni-heidelberg.de/fileadmin/neurologie/pdf_downloads/ANIM2013/ANIM2013_Cassier-Woidasky.pdf

Chu, K. M., Jayaraman, S., Kyamanywa, P., & Ntakiyiruta, G. (2014). Building research capacity in Africa: Equity and global health collaborations. *PLoS Medicine, 11*(3), e1001612. doi:10.1371/journal.pmed.1001612

Gully, S. M., Incalcaterra, K. A., Joshi, A., & Beauien, J. M. (2002). A meta-analysis of team-efficacy, potency, and performance: Interdependence and level of analysis as moderators of observed relationships. *Journal of Applied Psychology, 87*(5), 819–832.

Guzzo, R. A., & Dickson, M. W. (1996). Teams in organizations: Recent research on performance and effectiveness. *Annual Review of Psychology, 47,* 307–338. doi:10.1146/annurev.psych.47.1.307

Holzemer, W. L. (2007). University of California, San Francisco International Nursing Network for HIV/AIDS Research. *International Nursing Review, 54*(3), 234–242. doi:10.1111/j.1466-7657.2007.00571.x

Institute of Medicine (IOM). (2014). *Workshop: Evaluation methods for large-scale, complex, multi-national global health initiatives.* Retrieved from http://www.iom.edu/Activities/Global/EvaluationMethodsGlobalHealth/2014-JAN-07.aspx

International Federation of Pharmaceutical Manufacturers and Associations. (IFPMA). (2014). *Consensus framework for ethical consideration.* Retrieved from http://www.ifpma.org/news/news-releases/news-details/article/putting-patients-first-five-global-healthcare-org.html

James, C. (2013). NYU's Shedlin publishes study on the health of Colombian refugees in Ecuador. Retrieved from http://www.eurekalert.org/pub_releases/2013-02/nyu-nsp021913.php

Masiello, I. (2009). Learning to succeed in European Joint Projects: The role of the modern project manager—the flow keeper. *Journal of Interprofessional Care, 23*(5), 498–507.

Mullan, F., Chen, C., & Steinmetz, E. (2013). The geography of graduate medical education: Imbalances signal need for new distribution policies. *Health Affairs (Millwood), 32*(11), 1914–1921. doi:10.1377/hlthaff.2013.0545

National Academy of Sciences (NAS). (2014). *The science of team science.* Retrieved from http://sites.nationalacademies.org/DBASSE/BBCSS/CurrentProjects/DBASSE_080231

Polit, D. F., & Beck, C. T. (2014). *Essentials of nursing research: Appraising evidence for nursing practice* (8th ed.). Philadelphia, PA: Lippincott.

Reeves, S., Zwarenstein, M., Goldman, J., Barr, H., Freeth, D., Hammick, M., & Koppel, I. (2008). Interprofessional education: Effects on professional practice and health care outcomes. *Cochrane Database of Systematic Reviews* (1), CD002213. doi:10.1002/14651858. CD002213.pub2

Shedlin, M., Decena, C. U., Noboa, H., Báez, M., Betancourt, S., Villalobos, J., . . . Betancourt, O. (2014). *Salud y condiciones de vida de los refugiados Colombianos en Ecuador (The health and living conditions of Colombian refugees in Ecuador).* Quito, Ecuador: Abya Yala Press.

Thistlethwaite, J., & Grin Working Group. (2013). Introducing the Global Research Interprofessional Network (GRIN). *Journal of Interprofessional Care, 27*(2), 107–109. doi:10.3109/13561820.2012.718814

Wang, D., Waldman, D. A., & Zhang, Z. (2014). A meta-analysis of shared leadership and team effectiveness. *Journal of Applied Psychology, 99*(2), 181–198. doi:10.1037/a0034531

Wuchty, S., Jones, B. F., & Uzzi, B. (2007). The increasing dominance of teams in production of knowledge. *Science, 316*(5827), 1036–1039. doi:10.1126/science.1136099

Index

Printed in the United States
By Bookmasters